Therapeutic Plasmapheresis (XII)

Proceedings of the 4th International Congress of the World
Apheresis Association and the 12th Annual Symposium of the
Japanese Society for Apheresis, 3 - 5 June 1992, Sapporo, Japan.

This Congress has been executed with a grant from the
Commemorative Association for the Japan World Exposition.

T. Agishi, A. Kawamura and M. Mineshima

Therapeutic Plasmapheresis (XII)

Proceedings of the 4th International Congress of the World
Apheresis Association and the 12th Annual Symposium of the
Japanese Society for Apheresis, 3 - 5 June 1992, Sapporo, Japan

Edited by
T. Agishi
A. Kawamura
M. Mineshima

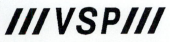

Utrecht, The Netherlands, 1993

VSP BV
P.O. Box 346
3700 AH Zeist
The Netherlands

© VSP BV 1993

First published in 1993

ISBN 90-6764-151-0

Printed in The Netherlands by ICG Printing, Dordrecht.

Contents

Contents

3. Autoimmune Diseases

5. Hepato–digestive Organs Diseases

11. Emergency Apheresis

12. Immunoadsorption

22. Donor Apheresis

23. Miscellaneous

1
Invited Lectures

Therapeutic Plasmapheresis (XII), pp. 3-11
T. Agishi *et al*. (Eds)
© VSP 1993

Cryopreservation of Human Blood Cells

S. SUMIDA

Department of Cardiovascular Surgery, National Fukuoka Central Hospital, Jonai 2–2, Chuoku, Fukuoka, 810 Japan

Key words: cryopreservation; erythrocyte; red cell; bone marrow; platelet; autologous transfusion; Arrhenius equation; colony forming unit in culture; CFU-C; BFU-E.

INTRODUCTION

Since 1965, I have cryopreserved human blood and bone marrow cells, several tissues and organs. After thawing, I have transfused or transplanted them to treat patients complaining of anemia, bleeding tendency and symptoms of acquired immunodeficiency and of organ failure.

From my experience of cryopreservation of human parts, I would like to report several fundamental and practical items concerning blood cell freezing.

MATERIALS AND METHODS

Erythrocytes

Seventeen thousands and forty-eight units of concentrated red cells (packed cells) were cryopreserved for up to 24 years at either -80 or $-196\,°C$. The 60–80% glycerol- slow freezing and the 28–30% glycerol-rapid freezing methods were used [1–4] . The thawed and deglycerolized concentrated red cells (TDCRC) have been used to treat anemia. The side-effects and complications have been checked as long the recipients lived.

The regression equation of recovery rate (RR) and preservation period (PP) for up to 23 years was derived by the degree of hemolysis after thawing.

The morphology of TDCRC was studied by scanning and transmission electron micrographs (SEM and TEM).

The osmotic fragility of TDCRC was measured by Ribiere's method as modified by Giffin–Sanford.

The membrane fluidity of TDCRC was deduced from electron spin resonance (ESR) signals for 12-nitroxide stearic acid (12NS) and 16NS of thawed red cells.

Adenosinetriphosphate (ATP) and 2,3-diphospho-glycerate (DPG) or TDCRC were measured by the enzyme method. ^{31}P-nuclear magnetic resonance (NMR) spectroscopy was used to identify phosphorous compounds and to record metabolic changes of TDCRC.

The optimal preservation temperature and constitution of cryoprotective solution was also investigated. In addition to glycerol, dimethyl sulfoxide (Me$_2$SO), ethylene glycol and sucrose were experimentally used to examine the optimal constitutions of cryoprotective solutions for red cells at either -80 or $-196\,°C$ and the recovery rates after thawing.

Platelets
Platelets were frozen with a 28% glycerol solution at $-80\,°C$ or by either 10% glycerol or 10% Me_2SO in either a 0.9% saline or in the donor's own sera at $-196\,°C$ from day 0 to 22 years. The thawed platelets were immediately and intravenously infused without further processing. Increments of platelet counts and bleeding time of the recipients were studied. Aggregability and morphology were also examined by TEM and SEM.

Bone marrow
Bone marrow was collected 301 times from 229 patients of advanced solid cancer for autologous transplantation. Approximately 1.4×10^{10} nucleated cells were obtained and frozen with 20% Me_2SO in medium 199 or in patients' own sera for periods up to 18 years at $-196\,°C$. Most marrow cells were thawed after 3–5 years, and immediately infused into the original patients without any further processing. About 30% of those marrow cells have remained in the frozen state without thawing, as the patients died from the acute progress of original cancer. Small samples of the thawed marrow cells were used to study the colony forming unit in culture (CFU-C). The regression equation of CFU-C recovery and preservation periods, and of CFU-C recovery and patients' age were derived.

RESULTS

Erythrocytes
Transfusion of TDCRC cryopreserved for up to 18 years completely improved anemia of a patient with uterine myoma without any side-effects. From then on, the patient had a hysterectomy and was discharged from hospital.

The transmission of transfusion related diseases has been controversial, even if TDCRC have been used. The incidence rate of post-transfusion hepatitis has remained zero since 1975.

HLA alloimmunization was nearly zero in recipients of TDCRC. Some patients who had complained of life-threatening allergic reactions including fever, shaking chill, dyspnea and hypotension by the banked whole blood and CRC, tolerated well the transfusion of TDCRC.

The regression equation of Y (RR: percentage) on X (PP: years) at $-80\,°C$ was derived as

$$Y = 85.6915 - 1.0642\,X \tag{1}$$

and that of Y on X at $-196\,°C$ was derived as

$$Y = 91.6512 - 0.3046\,X \tag{2}$$

Spherocytes and microspherocytes appeared more in the TDCRC $(-80\,°C)$ than in the TDCRC $(-196\,°C)$.

The osmotic fragility curves of TDCRC $(-80\,°C)$ shifted to the left side (hypo-osmotic side) and those of TDCRC $(-196\,°C)$ mostly overlapped on those of non-frozen fresh red cells.

The outer hyperfine splitting (T_{II}) value of the ESR signal for 12NS, as a measure of membrane fluidity, changed by 1.01 gauss in TDCRC $(-80\,°C)$ and by 0.29–0.68 gauss in TDCRC ($-196\,°C$) in comparison with those of fresh red cells. The T_{II} for 16NS showed the same tendency.

The normal values of ATP and DPG of fresh red cells were $2.57 \pm 0.32\ \mu mol/gHb$ ($n = 20$) and $12.8 \pm 1.6\ \mu mol/gHb$ ($n = 14$), respectively. After thawing, the ATP and DPG values of TDCRC ($-80\,°C$) changed to 2.19 ± 1.01 ($n = 28$) and 2.96 ± 2.77 ($n = 28$), respectively, and those of TDCRC ($-196\,°C$) 2.35 ± 1.61 ($n = 31$) and 2.71 ± 1.12, respectively. Therefore, the necessary amount of ATP was preserved in TDCRC. The DPG values decreased remarkably, but they can recover to the normal values in the recipient's circulation. The ^{31}P chemical shifts of ATP (alpha, beta and gamma fractions), ADP and inorganic phosphate of TDCRC showed interesting changes in comparison with those of fresh red cells. These changes would be caused by the effects of bounding hybridization and of neighboring bonded atoms of varying electronegativity.

The relationship between the various factors involved in recovery rates of red cells after freezing at either -80 or $-196\,°C$ in different suspending solutions consisting of different amounts of cryoprotectant and NaCl in water are summarized in the recovery rate–glycerol–NaCl three-dimensional surfaces (Figs 1 and 2). They show the following evidences. The $-196\,°C$ TDCRC yielded the more spread area of the surface clipped at the recovery rate of 90% than the $-80\,°C$ TDCRC. The red cell preservation at $-80\,°C$ needs a higher concentration of cryoprotectant than that at $-196\,°C$.

Platelets

Electron microscopy showed that 40% of the cells in 5% glycerol and 60% of the cells in 5% Me_2SO retained their disk form. ADP and collagen aggregability of frozen-thawed platelets were very weak, but bleeding tendency of the patients showed marked improvement in the clinical condition after the transfusion of frozen platelets. Preservation in 14% glycerol yielded *in vivo* survival of only 5% of control whereas the 5% Me_2SO procedure yielded significant elevation of platelet counts.

Bone marrow

All bone marrow, including bone marrow preserved for up to 18 years, showed colony formation *in vitro* after thawing. The colonies consisted of granulocytes, macrophages and erythroides.

Recovery percentage of 10% Me_2SO-protected marrow cells frozen up to 9 years was about 0.2. The regression equation of CFU-C recovery percentage (Y) and preservation period (X: year) was derived as

$$Y = 0.21 - 0.008\,X \tag{3}$$

The regression equation of CFU-C recovery percentage (Y) and age (X) of advanced solid cancer patients was derived as

$$Y = 0.26 - 0.002\,X \tag{4}$$

Marrow cells of digestive canal advanced cancer patients showed a significant decrease of CFU-C recoveries ($P < 0.01$).

Ninety-six (76%) of 126 patients showed subjective and/or objective improvement of the original cancer, 55 (44%) from the acquired hematopoietic suppression, and the

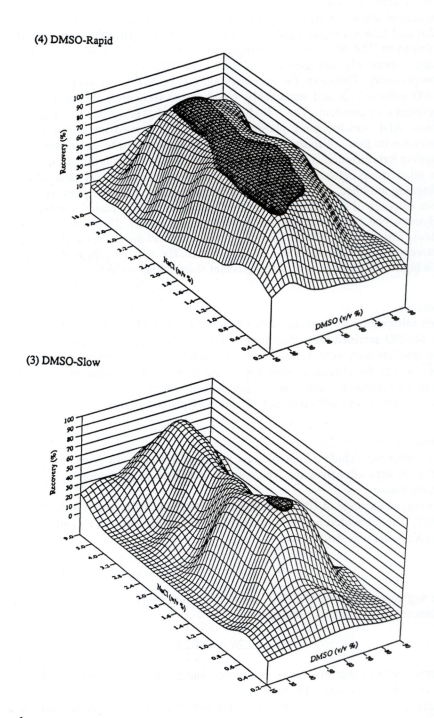

(4) DMSO-Rapid

(3) DMSO-Slow

Figure 1.

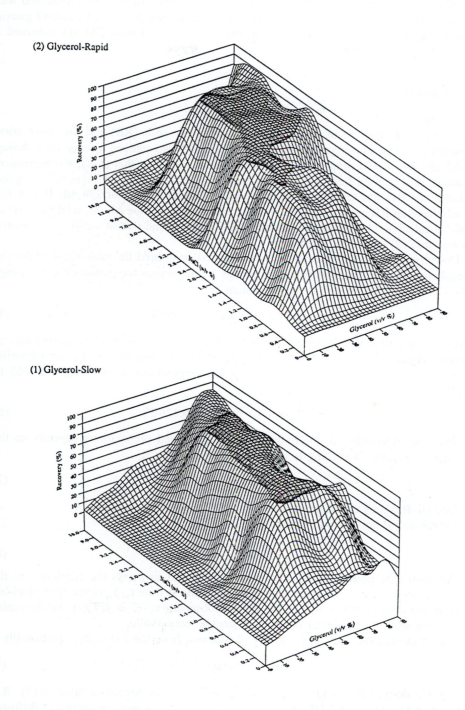

Figure 2.

remaining 103 cases died in a year from the original cancer without frozen autologous bone marrow transplantation (FABMT). An interesting case of complete remission was a case of osteosarcoma with bilateral pulmonary metastasis. Seven (14%) of 47 gastric cancer patients given megadose of chemotherapy combined with FABMT survived a year or longer.

DISCUSSION

Erythrocytes

The regression equation of the recovery rate of viable cells (RR) and the observation time (PP) is very important to determine the possible guaranteed storage time during which the RR would drop to the lowest threshold value. In this study, the regression equation was derived from the actually measured RR for up to 23 years. The regular volume of CRC was cryopreserved in this study, which was about 250 ml. If TDCRC should have an RR more than 80%, the guaranteed storage time (the term of validity) at $-80\,°C$ calculated by equation (1) would be 5.35 years and that at $-196\,°C$ calculated by equation (2) would be 38.25 years.

Dowell and Rinfret [5], using X-ray diffraction, measured the time required for the completion of devitrification from amorphous ice at various temperatures in the range of $-135\,°C$ to $-160\,°C$ and derived equation (5)

$$t = 2.04 \times 10^{28} \times \exp(-0.465\,T) \tag{5}$$

where t is the time in minutes for the conversion and T is the absolute temperature in Kelvin. Again, they observed the time required for the completion of recrystalization from cubic to stable hexagonal ice at various temperatures in the range of -65 to $-120\,°C$, and derived equation (6)

$$t = 2.56 \times 10^{12} \times \exp(-0.126\,T) \tag{6}$$

The loss of viability of freeze-dried or cryopreserved preparations depends on the storage temperature according to the Arrhenius equation (3)

$$k = A\,\exp(-E/RT) \tag{7}$$

Dowell–Rinfret's equations will be modified forms of this equation.
Sidyakina [6] applied the Arrhenius equation as

$$Yt = Y_0 \cdot e^{-Kt} \tag{8}$$

to determine the possible time of storage at 4°C and to assess the efficiency of the protective media used. Yt is the titer of viable cells at time t, Y_0 is the titer of viable cells in the control at $t = 0$, t is the time of observation, $K = f(T)$ is the Arrhenius coefficient which is the linear function of storage temperature.

The three-dimensional surface in Fig. 3 is drawn from the following equation (9)

$$R = 1 - t\,\exp(-T_0/T) \tag{9}$$

which was derived from equation (1) and (2) on the base of Arrhenius equation (7). R is recovery rate, and $T_0 = E/R_B$, in which E expresses the activation energy of diffusion and R_B is Boltzmann's constant. Figure 3 was drawn by $T_0 = 800$. However, we shall

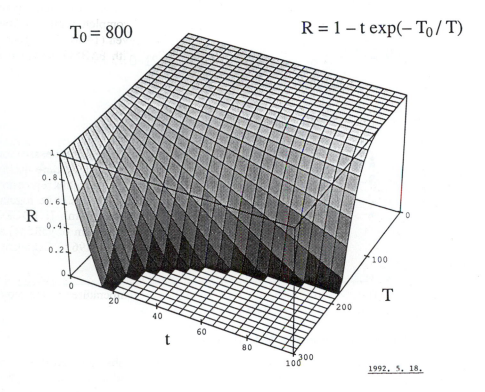

$T_0 = 800$

$R = 1 - t \exp(- T_0 / T)$

1992. 5. 18.

Figure 3.

be satisfied practically with the equation (1) and (2) to determine the guaranteed storage time at a destined temperature.

The rationality of equations (1) and (2) is supported by the results of electron micrographs, osmotic fragility, ESR and NMR. Figures 1 and 2 will be useful to make cryoprotective solutions of new constitutions.

Platelets
The platelet is a very delicate blood cell. The procedure introduced in this paper has been repeated by Thompson [7], and Hocking [8] reported a procedure using 10% glycerol as a simple routine. If we need to preserve platelets for 2 days or more, we should freeze them by the 10% Me_2SO procedure.

Bone marrow
Equation (3) will be useful to determine the guaranteed storage time, and equation (4) to determine the guaranteed age to apply FABMT to the patients with advanced solid cancer (Figs 4 and 5).

Cryopreservation of the autologous stem cells should be recommended to the workers around the nuclear reactors of atomic plant, as the proverb says, "No man knows his own future, He is wise that is ware in time".

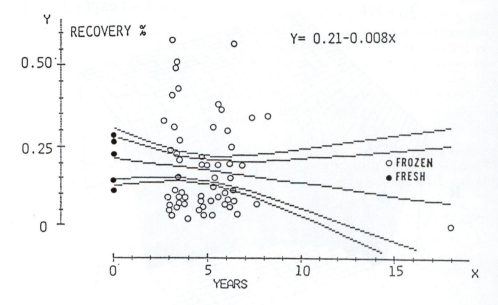

Figure 4. CFU-C recovery of bone marrow: fresh and frozen.

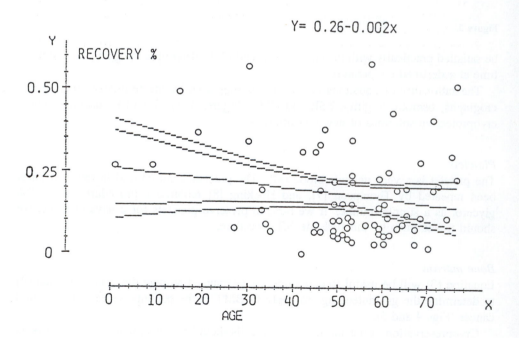

Figure 5. Aging and CFU-C recovery of frozen bone marrow.

CONCLUSION

Red cells, platelets and bone marrow cells have been cryopreserved for up to 23 years and several equations derived from the recovery rates of frozen cells, holding temperature, period and constitution of protective solution were introduced. These equations will be used to determine the guaranteed storage time of red cells and of marrow cells at -80 or $-196\,°C$.

Frozen cells have played an important role in treating anemia, bleeding tendency and acquired immunodeficiency. The clinical results were briefly introduced.

Acknowledgment
The author expresses great gratitude to Professor Y. Suezaki, who instructed me to derive the equations introduced in this study and to draw the three dimensional surfaces.

REFERENCES

1. C. E. Huggins. Frozen blood. *Ann. Surg.*, **160**, 643–649 (1964).
2. A. W. Rowe, E. Eyster, F. H. Allen and A. Kellner. Freezing of erythrocytes for transfusion by a glycerol–liquid nitogen procedure. *Transfusion*, **6**, 521 (1966).
3. S. Sumida, Y. Okuyama and T. Kamegai. Serum hepatitis form frozen blood. *Lancet*, **2**, 1255–1256 (1967).
4. S. Sumida. *Transfusion of blood preserved by freezing*. Igaku-shoin, Lippincott (1973).
5. L. G. Dowell and A. P. Rinfret. Low-temperature forms of ice as studied by X-ray diffraction. *Nature*, **188**, 1144–1148 (1960).
6. T. M. Sidyakina and N. D. Lozitskaya. The viability of microorganisms: *Pseudomonas denitrificans* VKM B-892 subject to lyophilization and cryopreservation in various protective media. *Problems of Cryobiol.*, **1**, 32–38 (1991).
7. R. Thompson. Reported at *Congress of the International Society of Blood Transfusion*, Helsinki (1975).
8. D. Hocking and R. E. Olsen. Platelet cryopreservation — a simple routine. *Australian J. Med.*, **1**, 537–538 (1980).
9. A. U. Smith. *Biological effects of freezing and supercooling*. Edward Arnold, London (1961).

Therapeutic Plasmapheresis (XII), pp. 13-20
T. Agishi *et al.* (Eds)
© VSP 1993

Experience with and Conclusions from Three Different Trials on Low Density Lipoprotein Apheresis

H. BORBERG[1] and K. OETTE[2]

[1]*Haemapheresis, Department of Medicine and* [2]*Institute of Clinical Chemistry, University of Köln, Germany*

Key words: LDL apheresis; atherosclerosis; regression; delipidation; prevention.

The term low density lipoprotein (LDL) apheresis was introduced in 1981 for the therapeutic application of immunespecific affinity chromatography [1, 2]. Since then other upcoming technologies have used our terminology, claiming to be superior. However, after 11 years of application no convincing evidence of superiority to the original system in terms of specificity, capacity and versatility has been demonstrated. Furthermore it was shown that, not unexpectedly, the closely related lipoprotein A (Lp(a)) is removed to virtually the same extent as LDL (66%), which, if Lp(a) is accepted as an additional risk factor, also supports the potency of the system.

As LDL apheresis columns are now derived from different sources, potential variations in the production process leading to better or worse quality have to be taken into consideration when observations on the principle are reported.

Our first trial, comprising 10 patients with familial hypercholesterolaemia type IIa (FH), was initiated with the introduction of LDL apheresis to investigate the capacity, the safety and the clinical relevance of the procedure, and was terminated in 1986. Originally designed to investigate whether a reduction of total cholesterol to post-treatment levels of 150–200 mg/dl could lead to secondary prevention with patients in whom ineffective lipid lowering therapy proved ineffective, primary prevention and, surprisingly, regression of coronary heart disease occurred. However, regression was mainly observed in young, homozygous patients and later on, though delayed, also in some heterozygous individuals [3]. Cardiac symptoms disappeared in eight out of 10 patients. Since this was observed earlier than the disappearance of skin and tendon xanthomae and also regression of coronary stenosis and sclerosis, the question arose whether delipidation led to a sequence of events initiated in small cardiac vessels. Also, improvement of rheology might contribute to the disappearance of symptoms. In contrast, the very slow regression of pathologically altered coronary morphology after years of therapy, mainly observed in patients under 35 years of age, might depend upon other factors such as plaque fibrosis or deposition of matrix substance not solely dependent on delipidation. Though unexpected, it was observed over a period of time that stenoses did not reoccur after angioplasty (PTCA), and bypasses also remained open, although at that time the number of patients was limited and the duration of observation was not long enough.

To extend these observations, a second trial was initiated with the support of the German Ministry of Research and Development. The original design, presented in

1985, compared one of the first HMG-CoA-reductase inhibitors with LDL apheresis and assessed the combination of both. This approach, now considered to be the therapy of choice, had to be abandoned, as the grant review board considered it unethical and the manufacturer of the drug withdrew his consent. As an alternative, suggesting the application of conventional drugs, was equally not accepted, the study had to be performed as an open longitudinal trial, embracing 30 patients with FH type II, according to the classification of Fredrickson (including an estimated five potential dropouts) to be treated at weekly intervals for a period of 3 years. The post-treatment total cholesterol was to be in a range of 100–150 mg/dl. The estimated average total cholesterol between two treatments (calculated by dividing the post- plus pretreatment cholesterol by 2) was supposed to be about 210 mg/dl. All detected homozygous patients with FH were supposed to be recruited. Heterozygous patients were recruited as well; if following strict diet and expert lipid lowering drug therapy including drug combinations the total cholesterol still exceeded 250 mg/dl total cholesterol.

The general data about the number of participating centers, recruited patients, number of dropouts, age and sex distribution are given in Table 1. It is noteworthy that only two homozygous patients were recruited during the phase II trial as compared with five in the phase I trial (total number of 10 patients) and that the average age of 43 years (ranging from 15 to 63) at the time of recruitment was 14 years higher as compared with the phase I trial (average age of 29 years with a range from 11 to 54 years). The mean number of treatments performed was 138 per patient (range 121–155). An average total cholesterol between treatments supposed to be slightly higher than 200 mg/dl was generally achieved. The average total cholesterol after treatment was 138 mg/dl and the average post-treatment LDL-cholesterol was 83. The average LDL-cholesterol/HDL-cholesterol ratio of 6:1 prior to apheresis, improved to 2.6:1 after apheresis and was 4.5:1 following therapy. Thus the average reduction was 188 mg/dl (57%) for the total cholesterol and 166 mg/dl (67%) for the LDL-cholesterol, with some difference from one center to the other.

The average decrease in tendon thickness was 1.9 mm for the right Achilles tendon and 2.1 mm for the left measured following the procedure of Blankenhorn and Meyers [4].

Cardiological evaluations were performed partly as published earlier [3] and partly closely related to that of the CAST trial [5]. A moderate subjective improvement was observed in all patients suffering from clinical cardiological symptoms.

Exercise ECGs were classified in four categories: improvement, questionable improvement, without change and deterioration. The detailed definitions will be published with the final report of the study. The results were correlated with the LDL-cholesterol level (< or > 150 mg/dl), the HDL-cholesterol level (< or > 150 mg/dl) and the LDL-cholesterol/HDL-cholesterol ratio (< 3.5 or > 3.5). As can be seen from Table 2, there was no deterioration; in seven patients (29.2%) a debatable improvement was found in eight patients (33.3%) and improvement was beyond any doubt in nine patients (37.5%). A significant correlation existed to a low LDL-cholesterol, a high HDL-cholesterol and a low LDL-cholesterol/HDL-cholesterol ratio.

The anonymous coronary angiography films were independently judged by a cardiological representative of each center at a joint final meeting arranged for the evaluation of all cardiological data. The Ramus Interventricularis Anterior (RIVA), the Ramus Coronarius Anterior (RCA) and the Ramus Circumflexus (RCX) were judged for both

Table 1.

German multicenter LDL apheresis trial: final general data

Center recruitment planned	5
Centers at time of termination	4
Patient recruitment planned	30
(including dropouts)	
Patients recruited	32
'Dropouts'	9
death due to myocardial infarction	2
inadequate treatment	2
unknown reasons (compliance?)	3
refusal of control coronary angiography	2
Average age (years) at start of study	43.2
(range)	(15–63)
Sex distribution	
female/male	19/13
Genetic background of familial hypercholesterolaemia	
homozygous/heterozygous	2/30

Table 2.

German multicenter LDL apheresis trial: first evaluation of exercise ECGs ($N = 24$)

LDL-cholesterol (mg/dl)	Pathological at start	Improved	Improvement questionable	No change	P
< 15		5	2	1	
	24				0.183
> 15		4	6	6	
HDL cholesterol (mg/dl)					
> 40		6	1	2	
	24				0.06
< 40		3	7	5	
RATIO					
< 3.75		4	0	1	
	24				0.07
> 3.75		5	8	6	

stenosis and sclerosis in angiograms performed prior to and at the end of the trial after 3 years. As Table 3 shows, there was no change over a 3 year period; however, in some cases a deterioration could be noted (one out of 25 in the RIVA, three out of 25 in the RCA and three out of 25 in the RCX).

The general conclusion to be drawn from this study is that in severe FH patients

H. Borberg and K. Oette

Table 3.

German multicenter LDL apheresis trial: first evaluation of coronary angiographies ($N = 25$)

Degree of stenosis	RIVA		RCA		RCX	
	initial	final	initial	final	initial	final
0	2	2	2	2	3	3
1	12	11	8	8	15	12
2	7	8	7	5	5	7
3	1	1	1	0	1	1
4	2	2	7	10	1	2

RIVA: (1)
RCX: (2), (1)
RCA: (2), (1)

Not evaluable, 1.
Numbers in brackets ( ) = number of patients with increase of stenosis.

without therapeutic alternative regression of xanthomas can be demonstrated, improvement of cardiac symptoms appears to occur, whereas the coronary morphology shows secondary prevention not excluding the possibility of partial progression. As mentioned before, the apparent discrepancy between subjective and functional improvement and secondary prevention may be due to an as yet unknown sequence of events following cellular delipidation. However, it is clear from these data that the process of improvement is rather slow.

The third trial was performed to determine the role of HMG-CoA-reductase inhibitors. As published earlier [6–8] we found that the combination of LDL apheresis with an HMG-CoA-reductase inhibitor could considerably lower the pretreatment LDL-cholesterol level as well as the average daily cholesterol increase in heterozygous patients, whereas homozygous patients scarcely responded. If, provided the patient complied, a bile acid binding resin such as cholestyramine was added, a further decrease of approximately 2/3 of the daily increase was observed (Table 4). Twenty patients were treated over a period of 16 weeks in a way that the treatment with LDL-apheresis was performed over 4 weeks. subsequently LDL apheresis plus Simvastatin in the standard dosage (20 mg/day) over another 4 weeks, LDL apheresis plus Simvastatin twice the standard dosage (40 mg/day) over 4 weeks and, finally, LDL apheresis again applied as the only treatment regimen for the last 4 weeks. An additional average decrease of 27% was found adding the standard dose of Simvastatin to the LDL apheresis, whereas twice the dosage led to a further decrease of only 29% in contrast to a decrease of 35% when the maximal dosage of Simvastatin was combined with colestyramin (Table 4).

Apart from the data from the three trials, additional information is of interest. During the phase I trial it appeared that patients after percutaneous transluminal coronary angioplasty (PTCA) or bypass operation did not need further invasive therapy. However, not enough time had elapsed to ascertain whether or not this was conclusive. Of six patients treated with PTCA, one refused a control coronary angiography. Neither this one nor the other five subsequently controlled needed a second intervention within a period of 6.3 years (range 4–8 years) (Table 5). Of 12 patients after the bypass operation, two died from myocardial infarction, one did not comply and left the treatment and two refused to undergo control coronary angiography. Neither these two nor the remaining eight who were angiographically controlled needed a second intervention after an average of

Table 4.

Combination of LDL apheresis and drug therapy: additional decrease of LDL-cholesterol under LDL apheresis applying different regimens

	No, of FH patients	Additional decrease of LDL-cholesterol (range)	
Simvastatin (20 mg/day)	8	27%	(11–49)
Simvastatin (40 mg/day)	8	29%	(14–49)
Simvastatin (40 mg/day) + Cholestyramine (8 g/day)	4	35%	(26–41)

Table 5.

FH patients after PTCA under long-term LDL apheresis

Total	6
Homozygous	2
Heterozygous	4
Refusal of control-coronary angiography	1
Evaluable	5
Average duration (years) of LDL apheresis following invasive intervention (range)	6.3 (4–8)
Number of restenosis	0
Second PTCA	0

5.4 years (range 0.5–10 years) (Table 6). From these data the claim that LDL apheresis may render further invasive intervention unnecessary gains additional support. Finally the survival of six homozygous patients is about to be extended beyond a critical age. According to Goldstein and Brown [9] only a few homozygotes survive past an age of 30 years. They usually develop angina pectoris and display myocardial infarction or sudden death between the ages of 5 and 30. Of six homozygous patients treated for 6–11 years at regular weekly intervals, lately some at biweekly intervals, all are alive. Two were treated for maintaining primary prevention. They had tendon xanthomas, but no coronary lipid deposits, in coronary angiograms. Another two demonstrated regression, as shown by control coronary angiography. Another patient, refusing control angiography, appears to be in regression according to clinical parameters. One patient poorly treated before being referred to us had to undergo heart surgery (implantation of artificial valves) and has since been in a state of secondary prevention. These survival data, as well as the data on PTCA an bypass follow-up, strongly support the value of regular LDL apheresis therapy for both secondary prevention and regression.

Summarizing the experience of these three trials it appears to be necessary prior to the initiation of any treatment in patients with FH to lay down the general aim of the

Table 6.

FH patients with aorto-coronary venous bypass under long-term LDL apheresis

Total	12
Homozygous	3
Heterozygous	9
Refusal of control-coronary angiography	2
Deaths or missing compliance (dropouts)	2
Evaluable	8
Average duration (years) of LDL apheresis following surgical intervention (range)	5.4 (0.5–10)
Number of restenosis	0
Second PTCA	0

therapy, e.g. primary prevention, secondary prevention or regression. Before extracorporeal therapy is taken into consideration one has to exclude whether any conventional lipid-lowering therapy with diet and drugs (including HMG-CoA-reductase inhibitors and appropriate drug combinations) is able to decrease the cholesterol level to an extent that titers set by the consensus conferences [10] will be obtained. However, this statement needs a more differentiated consideration, for instance including the serum HDL-cholesterol. If not, and if regression appears to be feasable, the variables, which others and we ourselves have postulated for many years [3, 6–8, 11] should also be considered.

Drawing from our present experience homozygous patients are not only diagnosed early but are young (average age generally not exceeding 29 years) and have good compliance. In contrast, the majority of our heterozygous patients have an average age of 43 years when entering long-term LDL apheresis and may not be convinced to undergo extracorporeal therapy as long as they do not really suffer from a significantly decreased quality of life, although xanthomas and alterations of the coronary system can already be demonstrated. The point that younger patients are more likely to regress is often not considered from the patients. Alternatively, additional factors determining the expression of the disease at higher age such as increased fibrosis, calcification, ulceration of plaques, etc., may have a negative impact on the beneficial influence of cellular delipidation.

It appears reasonable that with increasing age the disease is quite often also progressed and the chances for obtaining regression may be decreased with the extent of the disease. One should not anticipate a short-term clinical effect from any lipid lowering therapy in a condition which has developed over 30 or more years. The presence of other risk factors will most likely decrease the chance for potential regression. We have not found additional risk factors in our patients except for two, one of whom smokes, and another who smokes, has high blood pressure and is irregular with medication.

The period of time a patient is treated as well as the decrease of the LDL-cholesterol levels during the treatments performed, also leading to lower average LDL-cholesterol levels, are variables, which gain importance if our first trial can now be compared with the multicenter phase II trial. Beyond the fact that the phase I trial comprised more homozygous and also younger patients, it is clear that within a period of 3 years, though with average LDL-cholesterol levels of 166 mg/dl, it was not possible to obtain regression of coronary heart disease in heterozygous patients with an average age of 43 years. Although significant, regression of xanthomas, which preceeds that of the coronaries, was limited.

Based on this information and experience we recommend that if regression is desired, the therapeutic guidelines as given in Table 7 should be followed.

Table 7.
Therapeutic strategies for regression of coronary heart disease in patients with FH

I. Elimination of risk factors

1. Major risk factor: increased LDL-cholesterol

   aggressive: 50–100 mg/dl total cholesterol after therapy
   (30–70 mg/dl LDL-cholesterol after therapy)

2. Additional risk factors

   increased Lp(a)
   modified LDL (oxidized, aggregated and immunecomplexed LDL)

II. Change of the cholesterol kinetics

1. HMG-CoA-reductase inhibitors (decrease of cholesterol synthesis)

2. If necessary in combination with other lipid-lowering drugs

III. Increase of HDL

1. Post-treatment LDL-cholesterol/HDL-cholesterol ratio of 2.0

2. Infusion of 'artificial HDL'

As apolipoprotein A-I (apo A-I) is the main carrier protein of HDL it is prerequisite to have biocompatible apo A-I available. So far we have performed three studies with apo A-I. In a first trial on three healthy male volunteers the clearance of apo A-I was investigated infusing 4 g within 40 min. As anticipated the half-life was below 3 h. In a subsequent study, 10 healthy male volunteers were infused with a mixture of phosphatidylcholine (PC) and sodium deoxycholate (SDC) to form liposomerelated particles. This, in fact, prolonged the half-life in such a way that stable lipoprotein A-I particles were shown to have a half-life of about 9 h. Both trials were performed to demonstrate the safety of the apo A-I infusion as well as the combined infusion. In a third trial, apo A-I was infused with PC-SDC in three patients during LDL apheresis and into one patient with a severe HDL-deficiency syndrome. The catabolism of HDL was high in the HDL-deficient patient as compared with the patients with FH, who demonstrated an increase in lipoprotein A-I particles. This was encouraging enough for us to proceed with this development in the future, as it might well influence the process of regression using a different approach. Whereas in the past the elimination of risk factors was considered to be the major aim of the developments, emphasis may now be placed on the reversal of the cholesterol transport expected to contribute to the process of regression using a different mechanism.

Acknowledgments

The phase II trial was performed at the Universities of Köln (H. Borberg, J. Kadar and K. Oette), München (P. Schwandt and W. O. Richter), Tübingen (M. Eggstein, D. Knisel and H. Pfohl) and Würzburg (D. Wiebecke, H. Ullrich and W. Keller). The statistical analysis was performed at the Biometrical Unit, Department of Thoracic Surgery, University of Düsseldorf (E. Godehardt, H. Hermann and J. Kunert). The cardiological evaluation of the phase II trial was coordinated by V. Hombach and H. W. Höpp, Department of Medicine III (Cardiology), University of Köln.

REFERENCES

1. W. Stoffel and T. Demant. Selective removal of apolipoprotein B-containing serum lipoproteins from blood plasma. *Proc. Natl. Acad. Sci. USA*, **78**, 611–615 (1981).

2. W. Stoffel, H. Borberg and V. Greve. Application of specific extracorporeal removal of low density lipoprotein in familial hypercholesterolaemia. *Lancet*, **i**, 1005–1006 (1981).

3. V. Hombach, H. Borberg, K. Oette and W. Stoffel. Regression der Koronarsklerose bei familiärer Hypercholesterinämie IIa durch spezifische LDL-Apherese. *Dtsch. Med. Wschr.*, **111**, 1709–1715 (1986).

4. D. H. Blankenhorn and H. I. Meyers. Radiographic determination of Achilles tendon xanthoma size. *Metabolism*, **18**, 882–886 (1969).

5. Cardiac arrhythmia suppression trial (CAST). *N. Engl. J. Med.*, **321**, 406–412 (1989).

6. H. Borberg, A. Gaczkowski, K. Oette and W. Stoffel. Immunosorptive apheresis of LDL. In: *Apheresis*, G. Rock (Ed.), pp. 163–167, Wiley-Liss, Toronto (1990).

7. K. Oette and H. Borberg. Variables in regression of atherosclerosis in familial hypercholesterolaemic patients under longterm LDL-apheresis. *Plasma. Ther. Transfus. Technol.*, **9**, 17–23 (1988).

8. K. Oette, H. Borberg, J. Kadar and E. Godehardt. Longterm extracorporeal LDL elimination in the treatment of hypercholesterolaemia. Effects and clinical relevance. In: *Advances in Lipoprotein and Atherosclerosis Research, Diagnosis and Treatment*, M. Hanefeld, W. Jaroß and H. Dude (Eds), G. Fischer, Jena (1991).

9. J. L. Goldstein and M. S. Brown. Familial hypercholesterolaemia. In: *The Metabolic Basis of Inherited Disease*, Ch. R. Scriver, A. L. Beaudet, W. S. Sly and D. Valle (Eds), pp. 1212–1250, McGraw Hill, New York (1982).

10. Nationale Cholesterin Initiative. *Dt. Ärztblatt*, **87**, 991–1010 (1990).

11. A. Yamamoto. Regression of atherosclerosis. *Plasma. Ther. Transfus. Technol.*, **9**, 11–16 (1988).

Therapeutic Plasmapheresis (XII), pp. 21-23
T. Agishi *et al.* (Eds)
© VSP 1993

Apheresis, Immunoreconstitution and AIDS

H. G. KLEIN

*Department of Transfusion Medicine, Warren G. Magnuson Clinical Center,
National Institutes of Health, Bethesda, MD 20892, USA*

The acquired immunodeficiency syndrome (AIDS) is a protean illness resulting in severe immune suppression and death from opportunistic infections or neoplasia. Since the initial clinical reports in 1981, more than 250 000 cases of AIDS have been diagnosed in the US and almost half of these have died as a result of this illness. The World Health Organization estimates that 6–8 million people are currently infected with the human immunodeficiency virus type 1 (HIV-1) and an estimated 15–20 million people will be infected by the virus by the year 2000 [1].

The human CD4+ T lymphocyte and monocyte are the major targets for HIV-1 infection. The CD4 membrane antigen is a high-affinity receptor for this virus. After entry into the cell, the virus is uncoated and reverse transcription of viral RNA takes place, resulting in double-stranded DNA. An HIV-1 integrase promotes insertion of the DNA into the host genome. The provirus may remain dormant or HIV-1 gene expression may be stimulated by the action of inducible and constitutive host transcription factors. The result is sequential production of various viral mRNAs that result first in regulatory proteins (Tat, Rev, Nef) and eventually in viral structural proteins resulting in assembly of virions. Free HIV-1 virions that are produced by viral budding then continue the retroviral cycle by infecting additional target cells.

Death of the CD4+ subset of lymphocytes appears to be the critical event underlying the severe immunodeficiency of clinical AIDS. These 'helper' lymphocytes ordinarily regulate the normal immune response. Monocytes, macrophages, glial cells and bone marrow cells may also harbor virus. There may be receptors other than CD4 as well.

Before HIV-1 had been recognized as the agent responsible for AIDS, investigators at several collaborating institutes of the National Institutes of Health reasoned that one strategy for investigating this illness might involve immune reconstitution of infected patients [2]. The initial protocol involved a set of monozygotic twins, one a 35 year old homosexual male who had clinical AIDS and a T4 cell count below 10/mm^3, the other his identical, healthy twin brother. Both subjects were immunized with keyhole-limpet hemocyanin (KLH). Peripheral blood lymphocytes (10×10^9 to 20×10^9) were collected by a 4 h continuous flow lymphocytapheresis procedure from the healthy sibling and infused into the patient in monthly intervals. After 2 months, 10^{10} nucleated bone marrow cells were harvested from the iliac crest of the healthy sibling. The affected twin received the bone marrow without a conditioning regimen; lymphocyte infusions were continued (Fig. 1). As can be seen from Fig. 1, peripheral blood lymphocytes increased; however, the patient developed a maculopapular cutaneous eruption and temperature elevation, which recurred after most lymphocyte transfusions. Skin biopsy

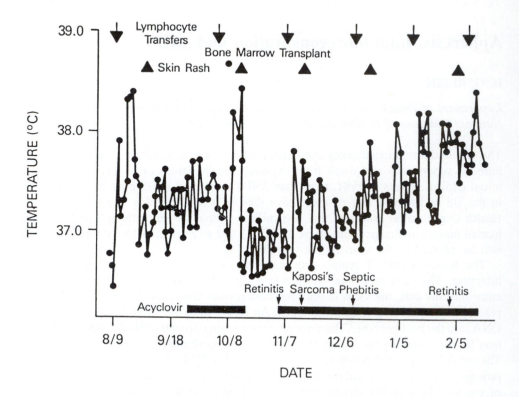

Figure 1. Clinical course of an AIDS patient treated with syngeneic lymphocyte transfers and bone marrow transplantation. Fever occurred with most infusions. Despite increased T4 cell counts and partial immune reconstitution, the clinical course deteriorated. Adapted from [2].

revealed nonspecific changes; however, on at least one occasion, the histopathology was consistent with graft-versus-host disease.

In the months after transplantation, the peripheral blood T4 cell numbers increased, peaking at three months post transplant. The patient had no skin response to KLH antigen before immunotherapy, while the twin had a 90 mm induration. After infusion, the patient was able to mount a substantial delayed cutaneous response which persisted for months. Nevertheless, he developed no serologic response nor an *in vitro* proliferative response to this antigen. Despite this immunologic improvement, the patient's clinical condition continued to deteriorate and he developed CMV retinitis, Kaposi's sarcoma, bacteremia with *Mycobacterium avium-intracellulare* and terminal CMV pneumonia. The partial immune reconstitution was encouraging, but the patient was not corrected to a clinically important degree.

The next strategy involved combining one or more chemotherapeutic agents with immune reconstitution in an effort to inhibit HIV-1 concurrent with immune reconstitution [3]. Sixteen subjects, 15 asymptomatic and one symptomatic HIV-1 infected patients with healthy monozygotic twins, were treated with zidovudine (AZT) to inhibit viral reverse transcription, treated with six peripheral blood lymphocyte infusions, transplanted with bone marrow from the healthy twin and subsequently randomized to receive either continued AZT or placebo after transplant. Subjects were monitored for CD4 cell counts, and sensitivity to tetanus toxoid and KLH. Immediately after marrow transplant and lymphocyte infusions the CD4 percentage rose 9% and increased delayed hypersensitivity (tetanus 4/13 to 11/13, KLH 8/12 by passive transfer) but there was no sustained immunologic improvement and no significant clinical improvement. The AZT-treated cohort did not differ from the placebo-treated group after immune reconstitution. These studies indicated that benefits from such combination therapy are transient, but suggest that future studies may need to combine cellular immune reconstitution with improved retroviral regimens, possibly involving several sites of attack (reverse transcriptase, uncoating, DNA insertion, activation, etc.). Additional strategies might involve ablation of the infected reservoir of virus, use of a soluble CD4 infusion, or immunization of the donor with HIV-specific antigen such as gp160. Finally, the advent of techniques applicable to somatic cell gene therapy suggest that autologous lymphocytes might be harvested from infected patients, and cytotoxic T cell clones might be expanded and even gene modified for specific cellular therapy combined with immune reconstitution. Apheresis technology will play a central role in these approaches.

REFERENCES

1. W. C. Greene. The molecular biology of human immunodeficiency virus type 1 infection. *N. Engl. J. Med.*, **324**, 308–317 (1991).
2. H. C. Lane, H. Masur, D. L. Longo, H. G. Klein *et al.* Partial reconstitution in a patient with the acquired immunodeficiency syndrome. *N. Engl. J. Med.*, **311**, 1099–1103 (1984).
3. H. C. Lane, K. M. Zunich, W. Wilson *et al.* Syngeneic bone marrow transplantation and adoptive transfer of peripheral blood lymphocytes in human immunodeficiency virus (HIV) infection. *Ann. Int. Med.*, **113**, 512–519 (1990).

Therapeutic Plasmapheresis (XII), pp. 25-28
T. Agishi *et al*. (Eds)
© VSP 1993

Randomized Trial of Low Density Lipoprotein Apheresis to Treat Coronary Artery Disease in Familial Hypercholesterolaemia

Y. KITANO and G. R. THOMPSON

MRC Lipoprotein Team, Hammersmith Hospital, London, UK

Key words: randomized trial; angiographic regression; combination therapy; LDL apheresis; integrated mean.

INTRODUCTION

It has been established that low density lipoprotein (LDL) apheresis is a safe and effective means of improving prognosis in homozygous familial hypercholesterolaemia (FH) and that this therapy should be started before atherosclerosis becomes apparent [1]. The other main indication for LDL apheresis is the far commoner condition of heterozygous FH although it remains to be shown whether this procedure has any advantages over modern drug therapy.

In order to establish the optimal therapy for heterozygous FH with coronary artery disease (CAD) a randomized trial, the FH Regression Study, is currently being undertaken in Britain.

PATIENTS AND METHODS

The FH Regression Study is a two-centre collaborative trial (London and Cardiff) into which FH heterozygotes of both sexes with documented CAD have been enrolled. The inclusion and exclusion criteria are as follows:

Inclusion criteria:

(i) Cholesterol > 8 mmol/l (310 mg/dl) plus tendon xanthomata in patient or first degree relative, or plus hypercholesterolaemia or MI < 60 years in first degree relative, or plus cholesterol > 8 mmol/l or MI < 50 years in second degree relative.

(ii) Both sexes, 20–64 years.

(iii) At least two abnormal coronary segments (excluding total occlusions) on angiography.

Exclusion criteria:

  (i) Previous CABG.

 (ii) Diabetes Mellitus.

(iii) Uncontrolled hypertension.

(iv) Hormone replacement therapy.

 (v) History of viral hepatitis.

(vi) Partial ileal bypass.

(vii) Anticoagulant drugs except aspirin.

(viii) Potentially fertile female.

(ix) Gross obesity.

Patients are randomized to two treatment groups, one of which undergoes bi-weekly LDL apheresis using dextran sulfate/cellulose columns (Kaneka) to treat one plasma volume per procedure, plus simvastatin 40 mg/day; the other group receives simvastatin 40 mg/day plus colestipol 20 g/day (or Questran 16 g). Changes in serum lipids and lipoproteins are monitored during the trial. Mean lipid levels between procedures in patients on apheresis/statin are calculated by integrating the area under the rebound curve and dividing by time. Patients also undergo exercise ECG tests every six months and coronary angiography before and after two years in the trial. Quantitative angiography analysis will be performed using a computer assisted method, the Cardiovascular Angiography Analysis System (CAAS).

RESULTS

All told, 42 patients have been randomized. The lipid values at screening visit 2, when all patients were on an anion-exchange resin alone, are shown in Table 1.

The differences between mean follow-up values and values during run-in period on resin (Table 1) are presented in Table 2.

The results of serial exercise ECG tests showing time taken to reach 1 mm ST segment depression are summarized in Table 3.

Table 1.
Baseline data (means) during run-in period on colestipol (20 g/day) or Questran (16 g/day)

Group		Apheresis	Drug
n		20	22
Male		14	16
Female		6	6
Total cholesterol ⎫		9.0	7.9
Triglyceride ⎬ mmol/l		2.7	2.0
HDL-cholesterol ⎭		1.1	1.1
ApoB ⎱ mg/dl		6.8 (19)	137 (15)
Lp(a) ⎰		43	37 (21)

Table 2.

Percentage change in lipids during trial compared to the baseline data

Group	Apheresis (interval mean)[a]	Drug (mean)
Total cholesterol	−48	−33
Triglyceride	−63	−15
HDL-cholesterol	+9	+9
LDL-cholesterol	−53	−42
ApoB	−40	−26
Lp(a)	−23	+22

[a] Estimated by integrating under rebound curves = mean preapheresis value ×0.77.

Table 3.

Serial exercise tests (Bruce protocol) showing minutes taken to 1 mm ST depression

Months	Apheresis/statin			Resin/statin		
	W	NC	I	W	NC	I
6	3	8	7	1	7	7
12	2	3	9	2	2	6
18	1	3	6	0	1	8
24	1	0	3	0	1	7

Worse (W) =⩾ 10% decrease in time; no change (NC) =< 10% change in time; improved (I) =⩾ 10% increase in time.

DISCUSSION

Several studies have demonstrated the ability of LDL apheresis to induce regression of CAD in hyperlipidaemic patients [2–6]. However, no data exist at present which show whether LDL apheresis is any more efficient in this respect than dual or triple combinations of lipid-lowering drugs such as colestipol, nicotinic acid, probucol and HMG CoA-reductase inhibitors.

The results of our FH Regression Study are expected to reveal (i) whether marked reductions in LDL-cholesterol can induce angiographic regression of coronary atherosclerotic lesions in patients with heterozygous FH; (ii) whether the combination of LDL apheresis and simvastatin is superior in this respect to simvastatin plus an anion exchange resin and (iii) whether reduction of both Lp(a) and LDL in patients with high levels of Lp(a) is more advantageous than reduction of LDL alone.

The overall results of changes in serum lipids and angiographic analysis will not be available until the first half of 1993. But as shown in Table 2, the reduction in serum lipids and lipoproteins, especially LDL, apoB, triglyceride and Lp(a), all appear to be more marked in the apheresis/statin group than in resin/statin group, despite the fact that serum lipid levels were slightly higher in the apheresis/statin group than in the resin/statin group at screening visit 2 (Table 1). However, serial exercise ECG tests show similar rates of improvement in each group (Table 3).

Although the combination of simvastatin with resin achieved a remarkable 42% reduction in LDL-cholesterol neither of these drugs lowers Lp(a), which is known to be associated with premature CAD in FH [7]. In contrast, LDL apheresis removes Lp(a); the addition of an HMG CoA reductase inhibitor appears to be effective in reducing the tendency for cholesterol synthesis to increase after LDL apheresis as evidenced by measurement of urinary mevalonic acid excretion [1].

It will be of particular importance to ascertain whether LDL apheresis plus simvastatin offers any advantage over combination drug therapy, especially in FH patients with raised levels of Lp(a).

SUMMARY

The FH Regression Study is a collaborative two centre trial in which 42 FH heterozygotes with CAD have been randomly allocated to receive bi-weekly LDL apheresis (dextran sulfate/cellulose gel) plus simvastatin or anion-exchange resin plus simvastatin. Coronary angiography is performed before and after 2 years of treatment and will be analyzed by a computer-assisted method.

Interim results as of May 1992 show that reductions in LDL-cholesterol, apoB and Lp(a) are slightly more marked in the apheresis/simvastatin group than in the colestipol/simvastatin group, especially in patients with raised levels of Lp(a). Serial exercise tests show improvement in similar numbers of patients in each group. However, the final results including angiographic analysis will not be available until 1993.

REFERENCES

1. Y. Kitano, C. Neuwirth, V. Maher *et al.* LDL apheresis — state of the art. In: *Treatment of Severe Dyslipoproteinaemia in the Prevention of Coronary Heart Disease 3*, A. H. Gotto Jr, M. Mancini and W. O. Richter (Eds), pp. 319–326, Karger, Basel (1992).

2. V. Hombach, H. Borberg, A. Gadzkowski *et al.* Regression der Koronarsklerose bei familiarer Hypercholesterinamie IIa durch spezifische LDL-apherese. *Dtsch. med. Woch.*, 111, 1709–1715 (1986).

3. W. O. Richter, K. Sühler and P. Schwandt. Extracorporeal LDL elimination by immunoabsorption: side effects and influences on other serum lipoproteins and serum parameters. In: *Treatment of Severe Hypercholesterolaemia in the Prevention of Coronary Heart Disease 2*, A. H. Gotto Jr, M. Mancini and W. O. Richter (Eds), pp. 183–187, Karger, Basel (1990).

4. D. Seidel, V. W. Armstrong, P. Schuff-Werner, for the HELP Study Group. The HELP-LDL-apheresis multicentre study, an angiographically assessed trial on the role of LDL-apheresis in the secondary prevention of coronary heart disease. 1. Evaluation of safety and cholesterol lowering effects during the first 12 months. *Eur. J. Clin. Invest.*, 21, 375–385 (1991).

5. N. Koga and Y. Iwata. Pathological and angiographic regression of coronary atherosclerosis by LDL-apheresis in a patient with familial hypercholesterolaemia. *Atherosclerosis*, 90, 9–21 (1991).

6. A. Yamamoto. Regression of atherosclerosis in humans by lowering serum cholesterol. *Atherosclerosis*, 89, 1–10 (1991).

7. M. Seed, F. Hoppichler, D. Reaveley *et al.* Relation of serum lipoprotein(a) concentration and apolipoprotein(a) phenotype to coronary heart disease in patients with familial hypercholesterolaemia. *N. Engl. J. Med.*, 322, 1494–1499 (1990).

Therapeutic Plasmapheresis (XII), pp. 29-35
T. Agishi *et al.* (Eds)

Plasmapheresis and Cytotoxic Drugs in the Treatment of Systemic Lupus Erythematosus

H. H. EULER, J. O. SCHROEDER, U. M. SCHWAB, P. HARTEN,
H. J. GUTSCHMIDT[1] and J. D. HERRLINGER[2]

2nd Medical University Clinic, Kiel,
[1]*Department of Dialysis, Municipal Hospital, Kiel and* [2]*Department of Internal Medicine, Rendsburg, Germany*

Key words: plasmapheresis; cytotoxic drugs; cyclophosphamide; treatment; systemic lupus erythematosus.

INTRODUCTION

The role of apheresis treatment in managing patients with systemic lupus erythematosus (SLE) is a matter of considerable dispute. According to several controlled clinical trials, plasmapheresis as a short-term adjunct to long-term p.o. immunosuppression is no longer justified. According to uncontrolled reports a possible role for plasmapheresis in SLE remains (i) for rapid disease control in critically ill patients, (ii) for rapid complement substitution in severe SLE due to congenital complement-deficiency, (iii) as a long-term adjunct to conventional immunosuppression, and (iv) in the context of the 'synchronization' protocol, i.e. plasmapheresis with subsequent pulse cyclophosphamide, aiming at increased clonal deletion by applying pulse cytotoxic drugs during the period of depletion-induced increased activity — and, thus, increased vulnerability — of pathogenic clones. This review summarizes previous and more extensive reports on the topic of plasmapheresis and cytotoxic drugs in SLE, focusing on the 'synchronization' approach [1].

CYTOTOXIC DRUGS IN SLE

Te 10-year mortality rate in SLE is still as high as 10–20% [2, 3]. Standard therapy includes long-term application of glucocorticosteroids (Prd) and cyclophosphamide (Ctx). To date, no treatment protocol has been able to achieve lasting treatment-free remissions in SLE. Ctx has been applied in SLE since 1964. Since then, several reports have described Ctx as effective for most SLE manifestations. It is usually given p.o., either in a constant dosage (e.g. 100–150 mg/d) or adjusted to reduce the WBC count to about 2.0–4.0/nl. Intravenous pulse Ctx ($0.5–1$ g/m^2 every 4–12 weeks) is replacing p.o. Ctx in some centers [4, 5], but not in all [6]. Uncontrolled studies in which pulse Ctx was applied have led to positive results e.g. in CNS-lupus [5] and in SLE-associated thrombocytopenia. In a controlled long-term study in lupus nephritis [4], pulse Ctx tended to induce better long-term results and fewer side effects (neoplasia and infection). The latter may have been due to the lower cumulative Ctx dosage. The survival rate was not higher in patients treated with pulse Ctx [4]. An advantage of pulse Ctx is its more rapid initial effect. A drawback might be the necessary intervals between subsequent pulses. During these intervals not only the bone marrow but also disease might recover. It has not yet been evaluated in detail, whether the concomitant application of supplementary drugs may influence the efficacy of pulse Ctx. Since Ctx has its most obvious effect on proliferating lymphocytes, the presence of Prd might retard this proliferation [1, 7]. The efficacy of Ctx might possibly be increased by avoiding Prd prior to, during, and immediately after pulse Ctx.

PLASMAPHERESIS IN SLE

Plasmapheresis (PP) was applied in a large number of case reports and small patient series. The prevailing result was that the treatment was beneficial in the short term, but without accompanying immunosuppression relapses occurred soon. In a randomized trial [8], better results tended to be achieved in 39 patients with lupus nephritis by combining Prd and cytotoxic drugs with Pl and by substitution with human albumin. A controlled double-blind study [9] revealed no difference between Pl and sham Pl with continued immunosuppression in 20 cases of mild lupus. A French trial [10] compared Prd plus Pl versus Prd alone in 39 patients over a period of 29 months and did not detect a significant difference. In a Dutch trial 20 patients were treated either with Prd and Pl or with Prd and cytotoxic drugs: neither protocol was superior [11]. Wallace analyzed a number of variables in 27 patients with severe lupus nephritis. Compared with treatments that did not involve Pl, Pl was associated with a more rapid improvement of laboratory parameters, and all seven patients who had the best response (resolution of nephrotic syndrome and normalization of creatinine) had been subjected to Pl [12]. Finally, Lewis and colleagues reported that treatment with Pl plus an 8-week standard regimen of Prd and p.o. Ctx did not improve the clinical outcome of severe lupus nephritis as compared with the standard regimen alone [13]. They conclude that Pl cannot be recommended for patients with severe lupus nephritis. This conclusion might be premature. The negative results might be due to the design of these previous trials. The aim of Pl treatment is to eliminate pathogenic antibodies (ab's) and circulating immune complexes. It has repeatedly been shown that Pl without concomitant immunosuppression induces a compensatory, sometimes overshooting ('rebound') synthesis of auto-ab's or immune complexes [1]. This is preceded by an increased activity — and thus increased vulnerability — of ab-producing lymphocyte clones to Ctx. To fully exploit this mechanism, combined Pl and Ctx requires an optimum sequencing: High-dose Ctx should be applied shortly after but not before or during Pl. In this concept, Pl is used to achieve rapid relief from pathogenic substances and to enhance the susceptibility of ab-producing clones to Ctx. In contrast to the conventional approach (Pl as an adjunct to long-term p.o. immunosuppression) this combined schedule attempts to utilize the rebound mechanism instead of suppressing it. This approach has been applied successfully in a pilot trial in SLE [14]. Pl with subsequent pulse Ctx has led to rapid improvement of clinical symptoms. In addition, treatment-free remissions have repeatedly been achieved for periods now amounting to several years [1]. To our knowledge, comparable long-term results are not reported elsewhere. Thus, previous trials on Pl in SLE possibly have not taken sufficient account of the concept of stimulation and subsequent deletion of pathogenic clones. Caution should be exercised in making definitive statements regarding the value of Pl in SLE, before thorough evaluations of this approach have been completed.

ANTIBODY KINETICS FOLLOWING ANTIBODY DEPLETION

In previous investigations on Pl in SLE, long-term reduction of auto-ab levels generally was not possible [15], although each exchange of one plasma volume eliminates about 50% of circulating IgG. When no long-term depletion is achieved, despite multiple repetitions and parallel immunosuppression, it must be assumed that there is a potent feedback cycle that counterbalances the losses. Within the feedback between ab's and their resynthesis, the term 'ab rebound' is used to describe enhanced ab synthesis (or excretion) following ab depletion [15–17]. This mechanism might have played a crucial role in previous negative results with therapeutic Pl. It might be possible to utilize it to increase clonal deletion, if pulse Ctx is applied during the period of increased lymphocyte activity and vulnerability. In closed biological systems a feedback between a product and the producing cell is the rule. The opposite — production that is not influenced by its product — has rarely been demonstrated in non-neoplastic diseases. It can be assumed that ab production is subject to a regulatory mechanism, since it does not end abruptly with disappearance of the ag stimulus. Another argument favoring a regulatory mechanism is the observation that initial titers are reached again within a short period of time. This becomes evident if we consider the individual components of ab resynthesis following ab elimination. One component is redistribution from the extravascular space. About 50% of IgG is distributed extravascularly [18]. Redistribution is largely completed within 24 h [19]. Thus, following exchange of one plasma volume eliminating 50% of intravascular IgG [20], a rapid reincrease to 75% of the initial titer can be expected. Another component is the basic synthesis rate. Assuming a steady state and a 50% turnover rate of human IgG of 20 [18–23] days [18], 1/40th (2.5%) will be resynthesized within 1 day. A further component is decreasing catabolism. Normally, resynthesis is balanced by the respective catabolism rate. Catabolism diminishes to compensate for protein depletion [18, 19]. Assuming catabolism were to halt completely, decreased catabolism might induce a daily IgG increase of up to 2.5%. Finally, enhanced clearance of the reticuloendothelial system following Pl [21] represents another component. In contrast to the mechanisms described above, this aspect tends to reduce ab levels. Any further increase indicates enhancement of neosynthesis or excretion. There is still a considerable difference between the renewed increase due to redistribution, basic resynthesis and altered catabolism on the one hand and the initial titer on the other. This difference represents the scope in which enhanced compensatory synthesis, i.e. the 'rebound' can take place. Although rebound kinetics overshooting the baseline have been described [22–24], rebound without overshoot should be more frequent. The basic synthesis rate of an IgG ab is about 2.5% of its circulating amount. A 100% increase in the synthesis rate represents a scarcely measurable 2.5% increase in the ab titer. However, the 100% increase should correspond to a 100% increase in lymphocyte proliferation and, thus, in vulnerability. Experimental evidence suggesting that circulating ab's are a component of a feedback mechanism regulating ab synthesis has long been available [22, 25]. Ab synthesis can be specifically suppressed by passive administration of complete ab's or Fab' or F(ab')2 of the same specificity before or during immunization with various ag's [25]. The reverse effect, i.e. stimulation of resynthesis following ab depletion, was demonstrated by means of immunoadsorption [26]. This was confirmed to be clonally specific by reduction of specific ab's [16]. In recent studies, ab's could not be decreased to below 50% of the values of untreated controls despite elimination of several plasma volumes [27]. As early as 1957 it was noticed that in immunized plasma donors specific ab levels remained more clearly elevated than in controls without plasma donation [28]. This is in accordance with routine laboratory knowledge that high ab titers are best obtained by starting bloodletting shortly after immunization. Activation by ab depletion at the cellular level has been reported [29]. The molecular mechanism controlling lymphocyte activation following ab depletion is only partially known (reviewed in [1]). It may include clonal stimulation through ag liberation [17], shifting ag/ab ratios within circulating immune complexes towards ag-rich, B cell stimulating complexes, and/or co-elimination of suppressive anti-idiotypes [30]. In SLE, increased production of immune complexes and auto-ab's following depletion has been reported [31–33]. This led to a warning against Pl without accompanying immunosuppression [32, 33].

'SYNCHRONIZATION'

The efficacy of Ctx rests on the principle that slowly proliferating cells are not injured as much as rapidly proliferating cells. Inducing maximum proliferation of pathogenic clones should improve the chances that they will be eliminated semiselectively by high-dose Ctx. Ctx inhibits B cell activity, if it is applied early following stimulation and at high doses [34]. This has been documented in studies inducing proliferation by ab-reapplication and subsequent Ctx [34, 35], enabling induction of immunological tolerance [36]. Critical factors for Ctx-induced tolerance have been determined [34]: high doses of ag [34], an exact schedule, calling for administration of Ctx in the brief 'window' a few days before or after clonal stimulation [34], a high Ctx dosage [34], and absence of Prd [7]. Clinically, this principle is seldom applicable. Pathogenic ag's are seldom known, and ag-reapplication would pose major problems. An exception is the successful combination of reimmunization with factor VIII and subsequent Ctx in F-VIII ab hemophilia [37]. Similar approaches have attempted to improve transplant tolerance in allogeneic transplantation by clonal stimulation with donor ag's prior to immunosuppression, excellently reviewed in [36]. Applied to stimulation by means of ab depletion this 'stimulation/deletion' [31] or 'synchronization' [14, 38] concept was applied experimentally [16, 24], and it was repeatedly discussed as an improved therapeutic option [31, 39, 40]. In a case report on myasthenia gravis [41] Pl with subsequent pulse Ctx led to remission under Prd for 10 weeks. In SLE [32], Pl and subsequent pulse Ctx (1 g) induced a symptom-free remission under Prd and azathioprine for 2 years. In 26 cases of refractory SLE, Robinson applied Pl and subsequent pulse Ctx (up to 1 g/m^2). Stable remissions occurred in 58%. In three patients ANA could no longer be demonstrated [40]. Similar positive results have been reported in small patient series by other groups [42]. However, the details of the protocols vary considerably. A schedule that aims at optimum utilization of the ab rebound should include the following principles:

(i) The basic rationale combines ab depletion with subsequent pulse Ctx.

(ii) Multiple repeated initial large volume plasmaphereses at short intervals achieve extensive elimination of intravascular and extravascular ab's [18].

(iii) Any influence that might retard lymphocyte proliferation should be avoided. Thus, Prd [7, 43] and other substances (e.g. morphins [1]) should be withdrawn during the period of Pl and pulse Ctx.

(iv) To accomplish maximum lymphocyte proliferation, substitution fluids containing immunoglobulin should be avoided [30].

A proposal for the comprehensive utilization of these principles is the following protocol. Initially, it starts with withdrawal of immunosuppressive drugs (cytotoxic agents 3 weeks prior to the first Pl, Prd 2 days before). This is followed by 360 ml/kg plasmaphereses on subsequent days. Pulse Ctx (3 days 12 mg/kg/d, total dose: 36 mg/kg) is started 6 h after the third Pl. Prd is reapplied after the Ctx pulse. During the next 6 months Ctx and Prd are given p.o. The Ctx dosage is modified, aiming at maintaining WBC counts between 2.0/nl and 4.0/nl. This protocol was applied in a pilot study [1, 14] in 14 patients (female, 18–56 years) with severe and refractory SLE. Disease activity, as measured by the SLAM [44] was 28.4 (13–37) points. All patients improved within 6 months. The mean SLAM had decreased to 8.9 (2–13) points. In 12 patients clinical remission was extensive, and immunosuppression (including Prd) was stopped. Currently, 8 patients continue to be under treatment-free observation. The mean treatment-free follow-up is 29 months, with the longest remission (residual SLAM: 1) now stable for 54 months without treatment [1, 14]. Comparison of IgG-ANA with total serum IgG showed a rapid drop in both parameters during Pl followed by a subsequent rise to near pretreatment levels. At 3–5 months later total serum IgG returned to nearly normal, whereas the ANA-IgG titers decreased. The synchronization concept may have to be extended by the assumption that active or disease-associated clones are more clearly subject to stimulation/deletion kinetics than resting clones, which comprise the larger portion of the total IgG pool. This semiselective principle may explain why the treatment does not induce severe humoral immunodeficiency.

Thus, in SLE the optimized combination of Pl with subsequent pulse Ctx led to rapid relief and to long-term treatment-free remissions in some patients. Some aspects of this protocol are currently being investigated in a randomized trial by the Lupus Plasmapheresis Study Group [45].

REFERENCES

1. H. H. Euler and J. O. Schroeder. Antibody depletion and cytotoxic drug therapy in severe systemic lupus erythematosus. *Transfus Sci.*, **13**, 167–184 (1992).

2. J. H. Klippel. Survival in SLE. In: *Proc. Second Int. Conf. on Systemic Lupus Erythematosus*, Professional Postgraduate Services, Singapore (1990).

3. J. D. Reveille, A. Barolucci and G. Alarcón-Segovia. Prognosis in systemic lupus erythematosus. Negative impact of increasing age at onset, black race, and thrombocytopenia, as well as causes of death. *Arthritis Rheum.*, **33**, 37–48 (1990).

4. A. D. Steinberg and S. C. Steinberg. Long-term preservation of renal function in patients with lupus nephritis receiving treatment that includes cyclophosphamide versus those treated with prednisone only. *Arthritis Rheum.*, **34**, 945–950 (1991).

5. D. A. Fox and W. J. McCune. Immunologic and clinical effects of cytotoxic drugs used in the treatment of rheumatoid arthritis and systemic lupus erythematosus. In: *Therapy of Autoimmune Diseases*, Karger, Basel (1989).

6. D. J. Wallace. A critique of the NIH lupus nephritis survey. *Arthritis Rheum.*, **35**, 605 (1992).

7. P. Dukor and F. M. Dietrich. Prevention of cyclophosphamide-induced tolerance to erythrocytes by pretreatment with cortisone. *Proc. Soc. Exp. Biol. Med.*, **133**, 280–285 (1970).

8. W. F. Clark, J. W. Balfe, D. C. Catttran *et al.* Long-term plasma exchange in patients with systemic lupus erythematosus and diffuse proliferative glomerulonephritis. *Plasma Ther. Transf. Technol.*, **5**, 353–360 (1984).

9. N. Wei, J. H. Klippel, D. P. Huston *et al.* Randomised trial of plasma exchange in mild systemic lupus erythematosus. *Lancet*, **1**, 17–22 (1983).

10. French Cooperative Study Group. A randomised trial of plasma exchange in severe acute systemic lupus erythematosus. *Plasma Ther. Transfus. Technol.*, **6**, 535–539 (1985).

11. R. H. Derksen, R. J. Hene, C. G. Kallenberg *et al.* Prospective multicentre trial on the short-term effects of plasma exchange versus cytotoxic drugs in steroid-resistant lupus nephritis. *Neth. J. Med.*, **33**, 168–177 (1988).

12. D. J. Wallace, D. Goldfinger, G. Savage *et al.* Predictive value of clinical, laboratory, pathologic, and treatment variables in steroid/immunosuppressive resistant lupus nephritis. *J. Clin. Apheresis*, **4**, 30–34 (1988).

13. E. J. Lewis, L. G. Hunsicker, S. P. Lan *et al.* A controlled trial of plasmapheresis therapy in severe lupus nephritis. *N. Engl. J. Med.*, **326**, 1374–1379 (1992).

14. J. O. Schroeder, H. H. Euler, H. Löffler. Synchronization of plasmapheresis and pulse cyclophosphamide in systemic lupus erythematosus. *Ann. Intern. Med.*, **107**, 344–346 (1987).

15. J. C. Bystryn. Plasma exchange in pemphigus. *Arch. Dermatol.*, **124**, 1702–1704 (1988).

16. J. C. Bystryn, I. Schenkein and J. W. Uhr. A model for regulation of antibody sythesis by serum antibody. In: *Progress in Immunology*, Academic Press, New York (1971).

17. J. W. Uhr and G. Moeller. Regulatory effect of antibody on the immune response. *Adv. Immunol.*, **8**, 81–127 (1968).

18. G. C. Kramer, B. I. Harms, R. H. Demling *et al.* Mechanisms for redistribution of plasmaproteins following acute protein depletion. *Am. J. Physiol.*, **243**, 803–809 (1982).

19. B. Charlton, K. Schindhelm, L. C. Smeby *et al.* Analysis of immunoglobulin G kinetic in the non-steady-state. *J. Lab. Clin. Med.*, **105**, 312–320 (1985).

20. R. M. Kellogg and J. P. Hester. Kinetics modelling of plasma exchange. *J. Clin. Apheresis*, **4**, 183–187 (1988).

21. C. M. Lockwood, S. Worlledge, A. Nicholas *et al.* Reversal of impaired splenic function in patients with nephritis or vasculitis (or both) by plasma exchange. *N. Engl. J. Med.*, **300**, 524–530 (1979).

22. J. C. Bystryn, M. W. Graf and J. W. Uhr. Regulation of antibody formulation by serum antibody. II. Removal of specific antibody by means of exchange transfusion. *J. Exp. Med.*, **132**, 1279–1287 (1970).

23. R. H. W. M. Derksen, H. J. Schuurman, G. F. H. J. Meyling *et al.* Rebound and overshoot after plasma exchange in humans. *J. Lab. Clin. Med.*, **104**, 35–43 (1984).

24. D. S. Terman, R. Garcia-Rinaldi, B. Dannemann *et al.* Specific suppression of antibody rebound after extracorporeal immunoadsorption. I. Comparison of single versus combination chemotherapeutic agents. *Clin. Exp. Immunol.*, **34**, 32–41 (1978).

25. J. W. Uhr and J. B. Baumann. Antibody formation: the suppression of antibody formation by passively administered antibodies. *J. Exp. Med.*, **113**, 935–957 (1961).

26. M. W. Graf and J. W. Uhr. Regulation of antibody formation by serum antibody: I. Removal of specific antibody by means of immunoadsorption. *J. Exp. Med.*, **130**, 1175–1186 (1969).

27. B. Vendeville, D. Baran, F. Imbert *et al.* Plasma exchange in a rat model of autoimmune glomerulonephritis. *Nephrol. Dial. Transplant.*, **3**, 405–411 (1988).

28. J. Smolens, J. Stokes and A. B. Vogt. Human plasmapheresis and its effect on antibodies. *J. Immunol.*, **79**, 434–439 (1957).

29. B. C. Sturgill and M. J. Worzniak. Stimulation of proliferation of 19S antibody forming cells in the spleens of immunized guinea-pigs after exchange transfusion. *Nature*, **228**, 1304–1305 (1970).

30. F. Rossi and M. D. Kazatchkine. Antiidiotypes against autoantibodies in pooled normal polyspecific IgG. *J. Immunol.*, **143**, 4104–4109 (1989).

31. J. V. Jones. Plasmapheresis in SLE. *Clin. Rheum. Dis.*, **8**, 243–260 (1982).

32. J. V. Jones, M. F. Robinson, R. K. Parciany *et al.* Therapeutic plasmapheresis in systemic lupus erythematosus. Effect on immune complexes and antibodies to DNA. *Arthritis Rheum.*, **24**, 1113–1120 (1981).

33. R. Schlansky, R. J. deHoratius, T. Pincus *et al.* Plasmapheresis in systemic lupus erythematosus. A cautionary note. *Arthritis Rheum.*, **24**, 49–53 (1981).

34. A. C. Aisenberg. Studies on cyclophosphamide-induced tolerance to sheep erythocytes. *J. Exp. Med.*, **125**, 833–845 (1967).

35. J. D. Herrlinger and W. Müller-Ruchholtz. Different suppressive effects of combined cyclophosphamide-antigen treatment compared with exclusive cyclophosphamide treatment of primary and secondary humoral immune reactivity. *Int. Arch. Allergy Appl. Immunol.*, **57**, 82–89 (1978).

36. H. Mayumi and K. Tokunaga. Cyclophosphamide-induced chimera-type tolerance to allografts: an overview of drug-induced immunological tolerance. *Fukuoka Acta Med.*, **81**, 20–40 (1990).

37. I. M. Nilsson, E. Berntorp and O. Zettervall. Induction of immune tolerance in patients with hemophilia and antibodies to factor VIII by combined treatment with intravenous IgG, cyclophosphamide, and factor VIII. *N. Engl. J. Med.*, **318**, 947–950 (1988).

38. H. H. Euler, H. Löffler and E. Christophers. Synchronization of plasmapheresis and pulse cyclophosphamide in pemphigus vulgaris. *Arch. Dermatol.*, **123**, 1205–1210 (1987).

39. P. C. Dau, J. M. Lindstrom, C. K. Cassel *et al.* Plasmapheresis and immunosuppressive drug therapy in myasthenia gravis. *N. Engl. J. Med.*, **297**, 1134–1140 (1977).

40. W. G. Barr, E. A. Hubbell and J. A. Robinson. Persistently active lupus erythematosus treated with intermittent plasmapheresis and bolus cyclophosphamide. In: *Therapeutic Plasmapheresis* (IV), ISAO Press, Cleveland (1987).

41. P. C. Dau. Plasmapheresis therapy in myasthenia gravis. *Muscle Nerv.*, **3**, 468–482 (1980).

42. C. Zielinski, C. Mueller and J. Smolen. Plasmapheresis in the treatment of systemic lupus erythematosus: a controlled study. *Acta Med. Austriaca*, **15**, 155–158 (1988).

43. G. J. Dennis and J. J. Mond. Corticosteroid-induced suppression of murine B cell immune response antigens. *J. Immunol.*, **136**, 1600–1604 (1986).

44. M. H. Liang, S. A. Socher, M. G. Larson *et al.* Reliability and validity of six systems for the clinical assessment of disease activity in systemic lupus erythematosus. *Arthritis Rheum.*, **32**, 1107–1118 (1989).

45. Lupus Plasmapheresis Study Group, W. F. Clark, P. C. Dau *et al.* Plasmapheresis and subsequent pulse cyclophosphamide versus pulse cyclophosphamide alone in severe lupus: design of the LPSG trial. *J. Clin. Apheresis*, **6**, 40–47 (1991).

Therapeutic Plasmapheresis (XII), pp. 37-43
T. Agishi *et al.* (Eds)
© VSP 1993

Plasma Self-sufficiency and Donor Plasmapheresis in Japan

S. SEKIGUCHI

Hokkaido Red Cross Blood Center, Japanese Red Cross Fractionation Center, Sapporo, Japan

Key words: plasma self-sufficiency; plasmapheresis.

INTRODUCTION

The blood program in Japan has been carried out completely by donated plasma; how-ever, most of source plasma for plasma derivatives have been imported. In these situations, the unfortunate event happened that hemophilia patients have been infected with human immunodeficiency virus (HIV) through imported coagulation products. The Ministry of Health and Welfare (MHW) decided on a new policy to process national self-sufficiency of blood coagulation factors with donated plasma, and then aimed to start the self-sufficiency of albumin and immunoglobulin products by degrees. Based on this schedule in 1991, the Japanese Red Cross (JRC) were going to achieve the procurement of about 500 000 l of source plasma in a year. To accomplish this pur-pose, about 800 000 donations, i.e. 10% of all donations, were planned to be collected through plasmapheresis. So, the JRC has prepared 75 donating rooms, 400 mobiles and 1800 apheresis machines at a total of 77 blood centers to manage the apheresis procedures.

At present, source plasma has been collected as scheduled and the 100 000 000 units of coagulant factor required per year in Japan are now being processed both by the Japanese Red Cross Plasma Fractionation Center (70% of all products) and other non-profit institutions.

DISCUSSION

In 1952, the JRC established the Tokyo Blood Bank, as well as the Hokkaido Blood Bank, which was the first public bank, and started to accept voluntary blood donation.

However, at that time, active commercial blood banking was still carried on and post-transfusion hepatitis using contaminated low-quality blood had become a serious problem. These circumstances finally led to 'the Cabinet Resolution' issued by the gov-ernment in 1964, entitled "Promotion of Voluntary Non-remunerated Blood Program." After the Cabinet Resolution, the number of voluntary blood donors increased year by year, and finally commercial blood banking was eliminated for whole blood supply in 1968. Meanwhile more and more plasma derivatives have been used and the Japanese

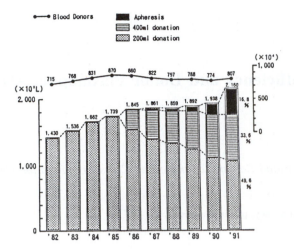

Figure 1. Yearly change of blood donation — total number of donors and collected volumes categorized.

consumption of albumin products came up to the one third of world use in 1980s. And in 1983, the JRC established a Plasma Fractionation Center and started operation to produce albumin and gammaglobulin products. Furthermore, to correspond to supply enough source plasma, in addition to conventional 200 ml donation, we started 400 ml and apheresis donation in 1986.

Figure 1 shows the yearly change in the number of voluntary donors and the volume of blood donations for the past 10 years. Bars in this figure shows three types of blood donations: 200 ml of whole blood, 400 ml of whole blood and apheresis. As the number of donors, about 8 000 000 people offered their valuable blood in 1991. The volume of blood or plasma collected in 1991 was 1 072 000, 725 000 and 362 000 l as 200 ml whole blood donation, 400 ml whole blood donation and apheresis, respectively. The percentage of them in the total was 49.6, 33.6 and 16.8%, respectively. The proportion of 200 ml whole blood donation has been decreasing year by year from 1985. On the contrary, 400 ml donation and apheresis has been growing more and more. As to the apheresis donation, we introduced this system in 1986 and it grew rapidly as the amount of plasma in 1991 was 2.5 times that in 1986. The volume of collected blood also has been increasing by degrees in spite of no increase of voluntary donors in these years. It means that the effective collection of plasma by apheresis systems and of 400 ml donation have been working well. The blood products needed in Japan are completely supplied by the JRC from voluntary donated blood at present.

The use of albumin product has increased rapidly from 1979 to mid-1980s and reached to a peak 3 840 000 l source plasma in 1985 (Fig. 2). In this situation, it was regrettable that donated blood as the source plasma has been very small as indicated in the lower part of bars.

In 1986, MHW produced a guidelines on adequate use of blood products. The volume of consumption was decreased momentarily, but it has not been continued and showed a plateau level of about 2 800 000 l from 1988 to now. Up to 2 years ago, paid donation for plasma fractionation continued in Japan. It has now been banned and the paid source plasma has been replaced by voluntary plasma.

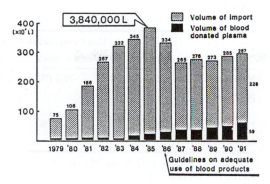

Figure 2. Volume of plasma fractionation products used in Japan (source plasma).

Items	Domestic Production Volume		Imported Products Volume
Volume of Production	1,987,000 * (67 × 10⁴L)		4,824,000 * (220 × 10⁴L)
Plasma Sources	Donated Plasma	Imported Plasma	
	59 × 10⁴L	8 × 10⁴L	
Rate of Donated Plasma	21%		79%

*UNITS 12.5g. EQV.

Figure 3. Use of albumin in Japan (1991).

Next, the amount of albumin is shown in Fig. 3. The domestic products corresponded to about 670 000 l as source plasma. The 590 000 l of it depends on donated blood, so the proportion of self-sufficiency was 21%. On the other hand, the imported products are 2 200 000 l as source plasma. Though the proportion of dependence on the imported products including the imported plasma tends to decrease, actually it is 79%.

The amount of intravenous immunoglobulin products used was about 3200 kg and Factor VIII was about 130 000 000 units. Factor IX used was 23 000 000 units, and IVIG, Factor VIII and IX were produced domestically, 74.7, 32.1 and 23.5%, respectively, but these products are mainly made from imported foreigner's blood.

AIDS shock through imported products has given us an another impact.

According to the data from February 1992, the MHW announced 458 people were recognized as AIDS patients and 324 of them, 70.7%, were infected through the coagulation products (Table 1). As to hemophiliacs, 1531 persons were infected with HIV through coagulation products at least. Most HIV patients in Japan are infected by the use of coagulation factor products. It is an unusual case in the world and very regrettable. In these situations, the Japanese government decided that coagulation factor products must be self-sufficient. According to this decision, the 'New Commission to Investigate Blood Programs' in the MHW planned a project to achieve this purpose. The first is the national self-sufficiency of blood coagulation factors with donated plasma in the near future. The second is the ratio of the self-sufficiency of albumin and immunoglobulin products to increase by degrees in the future. The peak of albumin consumption

Table 1.
Number of Japanese AIDS patients

	Total	By blood coagulation factor concentrates	
Number of AIDS patients	458	324	70.7 (%)
Number of persons infected with HIV	2008	1531	76.2 (%)

The data of February 1992 by the Ministry of Health and Welfare.

in Japan was 3 840 000 l in 1985 as source plasma, as mentioned previously, and the volume decreased gradually to 2 760 000 l in 1988 (Fig. 4). The plan aimed to decrease consumption to the appropriate level on one side, and to increase the amount of voluntary donation to the sufficient level on the other side, to achieve self-sufficiency. Based on this schedule in 1991, we are going to achieve self-sufficiency of blood coagulation factor products. When we could collect 500 000 l of voluntary source plasma in 1991, we can produce the coagulation factor products on our own account. After the accomplishment of this step, we will be able to produce other plasma products step by step.

As the number of hemophiliacs in Japan, hemophilia A patients were 3500, von Willebrand disease patients were 750 and hemophilia B patients were 700. Since von Willebrand factor and Factor IX are able to be purified from the remaining part of plasma after fractionation of Factor VIII, the maximum volume of source plasma we need for these coagulation factor products is equal to the volume needed for Factor VIII.

A hemophilia A patient needs 30 000 units of Factor VIII in a year, so 3500 patients in our country need about 100 000 000 units of this factor products. Since, we can now purify about 20% of the Factor VIII from the source plasma, about 500 000 l of plasma is needed to sustain this volume of products. This is the reason for the above mentioned 500 000 l. To accomplish this goal, we had planned to collect plasma from 10% of blood donors, about 800 000 people, by plasmapheresis. There are three methods for the procurement of 500 000 l source plasma. The first is the reinforcement of blood collection by plasmapheresis. The second is an increase in blood collection

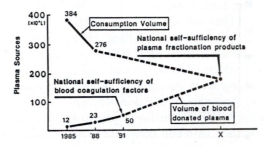

Figure 4. Scheme for national self-sufficiency of plasma fractionation products in Japan (Ministry of Health and Welfare).

rooms. The third is arrangement of the blood collecting mobiles and machines of plasmapheresis. Giving the real numbers in Table 2, we can see the situation of blood collecting facilities in the 77 blood centers all over Japan. As mentioned previously, we have 75 rooms as blood donation rooms and this number is 2.5 times that in 1986. Though the gross number (385) of travelling blood collection mobiles in 1991 was equal to 1986, there were big changes in the make-up; such as 47 buses used only for apheresis and 160 mobiles for both whole blood collection and apheresis. Furthermore, the number of apheresis machines was 1777 and this is about 11 times that of 1986.

Table 2.
The changes of maintenance conditions at each blood center

	1986	1987	1988	1989	1990	1991
Blood collection room	31	34	41	47	64	75
Blood collecting mobile (items)	359	356	351	359	375	385
whole blood	359	356	350	299	227	178
plasma pheresis	—	—	1	6	29	47
combination (WB, PP)	—	—	—	54	119	160
Machines for plasmapheresis	165	385	604	843	1341	1777

Figure 5 shows the actual data of source plasma collection for coagulant factor products for previous years. The total volume of source plasma (1991) was 505 000 l and we were able to achieve the goal of the year by the help of voluntary donors. This value was really 2.3 times that of 1990 and 4.8 times that of 1989. As the proportion of the plasma collected by apheresis, it extended to 63.4% of total. With this situation, it became a new problem of how we could transport these large masses of plasma from each blood center to the Plasma Fractionation Center safely and securely. To overcome this problem, we developed and introduced an intelligent transportation system (cooling container system). The characteristic of this cooling container is to keep the inner temperature below −30 °C. We distributed these containers to each blood center and have been collecting them regularly, then been gathering them to transport to the fractionation center by large trailers with electric power supplies. We

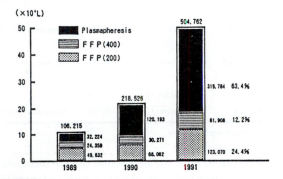

Figure 5. Volume of plasma sources for blood coagulation factors by year.

had used the procedure of putting frozen plasma in styrofoam boxes with dry-ice, and to transport by air. As to the cooling container system, it's advantages are as follows:

(i) Securely controlled temperature below −30 °C throughout the transportation system.

(ii) Needs no cooling materials like as dry-ice and cooling cases, and so increases the working efficiency.

(iii) Waste-less system as above.

(iv) Lower transport costs. About a half as usual.

(v) Fewer accidents of broken plasma bags. About a 60th as usual.

Like these, we have established a plasma collection protocol and transportation system.

We have taken advantage of this system and procured sufficient volume of source plasma, and also we have introduced an affinity purification system of Factor VIII with monoclonal antibody made by Baxter Ltd. So, we have been able to produce our Factor VIII products, 'Cross-Eight M.' The actual work started September 1991, and the products have been delivered from March 1992. Table 3 shows the variety and yearly amount of each plasma product planned for 1992. As to the Factor VIII products, we plan to produce 86 000 000 units. This value corresponds to about 70% of yearly demand and about 92% of these products will be made from voluntary blood. As to the Factor IX products, about 67% of them will be made from voluntary donated plasma. So, we will be able to produce more plasma products with international source plasma and hope to achieve self-sustaining production in the near future.

Table 3.
The kinds of product planned supply and product volume (1992)

Yearly use (×10³U)	Product and amount (×10³U)			Originated from	
Factor VIII products	Cross-Eight M	(Red cross)	86000	donated blood	92%
	Confact F	(Kaketsuken)	25000	donated blood	
120 000					
	Haemate P	(Hoechst)	9000	imported product	
Factor IX products	Novact F	(Kaketsuken)	5600	donated blood	67%
	Novact M	(Kaketsuken)	8000	donated blood	
27 000					
	PPSB	(Nichiyaku)	4500	donated blood	
	Proplex	(Baxter)	8900	imported product	

The Ministry of Health and Welfare.

Furthermore, we are trying to raise the proportion of self-sufficiency of albumin and gammaglobulin products and to supply the plasma fractionation products by voluntary donated plasma in our country.

REFERENCES

1. S. Sekiguchi and H. Tohyama. Current status of plasma formula supply and demand in Japan. In: *Therapeutic Plasmapheresis (II)*, T. Oda (Ed.), pp. 139–141, ISAO Press, Ceveland (1982).
2. *The Data of Blood Program in Japan*. Blood Products Research Organization, Japan (1982).
3. T. Kamiya. Blood Coagulation Factor Products. *Immunohaematology*, **9**, 453–457 (1987).

2
Angitis

Therapeutic Plasmapheresis (XII), pp. 47-51
T. Agishi *et al*. (Eds)
© VSP 1993

The Clinical Effects of Long-term Apheresis for Intractable Skin Ulcers in Immunological Diseases

M. HAYASHI, N. KOGA,[1] T. NAGANO[1] and H. SASAKI[1]

Hayashi Dermatological Clinic, Kurume City 830, Japan
[1]*Koga Hospital, Kurume City 830, Japan*

Key words: multiple skin ulcers; malignant rheumatoid arthritis; plasmapheresis.

INTRODUCTION

We have evaluated the clinical effects of apheresis therapy and compared there with laboratory data for patients with intractable skin ulcers.

METHODS

We applied various apheresis methods including double filtration plasmapheresis (DFPP), immunoadsorption (IMAP) and peripheral lymphocytapheresis (LCP). We employed either DFPP or IMAP once in 2 weeks session interval processing plasma at 2000–4000 ml/session, and 4000 ml of blood was processed by LCP once or twice a week. Pulse therapy (methylprednisolone, 1000 mg, continuously 3 days) was occasionally accompanied with apheresis.

CASES AND RESULTS

We have evaluated four patients with skin ulcers due to immunological disease (Table 1). All patients had a long clinical history of 7–17 years and the duration from the onset of skin ulcers to the initial apheresis session was 4–7 months. These patients were resistant to the conventional treatments.

Table 1.
Long-term apheresis for skin ulcers

Case no.	Diagnosis	Age (years)	Sex	Effectiveness	Number of sessions	Methods (sessions)	Period (months)	Side-effects
1	MCTD (PSS + SLE) + MRA	31	F	Good	129	DFPP (56) IMAP (73)	64	none
2	Sjögren's syndrome + MRA	48	F	Good	89	DFPP (77) IMAP (12)	51	none
3	MRA	37	F	Good	76	DFPP (38) LCP (20) IMAP (18)	41	none
4	MRA	69	F	Fair	97	DFPP (97)	49	none

Case 1 developed multiple skin ulcers in her lower extremities and hands. The symptoms deteriorated despite DFPP. We combined pulse therapy with DFPP and the symptoms subsided gradually. Since then, her symptoms were beneficially controlled with no use of pulse therapy.

Case 2 (Figs 1 and 2) refused steroid administrations but her symptoms significantly improved by apheresis. The ulcers in her lower extremities epitherized and no recurrence was observed for 4 years. However, during the period, laboratory data (Table 2) worsened.

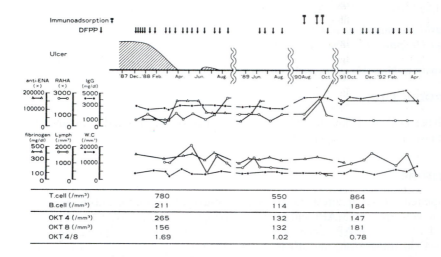

T.cell (/mm³)		780	550	864
B.cell (/mm³)		211	114	184
OKT 4 (/mm³)		265	132	147
OKT 8 (/mm³)		156	132	181
OKT 4/8		1.69	1.02	0.78

Figure 1. Clinical course and laboratory findings in case 2 (Sjögren's syndrome + MRA).

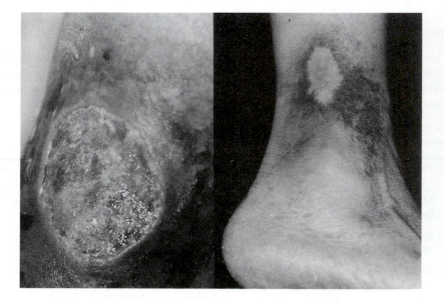

Figure 2. Clinical photo (Case 2). Left: recurrent tumor (4.5 × 4.5 × 0.3 cm) of the right lower extremities. Right: epithelization of the ulcer after the ninth session of apheresis.

Table 2.
Laboratory data

Case	Methods	Serum samples	Pre	Post	No. of samples
1	DFPP	Viscosity of Blood	3.610	3.245	8
	DFPP	Viscosity of Plasma	1.317	1.095	8
	DFPP	IgG	628.400	430.667	15
	DFPP	IgA	261.133	150.400	15
	DFPP	IgM	75.733	17.533	15
	DFPP	fibrinogen	320.818	106.091	11
2	DFPP	IgG	1712.238	1093.095	21
	IMAP	IgG	1753.077	1432.308	13
	DFPP	IgA	443.762	250.095	21
	IMAP	IgA	530.846	447.923	13
	DFPP	IgM	581.381	161.571	21
	IMAP	IgM	720.308	463.154	13
	DFPP	fibrinogen	339.125	105.500	8
	IMAP	fibrinogen	323.800	280.400*	5
	DFPP	RAHA	7275.789	1852.632	19
	IMAP	RAHA	6186.667	3413.333	12
	LCP	white cell	7846.154	6215.385	13
	LCP	Lymph	816.462	577.846	13
	LCP	T cell	713.668	505.565	10
	LCP	B cell	51.026	38.405*	10
	LCP	OKT 4	412.051	266.521	10
	LCP	OKT 8	157.680	124.888*	10
	LCP	OKT 4/8	2.536	2.239*	10
3	DFPP	Ig G	1494.812	1076.781	32
	IMAP	Ig G	1597.333	1241.000	3
	DFPP	Ig A	296.875	202.812	32
	IMAP	Ig A	271.667	220.667	3
	DFPP	Ig M	156.531	76.031	32
	IMAP	Ig M	155.667	117.000	3
	IMAP	fibrinogen	349.571	218.143	7
4	DFPP	Ig G	2899.229	1946.771	35
	IMAP	Ig G	3684.000	2946.750	4
	DFPP	Ig A	918.971	512.114	35
	IMAP	Ig A	1096.750	915.000	4
	DFPP	Ig M	188.229	77.000	35
	IMAP	Ig M	231.000	170.500	4
	DFPP	fibrinogen	357.143	155.500	14
	IMAP	fibrinogen	346.333	250.000	3
	DFPP	Anti-ENA Antibody	9414.815	82678.519*	27

Welch's two samples test, $*P > 0.05$.

Case 3 developed skin ulcers in her right lower extremities and her symptoms cor-related well with apheresis session intervals.

Case 4 had necrotic ulcers on the top of her fingers and feet which were defluxed and epithelized by apheresis once in 2 weeks intervals. No correlations were observed among clinical symptoms, thermography, and laboratory data (Table 2). Any apheresis methods significantly decreased immunological molecules but the levels returned to the previous values within 2 weeks.

No severe complications were observed among these patients.

DISCUSSION

Apheresis therapy is effective for skin ulcers. However, in patients with severe skin ulcers, the beneficial effects cannot be obtained only by apheresis. We accompanied immunological treatments with apheresis and obtained successful results [1]. Laboratory data and thermography showed that there were no correlations with the symptoms of skin ulcers. DFPP significantly decreased IgG, IgA and IgM rather than that of IMAP (Table 3). However, the values returned to the previous levels. The results suggest that DFPP may bring stronger rebound compared with that of IMAP or LCP. The limitation of the clinical effect of apheresis on the session interval (once in 2 weeks) was suggested. We are required to manage a more flexible apheresis method depending on the patient. There still remain many problems to clarify the mechanisms of apheresis and skin ulcers.

Table 3.
Welch's two samples test (case 3)

		Comparison of between the methods	
IgG	Pre	O — △	
		O — □	
		△ — □	
	Post	O — △	*
	R. R.	O — △	*
IgA	Pre	O — △	*
		O — □	
		△ — □	*
	Post	O — △	*
	R. R.	O — △	*
IgM	Pre	O — △	*
		O — □	*
		△ — □	
	Post	O — △	*
	R. R.	O — △	*
Fibrinogen	Pre	O — △	
		O — □	*
		△ — □	*
	Post	O — △	*
	R. R.	O — △	*
RAHA	Pre	O — △	
		O — □	
		△ — □	
	Post	O — △	*
	R. R.	O — △	*

DFPP : O
IMAP : △
LCP : □
R. R. : Removal Rate
* : P<0.05

REFERENCE

1. M. Hayashi, N. Koga and T. Nagano. Immunomoduration by apheresis in dermatological disease. In: *Extracorporeal Immunomodulation*, T. Agishi (Ed.), pp. 157–163, Nippon Medical Center, Tokyo (1990).

Therapeutic Plasmapheresis (XII), pp. 53-56
T. Agishi *et al.* (Eds)
© VSP 1993

The Effect of Plasmapheresis Therapy in Two Patients with Intractable Polyarteritis Nodosa

S. JODO, A. SAGAWA, N. OGURA, T. ATSUMI, T. NAKABAYASHI,
K. OHNISHI, A. FUGISAKU and S. NAKAGAWA

The Second Department of Internal Medicine,
Hokkaido University School of Medicine, Sapporo, Japan

Key words: polyarteritis nodosa; rheumatoid factor; double-filtration plasmapheresis; immunoadsorbent therapy.

INTRODUCTION

Polyarteritis nodosa (PN) is a well-known form of necrotizing angitis. Despite aggressive treatment of this disease with steroids and immunosuppressive agents, PN is a relapsable, recurrent disease with a poor prognosis. Recently, several studies have indicated that plasmapheresis is an effective treatment for PN accompanied with drug therapy. It can remove immune complexes effectively and facilitates clearance of these complexes by the reticuloendothelial system.

In our hospital, we found that three out of four patients with PN had high titers of rheumatoid factor (RF) in their serum. After sequential measurement of the level of RF in the sera of these patients, we found that the RF level paralleled the disease activity of PN.

In this study, we applied plasmapheresis therapy in two patients with PN who had high titers of RF, and after plasmapheresis the level of RF decreased selectively and clinical features improved. According to the results of our study, a combination of plasmapheresis with steroids and immunosuppressive agents is able to improve the course of intractable PN. Moreover RF is thought to be a disease-specific marker for PN, and measuring the level of RF might be helpful in obtaining diagnostic, prognostic and therapeutic information concerning PN.

DETECTION AND QUANTIFICATION OF RF

Most methods of detecting and quantifying RF, such as the commonly used sheep cell agglutination test and the latex fixation test, are only semiquantitative.

Recently, other methods have been applied to the quantification of RF, including radioimmunoassay (RIA), enzyme-linked immunosorbent assay (ELISA) and laser nephelometry (LN). RIA and ELISA, however, are not suitable for clinical laboratories, because they are time-consuming and costly. LN is a sensitive technique for measuring the degree of light scatter caused by the interaction of RF with latex particles. It is a simple and rapid method of measuring the total polyclonal RF level.

In this study, we applied LN to quantitative RF measurement and found it more reproducible and quantitative than the latex agglutination test. We also found that it can detect minor changes in RF levels reflecting the activity of RF-positive PN.

CASE REPORTS

Case 1: a 45 year old male

In March 1989, polyarthralgia developed and the patient consulted a hospital where he was given non-steroidal anti-inflammatory drugs and prednisolone (PSL), 30 mg daily. His symptoms failed to improve, and fever, polymyalgia and numbness of his lower extremities developed in addition. In March 1990, he was admitted to our hospital.

A biopsy obtained from the quadriceps femor demonstrated necrotizing vasculitis and the patient was diagnosed as having PN. He was then treated with PSL, 60 mg daily, and although most of his symptoms improved immediately, the numbness persisted, and he was given intravenous methyl-PSL, 1000 mg daily, for 3 days (pulse therapy), and oral azathioprine (AZP) was started. His numbness, however, failed to improve and the titers of RAHA and CRP remained high. Double-filtration plasmapheresis (DFPP) was then applied to remove high molecular factors, such as immune complexes (IC) and RF, which are thought to play an important part in pathogenic mechanism. Plasmacure (Kurare) was used as the plasma separator and Evaflux 2A (Kurare, pore size 0.01 μm) was used as the second membrane. The replacement fluid was 600 ml of 8% albumin. A total of 3000 ml of plasma was treated during each procedure, and it was performed 3 times. The level of RF markedly decreased and the level of immunoglobulins also decreased. This showed that RF in his serum was removed effectively by DFPP. There were no significant changes in the levels of total protein or albumin. No adverse effects were observed during or after each treatment. After the third DFPP, the patient was given intravenous methyl-PSL, 1000 mg daily, for 3 days, and oral AZP was increased to 100 mg daily. As a result of these treatments, his numbness improved immediately, CRP became negative and the RAHA titer declined.

In September 1989 when PSL was tapered to 20 mg daily, the level of RF measured by LN, and ESR and CRP increased. In October, polyarthralgia developed and a diagnosis of recurrent PN was made. The dosage of PSL was increased to 40 mg daily and oral cyclophosphamide (CYC), 50 mg daily, was added. AZP was stopped due to lack of efficacy. After these treatments, his symptoms abated and the levels of ESR, CRP and RF improved. PSL was tapered to 20 mg daily in addition to 100 mg daily of CYC, and the patient was discharged.

In this case, the patient's symptoms and the levels of RF and CRP were not improved by intravenous methyl-PSL 1000 mg daily, and oral AZP, but DFPP therapy 3 times accompanying with intravenous methyl-PSL, 1000 mg daily, was very effective. After this courses of treatment, his symptoms improved immediately, and the levels of RF and CRP decreased. It is concluded that DFPP accompanied with steroid therapy improved the patient's clinical condition by rapid removal of RF from the serum and improved the quality of the clinical response to steroids and AZP. When the patient suffered a relapse, the levels of RF measured by LN increased earlier than CRP, before the development of symptoms, and when the disease was treated and responded well to therapy, the levels of RF decreased in parallel with the decline in other inflammation variables, such as CRP and ESR, and the improvement in clinical course.

These findings suggested that RF levels were well correlated with disease activity in these two cases of PN and that RF levels could serve as a marker of therapy in this study.

Case 2: a 65 year old female

In October 1989, the patient was admitted to a hospital because of paralysis and sensory loss in the extremities, and skin ulcers on her legs. She was well until about 5 months earlier, when she experienced the onset of polyarthralgia. After admission, she began to experience arrhythmia, pleurisy and slight fever. Because biopsies of the leg ulcer and sural nerve revealed necrotizing vasculitis, she was diagnosed as having PN. PSL, 60 mg daily, was begun on November 10. Most of her clinical features improved, but paralysis of the extremities remained. In January 1991, she was transferred to our hospital.

After admission to our hospital, the dosage of PSL was gradually reduced according to RF levels and other inflammation variables. Oral AZP was stopped because of side effects. Her symptoms abated, and she was continued on steroid therapy alone.

In April 1990, the level of RF started to increase without any clinical manifestations. Three weeks later, the level of CRP and ESR also worsened, accompanied by the development of fever and pleurisy. A diagnosis of recurrent PN was made, and the dosage of PSL was increased to 40 mg daily, and 50 mg daily of CYC was added. Fever and pleurisy improved immediately, but general malaise, and the levels of RF, ESR and CRP did not improve. The patient was then given intravenous methyl-PSL, 1000 mg daily, for 3 days and immunoadsorbent therapy (IA) using a PH350 Immusorba column (Asahi Medical Co., Ltd, Tokyo, Japan), which consisted of polyvinyl alcohol with phenylalanine, was applied to remove IC and RF selectively. A total of 2000 ml of the patient's plasma was perfused in 120 min in one operation with no replacement fluid. The mechanism of this adsorption is related to the hydrophobic interaction between phenylalanine and RF. The level of RF decreased markedly from 469 to 283 IU/ml after this procedure.

The removal ratio of RF levels was 39.7%, but total protein, albumin, IgG, IgA, IgM, C3, C4 and CH50 did not decrease significantly. This showed that IA using a PH350 column selectively eliminated RF from the circulation of the patient compared with other proteins. No adverse effects were observed during or after each treatment. After two columns of IA, intravenous methyl-PSL, 1000 mg daily, for 3 days, was added. The levels of CRP and RF decreased immediately, and the patient experienced a clinical remission. PSL was gradually tapered to 25 mg daily and 50 mg daily of oral AZP was given in addition.

In this study, IA using a PH350 Immusorba column was very effective and is thought to have contributed to the patient's remission.

CONCLUSION

RF is an autoantibody against denatured IgG and consists largely of IgM. It is often found in the serum in RA. This antibody is presumed to be involved in the onset and progression of RA, and its level correlates well with the activity of RA. The mechanism of production and pathogenetic significance of RF are not understood, although many studies have been performed since 1940 when RF was reported by Waaler for the first time.

In this study, we measured the level of RF using LN in two RF-positive cases of PN. The results showed that the RF levels varied with the levels of ESR and CRP, and clinical manifestations of the patients. When steroid therapy or DFPP and IA were introduced, the RF level decreased, and the patient responded well to oral administration of steroids and immunosuppressive agents showing a favorable clinical course. Based on these results of our study, the level of RF was capable of serving as a marker of disease activity in RF-positive PN.

The standard therapy for patients with PN is steroids and immunosuppressive agents, such as CYC and AZP. Some patients in which plasmapheresis was useful in steroid-resistant cases have been reported, although the usefulness of plasmapheresis is controversial in the treatment of PN in general. In this study, we treated one patient with DFPP, and the other patient with IA using a PH350 Immusorba column. The level of RF decreased immediately after each procedure, and both patients improved in the quality of their clinical response to steroid and immunosuppressive agent therapy. As a result of these treatments, we concluded that DFPP and IA therapy can be effective in the treatment of patients with PN who have been resistant to steroid and immunosuppressive agent therapy, when applied accompanied with steroids and immunosuppressive agents.

Therapeutic Plasmapheresis (XII), pp. 57-60
T. Agishi *et al.* (Eds)
© VSP 1993

The Effect of Plasmapheresis in Systemic Lupus Erythematosus Patients with Antiphospholipid Antibodies

H. HASHIMOTO, M. YOKOYAMA, H. TSUDA and S. HIROSE

Department of Internal Medicine & Rheumatology, Juntendo University, Tokyo, Japan

Key words: SLE; antiphospholipid syndrome; antiphospholipid antibodies; double filtration plasmapheresis; adsorbent plasmapheresis.

INTRODUCTION

Recently, much attention has been focused on the antibodies (aCL), lupus anticoagulant (LAC) and false positive serological test for syphilis (STS) which has been considered as being associated with thrombosis, recurrent abortion and/or intrauterine death, central nervous system involvements, cardiovascular involvements, organ infarction and thrombocytopenia [1, 2].

On the other hand, plasmapheresis, including double filtration plasmapheresis (DFPP), has been used as a conservative treatment for SLE [3]. Plasmapheresis, which removes anti-DNA antibodies (anti-DNA), aPL and immune complexes from circulation, has been found to effective for patients with active SLE. Recently, an adsorbent dextran sulfate (DS) column which absorbs anti-DNA and aPL by utilizing negatively charged ions was developed [4, 5].

In this paper, the effect of plasmapheresis in SLE patients with aPL and clinical manifestations related to aPL was studied.

PATIENTS AND METHODS

Ten female patients with SLE having aPL who satisfied the ARA criteria for SLE were studied. Overlapping aPL antibodies were observed in five patients having aCL, nine patients having LAC and two patients having positive STS results. As for the clinical manifestations, six patients had thrombocytopenia, six patients had central nervous system (CNS) involvements including unconsciousness, emotional lability and cerebral infarction, one patient had a past history of recurrent abortion, one patient had thrombophlebitis and lung infarction, and one patient had renal failure. Adsorbent plasmapheresis using dextran sulfate columns (ADPP) was utilized in five patients and double filtration plasmapheresis (DFPP) was used in the remaining five patients. Two and a half liters of plasma were treated during each procedure. The frequency and the duration of plasmapheresis treatments varied from patient to patient. Plasmapheresis was performed 1–2 times per 1–2 weeks for a duration of 1–12 months. The number of plasmapheresis treatments in each patient varied from three to 198. Prednisolone (PSL) was administered in all patients in conjunction with the plasmapheresis treatment. Initial dose of PSL in each patient ranged from 10 to 100 mg/day.

The effects of plasmapheresis on the clinical manifestations and the changes in the laboratory findings were compared before and after plasmapheresis treatments. Paired t-tests were used to test significant differences.

RESULTS

Almost all of the clinical manifestations, including thrombocytopenia, unconsciousness, emotional lability, cerebral infarction, thrombophlebitis and lung infarction, improved after plasmapheresis with the exception of thrombocytopenia in one patient and renal failure in one patient. Concerning thrombocytopenia, five out of six patients with thrombocytopenia improved. Platelets increased more significantly after plasmapheresis in comparison to before plasmapheresis ($P < 0.05$). Four out of six patients with thrombocytopenia had positive platelet associated IgG (PA-IgG). The titers of PA-IgG in these patients also decreased after plasmapheresis, although the difference was not statistically significant.

A patient with three recurrent abortions and aPL was successfully treated by ADPP. The patient, a 34 year old female, was referred to our hospital during the 18th week of her fourth pregnancy. ADPP at the interval of once or twice/week was started during the 18th week of gestation in addition to low-dose therapy of PSL (5 mg/day) and aspirin (80 mg/day). During the 34th week of gestation, intrauterine growth retardation and fetal distress were observed and a baby girl (1600 g; Apgar 8) was delivered by Cesarean section.

Six out of nine patients with LAC showed negative LAC after plasmapheresis. The titers of aCL in five patients with aCL significantly decreased and normalized after plasmapheresis ($P < 0.025$). The titers of anti-DNA also decreased after plasmapheresis, although a statistically significant difference was not recorded. The dosages of PSL after plasmapheresis significantly decreased after plasmapheresis ($P < 0.05$).

DISCUSSION

It is evident that aPL including aCL, LAC and positive STS is significantly associated with the clinical features known as the antiphospholipid syndrome. Furthermore, there has been extreme concern in the past few years that some patients with aPL may present or develop an acute catastrophic or devastating syndrome characterized by multiple vascular occlusions which often results in death [6]. Although anti-DNA in SLE is thought to play an important role in the pathognomonic mechanism, aPL is also thought to be involved in the occurrence of recurrent thrombosis, thrombocytopenia and fetal loss among SLE patients [1, 2, 7]. On the other hand, plasmapheresis, which removes immune complexes, autoantibodies including anti-DNA, and aPL, and chemical mediators related to autoimmune mechanisms and inflammation, has been used for treatment of SLE. A DS adsorbent column was used in the ADPP in this study which has been widely utilized as a specific adsorbent for low density lipoprotein in familial hyperlipidemia [8], and has recently been refined and developed to adsorb not only anti-DNA but also aPL [4, 5]. In this study, 10 SLE patients with aPL and clinical manifestations related to the antibodies were treated with plasmapheresis in conjunction with PSL.

Five out of six patients with thrombocytopenia improved after treatment. Platelets in patients with thrombocytopenia significantly increased after plasmapheresis. The titers of PA-IgG which were thought to be associated with thrombocytopenia also decreased after plasmapheresis. CNS involvements including unconsciousness, emotional lability and cerebral infarction improved, thus the response coincides with the decline in titers of aPL and/or anti-DNA. Thrombophlebitis and lung infarction, which was thought to be due to embolism from the lower leg thrombophlebitis in one patient, also improved after plasmapheresis. In addition, the patient with SLE with recurrent abortion and aCL was successfully treated with ADPP. It is noted that a high dose of steroid (PSL 40–60 mg/day) and a low dose of aspirin suppressed LAC activity and proved to be a successful treatment for patients with LAC having a history of fetal intrauterine death [9, 10]. It is of value that a pregnant patient at risk with SLE can be successfully treated with a combination therapy of ADPP and low dose steroid. Concerning the serological findings, the titers of aCL significantly decreased after plasmapheresis. The titers of anti-DNA had a tendency to decrease after plasmapheresis.

CONCLUSION

Five out of six SLE patients with thrombocytopenia improved after plasmapheresis, showing a significant increase in the platelet count and decrease in the PA-IgG levels. CNS involvements including unconsciousness, emotional lability and cerebral infarction in six SLE patients improved after plasmapheresis. Thrombophlebitis and lung infarction in one patient also improved after plasmapheresis. However, renal failure in one patient did not improve. The titers of aCL in all five patients significantly decreased after plasmapheresis. Six out of nine patients with LAC showed negative LAC after plasmapheresis. A pregnant SLE patient with recurrent abortion and aPL was successfully treated by plasmapheresis.

Plasmapheresis, especially ADPP, is thought to be an influential strategy of treatment for patients with antiphospholipid syndrome as well as in SLE patients having aPL and related clinical manifestations.

REFERENCES

1. G. R. V. Hughes, E. N. Harris and A. E. Gharavi. The anticardiolipin syndrome. *J. Rheumatol.*, **13**, 486–489 (1986).

2. C. Ninomiya, O. Taniguchi, T. Kato *et al.* Distribution and clinical significance of lupus anticoagulant and anticardiolipin antibody in 349 patients with systemic lupus erythematosus. *Intern. Med.*, **31**, 194–199 (1992).

3. J. V. Jones. Plasmapheresis in SLE. *Clin. Rheum. Dis.*, **8**, 243–260 (1982).

4. M. Kinoshita, S. Aotsuka, T. Funahashi *et al.* Selective removal of anti-double stranded DNA antibodies by immunoadsorption with dextran sulphate in a patient with systemic lupus erythematosus. *Ann. Rheum. Dis.*, **48**, 856–860 (1989).

5. H. Hashimoto, H. Tsuda, Y. Kanai *et al.* Selective removal of anti-DNA and anticardiolipin antibodies by adsorbent plasmapheresis using dextran sulfate columns in patients with systemic lupus erythematosus. *J. Rheumatol.*, **18**, 545–551 (1991).

6. R. A. Asherson. The catastrophic antiphospholipid syndrome. *J. Rheumatol.*, **19**, 508–512 (1992).

7. E. N. Harris, A. E. Gharavi, M. L. Boey *et al.* Anticardiolipin antibodies: detection by radioimmunoassay and associated with thrombosis in system lupus erythematosus. *Lancet*, **2**, 1211–1214 (1983).

8. S. Yokoyama, R. Hayashi, M. Satani *et al.* Selective removal of low density lipoprotein by plasmapheresis in familial hypercholesterolemia. *Arteriosclerosis*, **5**, 613–622 (1985).

9. W. F. Lubbe, W. S. Butler, S. J. Palmer *et al.* Fetal survival after prednisolone suppression of maternal lupus-anticoagulant. *Lancet*, **1**, 1361–1363 (1983).

10. D. W. Branch, J. R. Scott, N. K. Kochenour *et al.* Obstetric complications associated with the lupus anticoagulant. *N. Eng. J. Med.*, **313**, 1322-1326 (1985).

Therapeutic Plasmapheresis (XII), pp. 61-65
T. Agishi *et al.* (Eds)
© VSP 1993

Thermography and Plasmapheresis in the Treatment of Raynaud's Syndrome

Y. KANAI, K. YAMAJI, T. KAWANISHI, M. TOUMYO, S. FUJITA,
M. YOKOYAMA, H. TSUDA, H. HASHIMOTO and S. HIROSE

Division of Rheumatology, Department of Internal Medicine, Juntendo University, Tokyo, Japan

Key words: Raynaud's syndrome; plasmapheresis; thermography; Hand Chilling Test; digital temperature.

INTRODUCTION

Raynaud's phenomenon described by Maurice Raynaud [1] in 1862 is characterized as episodic pallor or cyanosis on cold- or stress-induced vasoconstriction with suffusion and erythema on subsequent vasodilation. It is called Raynaud's syndrome, when the phenomenon is associated with several known causes, e.g. collagen disease, vibration tool exposure, trauma, neurological disorder, obstruction of flow to the thoracic outlet, obliterative arterial disease, vinyl chloride, etc.

We know that several factors are involved in the pathogenesis of Raynaud's syndrome. Especially, there is the condition of the walls of local blood vessels, peripheral nerve system and blood itself. Medication is the general treatment of Raynaud's syndrome, but there are some reports that plasmapheresis is effective [2, 3]. We treated patients with Raynaud's syndrome by plasmapheresis in an attempt to improve the quality of the blood. We used thermography to examine the efficacy of plasmapheresis.

MATERIALS AND METHODS

We performed plasmapheresis on three patients with Raynaud's phenomenon who had been admitted to our hospital. The patients were diagnosed as one case each of mixed connective tissue disease, progressive systemic sclerosis and dermatomyosis. There were one male and two females. Their ages ranged from 32 to 50 years, with a mean age of 42.7 years (Table 1). Six healthy persons served as the normal control group.

Table 1.
Patients' background data

No. of cases		Male:Female	Age (mean; years)
MCTD	1		
PSS	1	1:2	32–50 (42.7)
DM	1		

We performed double filtration plasmapheresis using a second filter having a membrane pore size of 0.02 μm. Plasmapheresis was 3 times at 10 days intervals. The total plasma volume treated each time was 2 l. Heparin was used as an anticoagulant: 2000 units at the start and 1500 units during the plasmapheresis. A 5% albumin solution was used for replacement.

As we judged the severity of Raynaud's syndrome and the efficacy of plasmapheresis, the digital temperature was measured by thermography. We examined improvement in the temperature by the Hand Chilling Test before and after each plasmapheresis (Fig. 1). The average temperature of the 2nd, 3rd and 4th digits of both hands were measured 'before chilling', 'after chilling at 0°C for 10 s' and at '6 and 12 min after chilling'. Furthermore, we calculated the recovery rate of the digital temperature 'after 6 and 12 min'. That is, the difference in the temperature at '6 or 12 min after chilling', and the temperature immediately 'after chilling' was divided by the difference between the temperatures 'before and after chilling' and then multiplied by 100.

We also examined clinical symptoms of Raynaud's phenomenon.

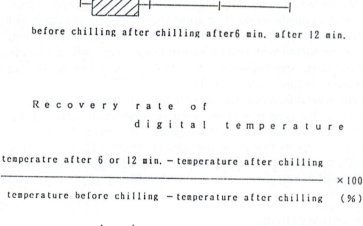

Recovery rate of digital temperature

$$\frac{\text{temperatre after 6 or 12 min.} - \text{temperature after chilling}}{\text{temperature before chilling} - \text{temperature after chilling}} \times 100 \; (\%)$$

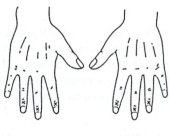

Measuring points

2nd. 3rd and 4th digits of both hands

Figure 1. Hand chilling test.

Figure 2 shows an example of thermography. Differences in temperature are shown by different colors. Pink and red is high temperature; blue color is low temperature. The digital temperature can be measured by thermography (Fig. 3). Figure 4 shows the change in temperature by the Hand Chilling Test 'before chilling', 'after chilling' and '6 and 12 min'.

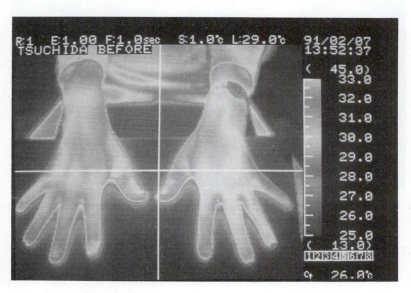

Figure 2. Thermography (before chilling).

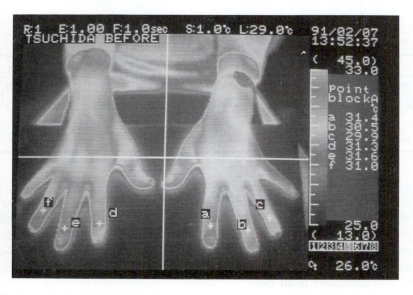

Figure 3. Measuring digital temperature (before chilling).

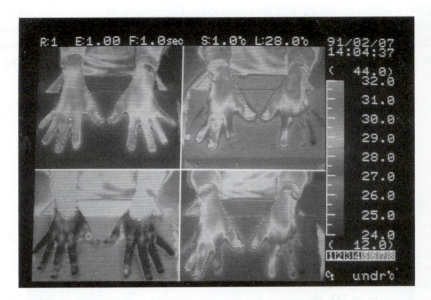

Figure 4. Change in digital temperature. Top left: before chilling. Bottom left: after chilling. Top right: after 6 min. Bottom right: after 12 min.

RESULTS

Table 2 shows the change in the average digital temperature before and after plasmapheresis. The average digital temperasture before and after plasmapheresis clearly dropped in comparison with the normal control 'before chilling' and 'after 6 and 12 min'. Though the difference in the digital temperature between before and after plasmapheresis was slight, the temperature tended to rise after plasmapheresis.

Table 2.

Change in the average digital temperature by thermography (°C)

	Before chilling	After chilling	After 6 min	After 12 min
Before PP	27.77 ± 3.41 ⎤ ns	22.03 ± 2.67 ⎤ ns	24.97 ± 3.98 ⎤ ns	26.33 ± 3.80 ⎤ ns
After PP	30.23 ± 2.71 ⎦	23.43 ± 0.76 ⎦	27.63 ± 3.27 ⎦	29.00 ± 3.93 ⎦
Normal control	32.32 ± 1.91	22.43 ± 1.43	31.00 ± 3.67	32.80 ± 1.56

Table 3 shows the recovery rate of the digital temperature 'after 6 or 12 min'. In the normal control, the recovery rate was higher. Especially 'after 12 min', the recovery rate was more than 100%, it means that the temperature was higher than 'before chilling'. Although a significant difference was not seen between before and after plasmapheresis, the recovery rate after plasmapheresis was a little better than that before plasmapheresis.

Clinical symptoms, especially color, cold, numbness and pain of fingers, were affected by plasmapheresis in all cases.

Cryoglobulins were not noted in any patient.

Table 3.

Recovery rate of digital temperature (see Fig. 1)

	After 6 min	After 12 min
Before PP	48.13 ± 13.22 ⎤ ns	72.43 ± 7.70 ⎤ ns
After PP	55.40 ± 31.33 ⎦	74.10 ± 37.95 ⎦
Normal control	86.40 ± 22.39	105.27 ± 6.30

DISCUSSION AND CONCLUSION

Regarding the etiology of Raynaud's syndrome, we considered mainly the roles of blood vessel factors and blood factors. The blood vessel factors include stenosis and occlusion of arteries, or spasms of arteries. On the other hand, the blood factors include reduced transformability of red blood cells, reduced fibrinolytic activity and increased blood viscosity.

Treatment of Raynaud's syndrome is chiefly drug therapy, e.g. vasodilators, fibrinolytic-enhancing drugs [4], defibrinated drugs and prostaglandin E_1 and I_2 [5]. However, we see that these are not useful in many cases. Some reports noted that plasmapheresis in the treatment of Raynaud's syndrome is useful [2, 3]. We noted an increase in blood viscosity, especially plasma viscosity, because we think that influence greatly the digital vessels in patients with Raynaud's syndrome. We treated patients with Raynaud's syndrome by plasmapheresis in an attempt to improve the quality of blood. As a result, improvement in digital temperature and clinical symptoms was noted after plasmapheresis.

In view of these observations, we surmise that plasmapheresis is useful for the treatment of Raynaud's syndrome. We intend to conduct further studies.

REFERENCES

1. M. Raynaud. *De l'asphyxie locale et de la gangréne symmetrque des extrémités.* Rignoux, Paris (1862).
2. G. Talopos, M. Horrocks, J. M. White *et al.* Plasmapheresis in Raynaud's disease. *Lancet,* **2,** 416–417 (1978).
3. M. J. G. O'Reilly, G. Talopos, V. C. Roberts *et al.* Controlled trial of plasma exchange in treatment of Raynaud's syndrome. *Br. Med. J.,* **1,** 1113–1115 (1979).
4. M. L. Ayres, P. E. M. Jarrett and N. L. Browse. Blood viscosity, Raynaud's phenomenon and effect of fibrinolytic enchancement. *Br. J. Surg.,* **68,** 51–54 (1981).
5. P. M. Dowd, I. B. Kovacs, C. J. H. Bland *et al.* Effect of prostaglandins I_2 and E_1 on red cell deformability in patients with Raynaud's phenomenon and systemic sclerosis. *Br. Med. J.,* **283,** 350 (1981).

3
Autoimmune Diseases

Therapeutic Plasmapheresis (XII), pp. 69-71
T. Agishi *et al.* (Eds)
© VSP 1993

Wegener's Granulomatosis and Plasma Exchange

A. M. SAKASHITA, A. MENDRONE Jr, M. A. MOTA, J. M. KUTNER,
P. E. DORLHIAC-LLACER and D. A. F. CHAMONE

*Fundação Pró-Sangue Hemocentro de São Paulo and Hematology Department,
University of São Paulo, São Paulo, Brazil*

Key words: Wegener's granulomatosis; systemic vasculitis; plasma exchange; ANCA; hemoptysis.

INTRODUCTION

Wegener's granulomatosis (WG) is a rare disease of unknown etiology, recognized as a distinct clinicopathological triad of necrotizing and/or granulomatous inflammation of the respiratory tract, glomerulonephritis and systemic vasculitis [1, 2]. Males and females are affected at approximately the same rate (M:F = 1.3:1), and WG can be seen in any age group from infancy to old age; the mean age of onset is 40.6 years [3]. The clinical manifestations of WG include a wide spectrum of different symptoms and organ related complaints, with upper and lower respiratory tracts and kidneys being the most often affected sites [4]. Anti-neutrophil cytoplasmic antibodies (ANCA), used for diagnosis and follow-up, are found in 93% of patients with active WG and in 13% of patients in remission [5, 6]. If untreated, the generalized form of the disease runs a lethal course with 80% mortality by the end of the first year [7]. Recommended therapeutic modalities include glucocorticoids, cytotoxic agents, antimicrobial compounds, cyclosporine A and local irradiation [7]. The drug considered to be most effective is cyclophosphamide (CPM). Plasma exchange (PE) is also a possible therapeutic modality, with a few reports in the literature describing its efficiency [7–9]. In this report we describe one case of WG treated with PE associated to CPM and corticosteroids.

CASE REPORT

A 26 year old woman was diagnosed with systemic vasculitis in 1985, when she presented with skin vasculitis (biopsy showed leukocytoclastic reaction), rapidly progressive glomerulonephritis and pharyngeal lesions (biopsy inconclusive). During the following 5 years she was treated with dexamethasone, prednisone and CPM, as necessary, on an outpatient basis, with disappearance of skin lesions and worsening of renal function. In 1987 hemodialysis began, 3 times a week.

In October 1990, she was admitted to the ICU with fever, pleuritic pain, hemoptysis and severe hypoxemia, necessitating orotracheal intubation and mechanical ventilation (MCV). On chest X-ray, a bilateral interstitial infiltrate could be seen. Classical anti-neutrophil cytoplasmic antibody (C-ANCA) was detected in the patient's serum and the diagnosis of WG was established. CPM (200 mg/day) and corticosteroids [methyl-prednisolone (1.0 g/day) for 3 days followed by prednisone (1.0 mg/kg/day)] were introduced.

On the 10th day, as hemoptysis and pulmonary function worsened, the Apheresis Department was contacted and it was decided to begin a PE program.

Eight PE sessions were performed during the next 20 days (the first three on consecutive days) using a continuous flow blood separator (Vivacell BT-798, Dideco, Italy) and ACD-A as anticoagulant. At each treatment, 1 plasma volume was exchanged for an equal amount of 5% albumin solution, performing a total of 18.5 l. During this period CPM and prednisone remained in use.

A few hours after the first PE, complete disappearance of hemoptysis was observed. Also, there was a significant improvement in pulmonary function. Over the next few days, red blood cell transfusion (RBC) needs decreased from 7 RBC units on the 10 days previous to PE to 1 unit on the 10 following days.

MCV could be discontinued on day 20 and the patient was discharged on day 55 (i.e. on the 10th and 45th day after first PE).

DISCUSSION AND CONCLUSIONS

This patient was followed for 5 years without diagnosis of WG, a rare disease that presents difficulties for its elucidation. Just when the clinical status worsened it was possible to perform serological testing that, associated to the previous and present clinical picture, established the diagnosis.

As no response was verified with the generally accepted therapy with CPM and corticosteroids, which is reported to be, at present, one the most efficient drug associations for WG [7, 10], and with progressive worsening of the clinical picture, alternative therapies had to be considered. PE has been referred as an useful option in a few reports [7–9].

Analyzing the patient's evolution, we can verify that PE was clearly effective in changing the clinical course. Improvement in pulmonary function and bleeding was directly related to PE. In addition, transfusion needs before and after PE significantly decreased.

The patient's clinical improvement cannot be attributed solely to PE, once CPM and corticosteroids were still in use. However, there is a clear correlation between this improvement and the beginning of PE sessions.

PE seems to be useful in those patients with WG considered to be resistant to regular therapy.

Acknowledgments
Supported in part by a grant from Fundação Banco do Brasil.

REFERENCES

1. R. Waldherr, M. Eberlein-Gonska and I. L. Noronha. Histopathological differentiation of systemic necrotizing vasculitides. *APMIS*, **98**, (Suppl. 19), 17–18 (1990).
2. W. L. Gross. Wegener's granulomatosis: new aspects of the disease course, immunodiagnostic procedures, and stage-adapted treatment. *Sarcoidosis*, **6**, 15–29 (1989).

3. A. S. Fauci, B. F. Haynes, P. Katz *et al.* Wegener's granulomatosis: prospective clinical and therapeutic experience with 85 patients for 21 years. *Ann. Int. Med.*, **98**, 76–85 (1983).

4. H. Lehman and B. Kiefer. Clinical manifestations of Wegener's granulomatosis. *APMIS*, **98**, (Suppl. 19), 19–20 (1990).

5. P. W. Mathiesson. Overview on systemic vasculitides other than Wegener's granulomatosis. *APMIS*, **98**, (Suppl. 19), 21–22 (1990).

6. A. Wiik. Current classification and definitions of autoantibodies to neutrophil granulocytes. *APMIS*, **98**, (Suppl. 19), 24–25 (1990).

7. K. Andrassy. Therapeutic modalities in patients with generalized Wegener's granulomatosis (WG) and related diseases. *APMIS*, **98**, (Suppl. 19), 47 (1990).

8. W. Szpirt, N. Rasmussen, B. Thomsen. Plasma exchange in patients with anti neutrophil cytoplasm antibodies (ANCA) and acute renal failure. *APMIS*, **98**, (Suppl. 19), 63 (1990).

9. D. R. W. Jayne, C. M. Lockwood. Intravenous immunoglobulin or plasma exchange alone can induce remission in systemic vasculitis. *APMIS*, **98**, (Suppl. 19), 64 (1990).

10. M. Ulmer, E. Reinhold–Keller, W. L. Gross. Alternative treatment strategies in Wegener's granulomatosis: First results of a prospective study. *APMIS*, **98**, (Suppl. 19), 51 (1990).

Therapeutic Plasmapheresis (XII), pp. 73-76
T. Agishi *et al.* (Eds)
© VSP 1993

Effect of Plasmapheresis Therapy for Progressive Systemic Sclerosis

T. SAKURAI, E. KUSANO, M. AMEMIYA, H. FURUYA, S. TAKEDA,
S. HOMMA, K. TABEI and Y. ASANO

Department of Nephrology, Jichi Medical School, Tochigi, Japan

Key words: progressive systemic sclerosis; plasmapheresis; plethysmography; thermography; peripheral circulation.

INTRODUCTION

Progressive systemic sclerosis (PSS) is a chronic disease involving peripheral vasculature and general collagenous tissue. It is widely accepted that immunological disorders contribute to the clinical manifestations of PSS. It is characterized by sclerotic skin lesions but also extends into multiple internal organs such as the intestine, lung, heart and kidney. Although no definite therapy has been established, plasmapheresis has been shown to be partly effective for this disorder.

Therefore, the present study was undertaken to evaluate plasmapheresis therapy with steroids and immunosuppressive agents on clinical symptoms and laboratory parameters of five cases with PSS.

PATIENTS AND METHODS

Four males and one female with PSS who ranged in age from 19 to 57 years old were treated with plasmapheresis including simple filtration, double filtration plasmapheresis and immunoadsorption. The duration of the disease varied from 0.5 to 20 years. Main signs and symptoms were systemic sclerosis, dyspnea, Raynaud's phenomenon and edema. Prior to plasmapheresis, all patients received immunosuppressive agents such as prednisolone, dexamethasone, cyclophosphamide and d-penicillamine. Before and after plasmapheresis, clinical findings, pulmonary function tests, immunological parameters, thermography and plethysmography were monitored. The plasmaflo AP08H, Cascadeflo AC1760 and Immusorber PH350 were used as the plasma separator, second separator and immunoadsorber, respectively.

RESULTS

In all cases, skin manifestations such as sclerosis, swelling, stiffness and Raynaud's phenomenon were improved. In particular, skin lesions improved dramatically in cases 2, 3 and 5. Improvements in the range of joint movement were also seen in all cases.

Muscle power and myalgia also improved except in case 2. However, dyspnea seen in cases 2, 3 and 4 improved moderately only in case 4 (Table 1).

Table 1.
Clinical features and treatment of five cases with PSS

Case no.	Sex	Age	Duration (Years)	Main signs and symptoms	Plasmapheresis PE	DFPP	IA	Drug
1	M	55	3.5	systemic sclerosis	3	5		PSL 40 mg; CYP 50 mg
2	M	51	20	systemic sclerosis, dyspnea, edema	6		3	Dexamethasone 4.5 mg; CYP 50 mg
3	M	57	2.5	systemic sclerosis, Raynaud's phenomenon	3	1	2	CYP 75 mg
4	M	44	4	systemic sclerosis, skin stiffness, dyspnea	4			PSL 20 mg
5	F	19	0.5	systemic sclerosis		6 (Sham1)		d-Penicillamine 100 mg

PE: simple filtration; DFPP: double filtration plasmapheresis; IA: immunoadsorption; PSL: prednisolone; CYP: cyclophosphamide.

Pulmonary function tests involving percent vital capacity, percent forced expiratory volume in 1 s, diffusing capacity of lung for carbon monoxide and arterial oxygen tension were not changed significantly before and after plasmapheresis.

Immunoglobulins and aDNA levels were elevated before the treatment. However, there was no significant decrease in IgG, IgA, IgM and aDNA levels after the treatments.

C3, C4 and CH50 did not differ from those in normal control. Plasmapheresis did not produce any significant changes in these complemental markers.

CD3 significantly increased after the treatment; however CD4, CD8 and CD4/CD8 did not change significantly before and after plasmapheresis therapy.

Since the most remarkable changes were improvements of skin manifestations, we also examined thermography and plethysmography.

Surface temperature of toes was elevated markedly, and distribution of the high-temperature area was expanded. The same trends were seen in all cases examined.

Almost all cases showed flat and low-amplitude plethysmography before plasmapheresis even in the area without definite skin lesions. Serial plasmapheresis brought dramatic improvement. Amplitude of plethysmography in the fingers and toes was significantly increased after the treatments (Fig. 1). Before the treatments, amplitude of

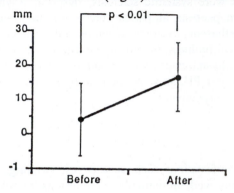

Figure 1. Amplitude of plethysmography.

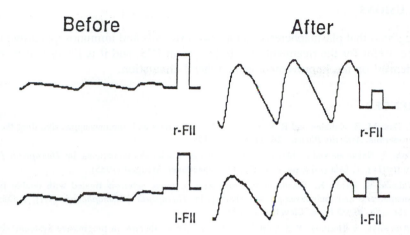

Figure 2. Changes in patterns plethysmography recorded before and after plasmapheresis.

plethysmography was flat and low. However, there was marked increase in amplitude of plethysmography after the treatments. A representative plethysmography is shown in Fig. 2.

Although data is not shown, there were no significant changes in the histologies of skin lesions after plasmapheresis therapy.

DISCUSSION

In the present study, various modes of plasmapheresis therapy combined with steroids and immunosuppressive agents resulted in improvements of skin lesions concomitant with improvement of thermography and plethysmography. Dau *et al.* [1] reported on 15 cases with PSS treated with a combination of steroid, immunosuppressive agents and plasmapheresis. They also noted clinical improvements in 14 of 15 cases with various degrees of skin and internal organ involvement. Oura *et al.* [2] found improvement of skin lesions after plasmapheresis in four cases with PSS. The presence of Raynaud's phenomenon in 95% of PSS patients called attention to a possible vascular pathogenesis of the disease. Although the precise mechanism remains to be elucidated, the present study, as well as others, indicates that restoration of peripheral circulation could lead to improvement of skin lesions.

However, the effects of plasmapheresis on internal organ involvement and immunological parameters are controversial. In this study, the pulmonary function tests used as parameters for internal organ involvement did not change significantly with plasmapheresis. Immunological parameters also did not change. The results of this study suggest that plasmapheresis therapy might be useful for the treatment of skin lesions in PSS and it is likely that its effects partly depend on the improvement of peripheral circulation [3, 4].

CONCLUSIONS

It is suggested that plasmapheresis therapy with steroids and immunosuppressive agents might be useful for the treatment of skin lesions in PSS, and it is likely that its effects partly depend on the improvement of peripheral circulation.

REFERENCES

1. P. C. Dau, M. B. Kahalen and R.W. Sagebiel. Plasmapheresis and immunosuppressive drug therapy in sclerodermia. *Arthritis Rheum.*, **24**, 1128–1136 (1981).
2. T. Oura, Y. Nakasone and G. Miura. Plasma exchange in scleroderma patients. In: *Therapeutic Plasmapheresis (IV)*, T. Oda (Ed.), pp. 269–272, FK Schauttauer, Stuttgart (1985).
3. S. Takeda, K. Tabei, K. Takeda *et al.* Progressive systemic sclerosis treated with double filtration plasmapheresis and immunosuppressive therapy. In: *Therapeutic Plasmapheresis (VII)*, T. Oda (Ed.), pp. 156–158, ISAO Press, Cleveland (1988).
4. M. Amemiya, S. Homma, Y. Sakairi *et al.* Plasmapheresis therapy in progressive systemic sclerosis. In: *Therapeutic Plasmapheresis (VIII)*, T. Ota (Ed.), pp. 97–100, ISAO Press, Cleveland (1990).

Therapeutic Plasmapheresis (XII), pp. 77-81
T. Agishi *et al.* (Eds)
© VSP 1993

Filter Leukapheresis for Rheumatoid Arthritis Patients

K. AMANO, H. EZAKI and K. AMANO[1]

*Kitakyushu General Hospital and [1]Shobara Red Cross Hospital,
Kitakyushu, Fukuoka, Japan*

Key words: rheumatoid arthritis; leukapheresis; immunomodulation; CD11b[+]CD8[+] cell.

INTRODUCTION

Controversy continues regarding the efficacy of apheresis on rheumatoid arthritis (RA) because its effectiveness has not been evaluated. Previous papers, however, demonstrated that this treatment proved feasible for RA patients without comparable laboratory parameters in blood samples according to clinical improvements [1–3]. This investigation was carried out to identify immunological parameters comparable with clinical improvements against RA, by changing the frequency of treatment or analyzing lymphocyte subsets using two-dimensional flow cytometory.

MATERIALS AND METHODS

Nineteen patients with RA; (stage II, four patients; stage III, 6 patients; stage IV, nine patients: class I, one patient; class II, three patients; class III, 13 patients; class IV, two patients) were treated with an Imugard leukocyte removal filter (Terumo Co., Japan). The schedule of treatment was once weekly for 3 weeks, the intensive treatment period, followed by a maintenance treatment period, twice monthly for 2 months (Fig. 1). Heparin was used as anticoagulant and 1400 ml of whole blood was processed with a blood flow rate of 20 ml/min in each procedure; the two filters were connected in parallel. Clinical and immuno-biochemical assessments were done before and at the intensive and maintenance treatment periods.

The laboratory tests performed were complete blood count (CBC), complements (C3, C4), immunoglobulins (IgG, IgA, IgM) and blood drawn at inlet of filter. Other laboratory tests were erythrocyte sedimentation rate (ESR; Westergern) and rheumatoid factor (RF). Two-dimensional study of lymphocyte subsets (CD3/HLADR, CD4/HLADR, CD8/HLADR, CD4/CD45R, CD4/CD8, CD11b/CD8) were added.

For the clinical assessment, numbers of swollen and tender joints and joints having limitation of range of movement (ROM) were counted. Duration of morning stiffness, mean grip strength and the time to walk 10 m were also included. Statistical analyses applied were the Wilcoxon signed-rank test or Friedman test.

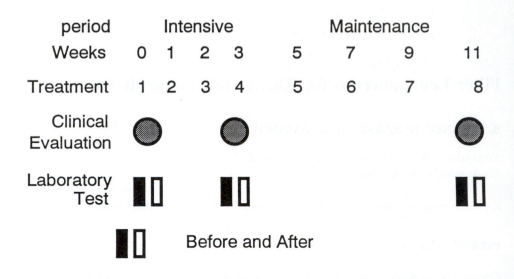

Figure 1. Treatment schedule.

RESULTS

Progressive clinical improvements were seen in all parameters during treatment. Statistically significant improvements treated with Imugard were seen in limitation of ROM, spontaneous pain, morning stiffness and swelling during the intensive treatment period, and additional pain on motion and the time to walk 10 m in the maintenance period.

Significant decreases occurred in RBC, platelets, compliments, immunoglobulins, RF and leukocyte after each filtration. Significant decreases were seen in the percentage of bands, monocytes in the classification of leukocytes and that of CD3$^+$HLADR$^+$, CD3$^-$HLADR$^-$, CD4$^+$(CD8$^+$, HLADR$^+$, CD45R), CD4$^-$(HLADR, CD8$^+$, CD45R), CD8$^+$(HLADR$^+$, CD11b), and increases in the percentage of HLADR$^-$(CD3$^+$, CD4$^+$, CD8$^-$), CD8$^-$(CD11b, CD4$^+$) in lymphocyte subsets after filtration.

In the intensive period, significant decreases were seen in leukocytes or red blood cell counts and in the percentage of CD3$^-$HLADR$^-$ cells and increases in CD3$^+$HLADR$^+$ or CD4$^+$HLADR$^-$ cells. In the maintenance period, significant decreases were seen in red blood cells counts, RF and in the percentage of CD8$^+$HLADR$^-$, CD4$^-$HLADR$^-$ or CD8$^+$CD11b$^+$ cells, and increases in platelets counts, ESR, CD4$^+$CD45DR$^+$ or CD8$^+$CD11b$^-$ cells.

Consistent decreases in RF and progression of anemia were observed with time. Consistent changes occurred in the following lymphocyte subsets; increase in the percentage of CD4$^+$HLA$^-$DR$^-$ and CD8$^-$CD11b$^-$, and decreases in CD8$^+$CD11b$^+$ with time (Table 1).

Table 1.
Laboratory data (mean)

	F	B	I	W	M	W	P
WBC ($\times 10^3$/mm^3)		7.065	6.094	*	6.28		
RBC ($\times 10^4$/mm^3)	*	371.4	340	*	337	*	*
PLT ($\times 10^4$/mm^3)	*	31.56	31.07		35.5	*	*
RF (IU/ml)	*	413.6	307		273	*	*
C3 (mg/dl)		78.81	80.33		79.5		*
C4 (mg/dl)		29.14	31.06		29.3		*
IgG (mg/dl)		1927	1872		1855		*
IgA (mg/dl)		418.3	402.4		472		*
IgM (mg/dl)		190.1	192.7		183		*
ESR (mm/h)	*	56.73	66.27		94.3	*	*
DR$^+$/L2a$^+$ (%)		9.182	12.26		9.5		*
DR$^-$/L2a$^-$ (%)		50.61	50.43		49.6		*
DR$^-$/L2a$^+$ (%)		16.27	13.42		15.3	*	*
DR$^-$/L3a$^-$ (%)	*	31.11	25.63		26.5	*	*
DR$^-$/L3a$^+$ (%)	*	35.15	36.78	*	37.1		
DR$^+$/L4$^+$ (%)		12.81	17.63	*	13.3		*
DR$^-$/L4$^-$ (%)	*	16.32	12.77	*	13.8		
2H4$^+$/L3a$^-$ (%)	*	47.83	47.32		47.7		*
2H4$^+$/L3a$^+$ (%)	*	17.42	20.94		20.4	*	*
L2a$^+$/Mo1$^-$ (%)		19.78	21.12		22.2	*	
L2a$^+$/Mo1$^+$ (%)		7.539	5.775		4.58	*	*
L2a$^-$/Mo1$^-$ (%)	*	58.64	59.26		61.3		*
ROM	*	10.84	8.875	*	6.73	*	
SP		2.167	1.25	*	0.85	*	
MP	*	12.37	10.06		6	*	
MS	*	107.1	33.75	*	45.5	*	
SW	*	3.158	1.438	*	2.6	*	
MG (kg)		8.487	10.06		11.3		
WALK (s)	*	11.58	11.27		9.16	*	
ADL		17.13	15.33		12.4		

B, before; I, intensive; M, maintenance; P, pre and post; F, Friedman test;
W, Wilcoxon signed-rank test.
* Significant ($P < 0.05$).

DISCUSSION AND CONCLUSION

Leukapheresis using filters proved feasible for autoimmune diseases as seen from the clinical improvement without severe side-effects. Though remarkable clinical improvements for RA patients treated by leukocyte removal filter were indicated in a previous paper, the clinical improvements were inconsistent throughout the treatment period and no comparable laboratory parameters were detected. To investigate appropriate treatment methods (processed volume and treatment frequency) and to identify laboratory parameters which change in relation to clinical improvements in RA patients, we increased the frequency and volume of leukapheresis and added measurements of lymphocytes subsets using two-color flow cytometory. By increasing the frequency of treatment from once to twice per month at the maintenance period and increasing the processed blood volume from 1000 to 1400 ml in each treatment, RA patients treated by this method showed consistent and progressive clinical improvements and comparable laboratory data without side-effects. Though clinical parameters improved with time, statistically different laboratory parameter changes were indicated between intensive and maintenance periods compared with the data before treatment. In the maintenance periods, statistically significant lymphocyte subset changes seen in the intensive period were not remarkable but the same tendency was observed. Laboratory parameter changes seen in maintenance period were progressive with time. This difference may be caused by the frequency of treatment. To evaluate long-term result of this treatment, the treatment schedule would be at most twice a month in frequency and 1400 ml in processed blood volume.

Among laboratory parameters were consistent decreases in RF and in the percentage of $CD8^+CD11b^+$ cells with time. $CD8^+CD11b^+$ cells have been thought to be suppresser T cells. Recently, they were considered to have pore forming protein [4] like killer cells, which is suggestive of destroying synovial cells.

This treatment is quite different from lymphocytapheresis or lymphocyte-plasmapheresis in terms of the removal rate of blood components or the effect on the immunological environments by contacting the blood with filters (gossypium barbadense cotton). The method is compared to the centrifugation method or thoracic drainage, and this method is more simple, safer and cost effective. Removal rates showed that these filters can remove not only WBC but platelets or even immunoglobulins, which might cause favorable effects on these diseases than simple removal of lymphocytes or plasma [1–3].

The comparison of lymphocyte subset changes in RA treated with Imugard between pre- and post-filtration suggested that activated T cells, double marker T cells or suppresser T cells are highly adhered to these filters, which conversely increases the percentage of suppresser inducer or helper T cells in the peripheral blood.

The percentage of $CD3^+HLADR^+$ cells decreased just after each filtration but, in turn, increased by the next filtration. Its tendency is particularly obvious in the intensive period. Immunomodulation by contacting the blood components with this filter may occur and may play an important role in ameliorating the activities of RA. We hypothesize that this treatment is effective by removing $CD11b^+CD8^+$ cells or by adhering blood components with gossypium barbadense cotton filters to modulate the immunological environment in RA patients.

REFERENCES

1. K. Amano, M. Imazu and H. Ezaki. Therapeutic on-line leukocyte removal for rheumatoid arthritis. *Artif. Organs*, **13**, 286 (1986).
2. K. Amano, M. Imazu and H. Ezaki. Therapeutic on-line fiber leukocyte filtration for rheumatoid arthritis. *Artif. Organs*, **14**, 163–166 (1990).
3. K. Amano, H. Ezaki, K. Fujimoto, H. Kadomoto and Y. Yokoyama. Leukapheresis for autoimmune diseases. In: *Therapeutic Plasmapheresis IX*, pp. 423–425, ISAO Press, Cleveland (1991).
4. M. J. Smyth, J. R. Ortaldo, Y. Shinakai, M. Nakata, H. Yagita, K. Okumura and H. A. Young. Interleukin-2 induction of pore-forming protein gene expression in human peripheral blood CD8[+] T cell. *J. Exp. Med.*, **171**, 1269–1281 (1990).

Therapeutic Plasmapheresis (XII), pp. 83-86
T. Agishi *et al.* (Eds)
© VSP 1993

Leukapheresis to Patients with Ophthalmic Graves' Disease

K. AMANO, H. EZAKI, M. MORI, K. SHINOZAKI, K. FUJIMOTO[1] and
H. KADOMOTO[1]

*Surgery and [1]Ophthalmology Divisions, Kitakyushu General Hospital, Kitakyushu,
Fukuoka, Japan*

Key words: leukapheresis; ophthalmic Graves' disease.

INTRODUCTION

Severe ophthalmopathy of Graves' disease afflicts only two or three percent of hy-
perthyroid patients [1]. The symptoms are distressing and no ideal treatment has been
reported. This paper reports on ophthalmic Graves' disease (OGD) patients successfully
treated through a new technology; leukapheresis.

MATERIALS AND METHODS

Seven patients with severe Graves' ophthalmopathy (six females and one male; mean
age of 38.5 years old) were treated by this method. All seven patients had distressing
subjective symptoms and exophthalmos. Six patients had received anti-thyroidal drugs.
Subtotal thyroidectomy had been done for three patients, and one total thyroidectomy
who developed thyroid cancer after administration of the radioisotope.

After obtaining the patient's informed consent leukapheresis was performed with
Cellsorba (Asahi Med., Japan) using an on-line filtration technique. Heparinized saline
was used for priming the filter before filtration. Access to both circulation outlet and
return lines was achieved by puncture of peripheral veins with 18 gauge needles. Systemic anticoagulation was maintained by the infusion of ACD (1:10) throughout the
procedure. The blood processed in a single therapy was 3000 ml with blood flow rates
of 30 ml/min.

For the clinical assessment of OGD, diplopia, proptosis and lagophthalmos were
evaluated by Hess's test or an exophthalmometer. We estimated a decrease of more
than 1 mm as an improvement of proptosis and lagophthalmos.

To evaluate the effect of this treatment on the peripheral blood, pre- and post-
treatment blood samples were drawn in each treatment from the inlet of the filter.
The laboratory tests performed were complete blood count (CBC), complements (C3,
C4), immunoglobulins (IgG, IgA, IgM), lymphocyte subsets or mitogens' stimulation

tests; phytohemagglutinin (PHA) and concanavalin (ConA). T cell subpopulation analysis was done using flow cytometry to distinguish and enumerate the cell populations
recognized by commercially available mouse monoclonal antibodies (Ortho Diagnostic
and Becton-Dickenson); OKT3, OKT4, OKT8, OKT11, OKM1, OKIa1, OKB7 and
Leu7.

Statistical analysis was performed using the Wilcoxon signed-rank test.

RESULTS

Subjective improvements were seen in all OGD patients treated by this method. Objective improvements were seen in five patients; improvement of diplopia (two of three),
proptosis (two of seven) and lagophthalmos (three of three). Two patients did not responded objectively, who had received total or subtotal thyroidectomy. Three patients
who were treated only by administration of drug all responded well, instead, the patients
previously treated by thyroidectomy tended to fail to respond (Table 1).

Table 1.
Materials and effectiveness

Case	Age	Sex	Ope	Drug	EXO	DV	LAG	Sub	Obj
NK	45	F	−	+	+	+	+	+	+
ST	21	F	−	+	+	−	+	+	+
IN	44	F	−	+	+	−	−	+	+
NT	20	F	+	+	+	−	+	+	+
KE	47	F	+	+*	+	+	−	+	+
KS	36	F	+	+*	+	−	−	+	−
ST	57	M	+	−	+	+	−	+	−
Effectiveness					2/7	2/3	3/3	7/7	5/7

EXO, exophthalmos; DV, double vision; LAG, lagophthalmos; Sub, subjective
symptoms; Obj, objective symptoms.
* Supplement thyroid drug.

In laboratory parameters, CBC, C3, C4, IgG, IgA and IgM decreased significantly
just after treatment, but 1 month later they all returned to the initial level. In lymphocyte
subsets, the percentage of OKM1, OKB7 and Leu7 decreased just after treatment. The
percentages of OKM1 and OKIa1 before treatment were abnormally high and tended
to decrease toward the normal range. The percentage of Leu7 consistently decreased
with time. No consistent changes were seen in the percentage of OKT3, OKT4, OKT8
and OKT11. In the mitogen stimulation test, both PHA and ConA, which started low
before treatment, showed no consistent changes, except that PHA increased just after
the first treatment. Among thyroid function tests, T_3 decreased significantly. TBII and
TSab decreased just after treatment, though not significantly; however, they showed a
tendency to return to initial values 1 month later. TSH increased 1 month later (Table 2).

Table 2.
Laboratory parameters changes

ID	B1	B2	A1	A2
WBC (10^3/mm^3)	6.41	4.94*	5.13	4.57
RBC (10^4/mm^3)	408	379*	421	393
Hb (g/dl)	12.7	11.7*	13.1	12.1
Plt (10^4/mm^3)	22.7	16.8*	26.7	23.4
C3 (mg/dl)	63.8	56.5*	64.1	51.5
C4 (mg/dl)	22.3	19.2*	21.7	19.8
IgG (mg/dl)	1161	970*	1216	1171
IgA (mg/dl)	212	169*	204	223
IgM (mg/dl)	145	120*	150	130
T3 (ng/dl)	116	95*	128	116
T4 (μg/dl)	7.81	6.78	8.23	6.70
TSH(μU/dl)	1.27	1.41	1.70*	0.65
TSH-R-AB	7.5	6.7	10.0	5.3
OKT3 (%)	69.9	71.8	69.8	70.2
OKT4 (%)	42.5	44.4	44.3	45.5
OKT8 (%)	29.4	28.1	28.0	24.3
OKT11 (%)	78.5	80.0	78.8	74.6
OKM1 (%)	33.1	27.3*	28.0	19.0
OKIa1 (%)	24.8	23.5	23.7	23.6
OKB7 (%)	16.6	13.8*	16.1	18.7
Leu7 (%)	18.6	15.2*	10.3*	6.3
PHABT (IU)	271	319*	289	252
CONABT (IU)	173	179	219	187
TBII (%)	9.9	5.6	8.5	
TSAB (%)	447	122	319	

B1, before first treatment; B2, after first treatment; A1, before second treatment; A2, after second treatment.
* Statistically significant ($P < 0.05$).

DISCUSSION

Current therapy for Graves' ophthalmopathy falls into three categories: (i) local measures to relieve symptoms, (ii) correction of thyroid over or under activity and (iii) suppression of immune response cells or removal of immune complexes or antibodies. Therapies (i) and (ii) are usually unsatisfactory and massive administration of predonisone [2], external irradiation to the orbit [2, 3] or pituitary gland, surgical decompression of the orbit [4, 5] and, rarely, cryosurgical destruction of the pituitary might be indicated. They are sometimes effective but also have severe side-effects or repeated surgeries are required.

Seven patients who had suffered from Graves' ophthalmopathy were successfully treated by leukapheresis using Cellsorba (Asahi, Japan) by an on-line filtration technique without side-effects. Clinical improvements were observed in a single treatment.

Cellsorba was made of a polyester fibre which utilizes the mechanism of adsorption by electrochemical binding. We speculate that this treatment brought favorable results by removing those cells which had the high adherent tendency.

Although T cell subsets in the peripheral blood have been studied in considerable detail in Graves' disease [6], there are few reports about the studies in Graves' ophthalmopathy. Weetman *et al.* [7] reported two cases with abnormal helper/suppressor T cell ratios and increased circulating activated T cells. An increase in numbers of Ia$^+$ (activated) T cells has been observed by Canonica [8] and Ludgate [9]. The profile of the T cell subset in our cases showed abnormality in the percentage of OKM1 and OKIa1, but others were normal including OKT4 and 8 or its ratio. After the first treatment, the profile of the T cell subset became normalized. It is comparable to the evidences that increased killer cells exist in the peripheral blood of Graves' patients or increased activated T cells were normal by the end of carbimazole treatment [9].

The optimal leukocyte (lymphocyte) volume to be removed is not known. It may also depend on the apheresis method mechanism. Using the centrifugation method, removed lymphocytes depend on their gravity, and by the filtration method, they depend on their chemical (immunological) character.

REFERENCES

1. R. D. Hamilton, W. E. Mayberry, W. M. McConahey and K. C. Hanson. Ophthalmopathy of Graves' disease: a comparison between patients treated surgically and patients treated with radioiodine. *Mayo Clinic Proc.*, **42**, 812–818 (1967).

2. G. D. Cavallacci, L. Baschieri and A. Pinchera. Orbital Cobalt irradiation combined with systemic corticosteroids for Graves' ophthalmopathy: comparison with systemic corticosteroids alone. *J. Clin. Endocrinol. Metabol.*, **56**, 1139–1144 (1983).

3. S. S. Donaldson, M. A. Bagshaw and J. P. Kriss. Supervoltage orbital radiotherapy for Graves' ophthalmopathy. *J. Clin. Endocrinol. Metabol.*, **37**, 276–285 (1973).

4. M. R. Hanabury, T. B. Cole, C. E. Clark, A. C. Chandler and N. C. Durham. Surgical treatment for malignant exophthalmos of endocrine origin. *Laryngoscope*, **94**, 1193–1197 (1984).

5. J. H. Ogura and S. E. Thawley. Orbital decompression for exophthalmos. *Otolaryngologic Clin. North Am.*, 29–38 (1980).

6. Y. Iwatani, N. Amino, H. Mori, S. Asri, Y. Izumiguchi, Y. Kumahara and K. Miyai. T lymphocyte subsets in autoimmune thyroid disease and subacute thyroiditis detected with monoclonal antibodies. *J. Clin. Endocrinol. Metabol.*, **56**, 251–254 (1983).

7. A. P. Weetman, A. M. McGregor, M. Ludgate, L. Beck, P. V. Milles and J. H. Lazarus. Cyclosporin improves Graves' ophthalmopathy. *Lancet*, **ii**, 486–489 (1983).

8. G. W. Canonica, M. Bagnasco and S. Ferrini. Circulating T-cell subsets in Graves' disease; differences between patients with active disease and in remission after ^{131}I therapy. *Clin. Immunol. Immunopathol.*, **28**, 265–271 (1983).

9. M. E. Ludgate, A. M. McGregor, A. P. Weetman, S. Ratanachaiyavong, J. Lazarus, R. Hall and G. W. Middleton. Analysis of T-cell subsets in Graves' disease; alternations associated with carbimazole. *Br. Med. J.*, **288**, 526–530 (1984).

Therapeutic Plasmapheresis (XII), pp. 87-91
T. Agishi *et al.* (Eds)
© VSP 1993

Synovial Estimation in Three Patients with Rheumatoid Arthritis Treated with Leukocyte Filtration

K. AMANO, Y. IKUTA,[2] T. MURAKAMI,[2] H. DAISAKU, M. ICHIKAWA, H. TANAKA and K. AMANO[1]

Department of Orthopaedic Surgery, Shobara Red Cross Hospital, Japan
[1]*Department of Surgery, Kitakyushu General Hospital, Japan*
[2]*Hiroshima University Hospital, Orthopaedics Division, Hiroshima, Japan*

Key words: rheumatoid arthritis; leukapheresis; CD11b+ CD8+ cell; arthoroscopic finding; roentgenographic finding.

INTRODUCTION

Though many double-blind controlled studies of lymphoplasmapheresis have been done on rheumatoid arthritis (RA), the efficacy of the treatment is still a matter of speculation.

Amano *et al.* [1–3] first experimented with using an Imugard (Terumo Co., Ltd, Japan); a leukocyte removal filter used in the treatment of autoimmune diseases. This leukapheresis was performed on three patients with RA. We evaluated its effects objectively by examining lymphocytes in the peripheral blood and in the synovial fluid aspirated from their inflamed knee joints using two-dimensional flow cytometory. Roentgenographic findings and arthroscopic findings were done to demonstrate the efficacy of the treatment.

PATIENTS AND METHODS

Case 1 was a 50 year old female with severe pain in the right shoulder. The pain began 7 years previous to our study. This patient was at anatomical stage IV and the functional class III. The synovial fluid was aspirated from the right knee joint at anatomical stage II. The joint was mildly swollen and tender. The visual analog pain scale (VAS) reading of this joint was 30%.

Case 2 was a 66 year old female with severe right shoulder pain that had begun 23 years previous to the treatment. The patient was at anatomical stage IV and functional class III. The synovial fluid was aspirated from the left knee joint at anatomical stage IV. The joint was moderately swollen and tender. The VAS reading was 90%.

Case 3 was a 41 year old male with pain in the metatarsal joints of all toes. The onset of the pain was 9 years prior to the study. The patient was at anatomical stage III and functional class II. The synovial fluid was aspirated from the right knee joint which was severely swollen and tender. The joint was at anatomical stage II with a VAS reading of 90%.

An Imugard filter, made of gossypium barbadense cotton, was used as the material for leukocyte removal in the on-line continuous filtration. Two parallel Imugard filters were connected to the patient. The blood was drawn continuously from the antecubital vein, filtered through the Imugard and returned to the other antecubital vein at room temperature. Anticoagulation was achieved by a bolus administration of 2000 U of heparin at initiation and maintained by constant infusion of 1000 U/h. About 700 ml of blood was processed through each Imugard at a blood flow rate of 20 ml/min.

The treatment schedule for Cases 1 and 2 was once a week for 3 weeks in an intensive treatment period, followed by maintenance treatment, twice monthly for 3 months. For Case 3, treatment was twice a week for the first 4 weeks, then twice a month for the following 3 months.

Blood samples were collected from the on-line circuit 15 min after initiation to evaluate the rate of removal of blood components.

Peripheral blood was checked periodically at the onset of treatment, and at 2 and 4 months of treatment. At the beginning of the study and at 5 days after the 2 and 4 month treatment periods, clinical and peripheral blood and synovial fluid parameters were assessed by counting the number of swollen and tender joints (including distal and proximal interphalangeal joints, metacarpophalangeal and metatarsophalangeal joints of all digits), recording the time to walk 10 m and performing HAQ and Lansubury index (duration of morning stiffness, grip strength, articular index, erythrocyte sedimentation rate (ESR) (Westergern)) determination. The following peripheral blood tests were performed: complete blood cell count, RA test and immunoglobulins (IgG, IgA, IgM) count. The peripheral blood and synovial fluid lymphocyte subsets CD3/HLA-DR, CD4/HLA-DR, CD8/HLA-DR, CD4/CD45RA, CD8/CD11b, CD8/CD11b bright, Leu4/HLA-DR, Leu3a/HLA-DR, Leu2a/HLA-DR, Leu3a/2H4, Leu2a/Mo1, Leu2a/Mo1 bright), were analyzed simultaneously using single and two-dimensional flow cytometory.

The radiographic and arthroscopic findings were also assessed. We attempted to maintain constant dosages of medications from a minimum of 8 months before treatment to 1 month after treatment. At 1 month after treatment, medication was decreased and clinical findings were evaluated by the attending doctor.

RESULTS

Removal rates of WBC, RBC, platelet and immunoglobulins were approximately 95, 6, 7 and 8%, respectively. Significant decreases occured in RBC, platelets and immunoglobulins after each filtration. Significant decreases were also seen in the percentages of $CD3^+HLA-DR^+$, $CD4^-HLA-DR^+$, $CD8^+HLA-DR^+$, $CD4^-CD45RA^+$, $CD4^-CD45RA^-$ and $CD8^+CD11b^-$ after filtration. Increases in the percentages of $CD3^+HLA-DR^-$, $CD4^+HLA-DR^-$, $CD8^+HLA-DR^-$, $CD4^+CD45RA^+$ and $CD8^-CD11b^-$ occurred after filtration.

Average clinical parameters at 2 and 4 months after treatment showed remarkable improvement in comparison with the results from the beginning of the study. The number of swollen joints decreased from eight joints to four and then to one. The time taken to walk 10 m went from 9.0 to 6.7 and then to 6.9 s. HAQ went from 1.93 to 1.04 and to 1.04. Lansbury index results were from 81 to 55 and then to 52%. Duration of morning stiffness dropped from 180 to 17 and then to 0 min. Grip strength increased from 112 to 141 and then to 137 mmHg. Articular index went from 113 to 27 and then to 39.

Comparable laboratory differences with clinical improvements were observed in $CD11b^+CD8^+$ cells in both the peripheral blood lymphocyte (PBL) and the synovial fluid lymphocyte (SFL) ratio. The average of $CD11b^+CD8^+$ went from 7.5 to 5.5 and then to 3.0% in PBL and from 7.7 to 1.4 and then to 3.0% in SFL.

No significant changes could be detected in laboratory parameters except in $CD11b^+CD8^+$ cells. (Table 1).

Table 1.
Laboratory parameters

	Before		2 months after		4 months after	
	PB	(SF)	PB	(SF)	PB	(SF)
WBC ($\times 10^3/mm^3$)	8500		8370		5870	
RBC ($\times 10^4/mm^3$)	394.7		332		343.3	
PLT ($\times 10^4/mm^3$)	44.2		49		48.1	
IgG (mg/dl)	1515		1402		1782	
IgA (mg/dl)	745.6		806		845.7	
IgM (mg/dl)	115		120.7		113	
ESR (mm/h)	79.7		102.7		96.3	
RA test	+		+		+	
$CD3^+HLA\text{-}DR^+$ (%)	6.8	61.9	6.5	58.9	5.4	54.3
$CD3^+HLA\text{-}DR^-$ (%)	61.5	24.3	50.3	27.8	56.6	29.3
$CD3^-HLA\text{-}DR^+$ (%)	11	3.2	18.9	5.7	14	5.1
$CD4^+45RA^+$ (%)	10.2	0.3	11.2	0.1	10.8	0.3
$CD4^+45RA^-$ (%)	34.6	37.4	27.8	34.3	30.8	38.7
$CD8^+11b^+$ (%)	7.4	7.7	5.5	2.2	3.4	2.7
$CD8^+11b^-$ (%)	19.1	30.9	18.7	50.5	19.1	38.2
$CD8^+dim11b^+$ (%)	5.2	1.4	4.6	1.8	3.1	1
$CD8^+bright11b^+$ (%)	2.2	6.3	0.9	0.4	0.3	1.7

PB: periferal blood (SF: synovial fluid); mean.

The average VAS reading of these aspirated knee joints decreased from 70 to 13 and then to 20%. In Case 1, after 4 months of treatment, there was almost no need to aspirate the synovial fluid.

Arthroscopic findings for Case 3 showed a decrease in synovial proliferation and fibrin deposits over time. Roentgenographic findings of Case 1 showed disappearance of periarticular bone atrophy in the interphalangeal joints of both great toes (Figs 1 and 2).

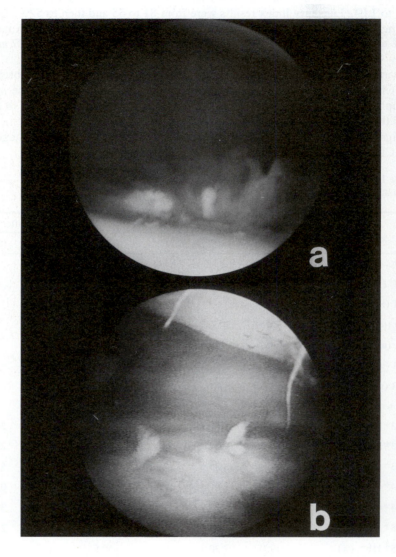

Figure 1. (a) Before treatment arthroscopic findings for Case 3 showed remarkable synovial proliferation. (b) After treatment the excess synovium has disappeared for the most part.

DISCUSSION

CD11b+CD8+ cells have been thought to be suppressor T cells. Recent studies, however, found that CD11b+CD8+ cells adhere to target cells and make pores in their membranes using cytotoxic particles called pore-forming protein (parforin) [4]. We hypothesize that the efficacy of our leukocyte filtration is due to decreasing CD11b+CD8+ cells from the peripheral blood and synovial fluid using a gossypium barbadense cotton filter.

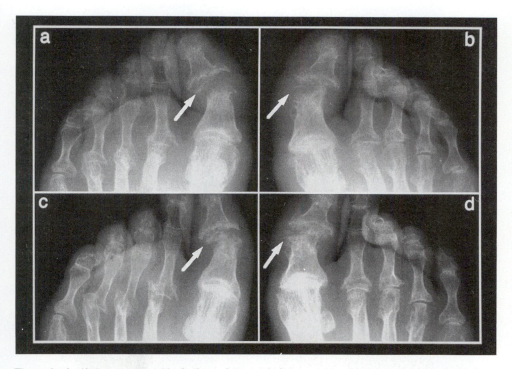

Figure 2. (a, b) Roentgenographic findings of Case 1 before treatment showed severe periarticular bone atrophy in interpharangeal joints of both great toes. (c, d) After treatment, the joints show significant improvement.

CONCLUSION

Results showed significant improvement after our leukocyte filtration treatment not only in several clinical parameters but also with respect to periarticular bone atrophy and synovial proliferation. Furthermore, this method is simple, safe and costs effective. Clinical improvement is related to the decrease in the number of $CD11b^+CD8^+$ cells of the blood and synovial fluid to a normal range.

REFERENCES

1. K. Amano, M. Imazu and H. Ezaki. Therapeutic on-line leukocyte removal for rheumatoid arthritis. *Artif. Organs*, **13**, 286 (1986).
2. K. Amano, M. Imazu and H. Ezaki. Therapeutic on-line fiber leukocyte filtration for rheumatoid arthritis. *Artif. Organs*, **14**, 163–166 (1990).
3. K. Amano, H. Ezaki, K. Fujimoto and Y. Yokoyama. Leukapheresis for autoimmune diseases. *Ther. Plasmapheresis*, **IX**, 423–425 (1991).
4. M. J. Smyth, J. R. Ortaldo, Y. Shinkai, M. Nakata, H. Yagita, K. Okumura and H. A. Young. Interleukin-2 induction of pore-forming protein gene expression in human peripheral blood $CD8^+$ T cell. *J. Exp. Med.*, **171**, 1269–1281 (1990).

Therapeutic Plasmapheresis (XII), pp. 93-99
T. Agishi *et al.* (Eds)

The Effect of Centrifugation-type Lymphocytapheresis or Lymphoplasmapheresis on the Activities of Rheumatoid Arthritis and Systemic Lupus Erythematosus

M. TOKUDA, A. MIZOGUCHI, I. KAWAKAMI, K. SETO, M. INOH, N. KURATA and J. TAKAHARA

First Department of Internal Medicine, Kagawa Medical School, Kagawa, Japan

Key words: centrifugation-type lymphocytapheresis; lymphoplasmapheresis; rheumatoid arthritis; systemic lupus erythematosus.

INTRODUCTION

The drugs which are commonly used for the treatment of rheumatic diseases have well-known side-effects. For example, disease-modifying antirheumatic drugs (DMARDs) may cause renal damage and corticosteroids also have deleterious metabolic complications which may severely affect patients' daily activities. Moreover, the patients whose diseases are refractory to conventional medical therapies may be treated by other immunosuppressive drugs (e.g. cyclophophamide, azathioprine) which may have more severe adverse effects such as myelotoxicity and mutagenicity.

Lymphocytapheresis (LCP) had been introduced as a hopeful strategy which might influence the disease activity via removing substantial numbers of lymphocytes from patients' peripheral circulation. In Japan, leukocyte-removal filters have been preferentially used in recent years because of the ability of removing leukocytes more efficiently than centrifugation-type LCP (c-LCP). However, we recognized that c-LCP could reflect a more pure effect of lymphocyte depletion than leukocyte-removal filters because significant numbers of neutrophils were contained in filtrated cells. Up to the present, several therapeutic trials of LCP for rheumatoid arthritis (RA) have been conducted but have shown conflicting results. On the contrary, limited information has been available concerning the effect of LCP on systemic lupus erythematosus (SLE).

In this study, we focused on the effect of c-LCP on the disease activity of RA and investigated whether c-LCP or lymphoplasmapheresis (LPP) could modify the activity of SLE.

PATIENTS AND METHODS

After informed consents were obtained, five patients were treated with c-LCP using continuous blood cell separator (CS-3000, Fenwall). To be eligible for the study, patients had to fulfill the following criteria (i). Fulfilling the ARA diagnostic criteria for RA. (ii) Having active diseases and being resistant to conventional antirheumatic drugs including non-steroidal anti-inflammatory drugs (NSAID) and DMARDs. (iii) Not having present or antecedent cardiovascular problems.

c-LCPs were performed once or twice a week for 6 weeks and 5000 ml of peripheral blood was processed in each procedure. Before and after each c-LCP, the patients were checked for the activity indexes (morning stiffness, the number of painful joints) and blood was withdrawn for testing blood cell count, erythrocyte sedimentation ratio, the value of C-reactive protein, serum immunoglobulin levels and the titer of RAHA. Circulating lymphocytes were classified by means of immunofluorescent staining using monoclonal anti-CD2, CD4, CD8 and surface IgG. Cells contained in removed fluids were also analyzed with routine hematological staining and the immunofluorescent technique.

In the study aimed at SLE, six patients who fulfilled the ARA diagnostic criteria for SLE were treated with c-LCP (in three patients) or LPP (in another three patients). All patients had experienced a couple of recurrences of disease activities and some had suffered from adverse effects of long-term treatment with corticosteroid. A discontinuous blood cell separator (Model V50, Hemonetics) was substituted for CS-3000 in the case of c-LCP. As a single procedure, Model V50 could remove half as many lymphocytes as CS-3000; c-LCPs by Model V50 were performed constantly twice a week for 6 weeks. LPP consisted of weekly c-LCP by CS-3000 and subsequent double filtration plasmapheresis (DFPP). Patients were evaluated before and after each LCP or LPP about the activity indexes (complement hemolytic activity, values of C3 and C4, titer of antinuclear antibody and anti-DNA antibody). Lymphocytes in both peripheral circulation and removed fluid were analyzed by the same procedures as in RA.

For statistical analysis, Wilcoxon rank sum test was employed.

RESULTS

RA
Mean disease duration of the patients was 6 years. Lymphocytes could be selectively removed via CS-3000 (purity; 87%) (Fig. 1). Although about 4.8×10^{10} of total lymphocytes were removed after 10 times LCP, both subjective (morning stiffness, joint score) and objective indexes (CRP, ESR) did not improve (Fig. 2). A decrease of the absolute number of circulating lymphocytes was observed in some cases but was statistically insignificant. Percentage of T cell, B cell and $CD4^+/CD8^+$ ratio did not alter (Fig. 3). Serum immunoglobulin levels and the titer of RAHA did not decrease except for IgM (Fig. 4). Lectin-induced blastogenesis of lymphocyte gave various results (Fig. 5).

SLE
Although about the same number of lymphocytes were removed as in RA, the titer of antinuclear antibody and anti-DNA antibody did not change after LCP or LPP (Fig. 6). Only in the case of LPP did the levels of circulating immune complexes and serum immunoglobulins decrease significantly (Fig. 7).

Adverse effects
No side-effects except for mild hypovolemia were encountered and all patients accomplished the predetermined schedules.

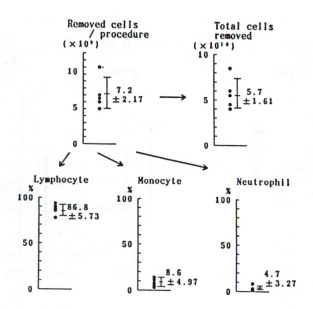

Figure 1. Analysis of removed fluid — patients with RA.

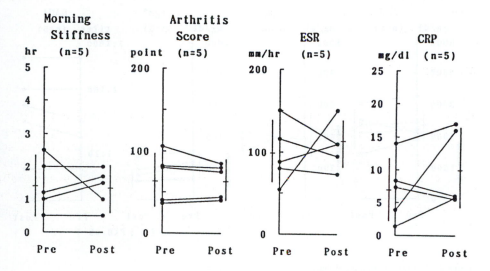

Figure 2. Effect of LCP on activity of RA.

DISCUSSION

In autoimmune disorders, the concept that sensitized lymphocytes might play an important role has prompted a number of investigators to use selective removal of lymphocytes in the management of patients refractory to standard medical therapy. As centrifuga-

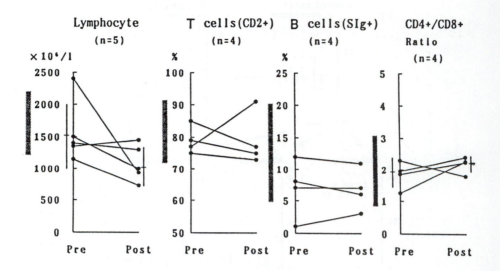

Figure 3. Change of peripheral blood cells.

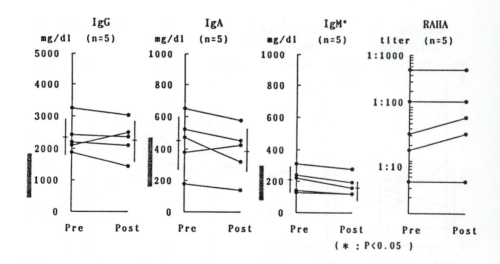

Figure 4. Change of immunoglobulins and rheumatoid factor.

tion cell separators could remove substantial number of lymphocytes more easily than thoracic duct drainage [1], many trials with c-LCP have been conducted, mainly for the treatment of RA, and have demonstrated that clinical improvements are widely variable both in degree and duration and that no correlation exists between the degree of clinical improvements and the number of cells removed [2–4]. In 1984, Karsh *et al.* [5] stated that c-LCP could not be recommended as a reliable strategy for RA until it could be performed in a comparable fashion to elucidate what kind of immunological changes

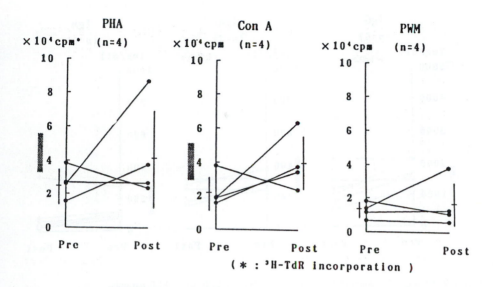

Figure 5. Change of lectin-induced blastogenesis.

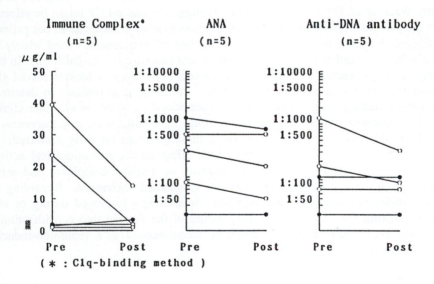

Figure 6. Change of immunological parameters after LCP (•) and LPP (o) — SLE patients.

could be anticipated. However, we think that c-LCP continues to be a good strategy in the treatment of rheumatic disease because c-LCP does not cause serious complications which may affect patients' well-being. On the other hand, limited information has been available concerning the effect of c-LCP on the activity of SLE.

In our present study, five RA patients and three SLE patients were treated with c-LCP. An other three patients with SLE were treated with LPP. Although about 4.8×10^{10} of

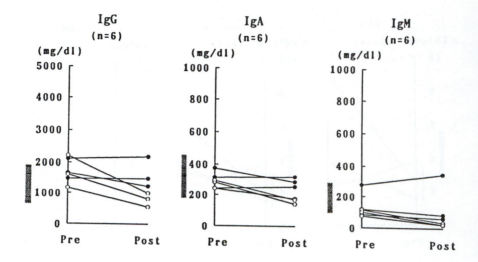

Figure 7. Change of immunoglobulins after LCP (•) and LPP (○) — SLE patients.

total lymphocytes were removed after 10 times LCP, either subjective indexes (morning stiffness, joint score) or objective indexes (CRP, ESR, RAHA) did not improve in RA patients. Wahl *et al.* [6] and Emery *et al.* [7] suggested that c-LCP might be effective only in the patients who showed hyporesponsiveness to soluble antigens. In our patients, the mitogenic response *in vitro* to lectins at the time of pretreatment varied widely but seemed to be enhanced at the time of post-treatment (statistically insignificant). In skin tests, two patients reacted to either purified protein derivatives or tetanus toxoid after treatment and other two patients did not react. Although it is difficult to determine whether these findings might argue for the observations by Wahl *et al.* other clinical factors than patients' immunological status could have influenced responsiveness to c-LCP. More data needs to be available before these questions are fully answered.

On the other hand, c-LCP or LPP had little effect on the immunological activity of SLE. LPP could remove a significant quantity of immune complexes and serum immunoglobulins but the titer of autoantibodies remained unchanged. Regarding the clinical manifestations, neither skin eruptions or arthralgia improved during or after treatment. Taking the acutely progressing nature of the disease into consideration, it seemed that neither c-LCP or LPP could be recommended as a remission-inducing strategy for SLE.

CONCLUSIONS

Our observations might strongly suggest that c-LCP could have no suppressive effect on disease activity of both RA and SLE.

REFERENCES

1. H. E. Paulus, E. I. Machleder, S. Levine *et al.* Lymphocyte involvement in rheumatoid arthritis: studies during thoracic duct drainage. *Arthritis Rheum.*, **20**, 1249–1262 (1977).

2. J. Karsh, J. H. Klippel, P. H. Plotz *et al.* Lymphapheresis in rheumatoid arthritis: a randomized trial. *Arthritis Rheum.*, **24**, 867–873 (1981).

3. T. W. Bunch, J. D. O'Duffy, A. A. Pineda *et al.* Lymphapheresis in rheumatoid arthritis. *J. Clin. Apheresis*, **2**, 127–134 (1984).

4. A. M. Boerbooms, D. J. De-Rooy, P. J. Geerlink *et al.* Lymphapheresis as compared with the rest period in treatment of severe rheumatoid arthritis. *Clin. Rheumatol.*, **3**, 21–27 (1984).

5. J. Karsh. An update on the status of the treatment of rheumatoid arthritis by lymphapheresis. *Int. J. Artif. Organs*, **8**, 35–38 (1984).

6. S. M. Wahl, R. L. Wilder, I. M. Katona *et al.* Leukapheresis in rheumatoid arthritis. *Arthritis Rheum.*, **26**, 1076–1084 (1983).

7. P. Emery, G. N. Smith and G. S. Panayi. Lymphocytapheresis — a feasible treatment for rheumatoid arthritis. *Br. J. Rheum.*, **25**, 40–43 (1986).

Therapeutic Plasmapheresis (XII), pp. 101-103
T. Agishi *et al.* (Eds)
© VSP 1993

A Long-term Follow-up Case of Dermatomyositis Treated with Apheresis Therapy

N. HIGUCHI, M. HAYASHI, N. KOGA,[1] H. SASAKI[1] and T. NAGANO[1]

Hayashi Dermatological Clinic, Kurume City, Japan
[1]*Koga Hospital, Kurume City, Japan*

Key words: dermatomyositis; plasmapheresis therapy; diabetes mellitus.

INTRODUCTION

Dermatomyositis (DM) has been recognized as a clinical type of polymyositis (PM) of the autoimmune disease. The differences of immunological mechanism and etiology between DM and PM have been discussed recently. The mainstay of the treatment for DM has been corticosteroid and immunosuppressive drugs. However, there are some steroid resistant cases and we should minimize steroid dosage because of side-effects and/or accompanying diseases such as diabetes mellitus.

We present here our clinical evaluation of the effects of apheresis therapy on a long-term follow-up case of DM complicated with diabetes mellitus.

PATIENT AND METHODS

A 48 year old male developed diffuse flash mainly on his chest and face with periorbital erythema like heliotrope in March 1985 (Fig. 1). Accompanying symptoms such as general malaise, fever and muscle weakness deteriorated despite receiving steroid administration. Six months after the onset, he became dystasia and was referred to us.

In October 1985, the first apheresis session was performed and a total of seven sessions including immunoadsorption (two sessions) and double filtration plasmapheresis (DFPP, five sessions) were performed over 16 months until March 1987. He had accompanied diabetes mellitus in March 1986.

We applied IMTR (Asahi Medical Co., Japan) for the immunoadsorption column. For DFPP, we used PS-05H (Toray Medical Co., Tokyo) as the first filter and QS-1250 (Toray Medical Co., Japan) for the second filter. We processed plasma at 2000–4000 ml/session on average and the mean time required per session was 211.6 min. We used the femoral vein for blood access and returned blood to the brachial vein. Between 3000 and 5000 units of heparin were injected initially and 2500 units/h of heparin were continuously injected.

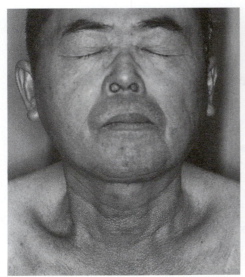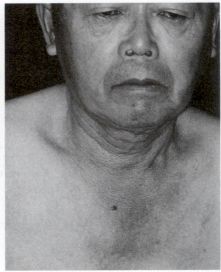

Figure 1. Clinical photo. Left: December 1985; right: October 1991.

RESULT

In October 1985, the first apheresis session was performed (Fig. 2). Significant improvement was obtained right after the initial session. He could flex and raise his upper extremities and he was able to walk after the second session. A total of seven sessions were performed over 16 months; the muscle symptoms, exanthema, and the complicated candidiasis improved gradually.

We obtained successful results by apheresis and we could control his condition with minimum use of steroids. OKT4/8 ratio also improved from 0.92 to 1.98 along with the clinical symptoms. From July 1990, he has needed no steroid administration and he has been in remission for 5 years to date.

DISCUSSION

Since the patient was steroid resistant accompanied with diabetes mellitus, we could not manage an adequate dosage of steroid to control the symptoms. However, apheresis brought significant improvements in the clinical symptoms with a minimum dosage of steroid. The results which we obtained suggest beneficial influences of apheresis in the immunological background. These days the investigation of the immunological mechanisms of DM has progressed, some literature has reported that there is no correlation between the clinical symptoms and T cell subsets in the peripheral blood. However, in this case, the clinical symptoms improved along with the improvement of the OKT4/8 ratio. We assume that apheresis brought some beneficial effects on cellular immunity on this patient. Further studies are required.

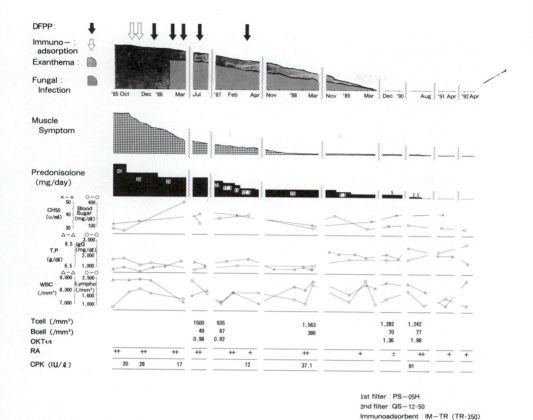

Figure 2. Clinical course.

CONCLUSION

Apheresis therapy brought beneficial results on steroid resistant DM with minimum use of steroids. The immunological mechanism which apheresis brings to the human body is not still clarified. We need to study specific antibodies including Jo-1 antibody and myosin autoantibody. Further investigations are needed.

REFERENCES

1. T. Agishi. *Extracorporeal Immunomodulation.* T. Agishi (Ed.). Nippon Medical Center, Tokyo (1990). (In Japanese).
2. K. Arahata, A. G. Engel and T. Sato. Monoclonal antibody analysis of the mononuclear cell in polymyositis. *Saishin Igaku*, **39**, 287–292 (1984). (In Japanese).
3. L. Murata and Y. Moroi. Significance and diagnostic evaluation of autoantibody. *Rinsho Derma (Tokyo)*, 217–227 (1986). (In Japanese).

Therapeutic Plasmapheresis (XII), pp. 105-107
T. Agishi *et al*. (Eds)

Long-term Remission in Rheumatoid Arthritis after Double Filtration Plasmapheresis

R. SRIVASTAVA, R. HOTCHANDANI and A. DAR

Nephrology Department, Safdarjang Hospital, New Delhi, India

Key words: rheumatoid factor; double filtration plasmapheresis; remission.

INTRODUCTION

Rheumatoid arthritis (RA) is a chronic crippling disease that often results in permanent disablement. Despite many modalities of treatment, including NSAIDs disease modifying drugs, immunosuppressants and medical and surgical synovectomy, many patients are left with significant residual deformities.

MATERIAL AND METHODS

Twenty one cases of seropositive RA with joint deformities who had not responded to appropriate medical treatment were taken up for the study.

These patients underwent PP at weekly intervals for 6 weeks. In addition to the PP, the patients received steroids (prednisolone, 1 mg/kg b.w.) which was tapered over a period of twelve weeks.

The patients were evaluated every week by a physical ability scale (including 15 ft walking time, duration of morning stiffness and functional improvement), C-reactive protein, ESR and rheumatoid factor, during the period of study; after completion of the study, the patients were followed up at 2 monthly intervals.

See Tables 1–3.

Table 1.
Sex wise distribution

Sex	No. of patients
Females	14
Males	7
No. of patients =	21.

Table 2.
Age distribution

Age group	No. of patients
11–20	3
21–30	4
31–40	9
41–50	3
51–60	0
61–70	2
Total no. of patients =	21.

Table 3.
Geographical distribution

State	No. of patients
A. P.	1
Bihar	1
Delhi	3
Haryana	1
Hong kong	1
MP	1
Orissa	2
Punjab	1
Rajasthan	3
UP	6
W Bengal	1
Total no. of patients =	21.

RESULTS

The results showed that all the patients improved significantly after starting DFPP. The improvement was sustained in 19 patients; however, two patients relapsed after 14 and 16 months.

DISCUSSION

RA is a common and crippling disease of the joints. Though initially it may manifest only as morning stiffness, the disease often progresses to fixed joint deformities and extra-articular manifestation. For the milder forms of the arthritis conventional drug therapy suffice, it is in the severe forms that DFPP has a role to play.

We believed that by removing the rheumatoid factor and the CIC not only will the progress of the disease be arrested but also some joints that have not yet undergone bony union may achieve some degree of mobility.

Laboratory investigations during the follow-up of these patients proved our point — when mask patients became seronegative during the follow up.

As shown in the results, 19 patients went into complete remission; however, all were able to achieve higher a degree of independence and this in itself was a considerable achievement.

It must be noted that the benefits of DFPP continued even after stopping the steroid use and that many of these patients had received steroids for prolonged periods prior to the DFPP.

RA is considered to be an immune complex disease [1]. Having failed with drugs, a new method of treatment for this disease has been tried, i.e. plasmapheresis [2]. This method is being extensively used all over the world [3–5]. At our centre this method has been in use extensively since 1985 [6]. The criteria for selection of patients was based on ARA classification (1958). One case of a child with RA was taken for study who could satisfy the diagnostic criteria of Kvin *et al.* [7]. Subjective improvement was studied and categorized, namely response with zero as base line and graded as +3 to −3 on a scale. How do you feel now in comparison to start of therapy? Much much worse is −3, and much much better is +3. Clinical improvement has been reported by various workers in RA with the use of PP [8].

CONCLUSION

From the studies conducted at our centre we conclude that wherever the patients can afford, DFPP is the best method for treatment of RA including long standing RA. Use of DFPP achieved long lasting remissions in comparison will any other treatment. The only limiting factor is cost, making it beyond reach of everyone needing it. RA is a crippling disease and further studies and research are required to make this treatment economical and for everyone.

REFERENCES

1. M. Ziff. Autoimmune process in rheumatoid arthritis. *Progr. Immunol. II*, **5**, 37–46 (1974).
2. D. J. Wallace, D. Goldfinger, R. Gatti *et al.* Plasmapheresis and lymphoplasmapheresis in the management of rheumatoid arthritis. *Arthritis Rheum.*, **22**, 703–710 (1979).
3. A. J. Wysenbeek, W. J. Smith and R. S. Krakauer. Plasmapheresis review of clinical experience. *Plasma Therapy*, **23**, 785–790 (1981).
4. H. Sakamoto, T. Takaoka, M. Usami *et al.* Apheresis: Clinical response to patients unresponsive to conventional therapy. *Trans. Am. Soc. Artif. Intern. Organs*, **31**, 704–708 (1985).
5. Council Report, Current Status of Therapeutic Plasmapheresis and Related Techniques. *J. Am. Med. Ass.*, **253**, 819–824 (1985).
6. R. Srivastava, G. K. Vishwakarma and S. Tyagi. Plasmapheresis therapy in rheumatoid arthritis in Indian patients. *JAPI*, **35**, 133-135 (1987).
7. R. Srivastava, G. K. Vishwakarma and S. Tyagi. Use of a new hollow fibre cellulose, diacetate plasma filter in rheumatoid arthritis in India. *IJN*, **3**, 127–131 (1987).
8. R. Srivastava, A. Dar and A. Pasricha. Rehabilitation of rheumatoid arthritis patients after DFPP. *Indian J. Apheresis*, in press.

Therapeutic Plasmapheresis (XII), pp. 109-111
T. Agishi *et al.* (Eds)
© VSP 1993

Double Filtration Plasmapheresis in Immune Complex Disorders in India

R. SRIVASTAVA, R. HOTCHANDANI and A. DAR

Nephrology Department, Safdarjang Hospital, New Delhi, India

Key words: single filtration plasmapheresis (SFPP); double filtration plasmapheresis (DFPP); immune complex disorders.

INTRODUCTION

Plasmapheresis was first started in India, at this centre, in 1985. Initially only SFPP was performed. However, since 1986, only DFPP has been done. DFPP was found to be more effective, associated with less number of side-effects and, hence, a more promising methods of plasmapheresis.

Patients with a diverse spectrum of immune complex (IC) disorders underwent DFPP. Improvement, both clinical and immunological, was recorded in the majority of the patients.

MATERIALS AND METHODS

Thirty-four patients underwent DFPP from 1986 to 1991. Of these 16 were males and 18 females. Their ages ranged from 8 to 65 years. All these patients underwent DFPP using PF-20 and Albusave filters. Plasmapheresis was performed at weekly intervals. On average six sittings of DFPP were given. Each sitting of DFPP was 80–120 min.

As the volume of the globulin fraction removed during DFPP was small, compensation resulted without giving replacement fluid.

See Tables 1–3.

Table 1.
Age distribution

Age group	No. of patients
0–10	1
11–20	8
21–30	5
31–40	11
41–50	5
51–60	1
61–70	3
Total no. of patients =	34.

Table 2.

Geographical distribution

State	No. of patients
AP	1
Bihar	1
Delhi	18
Hong Kong	1
Haryana	1
Orissa	1
Rajasthan	2
Thailand	1
UP	7
W Bengal	1
Total no. of patients =	34.

Table 3.

Diagnosis

Diagnosis	No. of patients
Rh. Arthritis	19
My. Gr.	1
RPGN	1
R. Tx. Rej.	2
CGN with CRF	4
ARF	5
SLE with CRF	2
Total no. of patients =	34.

RESULTS

Remarkable results were obtained using DFPP in immune complex disorder.

Conditions resulting due to an acute insult were completely cured in all patients and there were no residue or sequel. Chronic immune complex disorders, however, also showed a significant improvement, with longer remission periods.

No side-effects, except for arm pain in two patients, were observed.

DISCUSSION

As the science of immunology is making rapid advances many diseases which were initially classified as being of unknown etiology are known now to be due to immune complex disorders.

The treatment of these conditions used to be a long and tedious one, with the use of many toxic drugs, i.e. steroids and cytotoxic agents. Not only was the use of these drugs characterized by numerous side-effects, but they were not fully effective.

Plasmapheresis was attempted to remove not only the CIC, but also the pathogenetic globulin fraction and, therefore, attack the initial phase of the disease cycle. Once the CIC had been removed, their deposition in the tissues was decreased and, therefore, the progress of the disease stopped. This also resulted in the previously damaged organs having time to recover their function.

Presently, plasmapheresis is used for the treatment of CIC diseases [1]. Plasma exchange adsorption and filtration of plasma have been used as methods of removal of undesirable circulating substances [2]. Plasmapheresis is useful in the treatment of fulminant myasthenia gravis [3], lupus nephritis [4], polyarteritis nodosa [5], IC disorders in children [6], rheumatoid arthritis [7, 8], RPGN [9], HUS [10] and renal failure [11]. This is a method of extracorporeal cellular immunomodulation [12]. This has also been used in GP Syndrome [13].

CONCLUSION

In our set up in India, we found DFPP to be a very useful method of treating IC disorders with the minimum of side-effects and now are using DFPP as a treatment of choice in all such disorders baring individual economic limitations.

At our centre DFPP has more or less replaced SFPP.

REFERENCES

1. A. Geavlete *et al.* Plasmapheresis in treating circulating immune complex diseases. *Rev. Med. Int.*, **37**, 377–383 (1985).

2. G. Virella *et al.* Plasma exchange adsorption and filtration of plasma: four approaches to the removal of undesirable substances. *Biomed. Pharmachother.*, **40**, 286–296 (1980).

3. S. E. Levin *et al.* Successful plasmapheresis for fulminant myasthenia gravis during pregnancy. *Arch. Neurol.*, **43**, 197–198 (1986).

4. M. Amato *et al.* Can plasmapheresis improve Lupus Nephritis without its immunological markers? (Letter). *Nephron*, **48**, 252–253 (1988).

5. Y. Terada *et al.* Combined treatment of plasmapheresis and methyl prednisolone pulse therapy to polyarteritis nodosa with rapidly progressive glomerulonephritis. *Nippon Naika Gakkai Zassi*, **77**, 494–498 (1988).

6. I. E. Malakhovskii *et al.* Plasmapheresis in immune complex diseases in children. *Pediatriia*, **9**, 75–81 (1989).

7. R. Srivastava, G. K. Vishwakarma and S. Tyagi. Plasmapheresis therapy in rheumatoid arthritis in Indian patients: abstracts. *Xth International Congress of Nephrology*, London (1987).

8. R. Srivastava, G. K. Vishwakarma and S. Tyagi. Use of a new hollow fibre cellulose, diacetate plasma filter in rheumatoid arthritis in India. *Indian J. Nephrol.*, **3**, 127–131 (1987).

9. I. S. Milovanov *et al.* Plasmapheresis in the treatment of rapidly progressing glomerulonephritis. *Ter. Arkh.*, **61**, 78–81 (1989) (English abstract).

10. L. Camba *et al.* Hemolytic–Uraemic syndrome with renal failure: the effect of plasmapheresis. *Hemologica (Pavia)*, **70**, 341–344 (1985).

11. A. A. Mikhailov *et al.* Plasmapheresis in the treatment of patients of renal failure. *Klin. Med. (Mosk.)*, **65**, 117–121 (1987) (English abstract).

12. Y. Nose. A therapeutic plasmapheresis, extra corporlal cellular immunomodulation. *Artif. Organs*, **15**, 69 (1991).

13. A. Vasudev, R. Srivastava and R. N. Srivastava. Goodpasture's syndrome. *Indian Pediatr.*, **27**, 984–987 (1990).

Therapeutic Plasmapheresis (XII), pp. 113-115
T. Agishi *et al.* (Eds)
© VSP 1993

Reversal of Renal Failure with Double Filtration Plasmapheresis: An Indian Experience

R. SRIVASTAVA, R. HOTCHANDANI and A. DAR

Nephrology Department, Safdarjang Hospital, New Delhi, India

Key words: renal failure; double filtration plasmapheresis; reversal.

INTRODUCTION

End stage renal disease (ESRD) is generally believed to be a terminal, irreversible condition. Treatment options are limited to maintenance dialysis and renal transplant; the first, with its inherent complications and multiple side-effects and the second with its high failure rates. Moreover, these modalities do not act on the etiological agent/agents of the disease. We performed DFPP if four cases of ESRD, where the disease was believed to be immune complex in origin and then followed them up to determined permanency of the response.

MATERIALS AND METHODS

Four patients (Table 1) of ESRD underwent DFPP at our centre with PF-20 and Albusave filters of Dideco.

Table 1.
Patient distribution

No.	Sex	Age	Geographical distribution	Diagnosis
1	F	11	Delhi	CGN with CRF
2	M	58	Delhi	ICGN with CRF
3	M	52	Delhi	ICGN with CRF
4	M	17	UP	IGM with nephropathy

The patients were followed up for intervals from 5 months to 4.5 years, at each visit apart from history and clinical examination, the following were estimated: blood urea nitrogen (BUN), serum creatinine, immune profile, serum electrolytes and creatinine clearance.

DFPP was started without hemodialysis in all cases. PP at regular intervals was continued till 12 weeks.

Patients were observed for the following parameters for evaluation of results: (i) duration of follow up; (ii) results: (a) subjective, (b) objective and (c) biochemical; and (iii) treatment at present.

Each sitting of DFPP lasted for 80–120 min and no replacement fluid was given or needed.

RESULTS

The observations and follow up of this group of patients show that this treatment has
been very effective in reversing the process of renal failure. Two of these patients are
stable without drugs and diet, leading a normal life, while the third is stable with drugs
and diet. One case, however, expired due to acute myocardial infarction (AcMI) after
3 years of remission period. The periods of remission in these cases are shown in
Table 2.

Table 2.
Status and duration of remission

No.	Treatment of patients	Duration of remission
1	stable without drugs and diet	4.5 years
2	stable without drugs and diet	15 months
3	expired (due to AcMI)	3 years
4	stable with drugs and diet	5 months

DISCUSSION

Immune complex GN leads to chronic renal failure due to deposition of immune complexes in the glomeruli. This leads to inflammatory reaction resulting in fibrosis and
occlusion glomeruli.

It was with the intention of removing circulating immune complex and antibodies
that DFPP was done in these patients. Believing that removal of these complexes would
not only prevent further renal damage but also help in the recovery of partially damaged
nephrons, these were subjected to DFPP.

CONCLUSION

Our study shows that DFPP can be used as a modality of reversal of renal failure in
ESRD, especially where the etiology was of immune complex nature [1]. Its role in
other types of renal failure is yet to be determined. A study with a large number of
cases should be undertaken to fully determine the role of DFPP in chronic renal failure.
Various studies have been done for the treatment of renal failure caused by immune
complex renal diseases with the use of plasmapheresis as treatment of choice [2–4].
Apheresis is useful in the reduction of ESRD population and the reduction of complications of long-term hemodialysis [5]. Although recovery of useful renal functions is
normally unlikely by treatment but dialysis dependent patients may have it [6–8].

REFERENCES

1. H. Sakamoto, T. Takaoka, M. Usami *et al.* Apheresis: clinical response to patients unresponsive to
   conventional therapy. *Trans. Am. Soc. Artif. Intern. Organs*, **31**, 704–709 (1985).
2. L. Camba *et al.* Hemolytic–uraemic syndrome with renal failure: the effects of plasmapheresis. *Hemologica* (Pavia), **70**, 341–344 (1985).

3. J. E. Balow. Plsmapheresis: development and application in the treatment of renal disorders. *Artif. Organs*, **10**, 324–330 (1986).

4. A. A. Mikhailov *et al.* Plasmapheresis in the treatment of patients of renal failure. *Klin. Med. (Mosk.)*, **65**, 117–121 (1987) (English abstract).

5. Y. Nose, W. J. Smith and P. Malchesky. Plasmapheresis holds distinct advantages for twenty first century uremia therapy. *Kidney Int.*, **28** (Suppl. 17), 131–132 (1985).

6. A. V. Starikov. Plasmapheresis in the intensive therapy of renal insufficiency. *Vestn. Khir.*, **142**, 16–20 (1989) (English abstract).

7. A. P. Maxwell, W. E. Nelson and C. M. Hill. Reversal of renal failure in nephritis associated with antibody to glomerular basement membrane. *Br. Med. J.*, **4**, 844–850 (1989).

8. R. Srivastava, A. Dar and A. Pasricha. Treatment of renal failure with DFPP in India. *India J. Apheresis*, in press.

Therapeutic Plasmapheresis (XII), pp. 117-120
T. Agishi *et al.* (Eds)
© VSP 1993

Effect of Plasmapheresis for Severe Myasthenia Gravis Accompanied by an Enormous Thymus

Y. KINOSHITA, K. OKADA, S. TAKAHASHI, T. KUNO,
M. MAEJIMA and Y. NAGURA

*Second Department of Internal Medicine, Nihon University School of Medicine,
Tokyo and Nishi-Kofu National Hospital, Yamanashi, Japan*

Key words: myasthenia gravis; enormous thymus; immunoadsorption; acetylcholine receptor antibody; thymectomy.

INTRODUCTION

It has been suggested that anti-acetylcholine receptor (AChR) antibody plays an important role in the genesis of myasthenia gravis (MG), because removal of anti-AChR antibody due to plasmapheresis or administration of immunosuppressive drugs resulted in improving the symptoms of MG [1]. Since Pinching *et al.* reported plasmapheresis for the treatment of MG in 1976 [2], modified plasmapheresis, such as double filtration plasmapheresis and immunoadsorption, has been employed in order to selectively remove the causative substances if the disease [3]. We experienced a case of severe MG with an enormous thymus and high level of anti-AChR antibody refractory to conservative therapy and successfully treated it with plasmapheresis (immunoadsorption). The results are reported here.

CASE REPORT

A 14 year old female had an easy fatigability in late January, 1990 and MG was diagnosed in September, 1990. The patient was then administered prednisolone (20 mg/day), it did not show any improvement for the patient. Since dysphagia appeared in October, 1990, pyridostigimine bromide (100 mg/day) was administered instead of prednisolone. The symptom was temporarily improved, but disturbance of gait appeared in March, 1991. Then, the dose of pyridostigimine bromide was increased to 240 mg/day. However, her symptoms became gradually progressive and the patient was admitted to our hospital in July, 1991. The level of anti-AChR antibody was 1426 nmol/l. The levels of creatine phosphokinase and other laboratory data were within normal range. Neurological findings are shown in Table 1. Ptosis, dysphagia, dysstansia and decrease in strength of muscles were recognized, edrophorium test was positive, and muscle response to repetitive motor nerve stimulation was a warning phenomenon. Computerized tomography demonstrated an enormous thymus. Since myasthenic symptoms were severe and progressive, combined therapy (administration of prednisolone and pyridostigmine bromide) was performed. However, the effect on myasthenic symptoms was small despite the decrease in the level of anti-AChR antibody (930 nmol/l). Therefore, plasmapheresis (immunoadsorption) was employed (Fig. 1). The patient was cannulated by inserting a double-lumen catheter into the femoral vein.

Table 1.
Neurological findings on admission

Ptosis	(+)	
Diplopia	(−)	
Dysphagia	(+)	
Deep tendon reflex	normal	
Gait and stance	dysstansia	
Strength of individual muscles		
	Right	Left
deltoid	3/5	3/5
biceps	3⁻/5	4⁻/5
triceps	3/5	3/5
quadriceps femoris	3/5	3/5
hamstrings	4/5	4/5
tibialis anterior	5/5	5/5
tibialis posterior	5/5	5/5
hand grip	7 kg	7 kg
Electrophysiological tests		
edrophonium (Tensilon) test	(+)	
muscle response to repetitive motor nerve stimulation	waning	

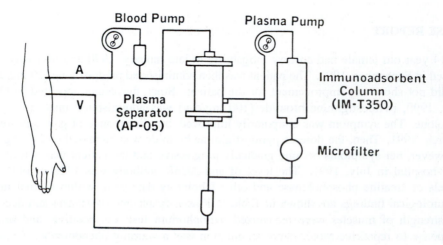

Figure 1. Method of plasmapheresis (immunoadsorption).

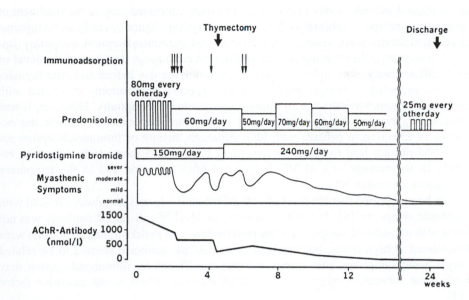

Figure 2. Clinical course.

Blood was separated through a polyethylene membrane (Plasmaflo OP-05, Asahi Medical Co.) as a first filter and the plasma was passed through a immunoadsorbent column (IM-T350, Asahi Medical Co.) for adsorbing anti-AChR antibody as a second filter using Plasauto 2500 (Asahi Medical Co.). Approximately 2 l of plasma per session was passed through the second filter with a 80–90 ml/min blood flow rate and a 20–25 ml/min plasma flow rate. After three sessions of immunoadsorption, both an improvement of myasthenic symptoms and a decrease in the level of anti-AChR antibody (696 nmol/l) were recognized. However, myasthenic symptoms were aggravated afterwards. Then extended thymectomy was performed on the 37th day after admission on next day of immunoadsorption to expect stronger effect. After thymectomy, myasthenic symptoms were not obviously changed despite a clear decrease in the level of anti-AChR antibody (279 nmol/l) because of the occurrence of respiratory infection. Since the symptoms became aggravating with continuation of infection, despite increases of doses of prednisolone and pyridostigimine bromide, two sessions of immunoadsorption were added. After immunoadsorption, the symptoms were improved with the disappearance of infection and the dose of prednisolone could be reduced to 25 mg every other day with 240 mg/day of pyridostigimine bromide. The patient was discharged in January, 1992 (Fig. 2).

DISCUSSION

It has been reported that approximately 15% of patients with MG have thymus and MG with thymus usually appears in patients aged more than 20 years [4]. In addition, it has been indicated that thymectomy leads to improvement of myasthenic symptoms without respect to the existence of malignant or benign tumors [5]. In the present case, MG with thymus was seen in a female patient aged 14 years and thymectomy was performed because severe myasthenic symptoms continued despite the treatment of conservative therapy combined with immunoadsorption. Since myasthenic symptoms before thymectomy were severe and systemic, and immunoadsorption temporary improved severe myasthenic symptoms in addition to continuous decrease of the level of anti-AChR antibody, we employed immunoadsorption the day before and after thymectomy and expected a stronger effect. As we expected, thymectomy combined with immunoadsorption was effective in improving myasthenic symptoms. However, it was transiently aggravated during infection. It is therefore important to prevent the occurrence of infection in patients with MG. Although therapy of immunoadsorption for severe MG did not lead to complete remission, this method seems to be effective, especially in the management of MG before and after operation and in the temporary management of severe MG.

It has been reported that the level of anti-AChR antibody was not always related with myasthenic symptoms [6]. In the present case, the level of anti-AChR antibody was not related with myasthenic symptoms when prednisolone and pyridostigimine bromide were administered at high doses, but the level of anti-AChR antibody seemed to be related to myasthenic symptoms after immunoadsorption. Therefore, immunoadsorption may adsorb some substances other than anti-AChR antibody which is one causative factor of MG.

CONCLUSION

It is suggested that immunoadsorption is effective in managing myasthenic symptoms before and after thymectomy in patients with severe MG refractory to conservative therapy.

REFERENCES

1. D. M. Linton and D. Philcox. Myasthenia gravis. *Dis. Mon.*, **36**, 593–637 (1990).
2. A. J. Pinching, D. K. Peters and J. Newsom-Davis. Remission of myasthenia gravis following plasma-exchange. *Lancet*, **ii**, 1373–1376 (1976).
3. K. Heininger, A. Gaczkowski, H. P. Hartung *et al.* Plasma separation and immunoadsorption in myasthenia gravis. In: *Therapeutic Plasmapheresis*, T. Oda (Ed.), pp. 3–10 Schattauer, Stuttgart (1986).
4. H. J. G. H. Oosterhuris. Myasthenia gravis and other myasthenic syndromes. In: *Clinical Neurology*, Churchill Livingstone, Edinburgh (1991).
5. G. K. Scadding, C. W. H. Havard, M. J. Lang *et al.* The long term experience of thymectomy for myasthenia gravis. *J. Neurol. Neurosurg. Psychiat.*, **48**, 401–406 (1985).
6. J. M. Lindstrom, M. E. Seybold, V. A. Lennon *et al.* Antibody to acetylcholine receptor in myasthenia gravis. Prevalence, clinical correlates, and diagnostic value. *Neurology*, **26**, 1054–1056 (1976).

Therapeutic Plasmapheresis (XII), pp. 121-123
T. Agishi *et al.* (Eds)
© VSP 1993

Effects of Plasma Exchange in a Nephrotic Syndrome as an Initial Manifestation of Thrombotic Microangiopathy

H. MORITA, T. SHINZATO, Y. FUJITA, I. TAKAI and K. MAEDA

The Branch Hospital of Nagoya University, Nagoya, Japan

Key words: thrombotic microangiopathy; HUS/TTP; plasma exchange; plasma infusion; nephrotic syndrome.

INTRODUCTION

A very uncommon case of thrombotic microangiopathy and nephrotic syndrome, occurring simultaneously, recently came to our attention.

Our primary interest in this case is to clarify whether or not the pathogeneses of the two diseases (thrombotic microangiopathy and nephrotic syndrome) were the same.

As there are no methods for proving this conclusively, we evaluated the effects of plasma infusion and exchange on each of the diseases and surmised whether or not the two were closely related in etiology.

CASE REPORT

A 42 year old male public servant was transferred to The Branch Hospital of Nagoya University with anemia, thrombocytopenia and nephrotic syndrome. Mass screening, which was performed 1 year prior to hospitalization, disclosed no abnormalities. He had been in excellent health up until 2 months before admission when he had caught a cold and consulted a physician.

Proteinuria was indicated by urine dipsticks but no quantification was performed. He had CCL and pronase for 3 days. When his common-cold-like symptoms subsided he stopped visiting the doctor.

One week before admission, he noticed peripheral edema over his lower extremities. On admission, his temperature was 37.3 °C, pulse 82, respirations 14 and blood pressure 134/80 mmHg.

The urinalysis showed 4+ protein and 5–6 RBC/high power field. Twenty-four-hour urine protein was 5.3 g and selectivity index was 0.27. The serum creatinine concentration was 1.2 mg/dl, albumin was 2.8 g/dl, lactic dehydrogenase 898 IU/dl, hematocrit 29.7% and the platelet count was 83 000/μl. The haptoglobin was low at 10 mg/dl, but both direct and indirect Coombs tests were negative. A large number of fragmented red cells were seen in the peripheral blood smear. The pro-thrombin and partial thrombin times were normal. Anti-nuclear antibodies and ANCA were negative.

The management of this case included the use of fresh frozen plasma and subsequent plasma exchange, which were effective in improving a variety of laboratory data, such as decreased serum hemoglobin levels (10.3 to 12.0 g/dl), decreased platelet counts (83 000 to 212 000), increased serum creatinine levels (1.48 to 1.28 mg/dl), increased serum lactic dehydrogenase levels (898 to 486 IU/l), and decreased serum haptoglobin levels (less than 10 to 50 mg/dl). Urinary protein excretion was still high at 3.1 to 8.7 g/24 h. At discharge, he was on dipyridamole, vitamin E, warfarin and cyclopyridine hydrochloride.

He had been followed as an outpatient for 2 months without any signs of exacerbation. Since nephrotic range proteinuria persisted, he was readmitted for a second kidney biopsy.

He was then treated with predonisone (0.9 mg/kg of body weight/day) for 4 weeks. The proteinuria resolved incompletely (from 5.0 to 2.0 g/day). For the next 4 weeks, 0.7 mg/kg of body weight/day of predonisone was administered, but proteinuria (from 1.0 to 2.0 g/day) persisted.

RENAL BIOPSY

First biopsy
Under the light microscope, the arterioles and extraglomerular small arteries showed elongation, wall thickening, endothelial proliferation and swelling. Intraglomerular involvements were minimal except for juxtaposition of the foot process of the podocytes, which was observed at the electron microscopic level. Tubulo-interstitial changes were unremarkable and direct immunofluorescence (IgA, IgG, IgM, C1q, C3) studies disclosed no abnormalities.

Second biopsy
Histopathological findings were essentially the same as those of the initial biopsy with the exception that the changes were mild in degree.

DISCUSSION

There are a few reported cases of thrombotic microangiopathy and nephrotic syndrome occurring in a single patient. They can be divided into two categories as follows.

(i) Nephrotic syndrome, with minor glomerular abnormalities, complicating thrombotic microangiopathy a few years after its initial onset [1].

(ii) Nephrotic syndrome with severe intraglomerular involvements and thrombotic microangiopathy, which occur simultaneously [2] or a few years after the onset of the former [3].

There have been no reported cases of thrombotic microangiopathy and nephrotic syndrome with minor glomerular abnormalities occurring simultaneously, such as that which we have observed.

In the present case, plasma infusion and subsequent plasma exchange were effective in improving thrombotic microangiopathy but not in nephrotic syndrome. This might indicate that the two diseases in this case have different pathogeneses.

REFERENCES

1. R. L. Siegler, E. D. Brewere, T. J. Pysher *et al.* Hemolytic uremic syndrome associated with glomerular disease. *Am. J. Kidney Dis.*, **13**, 144–147 (1989).
2. D. Salant *et al.* Case records of the Massachusetts General Hospital. Case 41–1990. *N. Engl. J. Med.*, **323**, 1050–1061 (1990).
3. A. Mariam, M. D. Friedlander, H. Gretta *et al.* Recurrent thrombotic thrombocytopenic purpura associated with membranous glomerulopathy. *Am. J. Kidney Dis.*, **17**, 83–85 (1991).

Therapeutic Plasmapheresis (XII), pp. 125-128
T. Agishi *et al.* (Eds)
© VSP 1993

Changes in Circulating Immune Complexes of Patients with Rheumatoid Arthritis after Plasmapheresis: Comparison of Monoclonal Rheumatoid Factor Assay, Anti-C3d Assay and C1q Solid Phase Assay

M. TOMYO, K. YAMAJI, Y. KANAI, T. KAWANISHI, S. FUJITA,
M. YOKOYAMA, H. TSUDA, H. HASHIMOTO and S. HIROSE

*Department of Internal Medicine, Division of Rheumatology, Juntendo University,
School of Medicine, Tokyo, Japan*

Key words: rheumatoid arthritis; plasmapheresis; mRF assay; anti-C3d assay; C1q solid phase assay.

INTRODUCTION

Recently, plasmapheresis (PP) has been used in the treatment of rheumatoid arthritis (RA) to eliminate rheumatoid factor and circulating immune complexes (CIC). We have already reported its efficacy.

In 1988, we examined RA patients treated by PP for using three methods, anti-C3, C1q solid phase and Raji cell assays, and compared the positive test rates and PP-associated CIC elimination rates from these assays. Of the three methods, the anti-C3 assay was most sensitive, i.e. the positive test rate and elimination rate were high, and correlation between the reaction and clinical findings was highest [1]. Subsequent studies showed that the Raji cell assay was not quite reliable because its sensitivity was low, while an assay utilizing the reaction with monoclonal rheumatoid factor (mRF) was introduced and found useful [2]. This time, we assayed CIC in RA patients using mRF, anti-C3 (AC3) and C1q solid phase (C1q SA) methods, and compared with positive tests and elimination rates. Further, we classified CIC by its molecular weight, then analyzed samples and compared assay data before and after PP.

MATERIALS AND METHODS

Sixteen RA patients who satisfied the ARA diagnostic criteria [3] participated in the study. They were seven men and nine women with a mean age at 56.7 years, who were in stage II–IV. These patients all received PP every 10 days–2 weeks in the past 1–4 years (2.8 years on average).

We use the double membrane filtration procedure for PP. In this PP, a constant flow of blood from the patient is passed through the primary membrane, where plasma is separated, then sent to the secondary membrane. The secondary membrane allows low molecular weight components such as albumin to pass through and return, to the patient together with the blood cells. The substances filtered out by the secondary membrane

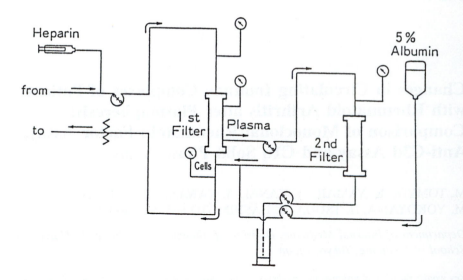

Figure 1. Double filtration plasmapheresis.

mRF	AC3	C1qSA
SP: mRF-F(ab)2	SP: anti-C3d	SP: C1q
100µl sample	100µl sample	100µl sample
| R.T., 1hr	| R.T., 1hr	| R.T., 1hr
ALP-anti IgG	POD-anti IgG	POD-anti IgG
| R.T., 1hr	| R.T., 30min.	| R.T., 30min.
Substrate	Substrate	Substrate
| R.T., 30min.	| R.T., 30min.	| R.T., 30min.
Color -reagent	Stopper.	Stopper
|	|	|
Read at 490nm	Read at 415nm	Read at 415nm

Figure 2. Methods of CIC detection.

are drained off, and the equivalent volume of 5% albumin is supplied. The volume of blood treated at one time was 2000 ml (Fig. 1).

CIC was identified by three methods, the mRF assay utilizing mouse IgG type mRF, AC3 and C1q SA. All assays were carried out by ELISA procedure with microplates and the values are shown in the heat agglutination titer of human IgG (Fig. 2).

RESULTS

Figure 3 shows the distribution of the positive CIC test before PP. The positive test rate was 63% with mRF, 63% with AC3 and 57% with C1q SA. Seven cases were positive and four cases negative, with all assays. No correlation was detected between the reaction and duration of morning stiffness, grasping power, duration of walking, joint score, ESR, CRP, rheumatoid factor, CH50, C3, C4, IgG, IgA or IgM.

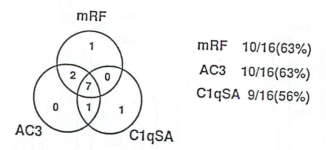

Figure 3. Number of CIC positive patients by three assays.

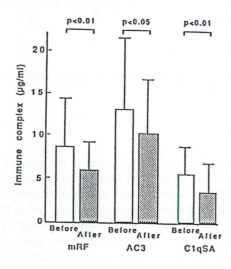

Figure 4. Changes in CIC after plasmapheresis.

Figure 4 shows the change in CIC due to PP in patients positive for CIC. The PP-associated CIC elimination rate was 34.1% with mRF, 27.5% with AC3 and 21.8% with C1q SA, i.e. its was highest with mRF. Compared with the elimination rate based on mRF, the elimination rate with C1q SA and that with AC3 were significantly reduced ($P < 0.01$, $P < 0.05$).

We analyzed the samples collected before and after PP from each patient positive for CIC. This involved gel filtration by high performance liquid chromatography, then dividing the effluents into the macromolecular fraction with the molecular weight above 10^6 (Fraction 1) and the $3–5 \times 10^5$ molecular fraction (Fraction 2), and estimating CIC in each fraction. mRF and AC3 gave higher values for Fraction 1 than for Fraction 2. The Fraction 1 value relative to the Fraction 2 value was higher with mRF than with AC3. PP eliminated CIC in Fraction 1 with a higher frequency than CIC in Fraction 2. When

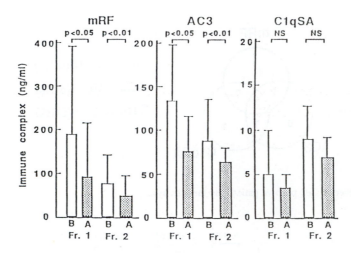

Figure 5. Changes in CIC after plasmapheresis.

the fraction was the same, mRF gave a relatively higher elimination rate as compared with AC3 or C1q SA (Fig. 5).

DISCUSSION

We used mRF for the first time in this study, but it has already been used by other authors, who reported that it can be used for monitoring of the patient's response to the treatment because it was highly sensitive and the reaction correlated with the clinical stage. However, there is little information as to the change due to PP. We carried out this study to evaluate the utility of mRF as compared with AC3 and C1q SA in determining the degree of CIC elimination by PP, and to estimate the molecular size of CIC most likely to be detected. The positive test rate was high with mRF and AC3, and the PP-associated elimination rate was highest with mRF. Besides, mRF tended to be more sensitive than the other assays to macromolecular CIC, and efficient in showing the elimination of CIC. From these results, we think the new mRF assay is highly sensitive and the reaction will serve as a good indicator for PP. The present patients examined for CIC were all on a long-term PP, but we are planning to apply mRF to patients newly introduced to PP and follow the course of the CIC assay simultaneously with the clinical course.

REFERENCES

1. M. Tomyo. Changes in circulating immune complexes of patients with rheumatoid arthritis after plasmapheresis: comparison of Raji cell assay, anti C3 assay and C1q solid phase assay. *Jpn. J. Clin. Immunol.*, **13**, 49–56 (1990).
2. H. Taguchi, M. Kanoh, N. Takubo *et al.* IgG isotype and isotype specificity of murine monoclonal IgG rheumatoid factors. *Clin. Exp. Immunol.*, **80**, 136–140 (1990).
3. F. C. Arnett, S. M. Edworthy, D. A. Bloch *et al.* The American Rheumatism Association 1987 revised for the classification of rheumatoid arthritis. *Arthritis Rheum.*, **31**, 315–324 (1988).

Therapeutic Plasmapheresis (XII), pp. 129-132
T. Agishi *et al.* (Eds) 125-128
© VSP 1993

Lymphocytapheresis in Multiple Sclerosis: Immunological and Clinical Effects

K. MATSUDA, Y. ISHIGAKI, T. KOMIYA, Y. FURUKAWA,
H. TSUDA[1] and T. SATO

Departments of Neurology and [1]Internal Medicine,
Juntendo University School of Medicine, Tokyo, Japan

Key words: multiple sclerosis; lymphocytapheresis; T cell.

INTRODUCTION

Multiple sclerosis (MS) in autoimmune disorders of the central nervous system is characterized by temporal and spacial multifocal demyelination and perivascular lymphocyte infiltration. The main neurological symptoms are visual, motor, sensory, and urinary disturbances, cerebellar ataxia and cerebral dysfunction. The most common treatment for acute attacks or active state exacerbation of MS is intravenous pulsed methylpredonine therapy followed by oral high-dose prednisolone therapy [1]. A number of studies on plasmapheresis have been carried out on MS patients. One double-blind study suggested that plasmapheresis may benefit patients who have already undergone long-term plasmapheresis in combination with oral cyclophosphamide and prednisolone therapy [2]. Lymphocytapheresis has also been used to treat MS patients, although, it is unclear whether the procedure was carried out using the centrifugation method [3]. Earlier, we released a preliminary report on a new lymphocytapheresis method that uses a lymphocyte adsorption column to treat MS patients who are in the active state [4]. The present paper reports the clinical efficacy and analyzes lymphocyte subsets in MS patients treated with the new lymphocyte adsorption column.

PATIENTS AND METHODS

Patients
Twenty-four patients with MS and four with acute retrobulbar neuritis during acute onset or in the active state of exacerbation of the disease were treated with lymphocytapheresis using the new method. Neurological symptoms in these MS patients were characterized by visual disturbances caused by retrobulbar neuritis, sensory and motor disturbances of the extremities and urinary disturbances caused by spinal cord lesions. Although all patients received intravenous pulsed methylpredonine therapy followed by oral high-dose prednisolone therapy, their clinical symptoms did not improve. Clinical symptoms were evaluated according to Kurtzke's expanded disability status scale (EDSS). Prior to treatment with lymphocytapheresis, the EDSS grades varied from 3.0 to 8.5.

Lymphocytapheresis

Lymphocytapheresis was carried out using a 'Cellsorba' lymphocyte adsorption column (Asahi Medical Co., Tokyo). The column employs non-woven fabric made of polyester fibers. Approximately 3000 ml of whole blood can be treated by this column. Blood withdrawn from an elbow vein at 50 ml/min was treated with the anticoagulant nafamostat mesilate and then passed through the column. The lymphocyte-reduced blood was immediately retransfused into the patient. Each lymphocytapheresis course lasted 60 min.

Lymphocyte subsets

Peripheral lymphocyte subsets were determined before and after lymphocytapheresis using the following monoclonal antibodies: anti-CD4; anti-CD8; anti-CD25 against the IL-2 receptor; and anti-CD20 against virtually all B cells. Anti-Ta1 monoclonal antibodies were produced against an IL-2-dependent human T cell line and immunoprecipitates produced a single, major 105-kd band. Unlike the antibody to IL-2R, anti-Ta1 does not inhibit T cell proliferative responses to antigen [6].

RESULTS

Eight of the 28 patients treated by lymphocytapheresis showed moderate or mild improvement. The eight patients ranged in age from 20 to 46 years with onset of the disease ranging from 2 weeks to 11 years. EDSS grades varied from 4.0 to 8.5 prior to lymphocytapheresis. Within 4–12 h following lymphocytapheresis eight patients

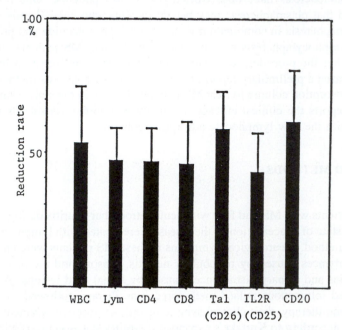

Figure 1. Reduction rate of blood cell counts before and after lymphocytapheresis.

showed EDSS grades improvements of 2 or more steps. Sensory disturbance and pyramidal tract signs caused by spinal cord lesions and visual disturbance responded very well to treatment. Details of the clinical symptoms will be described in a later paper.

Figure 1 shows the reduction rates in lymphocyte subsets as a percentage value following lymphocytapheresis. The mean reduction rates of white blood cell and lymphocyte counts were 52.0 and 46.9%, respectively. Reduction rates of CD4 and CD8 were 49.8 and 42.2%, respectively. Reduction rates of Ta1 and IL-2R were 59.2 and 39.9%, respectively. CD20 showed a reduction rate of 62.5%. Amongst the various lymphocyte subsets, Ta1-positive T cells and pan B cells displayed significantly higher reduction rates ($P < 0.05$). No difference was observed in the CD4/CD8 ratio before and after lymphocytapheresis, nor was there a significant reduction in the number of red blood cells or in immunoglobulin concentration in the serum.

We determined Ta1-positive T cell counts in the peripheral blood of MS patients in the active state of exacerbation and in remission. Ta1-positive T cells increased in number for those patients in the active state and decreased for those patients in remission. No serious complications were noted in any of the patients following lymphocytapheresis.

DISCUSSION

To treat MS patients, lymphocytapheresis was carried out in open trials rather than in blind. Although intravenous pulsed methylpredonine therapy failed in some MS patients in the active state, immediate improvement was observed following lymphocytapheresis using the lymphocyte adsorption column. In some patients, visual evoked potentials showed more rapid improvement than clinical symptoms. About 50% of the lymphocytes were adsorbed by the column. Amongst the lymphocyte subsets, Ta1-positive T cells and B cells showed higher adsorption than other lymphocytes subsets. Hafler *et al.* [6] demonstrated that the activation antigen Ta1 in the peripheral blood of patients with progressive MS was expressed more frequently than in patients with inactive MS. Treatment efficacy seems to be correlated with the removal of certain pathologically-activated lymphocytes, in particular, with Ta1-positive T cells.

In conclusion, lymphocytapheresis employing a lymphocyte adsorption column is effective in treating MS patients who did not respond to methylpredonine pulse therapy.

Acknowledgments
This study was supported in part by grants from the Japanese Ministry of Health and Welfare and the Tokyo Metropolitan Bureau of Health.

REFERENCES

1. H. L. Weiner and D. A. Hafler. Immunotherapy of multiple sclerosis. *Ann. Neurol.*, **23**, 211–222 (1988).
2. B. O. Khatri, S. M. Koethe and M. P. McQuillen. Plasmapheresis with immunosuppressive drug therapy in progressive multiple sclerosis. *Arch. Neurol.*, **41**, 734–738 (1984).
3. S. L. Hauser, M. Fosburg, S. V. Kevy and H. L. Weiner. Lymphocytapheresis in chronic progressive multiple sclerosis: immunologic and clinical effects. *Neurology*, **34**, 922–926 (1984).
4. Y. Ishigaki, T. Sato, S. Ikebe, T. Komiya and H. Tsuda. Effects of lymphocytapheresis with an immunoadsorptive column on 4 patients with multiple sclerosis. In: *Therapeutic plasmapheresis (VIII)*, T. Oda (Ed.), pp. 114–117, Schattauer, Stuttgart (1989).

5. J. F. Kurtzke. Rating neurologic impairment in multiple sclerosis: an expanded disability status scale (EDSS). *Neurology*, **33**, 1444–1452 (1983).

6. D. A. Hafler, D. A. Fox and M. E. Manning. *In vivo* activated T lymphocytes in the peripheral blood and cerebrospinal fluid of patients with multiple sclerosis. *N. Engl. J. Med.*, **312**, 1405–1411 (1985).

4
Hematological Diseases

Therapeutic Plasmapheresis (XII), pp. 135-138
T. Agishi *et al.* (Eds)
© VSP 1993

Correction of Bleeding Diathesis due to Factor XI Inhibitor by using On-line Plasma Filter Pheresis

G. A. SIAMI, M. A. SCHAPIRA and W. J. STONE

*Department of Medicine, Vanderbilt University School of Medicine and
the Department of Veterans Affairs Medical Center, Nashville, TN 37212, USA*

Key words: Factor XI; inhibitor; plasma filter; plasmapheresis.

INTRODUCTION

Factor XI (FXI), plasma thromboplastin antecedent, is one of the contact-phase co-agulation factors that mediates coagulation through its activation by FXIIa, followed by a direct action on FIX [1]. Inhibitors to FXI may develop following replacement therapy in patients congenitally deficient in FXI [2] or may be associated with drug administration such as procainamide and phenothiazines [1]. Inhibitors may arise spontaneously, especially in patients with autoimmune disorders [3]. Circulating inhibitors are immunoglobulins that either inactivate the coagulation factor or inhibit the function of phospholipids that mediate blood coagulation [4].

We report a patient with acquired FXI inhibitor and a bleeding diathesis who needed multiple colon polyps removed. He was treated successfully by using on-line plasma filter pheresis.

CASE PRESENTATION

A 59 year old man developed epistaxis, bleeding gums and hematuria in early 1990. He had previously undergone coronary artery bypass grafting, transurethral resection of prostate and penile implant surgery without hemorrhage. Later in 1990 GI bleeding prompted the discovery of colonic polyps. The patient also had a history of Type II diabetes mellitus, hypertension, gout, chronic renal insufficiency and anemia of chronic disease. He was admitted for elective colonic polypectomy. His prolonged bleeding time was thought to be secondary to his chronic renal insufficiency and it was corrected with DDAVP. His physical examination was remarkable for S4 gallop, trace pretibial edema, a glove/stocking neuropathy and heme positive stool. The following tests were normal: platelet count, prothrombin time, thrombin time, clot retraction, vWF antigen, lupus anticoagulant profile, anticardiolipin antibody, fibrinogen, FVIII screen, plasminogen and euglobulin lysis time. The APTT was prolonged and not corrected by addition of normal serum. Levels of FXI activity were 5 and 2% in serum and urine, respectively. Diagnosis of acquired FXI deficiency due to inhibitor was made.

MATERIALS AND METHODS

To prepare the patient for removal of the colonic polyps, eight plasmapheresis procedures were done over 10 days. Plasma was separated from blood by using a Haemonetic V-50 cell separator and on-line EVAL-2A Kuraray plasma filters were employed. A total of 4600 ml of plasma was processed per treatment. Only a total of 175 g of albumin was required for the eight procedures along with very low doses of heparin.

RESULTS

The result of coagulation studies are shown in Table 1.

Table 1.

Circulating anticoagulant:			
Control APTT	36 s	|	
Patient	52 s	| C/W inhibitors	
Patient + control	43 s	|	

Not corrected by increasing phospholipid

FXI activity	13%	Normal 50–150%	
vWF Ag	132%	45–150%	
PT	14	10–13	
APTT	51	25–40	
PLT	126	150–500 K	

Bleeding time	8 min	2·5–25 min
Plasminogen	111%	70–115
Euglobulin lysis time	5 h	2–8 h
Factor XIII screen	normal	
Fibrinogen	400	150–400

Lupus anticoagulant profile

Anticardiolipin Ab	negative	
Russells viper venom	1.1 ratio	
Reptilase time		
(Heparin independent)	Patient 29 s	normal
	Control 17 s	15–25
Dilute tissue		
thromboplastin	1.2 ratio	normal
		0.8–1.1

The results of PT, PTT, FXI activity and level of IgG (in mg/dL) pre eight pheresis, and PT and PTT for 7 days after eight pheresis are shown in Table 2.

Colonic polyps were removed on 8/17 and PTT remained normal after termination of plasmapheresis on 8/16 for 1 week and thereafter.

The results of percent reduction of IgG, IgA, IgM, fibrinogen and the volume of plasma processed in each plasmapheresis are shown in Table 3.

Table 2.

Date	PT	PTT	FXI	IgG		Date	PT	PTT
8/7	12.3	47.7	13%	2200		8/17[a]	11.9	30.7
8/8	12.4	48.5	5	1750		8/18	11.9	27.9
8/9	12.1	50.2	15	1240		8/19	13.1	30.9
8/10	12.9	45.8	15	1160		8/20	13.7	30.8
8/13	12.1	34.5	14	1300		8/21	13.4	28.8
8.14	11.6	29.3	13	1060		8/22	13.6	29.2
8/15	12.3	29.4	19	764		8/23	13.0	27.3
8/16	12.0	28	20	613				

[a] Day of polypectomy.

Table 3.

Date	Percent Reductions				Plasma processed
	IgG	IgA	IgM	fibrinogen	(ml)
8/7	27.8	27.7	34.6	32.5	2500
8/8	42.3	45.9	52.2	65.8	3175
8/9	40.9	50.4	42.0	73.1	4500
5/10	41.6	49.1	40.4	42.4	5090
8/13	50.0	50.6	52.4	60.4	5300
8/14	52.4	52.8	60.0	58.8	5276
8/15	52.6	50.7	—	39.1	5560
8/16	47.3	51.9	57.9	76.3	6000
Average	44.3 ± 8.1	47.4 ± 8.2	48.5 ± 9.2	56.6 ± 16.2	4675 ± 1223

FXI activity became 100% in 5 weeks. Cryoglobulins were negative. The FXI inhibitor was identified as a Protein A binding IgG. The patient underwent four surgical operations, i.e. creation of A–V fistula for hemodialysis, insertion of a peritoneal catheter, amputation of right great toe and right below knee amputation in the last 20 months with no bleeding.

DISCUSSION

FXI deficiency was not corrected with FFP. High dose prednisone was not tried in this diabetic patient. Plasmapheresis was the best therapeutic option to remove the inhibitor which was identified as a protein A binding IgG. Our patient had a high serum IgG. We used 2A-EVAL plasma filters which are shown to remove IgG efficiently while conserving albumin, other immunoglobulins, and fibrinogen compared to plasma exchange [5]. FXI activity below 20% is associated with major bleeding while activity of 20% or above usually does not cause bleeding. After eight procedures FXI activity rose to 20%. APTT normalized and stayed normal. FXI activity reached 100% in 5 weeks.

CONCLUSION

Intensive on-line plasma filter pheresis was effective in removing FXI inhibitor, in this case a Protein A binding IgG. It requires minimal albumin as replacement fluid and a high immunoglobulin level can be reduced to normal.

REFERENCES

1. R. Hoffman, E. J. Benz and S. J. Schattil (Eds). *Hematology, Basic Principles and Practice.* Churchill Livingston, New York (1991).

2. K. Morgan, S. Schiffman and D. Feinstein. Acquired FXI inhibitors in two patients with hereditary FXI deficiency. *Thrombo-Haemost.,* **51**, 371–375 (1984).

3. G. M. Vercellotti, and D. F. Mosher. Acquired FXI deficiency in systemic lupus erythematosus. *Thrombo-Haemost.,* **48**, 250–252 (1982).

4. E. A. Reece, L. P. Clyne, R. Romero *et al.* Spontaneous factor XI inhibitors. *Arch. Intern. Med.,* **144**, 525–529 (1984).

5. G. A. Siami, and W. J. Stone. Selective plasmapheresis using special secondary on-line filters in therapy of immune disorders. *Progr. Clin. Biol. Res.* (*Apheresis*), **337**, 355–358 (1990).

Therapeutic Plasmapheresis (XII), pp. 139-142
T. Agishi *et al.* (Eds)
© VSP 1993

A Randomized Clinical Trial Comparing Plasma Exchange and Plasma Infusion in the Treatment of Thrombotic Thrombocytopenic Purpura

G. A. ROCK, K. H. SHUMAK, N. A. BUSKARD, V. S. BLANCHETTE, J. G. KELTON, R. C. NAIR, R. A. SPASOFF and MEMBERS OF THE CASG*

Canadian Apheresis Study Group, Ottawa, Ontario, Canada

Key words: plasma exchange; plasma infusion; thrombotic thrombocytopenic purpura.

INTRODUCTION

Thrombotic thrombocytopenic purpura (TTP) is an uncommon disease but important because of its high mortality rate even when treated with a combination of drugs and plasma. In its classic form, this syndrome includes microangiopathic hemolytic anemia, thrombocytopenia, fever, and renal and neurological impairment. The cause of the syndrome is unknown as is the optimal treatment. Although both plasma exchange (PE) and plasma infusion (PI) are useful treatments, it is not clear whether they differ in effectiveness. Proponents of PI suggest that benefit is related to the administration of a substance deficient in TTP patients. Proponents of PE suggest that not only is a deficient factor replaced, but toxic substances are removed during the exchange procedure. In this report we describe a prospective randomized trial in which patients with TTP were treated with either PE or PI.

METHODS

All patients diagnosed as having TTP at any of 16 participating medical centres in Canada were eligible for consideration for entry into the trial which commenced in March, 1982. Specific eligibility criteria were: thrombocytopenia (defined as a platelet count of less than 100×10^9 per litre), microangiopathic hemolytic anemia as indicated by red cell fragmentation present on a peripheral blood film, no identifiable cause for the thrombocytopenia and microangiopathic hemolytic anemia such as disseminated intravascular coagulation, carcinoma or eclampsia, and no history of congestive heart

*The members of the CASG are as follows: Grenfell Adams, MD, Barrett Benny, MD, Noel A. Buskard, MD, Robert Card, MD, William F. Clark, MD, Peter Ford, MD, Philip Gordon, MD, Max Katz, MD, John Klassen, MD, Pierre Leblond, MD, Mariette Lepine-Martin, MD, Jack McBride, MD, Philip Mickelson, MD, Rama C. Nair, PhD, Harry Rayner, MD, Gail A. Rock, PhD, MD, Kenneth H. Shumak, MD, Robert A. Spasoff, MD, Marion Sternbach, MD, and David M. C. Sutton, MD

failure or of anuria which, in the opinion of the attending physician, rendered the patient unable to tolerate PI. Patients with a previous history of TTP were not excluded from the study. Informed consent was obtained from all patients before entry into the study.

Patients were randomized to receive either PE or PI with FFP, using a scheme which ensured a balanced allocation within each centre. One group received PE with FFP as replacement for a minimum of seven procedures over the first nine hospital days with treatment on the first three days being essential. The volume exchanged was 1.5 times the predicted plasma volume for the first three procedures and single volume PE thereafter. The other group received PI daily until the end of a cycle of treatment. The volume of plasma infused was 30 ml per kilogram over the first 24 h followed by 15 ml/kg each day thereafter. If patients became unable to tolerate this fluid load because of their cardiac or renal status, diuretics were used. A cycle of treatment was defined as the period from randomization to one of the following events: death, clinical deterioration to the extent that the patient was taken off protocol (which for PI patients usually meant crossing over to PE), early response or completion of seven days of treatment.

All patients received dipyridamole (400 mg per day) and aspirin (325 mg per day) by mouth for a minimum of 2 weeks following entry into the study. Outcome was assessed at the end of the first cycle of treatment following entry into the study and again at 6 months post-randomization.

The exact binomial test [1] was used to test the statistical significance of the difference in outcome between the two groups. The 95% confidence interval for the difference in proportion of responders and survivors between the two treatment regimes was also computed.

RESULTS

A total of 103 patients were entered into the trial over a 7 year period. One subject assigned to the PI group rapidly improved before receiving any treatment and never received either PI or PE. Attending clinicians decided that this patient did not have TTP and therefore the patient has been eliminated from the analysis. Of the remaining patients, 51 were randomly allocated to receive PE and 51 to receive PI. There were 67 females and 35 males in the study and the average age was 40.5 (SD 14.3) years. Eleven patients with a past history of TTP were entered into the study. All patients had thrombocytopenia; at the time of entry, the average platelet count was 23.3×10^9 per litre (SD 16.9) with a range of $1-94 \times 10^9$ per litre. Red cell fragmentation was seen on all of the 102 blood films. The average reticulocyte count was 324×10^9 per litre (SD 221.6).

Fluctuating neurological abnormalities were present in 64 of the patients at entry. An additional eight patients subsequently developed neurological signs during the course of the disease including one patient with classical TTP, as determined by gingival biopsy at entry, who did not present with neurological signs but subsequently showed transient confusion. Of the 38 patients who did not present with neurological signs, seven subsequently died with five of these patients developing neurological signs before death.

Fever was present in 24 of the 102 patients at entry. Renal abnormalities were present in 60 patients at entry with 53 having an elevated BUN and 47 an elevated creatinine.

A total of 1284 PE and 432 PI procedures were carried out on the 102 patients in the study. The PE patients received an average of 21.5 l (SD 7.8) of plasma whereas the PI patients received an average of 6.7 l (SD 3.3) by the end of the first cycle. Most patients tolerated the procedures well. Six PE patients and five PI patients had no complications during any procedure. Most complications were minor and occurred in less than one-quarter of the procedures.

The analysis at the end of the first cycle showed a higher rate of response (the platelet count rose to greater than 150×10^9 per litre and no new neurological events developed) in patients receiving PE than in patients receiving PI ($P = 0.025$). Twelve patients assigned to PI deteriorated rapidly and, on clinical grounds, were transferred to PE before the intended end of the first cycle of treatment. These patients were analyzed as PI failures. No PE patients transferred to PI.

Analysis was also carried out on patient outcome 6 months after entry into the study. At various times after the end of the first cycle of treatment, 19 additional patients in the PI group were crossed over to PE on clinical grounds. Fifteen of these patients had failed to respond at the end of the first cycle, and four had initially responded but later relapsed. These crossovers received PE according to the study protocol. Crossover from PE to PI did not occur.

In 10 of the patients who originally responded to PE, the platelet count again fell after an average of 5.3 days and they received an average of 15.4 (SD 8.2) further exchanges over 19.6 days before achieving a complete response with no further relapsed. Similarly, two of the PI patients relapsed after an initial response and received further PI with no further relapsed. Sixteen PE and two PI patients who failed treatment at the end of the first cycle eventually responded.

Thus in the final analysis, 51 patients received PE alone (40 survived), 20 received PI alone (10 survived), and 31 received PI first and then PE (22 survived).

Using predetermined response criteria, and regarding the early crossovers as PI failures, the results of the late analysis are again in favour of PE ($P = 0.002$). The results of this analysis are conservative, since they attribute to PI 15 eventual responses among the crossovers, although PI had already failed (11 patients) or the patients had incomplete responses (four patients). Using survival as the outcome with an intent-to-treat approach, the PE arm is still superior.

DISCUSSION

Analysis of response, as defined in our study, and of survival shows that PE is superior to PI in the treatment of TTP, both at the end of the first cycle and at the end of 6 months. The significantly lower death rate ($P = 0.036$) when plasma was exchanged suggests a possible role for the removal of some plasma constituent in addition to the supply of fresh plasma. However, our study was not designed to determine whether the improved outcome with PE was attributable to the removal of a toxic material by PE or to the administration of plasma in larger volumes by PE than is possible with simple PI. Furthermore, no attempt was made to define the optimal schedule either for PE or for PI. Instead, an empirical decision was made, by the clinicians at the 1981 Canadian Apheresis Study Group annual meeting, to adopt and adhere to the then standard PE and PI treatment regimens for TTP.

The eventual response to PE was not predictable from the platelet count at presentation or from the changes in the platelet count by day 9. Furthermore, the presence of neurological signs did not predict a poor outcome to either PE or PI. The fact that only 64 of the 102 patients presented with neurological findings and only 24 had fever may well reflect a relatively early presentation of these patients to the study, possibly contributing to the successful treatment responses. Approximately one-half of the patients tested had normal creatinine clearance and patients with poor or non-existent renal function were not eligible for randomization. Therefore this trial deals with a subset of patients with TTP who may be considered to have less severe disease.

Since neurological signs, fever and impaired renal function were not consistently present in the patients at entry, some might argue that not all patients met the criteria for a diagnosis of TTP. However, the validity of our diagnostic criteria is supported by the fact that eight patients developed neurological signs only after treatment was initiated. Our patients were comparable to patients, reported in the literature, who had variable presentations often without all of the classical signs of TTP. A review by Ridolfi and Bell [2] reported that 98% of patients with TTP had microangiopathic hemolytic anemia, 83% thrombocytopenic purpura, 84% neurological symptoms and 76% renal disease. Thus, clearly, the diagnostic pentad is not present uniformly in this syndrome.

We observed a substantial mortality rate in our patients with TTP indicating that while PE and combined drug therapy have considerable benefit and represent, likely, the best available treatment, TTP still remains a disease with less than optimal treatment. A better understanding of the pathophysiology of TTP should lead to more effective treatments. Until that time, PE with fresh frozen plasma should be used to treat patients with this disorder.

REFERENCES

1. S. Suissa and J. Shuster. Exact unconditional sample sizes for the 2 × 2 binomial trial. *J. R. Stat. Soc.*, **148** (A), 317–327 (1985).
2. R. L. Ridolfi and M. D. Bell. Thrombotic thrombocytopenic purpura: report of 25 cases and review of the literature. *Medicine*, **60**, 413–428 (1981).

Therapeutic Plasmapheresis (XII), pp. 143-146
T. Agishi *et al.* (Eds) 139-142
© VSP 1993

Treatment of Thrombotic Thrombocytopenic Purpura with Plasma Exchange: Plasma Cytokine Levels and Prognosis

H. WADA, T. KANEKO, M. OHIWA, M. TANIGAWA, S. TAMAKI,
N. MINAMI, K. DEGUCHI and S. SHIRAKAWA

*The 2nd Department of Internal Medicine, Mie University School of Medicine,
Tsu, Japan*

Key words: TTP; plasma exchange; cytokine; IL-1-b; IL-6.

INTRODUCTION

Thrombotic thrombocytopenic purpura (TTP) [1] is characterized by fluctuating aberrant neurological symptoms, consumptive thrombocytopenia and microangiopathic hemolitic anemia, as well as by renal dysfunction and fever. Perhaps because of the rarity of the disease, its pathogenic mechanism has not been clarified. The prognosis of patients with the disease has, therefore, remained poor. Although the therapeutic results in TTP have recently been improved by the increasingly widespread use of plasma exchange (PE), the disease occasionally manifests extreme refractoriness, and the effects of treatment vary in individual patients. More detailed analysis of each case is considered to be required. In this study, we evaluated the clinical results, therapeutic effects and plasma cytokine levels in 13 patients with TTP.

SUBJECTS

The subjects were 13 patients with TTP admitted to our hospital during the past 8 years. The clinical characteristics of the patients with TTP are shown in Table 1. Blood samples were obtained on admission (usually within a few days of onset) or at onset, and the examinations described below were carried out. Most patients underwent plasma exchange (PE) at 4000 ml/day 3 times a week and received anti-platelet agents (aspirin 300 mg/day + dipyridamole 300 mg/day) and/or steroids (methyl prednisolone 1000 mg/ml × 3 days).

METHODS

Tumor necrosis factor (TNF) level was determined by enzyme immunoassay using a monoclonal antibody provided by the Life Science Research Laboratories, Asachi Chemical Industry Co. [2]. Interleukin (IL)-1-β was determined with an IL-1-β RIA Kit (Medenix) [3] and IL-6 with an IL-6 EIA Kit (TFB), and soluble IL-2 receptor (SIL-2R) with an IL-2R Test Kit (T Cell Science, Inc.) Interferon (IFN)-α and -γ were assayed with a Sucrosep IFN-α Kit and IFN-γ Kit (Boots-Celltech Diagnostics, Ltd.), respectively, and IFN-β with an IFN-β EIA Kit (TFB).

Table 1.
Clinical characteristics of patients with TTP

Patient	Age	Sex	SLE	Auto-antibody	PAIgG	Micro-thrombus	PAF	vWF-HMW multimers	Therapy	Outcome	Survival period
1.	16	M	(−)	(+)	ND	(+)	(−)	ND	PE AT ST	death	2 weeks
2.	16	F	(+)	(+)	(+)	(+)	(+)	decrease	PE AT ST	CR	87 months
3.	32	F	(+)	(+)	ND	(+)	(−)	ND	ST	death	4 days
4.	61	M	(−)	(+)	(+)	(+)	(−)	decrease	PE AT ST	CR	60 months
5.	45	F	(−)	(+)	(+)	(−)	(+)	decrease	PE	CR	44 months
6.	81	M	(−)	(+)	(+)	(+)	(−)	decrease	PE AT ST	CR	>36 months
7.	16	F	(−)	(+)	(+)	(+)	(+)	decrease	PE AT ST splenectomy	CR	32 months
8.	59	M	(−)	(−)	(+)	(+)	(−)	decrease	PE AT ST	CR	31 months
9.	37	M	(−)	(−)	(−)	(+)	(−)	decrease	PE AT ST	death	4 days
10.	51	F	(−)	(+)	(+)	(+)	(+)	decrease	PE AT ST	death	6 weeks
11.	72	M	(−)	(+)	ND	(+)	(−)	decrease	PE AT	death	1 week
12.	66	F	(−)	(+)	(+)	(−)	(+)	ND	PE AT ST	CR	18 months
13.	67	M	(−)	(+)	(+)	(+)	(+)	increase	HD ST	death	3 days

PAIgG: Platelet associated immunoglobulin G. Autoantibody (+): antinuclear antibody, anti-DNA antibody or anti-cardiolipin antibody is positive. PAF: platelet aggregating factor. vWF-HMW multimers: high molecular weight multimers of von Willebrand factor. PE: plasma exchange. AT: anti-platelet drugs (aspirin 300 mg/day + dipyridamole 300 mg/day). ST: steroid therapy (methyl prednisolone 1000 mg/day × 3 days). HD: hemodialysis.

PATIENT CHARACTERISTICS AND RESULTS

Therapeutic effects

Complete remission (CR) was observed in seven patients, but the other six patients died. PE was effective in most patients, and good response without steroids was obtained in Patient 5. However, CR was observed after steroid pulse therapy in Patients 4 and 7, and Patient 8 also required concomitant pulse therapy. Patient 1 initially responded to treatments including PE, but exacerbation of symptoms was noted 2 weeks after onset. Patient 9 never responded to any of various treatments and died within several days. Patient 3 died prior to definitive diagnosis of TTP. Patient 10 initially responded to treatments, but showed recurrence 3 weeks after onset and died despite daily PE. The mean period until remission was about 7 weeks, and the range was 4–10 weeks. Seven patients are surviving at the time of writing.

Plasma cytokine levels

The mean plasma cytokine and SIL-2R levels for normal subjects and for the TTP patients at onset ($N = 13$) and at CR ($N = 7$) are shown in Table 2. At the onset of

TTP, the levels of most cytokines and of SIL-2R were increased compared with those in normal subjects, but these levels were decreased at the time of CR. In particular, TFN, IL-1, IL-6 and SIL-2R levels at onset were significantly higher than those at the time of CR. The plasma IFN-α level was increased in seven patients, but IFN-β and -γ levels were within the normal range in most patients. With respect to outcome, plasma SIL-2R and IL-6 levels were significantly higher in patients who died than in those who entered CR. While plasma TNF level was also higher in the group of patients who died, this difference, was not significant, and the two groups showed no difference in levels of other cytokines.

Table 2.
Plasma cytokine levels in patients with TTP

		Normal	CR ($N = 7$)	Onset ($N = 13$)	
SIL-2R	(u/ml)	225 ± 36	246 ± 45	819 ± 749	$P < 0.05$
TNF-α	(u/ml)	ND	0.02 ± 0.06	0.39 ± 0.35	$P < 0.01$
IL-1β	(ug/ml)	ND	0.05 ± 0.07	0.23 ± 0.13	$P < 0.01$
IL-6	(ng/ml)	ND	0.02 ± 0.02	0.42 ± 0.54	$P < 0.05$
IFN-α	(u/ml)	ND	0.31 ± 0.77	1.78 ± 1.66	
IFN-β	(u/ml)	ND	0.63 ± 1.08	1.09 ± 1.41	
IFN-γ	(u/ml)	ND	0.29 ± 0.45	0.31 ± 0.13	

Mean $\pm$SD.

DISCUSSION

As possible etiological factors in TTP, immune complex and autoimmune mechanisms, platelet aggregating factor, reduced production or disturbed stabilization of prostaglandin I_2, and quantitative and qualitative abnormalities of vWF have all been reported. However, examination results vary in individual patients, suggesting that the pathogenesis of TTP is heterogenous. Based on our observations that many patients were positive for auto-antibodies and/or had SLE as well, and that anti-platelet antibody was frequently positive, we consider some autoimmune process to be involved in the pathogenesis of TTP. All patients showed some response to PE, and the treatment was effective in some patients, especially in the one who received it in the absence of any other therapy. However, recurrence was observed in this patient, and in others large doses of methyl prednisolone were required. These differences among the patients also indicate heterogeneity in the etiology of TTP.

The immune system is activated in patients with infection, autoimmune disease or multiple organ failure (MOF), and IL-1, TNF, and IL-6 are considered to be involved in various inflammatory reactions. In these diseases, the development of procoagulant activity mediated by cytokines is considered to be a cause of disseminated intravascular coagulation (DIC) [2, 3]. Patients with TTP manifest some symptoms similar to those in patients with DIC, such as a bleeding tendency and organ failure caused by microthrombus. Our results suggest that an autoimmune process is involved in the pathogenesis of TTP. High levels of TNF, IL-1 and IL-6 were observed in patients with TTP, suggesting activation of an immunologic mechanism involving macrophages. Damaged endothelial cells and activated macrophages are known to release IL-1 and IL-6, and severe endothelial damage has been considered to be associated with TTP. Since IL-1 is involved in organ failure and endothelial cell injury, it may be related to the pathogenesis of TTP. SIL-2R level is considered to be increased in patients with autoimmune diseases, and activation of T cell subsets may be involved in the process of TTP. Therefore, cytokines such as IL-1 and TNF are considered to contribute to the pathogenesis of TTP. Of the patients in our study, those who died showed significantly increased plasma levels of SIL-2R and IL-6. This finding suggests that patients with a hyperactivated immune system may a poorer prognosis.

CONCLUSIONS

Although PE was effective in most patients with TTP, this effect was transient, and steroid therapy was required in some. Complete remission was observed in seven of the 13 patients, but the other six died. Since the outcome in patients with increased plasma cytokine levels was poor, immunological mechanisms, such as the activation of macrophages and endothelial cells, are considered to be involved in the pathogenesis of TTP.

REFERENCES

1. R. M. Bukouski. Thrombotic thrombocytopenic purpura. A review. *Prog. Hemost. Thromb.*, **6**, 287–337 (1982).
2. H. Wada, M. Ohiwa, T. Kaneko *et al.* Plasma level of tumor necrosis factor in disseminated intravascular coagulation. *Am. J. Hematol.*, **37**, 147–151 (1991).
3. H. Wada, S. Tamaki, M. Tanigawa *et al.* Plasma level of IL-1 in disseminated intravascular coagulation. *Thromb. Haemost.*, **65**, 364–368 (1991).

Therapeutic Plasmapheresis (XII), pp. 147-148
T. Agishi *et al.* (Eds)
© VSP 1993

Plasma Exchange and Plasma Infusion in the Treatment of Thrombotic Thrombocytopenic Purpura

K. ITO,[1] A. HATTORI, S. HIROSAWA, J. TAKAMATSU, E. KAKISHITA and
K. FUJIMURA (JAPANESE TTP STUDY GROUP)

[1]*Kyoto University Hospital, Kyoto, Japan*

Key words: thrombotic thrombocytopenic purpura; plasma infusion; plasma exchange; anti-platelet drug;
fresh frozen plasma.

INTRODUCTION

Thrombotic thrombocytopenic purpura (TTP) is a fulminant and fatal disease. However, plasma exchange (PE) and plasma infusion (PI) are effective and have decreased TTP mortality. The Canadian Apheresis Study Group has reported that PE is more effective than PI [1]. The Japanese Study Group has studied for 5 years to clarify which of PE and PI is preferable in the treatment of TTP. The number of entry patients is small, so a preliminary result is presented here.

PATIENTS

Entry of 20 patients with acute TTP was made. Seven were male and 13 were female. The age of the patients ranged from 15 to 79. Severe thrombocytopenia, severe anemia and very high values of LDH were found. Eighteen of 20 patients showed fluctuating neurologic abnormalities.

METHODS

Our protocol for TTP therapy was principally according to that of the Canadian Apheresis Study Group although the volume of infused fresh frozen plasma (FFP) in the PI therapy is smaller, as are the doses of anti-platelet drugs.

Dipyridamole was administered at 300 mg/day and acetylsalicylic acid at 80 mg/day.

In PI therapy, FFP was infused at 8 ml/kg of body weight/day, from day 1 to 7.

PE was not modified. PE was carried out from day 1 to day 3, and 4 times from day 4 to day 9.

PI or PE combined with the administration of anti-platelet drugs was selected alternatively. When a hospital was not equipped with any apheresis instrument to treat a patient with TTP, PI therapy was selected.

The Japanese TTP Study Group evaluated the therapeutic efficacy as did the Canadian Apheresis Study Group. Platelet counts more than 150×10^9 /l for two consecutive days, no deterioration in neurologic symptoms and an decrease in LDH were defined as indications of good response.

RESULTS

Seven patients were treated by PI and 13 patients by PE. The mean age of the patients in the PI group was higher by 14 years than that in the PE group. Six of seven patients in the PI group were female. Laboratory findings at entry of the patients in the PE and PI groups did not differ significantly in platelet, hemoglobin and lactate dehydrogenase.

The treatment number varies greatly in the PI and PE groups but averages 15 and 12, respectively. The average volume of FFP infused was 332 ml in PI and that of FFP exchanged in PE was about 3000 ml.

The clinical courses of patients treated by PI or PE were grouped into four patterns. Pattern A indicates an early (until day 10) good response which continues thereafter. Six patients were in pattern A. Pattern B indicates relapse after an early good response and subsequent good recovery. Four patients were in pattern B. Pattern C indicates no early good response but a subsequent increase in platelet count. Eight patients were in pattern C. Pattern D indicates no response to the treatments with resultant death. Two patients were in pattern D.

The patients were evaluated on day 10 just after the end of the 1st cycle of treatment. Four of seven patients in the PI group and six of 13 patients in the PE group were evaluated as good response. Four patients in the PE group with poor response were additionally treated by PI.

Six of seven patients in the PI group and 12 of 13 patients in the PE group survived on day 30. Ninety percent of the patients survived.

According to our protocol, the tapering therapy is carried out after good response has been obtained in the 1st cycle of treatment. Relapse of TTP occurred in four of 10 patients who were evaluated as good response on day 10. The frequency of the relapse was high.

CONCLUSION

PE and PI therapy were performed in 20 patients with acute TTP. The two therapies did not differ significantly in effectiveness as evaluated by the patient's response on day 10 and patient's survival on day 30.

The 1st cycle of treatment should be repeated to prevent the relapse of TTP after an early good response.

REFERENCE

1. G. A. Rock, K. H. Shumak, N. A. Buskard *et al.* Comparison of plasma exchange with plasma infusion in the treatment of thrombotic thrombopenic purpura. *N. Engl. J. Med.*, **325**, 393–397 (1991).

Therapeutic Plasmaphereses (XII), pp. 149-151
T. Agishi *et al*. (Eds)
© VSP 1993

Therapeutic Effects of Plasmapheresis on Hematological Disorders

K. TAKAYAMA, Y. SUGENOYA, S. KOJIRO, F. KOIWA, K. NIIKURA,
K. IIZUKA, E. KINUGASA, T. AKIZAWA and S. KOSHIKAWA

Internal Medicine, Showa University, Fujigaoka Hospital, Yokohama, Japan

Key words: plasmapheresis; hematological disease; multiple myeloma; acute renal failure; acute hepatic failure.

INTRODUCTION

About 130 patients were treated with plasmapheresis (PP) in Showa University Fujigaoka Hospital during the past 10 years. When we investigated the diseases of patients who were treated with PP, we knew that hematological disorder occupied an important position in the field of therapeutic PP. The total number of those patients was 27 (21%). In order to review the therapeutic effect of PP on hematological disease, patients with those disorders treated with PP were analyzed retrospectively.

PATIENTS

In total, 27 patients were treated with PP, consisting of 12 cases with multiple myeloma, four cases with acute leukemia, two cases with malignant lymphoma, two hemolytic uremic syndrome (HUS), two malignant histiocytosis, a case of thrombotic thrombocytopenic purpura (TTP), autoimmune hemolytic anemia (AIHA), aplastic anemia, paroxysmal nocturnal hemoglobinuria (PNH) and idiopathic plasmacytic lymphadenopathy with polyclonal hyperimmunoglobulinemia (IPL).

Main reasons, times of session and clinical effects of PP were analyzed.

RESULTS

Twelve patients with multiple myeloma were treated with PP because of a complication of one case with acute hepatic failure (AHF) and 11 cases with acute renal failure (ARF). PP was performed 6.5 ± 6.6 times (2–24), and five of 11 cases with ARF required hemodialysis. As a result, seven of 11 (64%) recovered from ARF, and two patients could be released from hemodialysis.

All the patients with malignant hematological disease such as acute leukemia, malignant lymphoma, malignant histiocytosis, complicated AHF. In spite of intensive care with plasmapheresis and hemodialysis or hemodiafiltration [1], only two patients recovered from AHF. In patients with other hematological disease, PP was conducted for treatment of ARF, hyperviscosity, consciousness disturbance and for removal of auto-antibody; consequently, four cases of those disorders were improved.

DISCUSSION

PP is now becoming an established therapy for hepatic failure, neurological and collagen diseases. From the present analysis of PP, it is clarified that PP has been applied not only for those diseases but also for hematological diseases.

In hematological disease, as expected, the most frequent indication was multiple myeloma. Acute or chronic renal failure represents one of the major complications of multiple myeloma, and has been considered an ominous prognostic factor. Though numerous factors are involved in renal damage such as dehydration, hypercalcemia, hyperuricemia, plasma hyperviscosity, the toxicity of the monoclonal immunoglobulin especially free immunoglobulin light chains plays a central pathogenic role. PP has been regarded the most efficient tool to remove large amounts of light chains rapidly. The total number of patients with multiple myeloma admitted to our hospital during the past 10 years was 52, and 23 of them (44.2%) had a complication of ARF, which was defined by a rapid increase of serum creatinine (> 2 mg/dl) without reversibility by correction of the water–electrolyte balance or previously normal renal function indices, when available. Out of the 23 patients, 11 with ARF and one with AHF were treated with PP (48%). The causes of renal failure consisted of two cases with hypercalcemia, a case with radiographic contrast agent, amyloidosis and the remaining seven were thought to be due to myeloma kidney. The serum value of not only creatinine but calcium and uric acid in patients treated with PP was significantly higher than in the patients whose renal function was normal.

All the patients with malignant hematological disease were treated with PP for a complication of AHF. The cause of AHF in two cases with malignant histiocytosis and a case with hairy cell leukemia was unknown, but according to the rapid progress on clinical course or the findings in autopsy that liver was infiltrated with malignant cells, the main cause was considered to be based on underlying disease. The cause in a case of a patient with leukemia was post-blood transfusion hepatitis. In the other four cases, AHF resulted from chemotherapy and immunosuppressive therapy. Immunosuppressive therapy and cancer chemotherapy have been reported to induce active hepatitis in asymptomatic HB carriers [2, 3]. This was the case in two patients with malignant lymphoma. Another two cases were thought to be induced by the same mechanism, because their hepatitis developed with the withdrawal of cyclosporin A after successful bone marrow transplantation. Patients receiving such an immunosuppressive therapy should be carefully monitored for such a complication.

Four cases with other hematological diseases had a complication of ARF. After the treatment with PP, two out of four recovered from their renal function.

Clinical effects of PP were summarized in Table 1. PP was clinically effective in 56% of patients.

CONCLUSION

Twenty percent of PP in our hospital was performed for hematological disease during the past 10 years. Among them, PP was mostly applied for patients with multiple myeloma. Of the patients with multiple myeloma, 44% had ARF. About a half of them were treated with PP, consequently renal function improved in 58% of them. All the patients with malignant hematological disease had complicated AHF. This complication

Table 1.
Clinical effects of plasmapheresis

	Case number	Clinical effects (+)	(−)
Multiple myeloma			
renal failure	9	6	3
hypercalcemia	1	1	
hepatic failure	1		1
hyperviscosity	1	1	
Acute leukemia, malignant lymphoma, malignant histiocytosis			
acute hepatic failure	7	2	5
renal failure	1		1
HUS, TTP			
renal failure	2	1	1
consciousness disturbance	1	1	
AIHA, aplastic anemia, PNH, IPL			
renal failure	2	2	
thrombocytopenia	1		1
hyperviscosity	1	1	
Total	27	15 (56%)	12 (44%)

was thought to result from the treatment with chemotherapy and immunosuppressive therapy for the underlying disease, and PP was insufficient for it.

In conclusion, 27 patients with hematological disease were treated with PP. PP was clinically effective in 56% of patients, especially for complications such as ARF.

REFERENCES

1. S. Kanesaka, K. Dehara, T. Taira *et al.* Combined detoxication system of a new hemodiafiltration and plasma exchange for fulminant viral hepatitis. *Artif. Organs*, **14**, 120–122 (1990).
2. R. M. Galbraith, A. L. W. F. Eddleston, R. Williams *et al.* Fulminant hepatic failure in leukemia and chorioncarcinoma related to withdrawal of cytotoxic drug therapy. *Lancet*, **ii**, 528–530 (1975).
3. J. H. Hoofnagle, G. M. Dusheiko, D. F. Schafer *et al.* Reactivation of chronic hepatitis B virus infection by cancer chemotherapy. *Ann. Intern. Med.*, **96**, 447–449 (1982).

Therapeutic Plasmapheresis (XII), pp. 153-155
T. Agishi *et al*. (Eds)
© VSP 1993

Inhibitor to Factor V in a Severe Factor V Congenital Deficiency: Successful Management of Bleeding by Platelet Transfusions

A. GIRARD, A. DERLON, B. GUILLOIS, P. BOUTARD and M. A. THOMAS

Centre Régional de Transfusion Sanguine, 14000 Caen, France

Key words: severe factor V deficiency; platelet transfusion.

INTRODUCTION

A 13 year old boy with a severe from of congenital factor V (F. V) deficiency and sporadic hemorrhagic episodes, appropriately controlled until then by intravenous infusions of fresh frozen plasma, was hospitalized following a severe hematuria associated with an hematoma of the buttock.

ANTECEDENTS

This boy had no hemorrhagic episodes until the beginning of 1991. His older brother, who has the same deficiency, has never shown hemorrhagic episodes. However, in January 1991 he suffered tongue hematoma after injury requiring the infusion of 2 units of fresh frozen plasma. In August 1991 he suffered hematoma of adductors muscles after a long mountain walk (4 units of fresh frozen plasma increase factor V to 25%). September 1991 he suffered thigh muscles hematoma treated by infusion of 2 units of fresh frozen plasma.

CASE PRESENTATION

October 1991:

> Severe hematuria
>
> Scanner reveals clot of blood in left ureter
>
> Hematoma of the buttock following hypodermic injection

The boy was hospitalized following this last hemorrhagic episode.
During the first 5 days, the patient received a treatment consisting of:

> Intravenous infusions of polyspecific immunoglobulins (400 mg/kg/day)
>
> Prednisone *per os* (1 mg/kg/day)
>
> Fresh frozen plasma (1.2 l/day)

On day 5, this regimen was ineffective with the sudden appearance of an extensive spontaneous hematoma of the abdominal wall associated with a permanent drop of the F.V titer under 1%, as a consequence of an inhibitor to F.V with a titer of 3 Oxford units/ml.

In addition, the patient became hyperhydrated as a consequence of the volume of plasma infused.

Consequently therapy with fresh frozen plasma and the immunoglobulines was discontinued but Prednisone *per os* was continued. Fresh frozen plasma was replaced by intravenous infusions every 12 h of one single donor deleukocyted platelet concentrate from day 8 to 12, to one single donor deleukocyted platelet once a day, day 13 to 15.

MATERIAL AND METHODS

Separation material
A COBE Spectra blood cell separator was used to collect platelets from a single donor. The COBE Spectra Blood Component Separator uses a continuous flow centrifugal method to separate whole blood into its major components, especially platelets.

Separation method
Whole blood was drawn from a donor, anticoagulated, pumped into the centrifuge and separated into components.

The platelets were collected into a bag and the other components were returned to the donor.

Anticoagulant: ACD.A 1 ml/kg/min.

Centrifuge speed: 2400 r.p.m.

Run time: 120 min.

The microprocessor calculated the blood flow rate and end point to have a platelet concentrate containing 200 ml of plasma and at least 5×10^{11} platelets.

Filtration material
A Sepacell PL 5 N filter was used for the deleukocyting platelet concentrate. Sepacell PL (Asahi Medical Co. Ltd, Japan) was made from 1.8 μm polyester non-woven fabric coated with a copolymer of hydroxyethylmethacrylate and diethylaminoethylmethacrylate.

Filtration method
A Sepacell PL 5 N filter was wet with serum 9‰. Platelet concentrate then flowed through the filter and about 30 ml of serum 9‰ pushed remained platelets. The flowspeed was about 50 ml/min. Residual leukocytes in the platelet concentrate was under 1×10^6 white cells.

RESULTS

Owing to this regimen the titer of F.V in the patient's plasma rose to 12% at 1 h after each infusion of the platelet concentrates and remained consistently at 4–5% for 12 h after these infusions.

Since the second day of treatment (D 10), the inhibitor to Factor V decreased and at D 12, the inhibitor was not discernable.

Moreover, we could notice a beneficial effect on the hematoma of the abdominal wall and on the hematoma of the buttock.

Hematuria was stopped.

OUT COME

Two months later:

No side-effects of transfusion treatment could be noticed.

No viral serological markers:

HBs Antigen
Hepatic C Antibody
HBc Antibody
Cytomegalovirus (CMV)
Human immunodeficiency virus (HIV)
EPSTEIN-BARR Virus

No alloimmunisation against leukocytes and platelets.

CONCLUSION

This observation shows that a F.V inhibitor may be observed after treatment with fresh frozen plasma in patients with severe congenital F. V deficiency and that a severe bleeding episode associated with this inhibitor may be successfully cured with single donor deleukocyted platelet concentrates.

5

Hepato–digestive Organs Diseases

Therapeutic Plasmapheresis (XII), pp. 159-162
T. Agishi *et al.* (Eds)
© VSP 1993

Chronic Intermittent Plasmapheresis for Recurrent Pancreatitis with Hypertriglyceridemia

R. HALLAC,[1] P. KORNFELD,[2] S. FOX[1] and K. MAIER[1]

[1]*Departments of Medicine of the Mount Sinai School of Medicine and Englewood
Hospital, Englewood, NJ 07631, USA*
[2]*Department of Medicine, Stanford University School of Medicine, Stanford,
CA 94305, USA*

Key words: pancreatitis; plasmapheresis; hypertriglyceridemia; diabetes mellitus.

INTRODUCTION

Plasmapheresis (PE) treatment of acute pancreatitis associated with hypertriglyceridemia has been reported previously [1–3]. We wish to present such a case and show that simple chronic intermittent PE was able to prevent subsequent recurrent bouts of pancreatitis and maintain serum triglyceride levels within the asymptomatic range.

CASE REPORT

A 45 year old obese woman presented with back pain of increasing intensity over the previous 5 days. One day before admission she began to experience generalized abdominal pains without nausea, vomiting, diarrhea or change in stools. The patient gave a history of at least 15 years of recurrent bouts of pancreatitis always associated with milky serum and hypertriglyceridemia. Within 2 years of onset of symptoms she underwent surgical removal of a mesenteric cyst, partial pancreatectomy and splenectomy. Postoperatively, the patient soon developed insulin dependent diabetes mellitus with subsequent development of documented retinopathy, neuropathy and nephropathy. She also gave a history of coronary artery disease with at least two myocardial infarctions in recent years. Three years prior to her present admission she underwent coronary artery bypass surgery. Her last hospital admission for acute pancreatitis had occurred 1 year previously. The current admission physical findings were benign except for a soft abdomen, normal bowel sounds but tenderness in epigastric and both hypochondria. The patient was in moderate distress. The vital signs were normal. Flat plate of abdomen showed a distended stomach, but no distension or air/fluid levels in bowel. There was no free air. The chest X-ray was normal. ECG showed old inferior and anterior wall infarctions. Neurological exam was negative. Pertinent laboratory values included: normal CBC; glucose 547 mg%, creatinine 1.5 mg%, acetone 15 mg%, cholesterol 499 mg%, amylase 433 u, lipase 992 u, LDH 585, alkaline phosphatase 197 IU, ALT

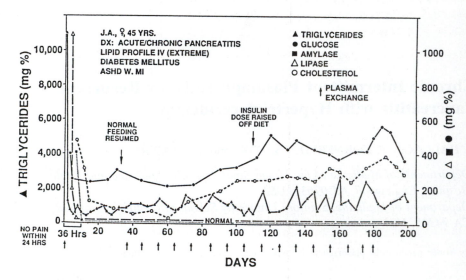

Figure 1. Clinical course.

964 u, AST 10 u, total bilirubin 1.0 mg% (direct), Ca 8.7 mg% and triglyceride of
5 750 mg%. Ultrasound showed a dilated gall bladder containing sludge and a normal common bile duct. Pancreas was not well visualized. Renal ultrasound showed
a smaller kidney on left. The patient became progressively more ill, complained of
severe low back pain and generalized abdominal crampy pains. Triglycerides rose to
9 340 mg%, glucose to 686 mg%, creatinine to 4.3 mg%, lipase to 10 992 u, WBC to
17 000 and Ca fell to 5.9 mg%. Fever spiked to 101°F. All cultures were sterile. The
patient was treated with i.v. fluids with insulin drip, nothing by mouth, antibiotics and
analgesics, and was plasmapheresed on day 1. One 3 l PE over 3 h resulted in complete
cessation of pain. Figure 1 demonstrates chemical changes immediately post-apheresis.
Triglycerides decreased to 959 mg% and gradually returned towards normal (283 mg%)
over the next 5 days. At this time the patient was placed on clear fluids by mouth. PE
was not repeated until 5 weeks later. During this interval the patient gradually resumed
a bland, low fat, diabetic diet which was accompanied by corresponding increases in
her serum triglyceride, glucose and cholesterol levels. Her insulin dose was increased,
Lovostatin was started and intermittent PE (see Fig. 1) was carried out at 1–3 week
intervals. Amylase and Lipase have remained normal since the initial 36 h. There has
been no pancreatitis recurrence during the past 18 months.

DISCUSSION

Most elevated serum triglyceride (TR) values reflect inadequate serum lipase values
needed to clear the plasma. Ordinarily such patients are treated with diet, alcohol in-
terdiction, insulin and drugs to decrease gastrointestinal absorption. Triglycerides are
esters of the alcohol glycerol and fatty acids (FA). Most are mixed acylglycerols. The
synthetic pathways of triglyceride metabolism overlaps that of phospholipids. Triglycerides are mainly stored in adipose tissue which is especially suited for esterification of

FA and their release. FA originate in the liver. To activate these FA and convert the resulting CoA-derivatives to glycerol, adipose cells must also have glucose to allow the reaction to proceed.

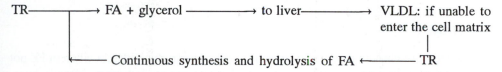

In diabetes there is unbridled mobilization of FA at a rate higher than the liver can oxidize leading to increased rate of lipoprotein and VLDL formation. Lipid clearance of VLDL and chylomicrons depends on the lipoprotein lipase which, in turn, is stimulated by glucose and insulin. In diabetes mellitus there is a relative lipoprotein deficiency which accentuates the hyperlipemia. Fluctuation in serum triglyceride levels in acute pancreatitis is most closely associated with hyperglycemia and insulin resistance.

In many laboratories PE treatment for hyperlipidemia involves double filtration and use of special affinity Sepharose or dextran sulfate cellulose adsorption columns. Scattered case reports in the literature point out that triglyceridemia due to causes other than pancreatitis also responded to PE [4–11]. Furthermore, a simple gravitational separator is all that is needed. As a matter of fact hollow fiber systems often clot and obstruct their ostia [9]. However, simple PE employing centrifugal separation has been known to be able to correct hypertriglyceridemia secondary to diabetes, pancreatitis, renal failure, isoretinoic acid, cyclosporins and congenital hyperlipoproteinemias [4–7]. These various reports all had similar experiences to ours, i.e. prompt clinical and chemical response to PE. Betteridge *et al.* [8] related the symptoms of hypertriglyceridemia to hyperviscosity of the blood plasma. Viscosity readings in our patient never exceeded 2, at which level patients are generally asymptomatic. In all the above instances, PE was used for acute attack treatments only. It is conceivable that PE affected cholecystokinin levels which may have been responsible, at best in part, for the decrease in serum triglyceride levels.

We believe this to be the first report of using chronic, intermittent plasmapheresis in a patient with chronically recurring acute pancreatitis with hypertriglyceridemia as a preventive as well as a therapeutic modality. It was our experience that one PE of one plasma volume removed about 70–85% of circulating triglycerides and about 30–33% of serum cholesterol. One to two PE treatments kept our patient's hypertriglyceridemia down and prevented clinical symptoms of acute pancreatitis. If blood glucose is well controlled with insulin, one to two PE will adequately depress serum lipid and lipoprotein levels for 2–3 weeks if patient is fasting and only receiving intravenous fluids. However, such depression of serum lipids lasts only 5–10 days when the patient is on oral feedings. Figure 1 shows that rising levels of triglycerides, glucose and cholesterol were always associated with the patient's periodic food 'binges'.

CONCLUSION

Periodic intermittent PE is a new additional treatment modality for recurrent pancreatitis with hypertriglyceridemia. It is not only effective during the acute episodes, but may actually be able to prevent recurrent bouts of pancreatitis. No untoward side effects from PE were observed. While it is known that pancreatitis may often be complicated by hypertriglyceridemia [12, 13] this case report suggests that the hyperlipemia itself may have been a causative factor.

SUMMARY

A case report of chronic recurrent pancreatitis with hypertriglyceridemia wherein PE not only shortened the acute episode and rendered it less severe, but where chronic intermittent PE was also able to prevent the disease from becoming clinically symptomatic during a 18 month period.

REFERENCES

1. W. J. Flynn, P. G. Freeman and L. G. Wickboldt. Pancreatitis with isoretinoin-induced hypertriglyceridemia. *Ann. Int. Med.*, **107**, 63 (1987).

2. M. V. Tobin and L. T. Fahy. Plasmapheresis and fulminant acute pancreatitis. *Br. Med. J.*, **297**, 979–980 (1988).

3. M. Larvin, M. R. J. Lansdown, M. J. McMahon *et al.* Plasmapheresis: a rational treatment for fulminant acute pancreatitis? *Br. Med. J.*, **297** 593–594 (1988).

4. M. Valbone, D. Occhini, C. Capra *et al.* Plasma exchange for the management of cyclosporin A-induced hypertriglyceridemia. *Int. Artif. Organs*, **11**, 209–211 (1988).

5. P. Vannini, G. Forlani, S. Giangiulio *et al.* Possible effectiveness of plasmapheresis and immunosuppressive therapy in reversing subcutaneous insulin resistance. A case report. *Diabetes & Metabolism*, **13**, 98–101 (1989).

6. R. Cantrina, O. Distefano, S. Spandrio *et al.* Double filtration plasmapheresis for hypertriglyceridemia. *J. Am. Med. Ass.*, **263**, 35 (1990).

7. H. E. Norbeck, L. Oro and C. A. Carlson. Serum lipid and lipoprotein concentration in chronic uremia. *Acta Med. Scand.*, **200**, 487–492 (1976).

8. M. Valbonesi, D. Occhini, R. Frisom *et al.* Cyclosporin-induced hypertriglyceridemia with prompt response to plasma exchange therapy. *J. Clin. Aph.*, **6**, 158–160 (1991).

9. H. Ito, C. Naito, H. Hayashi *et al.* Selective removal of triglyceride-rich lipoproteins by plasmapheresis in diabetic patients with active hypertriglyceridemia. *Artif. Organs*, **13**, 190–196 (1989).

10. D. J. Betteridge, M. Bakowski, K. G. Taylor *et al.* Treatment of severe diabetic hypertriglyceridemia by plasma exchange. *Lancet*, **1**, 1368 (1978).

11. W. Richter, G. Brahm and P. Schwandt. Type V hyperlipoproteinemia and plasmapheresis. *Ann. Intern. Med.*, **106**, 779 (1987).

12. A. B. Leibowitz, P. O'Sullivan and T. J. Iberti. Pancreatitis may often be complicated by hypertriglyceridemia. *Mt. Sinai J. Med.*, **59**, 38–42 (1992).

13. A. Bush, J. Bush, A. Carlsen *et al.* Hyperlipidemia and pancreatitis. *W. J. Surg.*, **4**, 307–314 (1980).

Therapeutic Plasmapheresis (XII), pp. 163-166
T. Agishi *et al.* (Eds)
© VSP 1993

Plasma Exchange Therapy in Multiple organ Failure

S. AGETA, S. OHIRA, T. KODAMA, S. NEGI, W. SHIMA, T. SAKAGUCHI,
S. OHASHI, T. MATSUO, K. UCHITA, Y. KITA and T. ABE

Wakayama Medical College, Kidney Center, Wakayama, Japan

Key words: multiple organ failure; plasma exchange; arterial ketone body ratio.

INTRODUCTION

Since the concept of multiple organ failure (MOF) was first proposed by Tilney [1] in 1973, it has become evident that this is a pathological condition with a poor prognosis in which functional disorders occur at the same time or in rapid succession in multiple organs. At present, the survival rate is quite low. In recent years, the efficacy of plasma exchange (PE) has been reported [2, 3].

In this paper, we report on our study of 29 patients with MOF in whom PE was performed over the past 7 years.

SUBJECTS AND METHODS

Table 1 shows the diagnostic criteria of MOF used at our center.

Our patients were 19 males and 10 females who met these criteria; therefore, we studied a total of 29 cases of MOF with a mean age of 57.9 years.

In all of the patients, PE was conducted by exchanging whole plasma by the membrane separation method. We used fresh frozen plasma as the replacement fluid. At the time of PE, we also conducted bicarbonate hemodialysis.

Table 1.
Criteria for organ failure

Heart failure	Necessiated high dose of the inotropic agents
Respiratory failure	Necessiated prolonged mechanical ventilation
Hepatic failure	Serum bilirubin greater than 3.0 mg/dl
Renal failure	Serum creatinin greater than 2.0 mg/dl or BUN greater than 50 mg/dl
Gastrointestinal bleeding	Necessiated transfusion
CNS failure	Only responded to pain stimulus
DIC	Serum FDP greater than 20 μg/ml and platelet count less than 5.0×10^4/mm^3

RESULTS

Table 2 shows the survival rate following PE. A total of 12 patients survived, including nine males and three females, so that survival rate was 41.4%. Therapeutic results showed that the survival rate was higher in patients with fewer dysfunctional organs. We were able to save five of six patients with failure of three organs, but we were only able to save one of the patients with failure of six or seven organs.

Among the 29 patients with MOF, Table 3 shows the cases accompanied by hyperbilirubinema that underwent PE during the past 2 years.

Table 2.
Survival rate after PE

Outcome	Number of organ failures					Total
	3	4	5	6	7	
Survival	5	3	3	1	0	12
Death	1	2	2	6	6	17
Total	6	5	5	7	6	29
Survival rate (%)	83.3	60.0	60.0	14.3	0	41.4

Table 3.
MOF patients treated with PE

Patient	Age	Sex	Disease	Outcome
1. Y. B	66	M	sepsis	death
2. Y. I	55	M	perforated cholecystitis	death
3. M. O	26	F	fatal distress	death
4. U. T	50	F	SMA thrombosis (post op.)	death
5. S. M	71	M	AAA (post op.)	survival
6. S. K	67	M	ruptured cecal cancer	survival
7. T. F	64	M	AAA (post op.)	survival
8. A. Y	73	M	AMI	survival

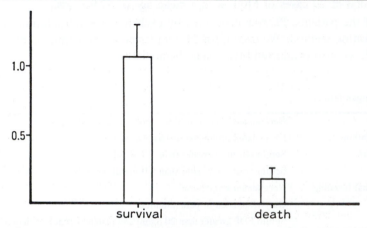

Figure 1. Comparison of AKBR before PE ($n = 8$, $P < 0.002$).

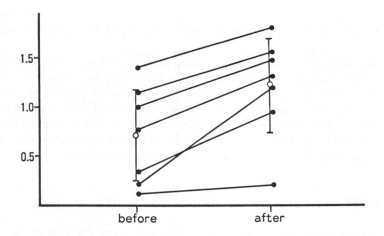

Figure 2. The changes of AKBR before and after PE ($n = 7$, $P < 0.01$).

Of these eight patients, four survived and four died. We conducted a comparative study of their total bilirubin, GPT, arterial ketone body ratio (AKBR), cyclic AMP and cyclic GMP before PE.

No significant difference in total bilirubin, GPT, cyclic AMP and cyclic GMP before PE was observed between the survivors and the fatal cases. However, AKBR was significantly lower in the fatal cases, and no patients with an AKBR of 0.4 or less before PE survived (Fig. 1).

Figure 2 shows the changes in AKBR before and after PE. Following PE, AKBR clearly rose.

DISCUSSION

MOF is a difficult disorder to treat because multiple organs undergo functional failure. Also, since septicemia is often the trigger, or since it may frequently appear as a complication during the course of illness, the condition of the patient often progresses from bad to worse. At present, as one of the methods of treating MOF, blood purification as artificial organ support is often applied. The therapeutic significance of blood purification is that it removes pathogenic and harmful substances. In addition, with PE, it is possible to supplement coagulation factors, albumin and other useful substances.

When we compared the four patients in whom PE was effective with the four in whom PE was ineffective, our results indicated that there were no significant differences before PE with regard to total bilirubin, GPT, cyclic AMP or cyclic GMP, but AKBR was significantly lower when PE was ineffective. It is said that AKBR reflects the function of the hepatic mitochondria. Ozawa *et al.* [4] reported that if AKBR falls postoperatively, the number of dysfunctional organs increases, and if AKBR fell below 0.25, all patients died. In our four patients who did not respond to PE, AKBR before PE was below 0.4, so our results showed a tendency similar to those of the above-mentioned report. On the other hand, before and after PE, AKBR showed a rise in all patients, suggesting that due to PE, energy metabolism in the liver is corrected. The reason for this is that with PE, toxic histological substances including bilirubin and endotoxins are removed, and moreover, by supplementing such useful substances as coagulation factors, albumin and fibronectin, the metabolic burden on the liver is thought to be reduced.

During this study, we found we were able to save the lives of 12 of 29 MOF patients (41.4%) by conducting PE, so we concluded that PE is a useful measure for preventing the progress of MOF. However, even when PE was repeatedly performed, many of the patients still could not be saved. PE uses massive amounts of fresh frozen plasma and is very costly, so it is necessary to cautiously consider its indications and the number of times it should be performed. Since PE was ineffective in patients with AKBR of less than 0.4, it may be a useful parameter in deciding the indication for PE.

CONCLUSIONS

(i) We conducted PE in 29 patients with MOF and saved the lives of 12.

(ii) AKBR before PE was significantly lower in the fatal cases than in the survivors.

(iii) AKBR rose significantly after PE, which suggests that PE corrects energy metabolism in the liver.

(iv) AKBR may be a useful parameter in deciding the indication for PE.

REFERENCES

1. N. L. Tilney, G. L. Bailey and A. P. Mrgan. Sequential system failure after rupture of abdominal aortic aneurysms. *Ann. Surg.*, **178**, 117–122 (1973).

2. P. McClelland, P. S. Williams, M. Yagoob *et al.* Multiple organ failure — a role for plasma exchange?. *Intensive Care Med.*, **16**, 100–103 (1990).

3. K. Kumon, K. Tanaka, N. Nakajima *et al.* Roles of plasma exchange in multiple organ failure. *Jpn. J. Artif. Organs*, **14**, 586–589 (1985).

4. K. Ozawa, H. Aoyama, K. Yasuda *et al.* Metabolic abnormalities associated with postoperative organ failure. *Arch. Surg.*, **118**, 1245–1251 (1983).

Therapeutic Plasmapheresis (XII), pp. 167-170
T. Agishi *et al.* (Eds)

A Case of Serious Hepatic Failure Treated through Metabolic Management and Plasma Exchange

H. ANDOH, Y. ASANUMA, H. KOTANAGI, S. OMOKAWA,
S. MIYAKATA and K. KOYAMA

Akita University, Akita, Japan

Key words: metabolic management; indirect calorimetry.

INTRODUCTION

Plasma exchange (PE) is now commonly used as a treatment for hepatic failure. However, in serious cases of hepatic failure, deciding when to perform the PE becomes a problem due to the effect on circulation and hepatic metabolism. We would like to report a serious case of hepatic failure treated by improving hepatic metabolism through metabolic and nutritional management measuring metabolic dosage used by indirect calorimetry and arterial ketone body ratio (AKBR) prior to performing the PE.

A CASE REPORT

A 48 year old male automobile accident victim underwent emergency operation for a laceration of the transverse colon and injury to the superior mesenteric vein, the bleeding was stopped and debridment and intestinal anastomosis was performed. However, leakage of the anastomosis took place and subsequently resulted in diffuse peritonitis. Total parenteral nutrition, 3000 kcal/day, was then initiated, but the jaundice gradually became worse and total bilirubin fluctuated around 10 mg/dl, showing the nutritional liver dysfunction after total parenteral nutrition. Furthermore, rebleeding from the superior mesenteric vein took place 1 month later and total bilirubin rose to 16.7 mg/dl. The patient was then transferred to our department.

With respect to liver functions, ALT was normal; however, AKBR was 0.23, blood sugar level was over 400 mg/dl and advanced metabolic disorder was presumed. Furthermore, the patient became septic due to intraabdominal abscess. After admission, the abscess was drained at first and the abdominal cavity was irrigated through an abdominal drain. Then energy expenditure (EE) and respiratory quontient (RQ) were measured by indirectory calorimetry, and the caloric dosage was decided to be the same as EE (500–600 kcal/day). The function of protein synthesis was assessed using rapid turnover protein (RTP) as pre-alubumin (PreAlb), transferrin (Tf) and retinol binding protein (RBP).

When the AKBR improved to 1.16, 3000 ml of PE was performed for three consecutive days. After the treatment, total bilirubin dropped from 27.8 to 10.3 mg/dl and AKBR improved from 0.23 to 1.75. Regarding metabolic condition, on admission, indirect calorimetry showed a carbohydrate metabolism disorder with an RQ of 1.18 and an EE/basal EE (%REE) of 124%. After the restriction of calorie administration at the level of EE, carbohydrate metabolism was gradually improved, and 4 days after PE became normal. With regard to energy balance, on admission, excess calorie administration caused hyperglucometabolism and depressed protein synthesis. Energy balance was corrected by restriction of calorie administration and PE. All RTPs were very low on admission. After metabolic management, RTPs were gradually improved and they became normal after PE. See Table 1 and Figs 1–5.

Table 1.
Measurements

Liver function
    AST, ALT, T-Bil, D-Bil, ALP, LDH, γ-GTP

Metabolic measurement
    RQ, EE, %REE, Energy balance, Urine urea

Protein synthesis
    TP, Alb, PreAlb, transferrin, RBP

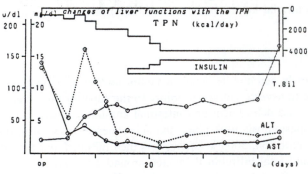

Figure 1. Changes of liver functions with the TPN.

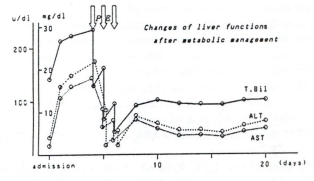

Figure 2. Changes of liver functions after metabolic management.

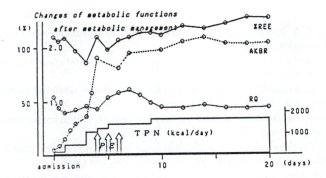

Figure 3. Changes of metabolic functions after metabolic management.

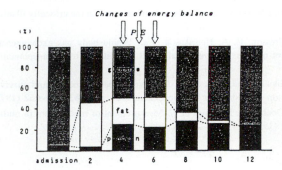

Figure 4. Changes of energy balance.

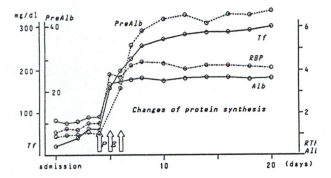

Figure 5. Changes of protein synthesis.

SUMMARY

In combination with the treatment for the abscess, PE has been very helpful in the presented case. However, PE seems to place a heavy burden on metabolism due to the mass movement of protein. We feel that metabolic management is important before, during and after PE.

REFERENCES

1. J. A. Harris and F. D. Benedict. *A biometric study of basal metabolism in man*. Carnegie Institute of Washington, Washington, DC (1919).
2. J. B. Weir. New methods for calculating metabolic rate with special reference to protein metabolism. *J. Physiol.*, **109**, 1–9 (1949).
3. K. Ozawa. Biological significance of mitochondrial redox potentials in shock and multiple organ failure: redox theory. *Proc. Clin. Biol. Res.*, **111**, 39 (1983).
4. M. Yamamoto *et al.* Significance of acetoacetate/b-hydroxybutyrate ratio in arterial blood as an indicator of the severity of hemorrhagic shock. *J. Surg. Res.*, **28**, 124 (1980).
5. K. Ozawa *et al.* Contribution of the arterial blood keton body ratio to elevate plasma amino acids in hepatic encephalopathy of surgical patients. *Am. J. Surg.*, **146**, 299 (1983).
6. T. Nakatani *et al.* Differences in predominant energy substrate in relation to the resected hepatic mass in the phase immediately after hepatectomy. **97**, 887 (1981).
7. M. Ito *et al.* Clinical study on postoperative intervenous infusion of fat emulsion. *J. Clin. Surg.*, 2248–2252 (1991).
8. K. Lakshman and G. L. Blackburn. Monitoring nutritionalstatus in the critically ill adult. *J. Clin. Monit.*, **2**, 114–120 (1986).
9. K. L. Svensson, H. Presson, B. A. Henriksson *et al.* Whole body gas exchange: amino acid lactate clearance as indicators of initial and early allograft viability in liver transplantation. *Surgery*, **105**, 472–480 (1989).
10. H. Hirasawa, I. H. Chaudry and A. E. Baue. Improved hepatic function and survival with adenosine triphosphate–magnesium chloride after hepatic ischemia. *Surgery*, **83**, 655–662 (1978).
11. R. H. Bartlett, R. E. Dechert, J. R. Mault *et al.* Measurement of metabolism in multiple organ failure. *Surgery*, **92**, 771–779 (1982).

Therapeutic Plasmapheresis (XII), pp. 171-174
T. Agishi *et al.* (Eds)
© VSP 1993

Clinical Experience of Plasmapheresis in a Patient with Abrupt Liver Damage

S. NAKAMURA, T. YAMANAKA, H. YAMADA, S. TAKIYA, M. KITANO, K. KATO, T. MITSUI, G. ITO, H. IKEDA and Y. SUZUKI

Aichi Medical University, Nagakute, Aichi, Japan

Key words: plasma exchange; anion exchange resin; BR-350; drug-induced hepatitis; intrahepatic cholestasis.

INTRODUCTION

This hemodialysis patient was receiving medication for rheumatoid arthritis but developed acute liver dysfunction. She underwent plasmapheresis to remove serum bilirubin, but died before treatment was complete.

CASE REPORT

This 68 year old female had been treated as an outpatient for renal failure and rheumatoid arthritis. She had received daily doses of dipyridamole (300 mg) and prednisolone (10 mg) for over 3 years. She was also taking methotrexate (2 mg) orally once a week for severe rheumatoid arthritis. One week after the administration of this oral agent, she visited the out-patient clinic with symptoms of vomiting, diarrhea, dehydration, severe anorexia and stomatitis accompanied by a sore throat. Laboratory findings showed WBC of only $1000/mm^3$, leading to a diagnosis of secondary agranulocytosis with stomatitis caused by methotrexate [1]. Other chemical data showed RBC of $281 \times 10^4/mm^3$, Hb 8.4 g/dl, Hct 25.7%, platelets $7.2 \times 10^3/mm^3$, BUN 48.0 mg/dl, creatinine 4.0 mg/dl, total bilirubin 0.44 mg/dl, GOT 15 mU/ml, GPT 40 mU/ml, alkaline-phosphatase 238 mU/ml, LDH 358 mU/ml, γ-GTP 45 mU/ml, cholinesterase 0.68 ΔPH, Na 140 mEq/l, K 6.1 mEq/l and Cl 101 mEq/l.

Methotrexate was immediately discontinued. She was treated on an out-patient basis for 5 days, and was then admitted to the hospital when WBC returned to normal at $4900/mm^3$ and other chemical data showed RBC of $255 \times 10^4/mm^3$, Hb 9.8 g/dl, Hct 22.7%, platelets $9.5 \times 10^4/mm^3$, BUN 41.2 mg/dl, creatinine 4.0 mg/dl, total bilirubin 0.23 mg/dl, GOT 32 mU/ml, GPT 29 mU/ml, alkaline-phosphatase 333 mU/ml, LDH 293 mU/ml, γ-GTP 57 mU/ml, total cholesterol 189 mg/dl, Na 136 mEq/l, K 5.9 mEq/l, Cl 112 mEq/l, Ca 8.1 mg/dl and Pi 4.5 mg/dl.

Over a 5 month period, WBC ranged from 5000 to $11\,000/mm^3$ under daily doses of prednisolone (10 mg) and a non-steroidal anti-inflammatory drug (NSAID, 25 mg). The clinical course was otherwise uneventful except for continuing symptoms of rheumatoid arthritis. However, hemodialysis was begun in March 1991 after the onset of uremia and increases in BUN and serum creatinine due to chronic renal failure.

Acute liver dysfunction arose 2 months after beginning hemodialysis. Plasma exchange was undertaken in two sessions after total bilirubin measured 22.2 mg/dl for 3 weeks. Plasmapheresis was also carried out in 14 sessions over 2 months using a BR-350 filter (Asahi Medical Co., Tokyo, Japan) with an anion exchange. Laboratory data of liver function for pre- and post-plasmapheresis are shown in Table 1. The patient continued daily treatments of either hemodialysis or plasmapheresis. Daily intakes of sodium chloride and water were restricted on days of hemodialysis therapy. She experienced dysorexia due to diet restriction and liver damage. Although hemodialysis and plasmapheresis were successful, she died of malnutrition before plasmapheresis treatment could be completed.

Table 1.
Changes in laboratory findings between pre- and post-plasmapheresis

BR350 / PE — plasma exchange (↓) and BR350 (↓) treatment markers along the timeline.

	April 15	20	30	May 5	10	25	30	June 5	10	15	20	25	30	July 5	10	15	20	25
T. B (mg/dl)	0.29			3.7	10.4	22.7	29.3	24.9	19.9	17.7	22.9	13.4	17.7	17.7		13.3	10.4	
D. B (mg/dl)				3.2	9.3		23.8				12.1						8.3	
GOT (mU/ml)	21			183	306	120	118	82	45	77	54	50	48	44		48		
GPT (mU/ml)	33			220	425	138	149	105	76	83	87	76	68	66		40		
LDH (mU/ml)	399			350	700	492		379	311					747		938		
AL-P (mU/ml)	198			354	530	1320	2000	3055	2644	2490	2877	2402	1915	1875		1530		
γ-GTP (mU/ml)	70			215	355	232	335	455		415			340	335		211		
CHE (ΔPH)	1.06			0.17	229	0.58	0.69	0.59	0.32	0.36	0.35	0.33	0.31					

(↑ died — at the far right of the timeline)

DISCUSSION

There were three primary complications in the clinical course of this patient. The first was agranulocytosis and stomatitis induced by methotrexate, but fortunately liver function, BUN and serum creatinine remained unaffected by the drug [2]. Symptoms disappeared shortly after discontinuation of the agent. The second incident arose after the introduction of hemodialysis due to BUN and creatinine elevations. The third, acute liver dysfunction, occurred 2 months after beginning hemodialysis, but the etiology could not be identified.

Plasma exchange therapy is a widely accepted treatment for such cases as hepatic failure and multiple organ failure [3]. Since abnormal liver function was detected and total bilirubin exceeded 20 mg/dl after 3 weeks of observation, plasmapheresis was undertaken in two sessions using massive amounts of fresh frozen plasma as the replacement fluid (Table 1). Plasma exchange is known to be effective in removing serum bilirubin; however, the disadvantage of this treatment is the massive amounts of blood preparations required for replacement. Plasmapheresis was thus carried out in 14 sessions using a BR-350 resin, a new brand of BR-601 with a secondary filter, which does not require any blood preparations for the replacement fluid.

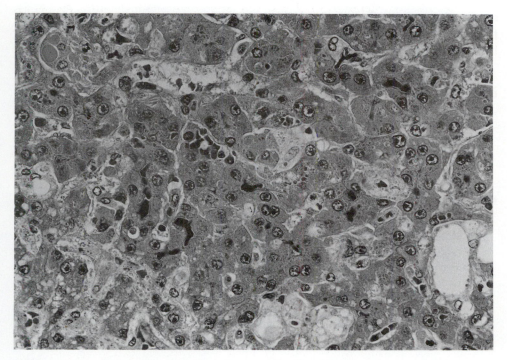

Figure 1. Autopsy findings of the liver suggesting congestive liver damage.

BR-601 is a strong basic anion exchange resin consisting of styrene divinylben-zen copolymer as its base with ammonium as the exchange radical [4]. When 3 l of blood were plasmapheresed in our patient, the average removal rate for total biliru-bin was 36.6% by plasma exchange and 42.7% by BR-350 filter. Total bilirubin re-moval (%) is reportedly higher with plasma exchange than with plasmapheresis using BR-601 [4]. In this case the BR-350 filter may have had the same or stronger ef-fects as plasma exchange in removing serum bilirubin. Liver function variations at pre- and post-plasmapheresis are shown in Table 1. Serum bilirubin fluctuated between 13.5 and 23 mg/dl, indicating the efficacy of plasmapheresis using the BR-350 filter. Cholinesterase, which markedly decreased at the onset of liver dysfunction, moderately improved along with GOT and GPT, although no such improvements were seen in the γ-GTP level. By contrast, the alkaline-phosphatase level rose gradually over the clinical course. The patient underwent plasmapheresis twice a week and hemodialyzed 3 times a week. However, she developed severe malnutrition and died due to diet restrictions of sodium chloride and water.

What caused the acute liver dysfunction in this case? The patient had been given 10 mg of prednisolone over three years and 25 mg of NSAID over 6 months. It is known that steroid hormones can sometimes induce congestive liver damage [5]. Serum viral examinations were all negative for hepatitis A, B and C. Judging from the increasing levels of such enzymes as GOT, GPT, alkaline phosphatase and γ-GTP, these elevations could have been caused by prednisolone, but not by NSAID. Autopsy findings of the liver revealed intrahepatic cholestasis and bile plugs in the canaliculi of the bile ducts although there was no evidence of hepatitis or liver cirrhosis. These findings suggested a case of congestive liver damage (Fig. 1). Based on the chemical data and autopsy findings, we believe prednisolone may have been responsible for the acute congestive liver damage in this case.

CONCLUSION

(ii) The anion exchange resin (BR-350) filter is useful for removing serum bilirubin without requiring blood preparations.

(ii) Prednisolone may have induced acute congestive liver damage.

REFERENCES

1. R. A. Novak and A. Kessinger. Methotrexate-induced colitis. *Nebr. Med. J.*, **61**, 84–87 (1976).
2. E. M. Hersh and V. G. Wong. Hepatotoxic effects of methotrexate. *Cancer*, **19**, 600–606 (1966).
3. Y. Ochiai and M. Baba. Removal of substance by two methods of plasma exchanges and the influence on respiratory function. *J. Intensive Care. Med.*, **10**, 587–592 (1986).
4. K. Sakagami and M. Miyazaki. Artificial liver support for postoperative hepatic failure with anion exchange resin (BR-601). *Acta Med. Okayama*, **40**, 249–255 (1986).
5. M. Hartleb and A. Nowak. Severe jaundice with destructive cholangitis after administration of methyl-testosterone. *Am. J. Gastroenterol.*, **85**, 766–767 (1990).

Therapeutic Plasmapheresis (XII), pp. 175-179
T. Agishi *et al.* (Eds)
© VSP 1993

Effect of Therapeutic Plasma Exchange and Bilirubin Absorption on Serum Bilirubin Subfractions in Hepatic Failure

M. SUENAGA, O. YOSHIKATSU, H. SUGIURA, Y. KOKUBA, S. UEHARA, K. MORI, S. YAMAGUCHI, N. YAMANAKA[1] and O. ODA

Surgical Service, Nagoya Memorial Hospital, Nagoya, Japan
[1]*The Bio-Dynamic Research Institute, Nagoya, Japan*

Key words: bilirubin subfraction; hepatic failure; hyperbilirubinemia; plasma exchange; bilirubin absorption.

INTRODUCTION

There is no established therapy for severe hepatic failure due to various causes. However, since hyperbilirubinemia might cause impairment in many organs, two treatments for reduction of serum bilirubin level, plasma exchange (PE) and bilirubin absorption (BA), have occasionally been performed. We examined here the effect of the two treatments on serum bilirubin subfractions.

PATIENTS AND METHODS

Fourteen patients who developed severe hepatic failure following surgery or variceral bleeding were treated by PE and/or BA. Five patients had postoperative hepatic failure, and two of them were under hemodialysis for chronic renal failure and another two had co-existing liver cirrhosis. Eight patients became hepatic failures following variceral bleeding caused by cirrhosis. One patient suffered from postoperative hepatitis which occurred 3 months after pancreato-duodenectomy for carcinoma of papilla Vater.

PE was applied in two patients, BA was applied in four patients and a combination of PE and BA was applied in eight patients. Numbers of courses of PE were 37 times and those of BA were 70 times.

Fresh frozen plasma (FFP) was used as the replacement fluid in PE and the volume replaced during each procedure ranged from 2400 to 2800 ml. BA was performed by using a Plasorba BR-350 (Asahi-Medical) which is an anion exchange resin column. Plasma flow rate in the column was 25 ml/min during the treatment (3 h). The bound bilirubin was eluted from the BR-350 column with 6N HCl–methanol or 6N HCl–methanol–chloroform.

Subfractionation of serum bilirubin was done by high performance liquid chromatography (HPLC) according to the method of Lauff *et al.* [1]. δ-Bil observed as the first peak in the HPLC system (retension time, 11 min) and followed in order by γ-Bil (13 min), β-Bil (15 min) and α-Bil (11 min).

Elimination ratio of bilirubin after treatment was calculated by following equation:

$$\frac{\text{Pretreatment bilirubin value} - \text{Post-treatment bilirubin value}}{\text{Pretreatment bilirubin value}} \times 100(\%).$$

RESULTS

Preceding BA treatment was performed for almost all the patients with PE. Total bilirubin (T.Bil) values before PE and BA were 13.3 ± 5.4 and 20.11 ± 9.02 mg/dl (mean $\pm$ SD),
respectively (Tables 1–4). T.Bil after PE decreased to 8.04 ± 3.45 mg/dl, and T.Bil was

Table 1.
Bilirubin subfractions in serum before and after PE and their elimination ratio

	Before (mg/dl)	After (mg/dl)	Eliminated (mg/dl)	Elimination ratio (%)
T.Bil	13.30 ± 5.40	8.04 ± 3.45	5.41 ± 2.47	40.33 ± 9.38[*1]
α-Bil	3.03 ± 1.87	2.40 ± 1.37	0.80 ± 0.76	22.33 ± 13.14[*2]
β-Bil	5.11 ± 2.45	2.71 ± 1.39	2.39 ± 1.32	45.79 ± 12.77
γ-Bil	2.15 ± 1.13	1.39 ± 0.72	0.82 ± 0.60	35.05 ± 16.10
δ-Bil	3.01 ± 1.50	1.54 ± 0.92	1.47 ± 0.76	49.36 ± 12.10[*3]

[*1, 2, 3] $P < 0.001$.

Table 2.
Percentage of bilirubin subfractions in serum before and
after PE

Subfraction	Before (%)	After (%)
α-Bil	23.13 ± 10.42	30.11 ± 10.76
β-Bil	37.59 ± 6.52	33.19 ± 5.86
γ-Bil	16.07 ± 5.49	17.29 ± 5.50
δ-Bil	23.20 ± 7.22	19.40 ± 6.75

lowered to 14.55 ± 6.85 mg/dl after BA. The elimination ratio of T. Bil was $40.33\pm9.38\%$
for PE treatment and $27.30\pm9.64\%$ for BA treatment. There was statistically significant
difference in the elimination ratios between PE and BA. In PE treatment the elimination
ratios did not show any significant difference among bilirubin subfractions except α-
Bil whose ratio was 22.33%. The elimination ratios of β-Bil and γ-Bil with BA were
similar to those with PE. On the other hand, the respective elimination ratios of α-Bil
and δ-Bil with BA were 12.33% and 9.65%, and they were half and one fifth compared
with PE treatment. Therefore, the significant difference of elimination ratios of T.Bil
between PE and BA was considered to be caused by more effective elimination of α-Bil
and δ-Bil with PE treatment (Tables 1–4).

Table 3.
Bilirubin subfractions in serum before and after BA and their elimination ratio

	Before (mg/dl)	After (mg/dl)	Eliminated (mg/dl)	Elimination ratio (%)
T.Bil	20.11 ± 9.02	14.55 ± 6.85	5.55 ± 3.14	27.30 ± 9.64[*1]
α-Bil	3.65 ± 2.12	3.26 ± 1.86	0.51 ± 0.53	12.33 ± 9.22[*2]
β-Bil	8.42 ± 3.98	15.03 ± 2.74	3.40 ± 1.84	40.54 ± 12.17
γ-Bil	3.51 ± 1.95	2.09 ± 1.17	1.42 ± 1.05	39.19 ± 13.65
δ-Bil	4.53 ± 2.14	4.17 ± 2.07	0.42 ± 0.34	9.65 ± 6.43[*3]

[*1, 2, 3] $P < 0.01$.

Table 4.
Percentage of bilirubin subfractions in serum before and after BA

Subfraction	Before (%)	After (%)
α-Bil	18.30 ± 6.60	22.73 ± 7.37
β-Bil	41.43 ± 5.27	33.77 ± 5.99
γ-Bil	16.96 ± 3.17	13.95 ± 2.68
δ-Bil	23.31 ± 6.28	29.54 ± 7.51

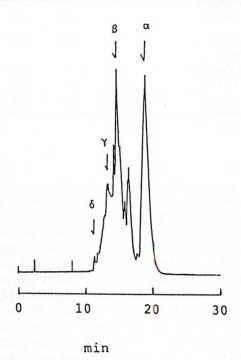

Figure 1. HPLC separation of bilirubin eluate from BR-350.

In order to examine the difference of elimination ratios among bilirubin subfractions with BA treatment, the material bound to the BR-350 column was eluted and analyzed. Figure 1 shows the very low content of δ-Bil in the eluate. The contents of bilirubin subfractions in the eluates were measured in four hyperbilirubinemic patients and are shown in Table 5. δ-Bil was eluted a little in all of four patients, but α-Bil was eluted satisfactorily from the column as well as β- and γ-Bil.

Table 5.
Comparison of the yield from the BR-350 column and the elimination of each bilirubin before and after BA

		α-Bil	β-Bil	γ-Bil	δ-Bil	T.Bil
1. H. O.	Concentration in eluated solution (mg/dl)	7.4	6.67	3.6	0.13	17.8
	BR-350 yield (mg)	148.0	133.4	72.0	2.6	356.0
	Bil before BA (mg/dl)	6.8	15.8	7.8	8.7	39.1
	Bil after BA (mg/dl)	8.0	8.5	3.0	8.5	27.9
2. K. I.	Concentration in eluated solution (mg/dl)	3.51	1.89	1.35	0	6.75
	BR-350 yield (mg)	70.2	37.8	27.0	0	135.0
	Bil before BA (mg/dl)	2.9	7.9	3.6	4.1	18.5
	Bil after BA (mg/dl)	2.6	5.2	2.5	4.0	14.3
3. T. Y.	Concentration in eluated solution (mg/dl)	2.85	4.26	2.1	0.15	9.36
	BR-350 yield (mg)	57.0	85.2	42.0	3.0	187.2
	Bil before BA (mg/dl)	6.6	14.5	5.9	8.5	35.5
	Bil after BA (mg/dl)	6.6	10.5	4.3	8.7	30.1
4. T. S.	Concentration in eluated solution (mg/dl)	8.54	4.94	4.4	0.13	18.01
	BR-350 yield (mg)	170.8	98.8	88.0	2.6	360.2
	Bil before BA (mg/dl)	2.6	14.7	7.5	4.8	29.6
	Bil after BA (mg/dl)	2.2	10.5	4.3	4.3	19.6

DISCUSSION

Although PE and BA treatments have been conducted to remove hepatic toxins such as bilirubin and other protein-bound substances in hepatic failure, the therapeutic significance of the treatments remains to be assessed precisely [2, 3]. In the present study we mesured the contents of bilirubin subfractions in hyperbilirubinemic patients before and after PE and BA, and found that PE and BA had dissimilar efficacy for reduction of bilirubin subfractions. Since all of the plasma components are exchanged with PE, it is logical that PE treatment reduced the levels of the four bilirubin subfractions evenly. On the other hand, BA treatment utilizes an anion-exchange resin [4, 5] and therefore efficiently eliminated the negative changed and hydrophilic bilirubin, β-Bil and γ-Bil [6]. δ-Bil has been known to bind strongly to albumin in serum [7, 8]. This strong binding may explain the low elimination ratio of δ-Bil in this study, for the albumin-binding form could not bind to BR-350. Although α-Bil also usually binds to albumin receptors, we detected α-Bil in eluate from the BR-350 column. This may be attributable to the fact that the affinity of α-Bil to BR-350 is higher than that to albumin. The elimination ratio of α-Bil with BA was lower than those of other bilirubin subfractions. This tendency was also observed even in PE treatment. Further studies are required to clarify the mechanism of the tendency.

CONCLUSION

(i) Although both PE and BA effectively reduced serum bilirubin levels in hyper-bilirubinemia due to hepatic failure, the magnitude of the reduction with PE was more than that with BA.

(ii) When the bilirubin subfractions were analyzed by HPLC, β-Bil and δ-Bil were shown to be eliminated satisfactorily. On the other hand, the eliminations of α-Bil and δ-Bil were not sufficient. The insufficient elimination of δ-Bil resulted in the observation that BA was less effective than PE in reduction of T. Bil.

(iii) The insufficient elimination of δ-Bil in BA was based on its higher affinity to albumin than that to BR-350 column.

REFERENCES

1. J. J. Lauff, M. E. Kasper and R. T. Ambrose. Separation of bilirubin species in serum and bile by highperformance reversed-phase lioquid chromatography. *J. Chromatogr.*, **226**, 391–402 (1981).

2. M. Miyasaka, S. Tokunaga, M. Terashima *et al.* Evaluation of therapeutic effects of plasma exchange therapy for acute hepatic failure. In: *Therapeutic Plasmapheresis (IX)*, pp. 66–70, ICAOT, Cleveland (1991).

3. M. Usami, Y. Takeyama, H. Nomura *et al.* Therapeutic plasmapheresis supporting hepatobiliary surgery. In: *Therapeutic Plasmapheresis (IX)*, pp. 71–76, ICAOT, Cleveland (1991).

4. T. Morimoto, M. Matsushima, N. Sowa *et al.* Plasma adsorption using bilirubin-adsorbent materials as a treatment of patients with hepatic failure. *Artif. Organs*, **13**, 447–452 (1989).

5. Y. Suzuki, T. Morita, H. Hasegawa *et al.* Clinical performance of an artifical liver support system in severe liver failure: evaluation of four systems. In: *Therapeutic Plasmapheresis (IX)*, pp. 77–80, ICAOT, Cleveland (1991).

6. J. Sone, T. Saibara, H. Himeno *et al.* Assessment of bilirubin clearance capacity of a newly developed ion-exchange adsorption column and its possible use as a supportive therapy in hepatorenal syndrome. *J. Clin. Apheresis*, **5**, 123–127 (1990).

7. J. S. Weiss, A. Gautan, J. J. Lauff *et al.* The clinical importance of a protein-bound fraction of serum bilirubin in patients with hyperbilirubinemia. *N. Engl. J. Med.*, **309**, 147–150 (1983).

8. T. W. Wu. Bilirubin analysis — the state of the art and future prospects. *Clin. Biochem.*, **17**, 221–229 (1984).

Therapeutic Plasmapheresis (XII), pp. 181-183
T. Agishi *et al.* (Eds)
© VSP 1993

Evaluation of Apheresis for the Removal of Bilirubin Fractions

K. UMIMOTO, T. NAKANO, T. SHIKANO, N. CHIKAMORI,
H. KITAMURA and H. ABE

Division of Hemodialysis and Nephrology, Osaka Rosai Hospital, Osaka, Japan

Key words: plasma exchange; plasma perfusion; double filtration plasma pheresis; bilirubin fraction; delta bilirubin.

INTRODUCTION

Jaundice is due to the accumulation of bilirubin. In direct bilirubin (D-B), the presence of delta bilirubin (Bδ), which forms covalent bonds with albumin and displays a different metabolism to conjugated bilirubin (Bc), has been reported [1]. Recently, it has become possible to measure Bδ simply [2]. The measurement of bilirubin fractions is useful for the diagnosis of jaundice and the investigation of the pathological course.

Bilirubin can be removed by apheresis. However, the removal of bilirubin fractions has not been investigated in detail. In this paper, three different apheresis procedures were used to remove bilirubin in patients with hyperbilirubinemia. We studied the ability of each procedure to remove different bilirubin fractions.

PATIENTS AND METHODS

All patients displayed hyperbilirubinemia whose total bilirubin (T-B) was greater than 6.0 mg/dl. Three patients with fulminant hepatitis were treated by plasma exchange (PE). One patient with liver cirrhosis and one patient with primary biliary cirrhosis (PBC) were treated by one course each of plasma perfusion (PP) and double filtration plasma pheresis (DFPP).

Blood samples were collected before and after each procedure and T-B, unconjugated bilirubin (Bu), Bc and Bδ were determined with an Ektachem dry chemistry automatic analyzer (Eastman Kodak) [2].

Results are expressed as percent removal rate (%).

$$\text{Removal rate } (\%) = (1 - B/A) \times 100\%$$

A = bilirubin fraction value before treatment. B = bilirubin fraction value after treatment.

PE was performed with a plasauto iQ (Asahi Medical, Japan) using plasmaflo OP-05 (Asahi Medical) for plasma separation and 4 l of the patient's plasma was replaced with fresh frozen plasma. PP was also performed with a plasauto iQ using plasmaflo

OP-05 for plasma separation and plasorba BR-350 (Asahi Medical) for plasma bilirubin absorption. In a single session of PP, 3 l of plasma was treated.

DFPP was performed with a KM-8800 (Kuraray Medical, Japan) using plasmacure 0.5 (Kuraray Medical) for plasma separation (first membrane) and Evaflux 2A (Kuraray Medical) for plasma fractionation (secondary membrane). In a single session of DFPP, 250 ml of plasma was replaced with 7% albumin solution.

RESULTS

The results are shown in Tables 1 and 2.

PE removed $56.3 \pm 4.9\%$ of Bc and $53.8 \pm 8.4\%$ of Bδ. However, Bu was removed as little as $22.5 \pm 5.4\%$.

PP removed $43.2 \pm 1.2\%$ of Bc. This removal rate was almost equal to that of PE; however, Bu and Bδ were removed only $7.5 \pm 7.5\%$ and 0%, respectively.

DFPP removed $48.5 \pm 4.5\%$ of Bδ. This removal rate was almost equal to that of PE. Bc was removed at a rate of $29.2 \pm 6.7\%$, which was less than the removal rates of PE and PP. Bu was removed only $7.1 \pm 4.1\%$.

Table 1.
Changes in bilirubin fractions before and after treatment with PE, PP and DFPP

Bilirubin fractions	PE		PP		DFPP	
	before	after	before	after	before	after
T-B (mg/dl)	7.5 ± 1.2	3.9 ± 0.7	21.1 ± 8.7	15.8 ± 5.4	20.8 ± 8.5	14.8 ± 7.6
D-B (mg/dl)	6.0 ± 1.5	2.6 ± 0.6	17.0 ± 6.2	12.1 ± 3.7	16.5 ± 6.8	11.6 ± 5.9
Bu (mg/dl)	1.6 ± 0.3	1.3 ± 0.1	4.1 ± 2.5	3.6 ± 2.0	3.5 ± 1.7	3.3 ± 1.7
Bc (mg/dl)	4.6 ± 1.3	2.0 ± 0.6	12.2 ± 7.2	6.9 ± 4.0	11.2 ± 4.8	8.3 ± 4.2
Bδ (mg/dl)	1.4 ± 0.4	0.6 ± 0.1	4.8 ± 1.0	5.2 ± 0.5	5.3 ± 1.9	3.3 ± 1.7

Table 2.
Comparison of removal rates of bilirubin fractions treated with PE, PP and DFPP

Bilirubin fractions	PE	PP	DFPP
	(%)	(%)	(%)
T-B	47.4 ± 2.9	22.7 ± 6.6	29.3 ± 8.2
D-B	55.7 ± 3.2	27.1 ± 4.9	33.1 ± 8.1
Bu	22.5 ± 5.4	7.5 ± 7.5	7.1 ± 4.1
Bc	56.3 ± 4.9	43.2 ± 1.2	29.2 ± 6.7
Bδ	53.8 ± 8.4	0.0 ± 0.0	48.5 ± 4.5

DISCUSSION

The measurement of serum bilirubin is useful for the diagnosis of jaundice. Its fraction was formerly divided into direct-bilirubin and indirect-bilirubin [3], but it later become evident that direct-bilirubin was Bc [4]; also, the presence of Bδ, which forms a covalent bond with albumin, was indicated by high performance liquid chromatography although it responds to the direct diazo reaction [1]. Moreover, in recent years, with regard to the clinical significance of Bδ, it has been reported that jaundice patients with a favorable course have high levels of Bδ/T-B, and jaundice patients with a poor course have low levels of Bδ/T-B [5], so that Bδ has become significant with regard to pathological course and bilirubin metabolism.

In treating PBC and hyperbilirubinemia with jaundice, PE [6] and PP [7] are being attempted. Although clinically transitory effects are observed, in looking at the removal of bilirubin, with regard to the removal of fractions Bu, Bc and Bδ, no detailed reports other than our own has appeared [8]. In this study, PE was able to remove all of the fractions at high rates, but this is accompanied with a risk of infection because of the use of fresh frozen plasma. PP was effective with the removal of Bc whereas DFPP was excellent in removing Bδ. Since BR-350 (Asahi Medical) used in PP consists of an anion exchange resin, it is thought that Bc has a strong negative charge. Also, since albumin is removed by DFPP, it is thought that Bδ bonded to albumin is also effectively removed. In the future, the apheresis procedure will be selected based on the bilirubin fraction values, and it is thought that this will permit the effective removal of bilirubin.

CONCLUSION

Five patients with hyperbilirubinemia and jaundice were treated by PE, PP and DFPP procedures. We studied the ability of each procedure to remove bilirubin fractions.

PE was able to remove all fractions at high rates. PP and DFPP was able to efficiently remove Bc and Bδ, respectively.

These results indicate that it is necessary to select the appropriate apheresis procedure according to the elevated bilirubin fractions in cases of hyperbilirubinemia.

REFERENCES

1. J. J. Lauff, M. E. Kasper and R. T. Ambrose. Separation of bilirubin species in serum and bile by high performance reversed phase liquid chromatography. *J. Chromatogr.*, **226**, 391–402 (1981).
2. T. W. Wu, G. M. Dappen, R. W. Spayd et al. The ektachem clinical chemistry slide for simultaneous determination of unconjugated and sugar-conjugated bilirubin. *Clin. Chem.*, **30**, 1304–1309 (1984).
3. H. T. Mallorg and K. A. Evelyn. The determination of bilirubin with the photoelectric colorimeter. *J. Biol. Chem.*, **119**, 481–490 (1956).
4. E. Talafant. Properties and composition of the bile pigment giving a direct diazo reaction. *Nature*, **2**, 312 (1956).
5. J. S. Weiss, A. Gautam, J. J. Lauff et al. The clinical importance of a protein-bound fraction of serum bilirubin in patients with hyperbilirubinemia. *N. Engl. J. Med.*, **309**, 147–150 (1983).
6. P. W. N. Keeling, J. Bull, P. Kingston et al. Plasma exchange in primary biliary cirrhosis. *Prostgrad. Med. J.*, **57**, 433–435 (1981).
7. B. H. Lauterburg, E. R. Dickson, A. A. Pineda et al. Removal of acids and bilirubin by plasma perfusion USP-charcoal-coated glass beads. *J. Lab. Clin. Med.*, **94**, 585–592 (1979).
8. T. Nakano, K. Umimoto, T. Shikano et al. Evaluation of procedures for the removal of bilirubin in hyperbilirubinemia. *Am. Soc. Artif. Intern. Organs*, in press.

Therapeutic Plasmapheresis (XII), pp. 185-188
T. Agishi *et al.* (Eds)
© VSP 1993

Clinical Trial of Plasmapheresis Therapy for Acute Encephalopathy with Reye's Syndrome

M. SUENAGA,[1] Y. NAKAMURA,[1] K. TANAKA,[1] T. YAMADA,[1] K. UJIIE,[1]
Y. NISHIJIMA,[1] T. MIGITA,[1] T. SHIBAMOTO,[2] H. OHBA,[3]
O. MATSUDA[3] and M. OKANIWA[3]

[1]*Kidney Center, Tokyo Metropolitan Bokuto General Hospital,*
 4-23-15 Koutoubashi, Sumida-Ku, Tokyo, Japan
[2]*Tokyo Medical and Dental University, Japan*
[3]*Musashino Red Cross Hospital, Japan*

Key words: Reye's syndrome; acute encephalopathy; plasmapheresis.

INTRODUCTION

Reye's syndrome is often complicated with acutely advancing lethal encephalopathy. The brain edema induced by both hepatic and cerebral function failure is thought to be the main cause of death, but the exact and established pathological mechanism of encephalopathy has not yet been elucidated. Though there are no established treatments of the disease, it is reported that blood purification is effective for the control of encephalopathy. We had tried several kinds of blood purification therapy in five cases of Reye's syndrome and will briefly discuss the clinical efficacy and indication.

CASES

Five cases of Reye's syndrome had been admitted to our hospital in the past 5 years. All of them were small infants (3 months to 7 years old) whose chief complaints were consciousness disturbances and convulsions succeeding some infections. Two of them had ingested aspirin. The laboratory data at admission showed highly elevated levels of transaminase, LDH, CPK and ammonia but no elevation of total bilirubin. In addition, blood prothrombin time was extremely prolonged. Their clinical courses, signs, neurological disturbances and these data suggested the diagnosis of Reye's (like) syndrome which was confirmed by examination of cerebro-spinal fluid and liver necropsy. We immediately started conservative therapy against cerebral edema and hepatic function failure but the degree of encephalopathy rapidly deteriorated. We then decided to perform blood purification therapy (Table 1).

Table 1.

Clinical profile of patients with Reye's syndrome (RS)

Case	Age (years)	Sex	Syndrome	Aspirin intake	Signs at onset	RS stage at onset
1	7	m	flulike	convulsion	−	2
2	11	f	—	convulsion	−	2
3	3	f	fever	fever	+	2
4	3	m	—	convulsion	−	4
5	3[a]	m	diarrhoea	convulsion	+	4

[a] month.

METHODS

We performed three types of blood purification therapy, i.e. plasma exchange (PE), direct hemoperfusion with charcoal (DHP) and blood exchange (BT). In plasmapheresis therapy, we constructed miniature blood circuits and primed them with fresh frozen plasma (FFP). The plasma separator (Plasmacure) and about 8 units of FFP was exchanged for the same amount of patient's on-line hemodialysis was combined with PE. These therapies were repeated intermittently until they came conscious or died.

RESULTS

In total, 16 procedures of PE, one of DHP and two of BT were performed. Of the five cases, three recovered and two died of cerebral herniation. By each procedure, intracranial pressure increased slightly but not significantly.

The consciousness level of the three recovered cases were in stage II to III and improved to I or II after only one or several procedures of blood purification therapy. On the other hand, those of the two lethal cases were in stage IV or more and no improvements were observed after any therapy. The examination of EEG revealed the same tendency. That is, the main background activity of EEG of the three were at the θ band and improved to the α band, but two the cases that died were in the δ band or flat and never improved (Tables 2 and 3, Figs 1–3).

Table 2.

Laboratory data of five patients

Case	GOT	GPT	LDH (IU/l)	CPK	Amylase	NH3 (μg/l)	T.Bil (mg/dl)	PT (sec.)
1	6650	3064	2326	9070	5795	98	0.9	20.9
2	5730	5040	1032	1032	625	104	1.8	24.9
3	1815	165	12390	16359	289	121	2.0	23.7
4	500	179	4166	2359	110	46	0.4	25.0[a]
5	8950	3610	9050	2630	3160	58	1.3	23.0[a]

[a] (%).

Table 3.
Prognosis and clinical state

Case	Consciousness level	Brain edema	Renal failure	Respiratory arrest	DIC	Prognosis	Consciousness disturbance
1	100	−	+−	+	−	alive	improved
2	20	−	+−	−	−	alive	improved
3	20	−	−	−	+	alive	improved
4	200	+	−	+	+	dead	unchanged
5	200	+	−	+	+	dead	unchanged

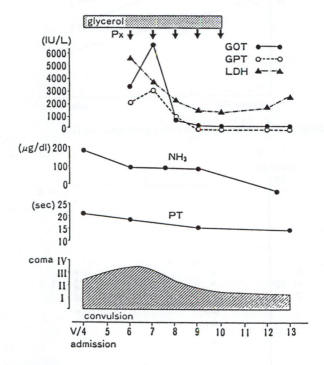

Figure 1. Case 1: clinical course.

DISCUSSION

We treated five Reye's syndrome with acute encephalopathy with blood purification therapy, mainly with plasmapheresis. Of the five cases, three recovered and two died. The consciousness levels and the main background activities of EEG of the three recovered cases were better than those of the two who died of cerebral herniation. In addition, the recovered cases responded well to the therapy and the two that died did not respond at all. These result suggests that blood purification therapy, especially plasmapheresis, is effective for the treatment of encephalopathy of Reye's syndrome in NIH stage II to III, but is not of value in more advanced cases. We recommend treating patients with Reye's syndrome as early as possible before they advance to stage III or more.

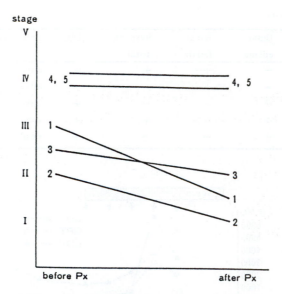

Figure 2. The change of the consciousness level after plasmapheresis (Px).

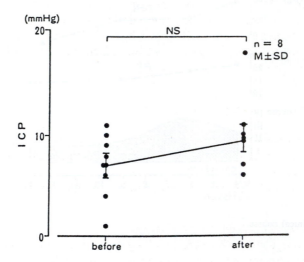

Figure 3. The change of intracranial pressure (ICP) during hemodialysis/hemodialysis + Px.

REFERENCES

1. R. D. K. Reye, G. Morgan and J. Baral. Encephalopathy and fatty degeneration of the viscera. *Lancet*, **2**, 749 (1953).
2. L. Corley, R. Rubin and W. Hattwick. Reye's syndrome: clinical progression and evaluation of therapy. *Pediatrics*, **60**, 708 (1977).
3. NIH Consensus conference. Diagnosis and treatment of Reye's syndrome. *J. Am. Med. Ass.*, **246**, 2441 (1981).
4. F. H. Lovejoy, A. Smith, M. Bresnan, J. N. Wood, D. I. Victor and P. C. Adams. Clinical staging in Reye's syndrome. *Am. J. Dis. Child*, **128**, 36 (1974).

Therapeutic Plasmapheresis (XII), pp. 189-192
T. Agishi *et al.* (Eds)
© VSP 1993

Basic Studies on a New Adsorbent for Hemoperfusion to Remove Bilirubin from Patients Blood

Z. YAMAZAKI, M. HIRAISHI, F. KANAI, T. TAKAHAMA, Y. IDEZUKI,
N. INOUE,[1] M. YOSHIDA,[2] Y. TAKENAKA,[2] N. TOMA[2] and K. IDE[2]

Second Department of Surgery, University of Tokyo, Tokyo, Japan
[1]*Social Insurance Medical Center, Tokyo, Japan*
[2]*Asahi Medical Co., Tokyo, Japan*

Key words: hemoperfusion; adsorbent; bilirubin.

INTRODUCTION

Plasma perfusion through an anion exchange resin (Current Adsorbent (CA)) column has been available as a technique for removing bilirubin and bile acids selectively from patients with hyperbilirubinemia [1, 2]. However, hemoperfusion appears to be an easier procedure than plasma perfusion. Therefore, a New Adsorbent (NA) for hemoperfusion which removes bilirubin has been developed.

MATERIALS, METHODS AND RESULTS

NA has an antithrombogenic surface coated with acrylate hydrophilic polymer to prevent platelet adhesion, making it available for hemoperfusion [3]. Moreover it adsorbs heparin much less than CA.

Charcoal adsorbent for hemoperfusion was also used in this experiment.

Preliminary in vitro *bovine blood hemoperfusion*
Bovine blood, anticoagulated with heparin (5000 IU/l), was passed through an NA (350 ml) and charcoal column at a flow rate of 60 ml/min respectively for 2 h. Blood cell analyses indicated that little change was observed in the red cell count level, however, there was a marked decrease in the white cell count and in the platelets in the initial stage of perfusion. This was then followed by a recovery during NA and charcoal hemoperfusion.

Batchwise adsorption studies
Heparin (5000 IU/l) in saline solution. The heparin solution and adsorbent were mixed at a volume ratio of 30:1. After shaking the mixture at 37°C for 3 h, the heparin concentration of NA was almost half the pre-adsorption level. While that of CA decreased markedly to less than 10%.

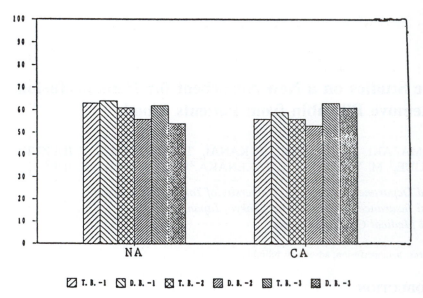

Figure 1. Reduction rate in plasma (%): *in vitro* test with patient plasma.

In vitro *adsorbent minicolumn plasma perfusion*

Plasma obtained from patients with hepatic failure was passed through the adsorbent column (packed with 1 ml of NA or CA), at the same passage of time as under *ex vivo* adsorbent plasma perfusion, and at a flow rate of 0.06 ml/min for 2 h.

Both NA and CA showed almost equal adsorption capacity for total and direct bilirubin during 2 h, as indicated in Fig. 1.

In vitro NA 350 ml column hemoperfusion with the use of volunteer human blood (fractionated red cells or platelet solution) showed a mild decrease in the level of platelets, while the red cell count remained constant. The level of platelets passed through the column 1 h after the perfusion measured over 60% of the pre-perfusion level (Fig. 2).

Ex vivo *NA hemoperfusion and CA plasma perfusion*

Four dogs, weighing 16–20 kg, with hyperbilirubinemia were used in these experiments 1 week after common bile duct–inferior caval vein shunt using a polyethylene tube.

NA hemoperfusion was carried out at a blood flow rate of 60 ml/min for 2 h. CA plasma perfusion, using OP-05 as a plasma separator, was performed at a plasma flow rate of 20 ml/min for 2 h. An initial heparin dose of 2000 IU was given at the start of the perfusion. Thereafter, heparin was continuously infused into the outflow site of the extracorporeal circuit for anticoagulation at a flow rate of 1000 IU/h. Hemoperfusion and the plasma perfusion were successfully carried out, in alternating order, in the same dogs during the one experiment.

All four dogs tolerated the procedure well and no serious side-effects were observed.

Blood and plasma samples were taken before and after the column every 30 min for blood and biochemical studies.

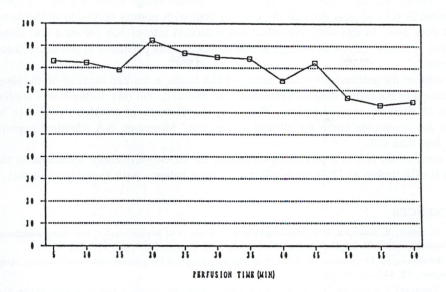

Figure 2. Recovery (human platelet): % of pre-perfusion level.

Reduction rate of NA for total bilirubin, calculated from the following formula, was almost the same as that of CA.

$$100 \times \frac{\text{TBC in outflow plasma from the dog} - \text{TBC in inflow plasma into the dog}}{\text{TBC in outflow plasma from the dog}}$$

where TBC is total bilirubin concentration. The reduction rate of both NA and CA remained almost constant throughout the experiment.

The levels of bilirubin, bile acid and glycocholic acids in the blood, markedly decreased with the passage of time during adsorbent perfusion. However, total protein and uric acids in the plasma were at almost the same levels during the experiment.

There was no marked change in the red cell count; however, after an initial decrease, the white cell count increased to a level similar to that observed during the adsorbent perfusion studies.

Platelets in the blood were not well analyzed because of aggregation of platelets in some samples.

Heparin in the outflow plasma from the CA column was at nearly zero level throughout the experiment, while that from the NA column was at almost the same level as that of the inflow blood into the NA column at 30 min after perfusion.

DISCUSSION AND CONCLUSION

The *in vitro* and *ex vivo* experimental results indicate that NA and CA have almost equal adsorbing capacity for bilirubin and bile acids. However, with respect to the handling technique and the expense involved, it is evident that hemoperfusion is superior to plasma perfusion. Moreover, hemoperfusion has the advantage in that a greater amount of plasma is able to pass through the column than with plasma perfusion at the same blood flow rate. In this way, the calculated reduction rate of NA for total and direct bilirubin is almost 1.5 times as high as that of CA plasma perfusion at the same blood flow rate.

In spite of the antithrombogenic coating of NA beads, a marked decrease in the level of platelets in the initial stage of perfusion was observed, and this decrease was similar to that of charcoal hemoperfusion. Therefore, the decrease in platelets seemed to be within the acceptable range for clinical application. Moreover, NA adsorbed heparin much less than CA.

In conclusion, NA is a promising adsorbent for an easy-to-handle technique in the removal of bilirubin and bile acids effectively from patients with hyperbilirubinemia.

REFERENCES

1. J. W. Smith, Y. Asanuma, P. S. Malchensky *et al.* Treatment of hepatic dysfunction using membrane plasmapheresis with sorptive plasma detoxication. *Artif. Organs,* **5** (Suppl.), 828–832 (1981).
2. T. Morimoto, M. Matsushima, N. Sowa *et al.* Plasma adsorption for patients with hepatic failure. *Artif. Organs,* **13**, 447–452 (1989).
3. Z. Yamazaki, F. Kanai, M. Hirashi *et al.* Immunoadsorption and adsorptive cell separation. *Mater. Res. Soc. Symp. Proc.,* **110**, 729–737 (1989).

Therapeutic Plasmapheresis (XII), pp. 193-196
T. Agishi et al. (Eds)
© VSP 1993

Plasma Exchange in Combination with High Performance Hemodiafiltration for the Treatment of Fulminant Viral Hepatic Failure

K. NIIKURA, Y. SUGENOYA, K. TAKAYAMA, E. KINUGASA, T. AKIZAWA,
S. KOSHIKAWA, K. DEHARA, M. YOSHIBA and F. SUGATA

Internal Medicine, Showa University, Fujigaoka Hospital, Yokohama, Japan

Key words: artificial liver support; plasma exchange; hemodiafiltration; fulminant viral hepatic failure; survival rate.

INTRODUCTION

Inspite of the clinical application of plasma exchange (PE), fulminant hepatic failure still remains a critical illness with a high mortality rate. As an artificial liver support (ALS), PE is effective to supplement plasma components such as coagulating factors; however, its eliminating capacity for toxic substances is insufficient, especially, for pathogenetic substances of hepatic encephalopathy including middle molecular substances or low molecular weight protein fractions.

For the removal of those substances, high performance hemodiafiltration (HDF) is the most reliable blood purification method [1]. In this study, to clarify the therapeutic effects of a combination system composed of PE and high performance HDF, patients with fulminant viral hepatic failure (FVHF) were reviewed with respect to the recovery of hepatic coma and survival rate.

SUBJECTS AND METHODS

The subjects were 32 patients (18 males and 14 females, mean age 48.3 ± 14.0 years old) with FVHF treated in our hospital from 1987 to 1991. Underlying diseases were hepatitis B in nine, and non-A non-B hepatitis in 23 patients. Hepatic coma grade before treatment was judged as grade I in eight patients, II in six, III in eight and IV in 10 patients. The definition of hepatic coma grade was based on Trey's classification [2].

The details of ALS are shown in Tables 1 and 2. PE was performed by membrane plasma separation. For HDF, a polymethylmethacrylate membrane was used during the first 2 years, then changed to cellulose triacetate membrane for the last 3 years. The cut-off points of these two membranes was estimated to be above 25 000 dalton. As an anticoagulant, nafamostat mesilate (NM), an ultra-short acting anticoagulant, was continuously infused at the rate of 20–30 mg/h.

Principally, PE and HDF was performed simultaneously not only to shorten the therapeutic time, but to correct acid–base and electrolyte disturbance caused by both FVHF and PE [3].

Table 1.

Method of ALS composed of PE and high-performance HDF

Blood access:	Double lumen catheter
Membrane for plasma separation:	Cellulose diacetate or Polyethylene
Membrane for HDF:	Polymethylmethacrylate or cellulose tri-acetate
Dialysate:	Kindaly AF-2 (HCO_3 30 mEq/l, K 3.5–4 mEq/l)
Substitution fluid:	HF-B (HCO_3 30 mEq/l, K 4.0 mEq/l)
Anticoagulant:	Nafamostat mesilate (NM)

Table 2.

Therapeutic conditions of ALS

PE	blood flow rate	100 ml/min
	plasma separation rate	30 ml/min
	replacement FFP volume	2.4–4.8 l
HDF	blood flow rate	150–200 ml/min
	ultrafiltration rate	30–60 ml/min
	dialysate flow rate	500 ml/min
	substitution fluid volume	10–30 l
Anticoagulant	NM	20–30 mg/h
Total therapeutic time		6–12 h

HDF was carried out every day until the consciousness level improved or deteriorated to grade IV coma. Substitution fluid volume was determined according to coma grade and the type of FVHF. When prothrombin time (PT) prolonged to less than 40% of control, PE was started to keep PT above 30% by replacing 2.4–4.8 l of fresh frozen plasma (FFP). As a consequence, total therapeutic time was 6–12 h depending on the volume of substitution fluid and FFP.

RESULTS

Twenty of 32 patients survived (survival rate; 62.5%), including eight out of nine patients (88.9%) with hepatitis B and 12 out of 23 patients (52.2%) with non-A non-B hepatitis.

Even in a non-survivor group, 10 of 12 patients (83.3%) transiently recovered from coma during PE and HDF.

Comparing survivors with non-survivors, survivors were significantly younger and took a shorter interval from the onset until the first ALS than non-survivors, though the initial grade of coma and frequencies of ALS were comparable (Table 3). From the point of laboratory data at the first ALS, survivors showed a higher ratio of direct bilirubin to total bilirubin, blood urea nitrogen and molar ratio of branched chain to aromatic amino acids than non-survivors (Table 4). Interestingly, PT did not become a determining factor for survival.

Table 3.
Comparison of background factors between survivors and non-survivors

	Survivors ($n = 20$)	Non-survivors ($n = 12$)	P value
Age (years)	44.5 ± 13.5	55.4 ± 12.7	< 0.03
HB/Total (%)	36.4	8.3	< 0.05
Coma grade (I:II:III:IV)	14:3:3:0	8:2:2:1	NS
Interval until ALS (days)	8.6 ± 4.8	20.1 ± 10.6	< 0.005
Total ALS (times)	12.2 ± 16.5	20.2 ± 31.5	NS

Mean ± SD.

Table 4.
Comparison of laboratory data between survivors and non-survivors

	Survivors ($n = 20$)	Non-survivors ($n = 12$)	P value
PT (%)	20.7 ± 10.8	15.3 ± 11.8	NS
T.Bil (mg/dl)	18.4 ± 9.4	28.3 ± 10.1	< 0.05
D.Bil/T.Bil	0.54 ± 0.37	0.12 ± 0.24	< 0.01
BUN (mg/dl)	9.9 ± 4.9	6.0 ± 5.3	< 0.03
BCAA/AAA	0.97 ± 0.57	0.59 ± 0.31	< 0.05
NH3 (μg/dl)	140 ± 68	131 ± 41	NS

Bil, bilirubin; BUN, blood urea nitrogen; BCAA, branched chain amino acid; AAA, aromatic amino acid. Mean ± SD.

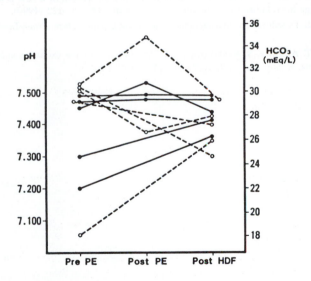

Figure 1. Changes in blood gas analyses during ALS: •, pH; o, HCO_3.

Figure 1 illustrates the changes in pH and bicarbonate in five patients who underwent PE and substantial HDF. Though these values were distributed widely before or after PE, they were directed toward normal after HDF.

DISCUSSION

FVHF still has remained a critical illness with a high mortality. Until present, we could not find reports which described a higher survival rate than 30%. With regard to survival rate, the present ALS system composed of PE and HDF exerted a better effect (overall survival rate; 62.5%) than the other methods. However, there exists some problems in this ALS system. One is the transient cytopenia which results from blood–membrane interaction. White blood cells and platelets transiently decreased during ALS and the possibility that these phenomenon may contribute to infection or bleeding could not be completely excluded. Second is the possibility of removal of essential substances for the regeneration of liver, including human hepatic growth factor (hHGF), by PE. Though the hHGF concentration was known to be much higher in FVHF than in acute hepatitis, a relative deficiency in hHGF after PE could not be ruled out. Careful attention should be paid to infection, hemorrhage and hypoalubuminemia during PE and HDF.

CONCLUSION

The main role of ALS for fulminant hepatic failure is considered to be in maintaining liver function and preventing complications until liver regeneration or transplantation. From our results, an intensive liver support system consisting of PE and high-performance HDF is effective for the treatment modality of FVHF.

REFERENCES

1. S. Kanesaka, K. Dehara, T. Taira *et al.* Combined detoxication system of a new hemodiafiltration and plasma exchange for fulminant viral hepatitis. *Artif. Organs,* **14**, 120–122 (1990).
2. C. Trey and C. S. Davidson. The management of fulminant hepatic failure. *Progr. Liver Dis.,* 3, 282–293 (1970).
3. N. Kanamori, T. Akizawa, S. Koshikawa *et al.* The effect of plasma exchange and hemodiafiltration for hepatic coma. *Kidney and Dialysis,* **23** (Suppl.), 56–59 (1987).

Therapeutic Plasmapheresis (XII), pp. 197-200
T. Agishi *et al.* (Eds)
© VSP 1993

Therapeutic Plasma Exchange in the Treatment of Acute Hepatic Failure

R. BAMBAUER and U. MARQUARDT

University of Saarland, Germany

INTRODUCTION

Acute hepatic failure (AHF) is the consequence of severe hepatic functional disorders, mostly leading to death. Although an adequate function is still ensured with a hepatic parenchym loss of 70–80% and although the unlimited hepatic regenerative ability can largely re-establish the hepatic function with regard to synthetic, regulation and detoxication, the acute hepatic coma usually ends lethally. However, if artificial detoxication can be provided as a support during critical hepatic failure, serious morphological and functional damage can be avoided thanks to the liver's extensive regenerative capacity.

Since therapeutic plasma exchange (TPE) in hepatic failure was first reported in 1967 by Lepore [1], many groups have examined TPE as a treatment for acute hepatic functional disorders, particularly by plasma separation using membrane separators.

METHOD AND PATIENTS

TPE was carried out using the single-needle method. For liver diseases, hollow-fiber membranes made of polypropylene were used. Easy vascular access for TPE was achieved by percutaneously puncturing the *V. jugularis int.* or the *V. subclavia*. For 3 years the back flow of blood was achieved over an arterial catheter in the femoral artery. Usually an anticoagulant, heparin, as a rule, was used in low doses (100–1000 U/l). The substitution solution was fresh frozen plasma, lyophilized plasma in 58.0%, plasma protein solution in 26.0%, and albumin in 16.0% of the treatments.

TPE was carried out in 115 patients with AHF: 62 patients suffering from severe hepatic failure after surgery, 26 patients suffering from decompensated liver cirrhosis, 10 from toxic hepatosis, a further three patients from hepatitis, another three patients from a Budd–Chiari syndrome and 11 patients suffered from miscellany like Cytomegaly infection, Gestosis, etc. (Table 1).

Only a small number of patients showed coma grade I or II of the hepatic encephalopathy; most of them, 86 out of 115 patients, showed coma grade III (50 patients) or IV (36 patients).

Table 1.
TPE in AHF

Diagnosis	n	TPE (n)	Duration days (x)	x	Course (x)	—
Post surgery	62	255	4.9	10	18	34
Liver cirrhosis	26	197	10.5	4	11	11
Toxic hepatosis	10	83	13.5	1	4	5
Hepatitis	3	10	2.0	1	—	2
Budd–Chiari syndrome	3	7	2.0	—	—	3
Miscellany	11	96	15.0	5	3	3
Total	115	648		21	36	58

RESULTS

The elimination of bilirubin in 80 patients over the whole treatment time varied between 15.0% in hepatitis and 71.0% in AHF with various primary diseases. Cholinesterase showed a contrary reaction under TPE. After TPE, cholinesterase serum concentrations increased in most of the cases. One of the reason is the substitution of cholinesterase with fresh frozen plasma and the other reason can be surely a part improvement of the liver function. See Fig. 1.

Only 21 (19.1%) out of 115 patients survived; 58 out of 115 patients died (50.4%) and 36 patients (30.5%) showed only a temporary improvement and then died after a short interval of 1–10 days after treatment (Table 1).

The following side-effects where observed in all patients: in 11.6% decrease of blood pressure during treatment, increasing bleeding tendencies in 7.5% and catheter sepsis in 1.8%. The most side-effects, 32.5%, which we observed were allergic reactions in dependence of the substitution solution like lyophilized (12.1%) or fresh frozen plasma (20.4%). The histological diagnosis of the liver of 52 out of 94 patients who died without any effect of the TPE treatment or died after temporary recovery is shown in Table 2. It was impressive that in most cases with complete liver cirrhosis, parenchym regenerates between small, medium or large modules were observed.

Table 2.
Liver histology of 52 patients with AHF

Cholestasis	$n = 30$
Liver cell necrosis	$n = 29$
Liver cirrhosis	$n = 23$
Cholangitis	$n = 11$
Toxic hepatosis	$n = 6$
Budd–Chiari syndrome	$n = 3$
Acute hepatitis	$n = 4$
Liver fibrosis	$n = 3$
No histology	$n = 42$

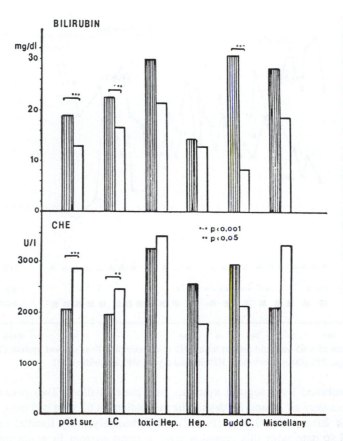

Figure 1. Bilirubin and cholinesterase (CHE) in 115 patients with AHF during plasmapheresis treatment.

DISCUSSION

The pathogenesis of AHF and hepatic encephalopathy are still unclear. AHF results from the simultaneous decrease in synthetic functions of the hepatocyte mass and a decrease in metabolic and excretory function. Numerous substances have been shown to accumulate in the brain and central nervous system in such patients. The precise role that each of all these substances plays in the genesis of hepatic coma is unknown.

All functions of the liver are interrupted in AHF. The three main functions of the liver can be reproduced with the help of TPE better than with any other therapeutic measures. The synthesis function is largely compensated by the large-bore substitution of fresh frozen plasma. The metabolic function is partly replaced by TPE, which relieves and restores the disturbed ratio of various amino acids and lipids. The detoxication function eliminates toxins, decay products and other blocking metabolic products. Among the different liver support systems proposed for acute hepatic failure, TPE now has the highest credit.

The survival rate was only 19.0% in our patients, therefore we introduced the complex liver support system which combines all detoxification methods like TPE, plasmaperfusion, hemodialysis and hemofiltration. Until the present we have treated five patients

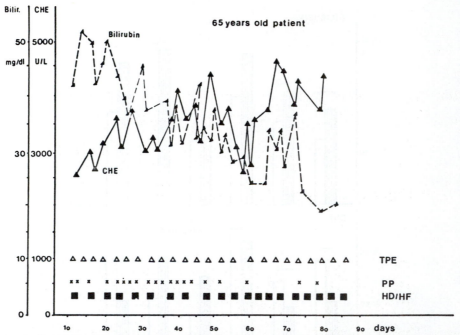

Figure 2. Course of a 65 year old patient with AHF under complex liver support system (TPE: therapeutic plasma exchange, PP: plasma perfusion, HD: hemodialysis, HF: hemofiltration).

with this combined liver support system. Two patients died. Two patients showed a temporary recovery of 15 and 30 days. The last patient, a 65 year old man, had survived acute hepatic failure for 90 days (Fig. 2). Unfortunately, only limited experience has been gained to date with this complex liver support system in acute hepatic failure, therefore definite conclusions are not yet possible.

We need more experience in the management of the complex liver support systems, which undoubtedly still require improvement. In conclusion the pathogenesis of AHF and hepatic encephalopathy are still unclear. Among the different liver support systems proposed for AHF, TPE has the highest credit. A complex liver support to influence better the complicated phenomenon of AHF is needed.

REFERENCE

1. M. J. Lepore and A. J. Martel. Plasmapheresis in hepatic coma. *Lancet*, II, 771–772 (1967).

Therapeutic Plasmapheresis (XII), pp. 201-205
T. Agishi *et al.* (Eds)
© VSP 1993

Strategy of Long-term Treatment by Plasma Exchange for Patients with Fulminant Hepatic Failure

Y. NAKAGAWA, S. TERAOKA, M. MINESHIMA, H. FUJIKAWA,
M. KIMIKAWA, I. NAKAJIMA, S. NAGANUMA, T. SUZUKI,
S. FUCHINOUE, K. ERA, T. AGISHI and K. OTA

Tokyo Women's Medical College, Kidney Center, Tokyo, Japan

Key words: fulminant hepatic failure; plasma exchange; bilirubin kinetics.

INTRODUCTION

It would be desirable to be able to predict the course and response to treatment of patients with fulminant hepatic failure (FHF) in a early phase from onset. Unfortunately in spite of many attempts to correlate clinical variables and laboratory data with prognosis, there are no reliable criteria that enable the clinician to determine whether an individual with FHF will die or regain consciousness and ultimately survive. In the present study, plasma bilirubin kinetics was investigated to predict the prognosis of individuals.

PATIENTS AND METHODS

From 1981 to 1991, 21 patients (11: male, 10: female, age: 9–78, average: 41.9 ± 15.2 years) with FHF treated with exchange transfusion (ExTf), hemoperfusion over charcoal (CHP) and plasma exchange (PE) were investigated. In 17 of the patients, the cause of FHF was related to a viral origin (HA: 1, HB: 5, non-A non-B: 3, non-B: 8) while it was related to drugs in two other patients. In the remaining two patients, FHF occurred immediately after the operation. The interval between the onset of diseases and coma was less than 10 days in 12 patients (designated as acute type), while it was more than 10 days in nine patients (designated as subacute type).

PE using 1.2–4.0 l of fresh frozen plasma was performed in 13 patients; in three out of these 13 patients, it was combined with CHP. Plasma separation was attained by a hollow-fiber membrane separator. Daily serum level of bilirubin, other laboratory data and coagulation tests were examined.

Plasma bilirubin kinetics was studied in seven patients treated with PE. The concept of bilirubin appearance rate (BAR) is proposed in order to investigate the relationship between the hepatic functional mass and the rate of the increase in plasma bilirubin after PE. BAR was calculated by the equation shown in Fig. 1.

$$BAR = \frac{Bil(t_2) - Bil(t_1)}{100} \times Vp/(t_2 - t_1)/Vp$$

$$(mg/min/ml)$$

Bil_2 : serum level of bilirubin at $t_2 (mg/dl)$

Bil_1 :   "   "   at $t_1 (mg/dl)$

Vp : circulating plasma volume (ml)

$$Vp = BW \times 1000/13(1 - Ht/100)$$

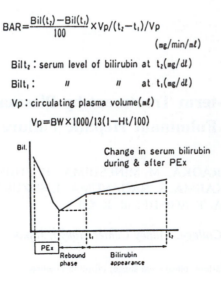

Figure 1. Concept of bilirubin appearance rate (BAR).

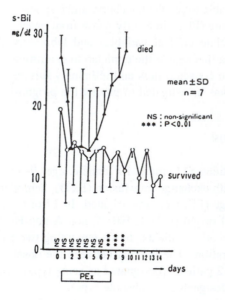

Figure 2. Changes in serum bilirubin level after the initiation of PE.

RESULTS

Overall recovery from coma and survival rate were 61.9% and 33.8%, respectively. In the acute type of FHF, eight out of 12 patients recovered from coma (66.7%) and six patients survived after the treatment (50.0%). On the other hand, recovery from coma and survival rate in the subacute type were 55.6% and 11.1%, respectively. Ten out

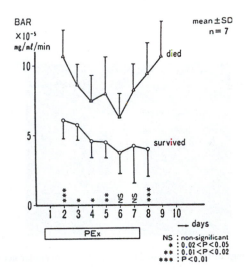

Figure 3. Changes in BAR after initiation of PE.

of 13 patients treated with PE recovered from coma (76.9%) and six patients survived (46.2%). In the acute type of seven patients treated with PE, recovery from coma and survival rate were 57.1% and 85.7%. On the other hand, recovery from coma and survival rate in the subacute type treated with PE were 66.7% and 33.3%, respectively.

Causes of death was divided into two categories. One was attributed to complications such as DIC, GI bleeding and sepsis while the other was related to so-called impaired regeneration. Two patients needed long-term PE for over 3 months due to the impaired regeneration syndrome. One died of sepsis 17 months after onset, and the other died of sepsis and DIC after 7 months.

When the maximum serum bilirubin level just before the next PE was less than the maximum level just before the previous PE, the base-line of serum bilirubin declined slowly and steadily by means of daily PE; in these situation, most patients survived. However, patients whose base-line serum bilirubin level was elevated despite daily PE did not survive (Fig. 2).

The relationship between BAR and the survival rate is demonstrated in Fig. 3. BAR in a non-survivor was greater than 6×10^{-5} mg/ml/min while BAR in a survivor was less than 6×10^{-5} mg/ml/min.

DISCUSSION

It is apparent that bilirubin is not a major toxic substance in FHF. However, the serum level of bilirubin can be a good index in predicting the prognosis of patients with FHF. The increase in the serum bilirubin level despite five to six sessions of PE may suggest a poor prognosis. BAR makes an earlier prediction of the prognosis possible, as shown in Fig. 3. BAR appears to reflect the net balance between production and excretion of bilirubin. BAR greater than 6×10^{-5} mg/ml/min may suggest a poor prognosis regardless of the serum bilirubin level [1].

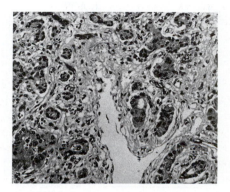

Figure 4. Pathological findings of the liver (case 21): massive hepatocellular necrosis.

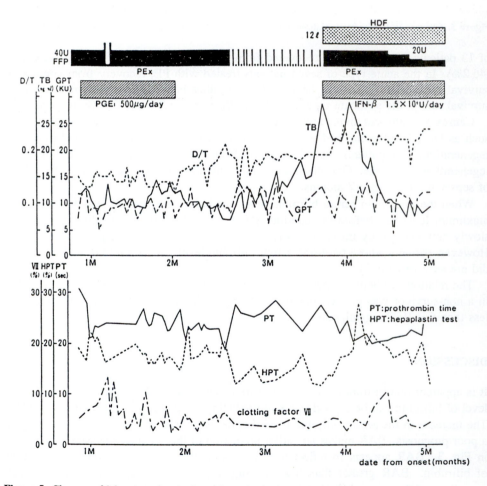

Figure 5. Changes of laboratory data in the patient with long-term PE treatment.

From a theoretical viewpoint, the clinical patterns of FHF were divided into three types. Type (a) is considered to comprise patients in whom liver functional mass does not decrease to less than survival limit. Type (b) is considered to comprise patients who would die because their liver function would fall below the survival limit; however, they have the potential for hepatic regeneration. Type (c) is the patients who have progressively deteriorating liver function and would die irrespective of any currently available therapy other than hepatic transplantation. In type (b′), the cause of death is attributed to complications such as DIC, sepsis and/or GI bleeding. The cause of death in type (b″) may be attributed to impaired regeneration despite the improvement during artificial liver support. In our study, two patients (type b″) died of impaired regeneration without any chance of hepatic transplantation despite long-term treatment by PE. Changes in laboratory data of one patient who died of sepsis 7 months after the admission despite long-term treatment by PE was shown in Figs 4 and 5. The rationale for the application of methods to provide temporary hepatic support in managing patients with FHF based on the assumption that the hepatic lesion is reversible provided that the patient can be kept alive sufficiently long for hepatic regeneration to take place. If the patients with FHF have progressively deteriorating liver function and would die without the hepatic transplantation, we need to perform temporary artificial liver support for bridge use until hepatic transplantation.

REFERENCE

1. S. Teraoka, T. Agishi, T. Sanaka *et al.* Efficacy and limitations of plasma exchange treatment for fulminant hepatic failure. In: *Therapeutic Plasmapheresis (VI)*, pp. 177–186, ISAO Press, Cleveland (1986).

Therapeutic Plasmapheresis (XII), pp. 207-210
T. Agishi *et al.* (Eds)
© VSP 1993

Indication of Plasmapheresis for Patients with Severe Hepatic Dysfunction

Y. OHTAKE, H. HIRASAWA, T. SUGAI, S. ODA, H. SHIGA, K. NAKANISHI, K. MATSUDA, N. KITAMURA and H. UENO

*Department of Emergency and Critical Care Medicine,
Chiba University School of Medicine, Chiba, Japan*

Key words: plasmapheresis; plasma exchange; plasma adsorption; redox state; arterial ketone body ratio.

INTRODUCTION

Plasmapheresis therapy has been one of the important treatments for patients with severe hepatic dysfunction. Plasma exchange (PE) and plasma adsorption (PA) have been applied to those patients. This study was undertaken to evaluate the changes in the parameters of hepatic function by PE or PA, and to investigate the efficacies of those modalities and the usefulness of those parameters in the selection of the modalities. The patients with severe hepatic dysfunction in this study included patients with hepatic failure and patients with hyperbilirubinemia diagnosed according to the criteria detailed below.

MATERIALS AND METHODS

Fifty-five hepatic failure patients and five hyperbilirubinemia patients were entered to the study. Sulflux 05 was used as a plasma separator and Bespore was used as a plasma adsorber. Fresh frozen plasma (FFP) in a volume of 3200 ml was replaced in PE and 3200 ml of separated plasma was perfused through the absorbent column in PA. Arterial blood samples were taken at the start of PE and PA, and 1 and 24 h after the end of PE and PA. T.Bil, total protein, HPT, acetoacetate (ACAC) and β-hydroxybutyrate (BOHB) [1] were measured. Those parameters of FFP were also measured. In addition, theoretical values of ACAC and BOHB in arterial blood after PE were calculated by the equation of the one pool model [2]. Ketone body ratio (KBR) was calculated with values of ACAC and BOHB [1, 3]. Criteria of hepatic failure (i) arterial ketone body ratio (AKBR)<0.7 and (ii) total bilirubin > 5 mg/dl or hepaplastin test < 30%. Criteria of hyperbilirubinemia are (i) AKBR > 0.7 and (ii) T.Bil > 20 mg/dl.

RESULTS

The reduction rate of T.Bil was over 40% with both PE and PA, and there was no significant difference in the reduction rate. The values of HPT increases significantly with PE. On the other hand, then decreased significantly with PA. Total protein and AKBR did not change significantly before and after PE and PA (Fig. 1).

Figure 2 shows changes in ACAC, BOHB and KBR in arterial blood and FFP. The values of ACAC, BOHB and AKBR did not change significantly with PE. The values of ACAC and BOHB in FFP were one tenth and half of those of arterial blood, respectively. Consequently, KBR in FFP was significantly lower than that of arterial blood.

Figure 3 shows actual and theoretical values of ACAC, BOHB and KBK before and after PE. Actual values of both ACAC and BOHB were significantly higher than theoretical values. The improvement in the production of ACAC compared with that of BOHB resulted in increased KBR.

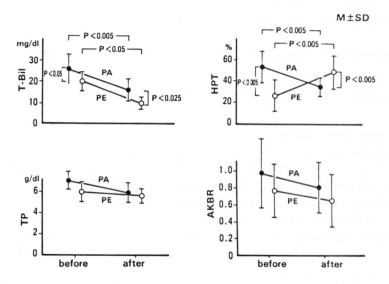

Figure 1. Changes in total bilirubin (T.Bil), total protein (TP), hepaplastin test (HPT) and arterial ketone body ratio (AKBR) values before and after PE and PA.

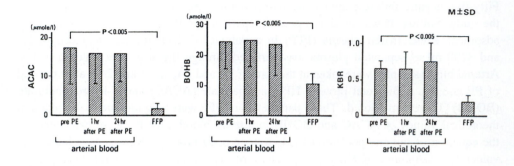

Figure 2. Changes in ACAC, BOHB and ketone body ratio (KBR) values in arterial blood and FFP.

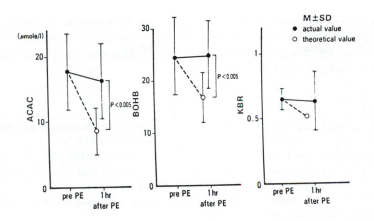

Figure 3. Actual and theoretical values of ACAC, BOHB and KBR before and after PE.

DISCUSSION

Since 1985, we have used AKBR [3] as the most important parameter in the criteria of hepatic failure. AKBR was proposed by Dr Ozawa in Kyoto University as redox theory in 1980. The redox theory was formulated on the basis of a relationship between redox state and AKBR [1, 3]. The hepatic mitochondria play an important role in the energy production of the hepatocyte. When the hepatic mitochondrial redox state shifts from an oxidized state to reduced state, the hepatic energy charge decreases. This shift in the redox state reflected by *in vivo* changes in AKBR. Therefore, through the measurement of AKBR, we can estimate hepatic mitochondrial function without taking a biopsy of hepatic tissue.

Liver is the most important organ in regulating energy metabolism and PE has been widely applied for treatment of hepatic failure. However, there are few reports concerning the effects of PE on hepatic cellular energy metabolism [4, 5]. Therefore, we investigate the effects of PE on hepatic cellular energy metabolism using AKBR as a parameter.

PE seemed not to affect the redox state of hepatocytes since KBR did not change significantly. However, since approximately 3200 ml of FFP was replaced, it seems to be reasonable to assume that those values decrease significantly after PE compared with those in arterial blood. However, no significant change in the values of ACAC, BOHB and KBR was observed with PE. These results suggest that the production of ACAC and BOHB in the liver could be increased significantly and that the increased KBR could be due to more improvement in the production of ACAC compared with that of BOHB. This hypothesis was supported by the *in vitro* experiment using the one pool model in this study.

The reduction rates of T.Bil with PA and PE were over 40% and there was no significant difference between PA and PE. However, PA decreased the HPT value significantly and also has no ability of supplementation of necessary substances such as coagulation factors. Therefore PA should not be applied to patients with depleted ABBR and HPT.

CONCLUSION

PE should be chosen as a first artificial liver support in the treatment of hepatic failure. Then, either PE or PA should be chosen according to the values of AKBR, T.Bil and HPT. Furthermore, PA should be preferred to PE in the treatment of hyperbilirubinemia without depleted AKBR and HPT.

REFERENCES

1. D. H. Williamson, P. Lund, H. A. Krebs *et al.* The redox state of free nicotinamide-adenine dinucleotide in cytoplasma and mitochondria of rat liver. *Biochem. J.*, **103**, 514–526 (1967).
2. J. A. Surgent and F. A. Gotch. Mathematic modeling of dialysis therapy. *Kidney Int.*, **18**, 2–10 (1980).
3. K. Ozawa, H. Aoyama, Y. Yasuda *et al.* Metabolic abnomalities associated with postoperative organ failure — a redox theory. *Arch. Surg.*, **118**, 1245–1251 (1983).
4. Y. Ohtake, H. Hirasawa, T. Sugai *et al.* Effect of plasma exchange and plasma perfusion on redox status of liver. *Jpn. J. Artif. Organs*, **18**, 1286–1289 (1989).
5. Y. Ohtake, H. Hirasawa, T. Sugai *et al.* The effects of plasma exchange on hepatic cellular metabolism. *Artif. Organs*, **14** (Suppl. 2), 182–184 (1990).

Therapeutic Plasmapheresis (XII), pp. 211-214
T. Agishi *et al.* (Eds)
© VSP 1993

Development of Poly-HEMA Coated Anion-exchange Resin Adsorbent for Removal of Bilirubin in Plasma Perfusion Treatment

S. NAKAJI, Y. INUKAI and K. TAKAKURA

Kuraray Co., Ltd, Kurashiki, Japan

Key words: adsorption column; plasma perfusion; anion-exchange resin; poly-HEMA; hyperbilirubinemia.

INTRODUCTION

Plasma exchange has been widely used for the treatment of liver failure to remove pathogenic or toxic substances. However, this method has the disadvantage that a large quantity of replacement fluid (fresh frozen plasma or albumin preparations) is required, consequently leading to possible risk of viral infection. Therefore, in recent years, the clinical usefulness of plasma perfusion using selective adsorbents has increasingly been recognized.

We have developed a new selective adsorbent for bilirubin, Medisorba BL, using a biocompatible poly-2-hydroxyethyl methacrylate (PHEMA) coated anion-exchange resin, which is highly effective for the clinical treatment of hyperbilirubinemia.

MATERIALS AND METHODS

Porous-type anion-exchange resin beads (diameter $400\,\mu$m), based on styrene–divinyl-benzene copolymer BPR (Mitsubishi Chem. Inc.) was chosen as an effective adsorbent [1]. To improve the blood compatibility of the adsorbent and to prevent the release of microparticles from the porous resin beads, the resin beads were coated by hydrophilic poly-HEMA containing 0.5% glycidyl methacrylate as a comonomer.

The *in vitro* study on the adsorption performance was carried out as follows. In batchwise test for bilirubin adsorption, 1 ml of saline was added to 0.1 g dry, coated adsorbent, and then treated with 1 ml of plasma from patients with hyperbilirubinemia for 1 h at 37°C, the concentrations of bilirubins were measured. In batchwise test for plasma protein adsorption, 1 ml of saline was added to 0.3 g dry, coated adsorbent, then treated with 1 ml of fresh plasma from healthy volunteers for 2 h at 37°C, and the concentrations of plasma proteins were measured. In column perfusion test, the column (300 ml) was packed with the adsorbent and patient plasma (3000 ml) was perfused through it at a flow rate of 30 ml/min for 3 h, at 37°C. The concentrations of bilirubins in the plasma were measured.

For clinical applications, the plasma perfusion column, Medisorba BL, which contains 300 ml of the coated resin beads, sterilized by autoclaving has been developed. The priming volume is 110 ml. The plasma perfusion treatment was performed by using a PVA plasma separator and KM-8800 monitor (Kuraray), at Toranomon hospital, Tokyo [2] and Okayama University Hospital [3].

RESULTS AND DISCUSSION

Figure 1 shows the comparison of the bilirubin adsorption rate of anion-exchange resins (porous and gel-type) and activated carbon. The porous type resin (BPR) exhibited excellent adsorptive property compared with the non-porous gel type one and activated carbon.

The effect of poly-HEMA coating of the porous resin on the adsorption rate of bilirubins and plasma proteins are shown in Figs 2 and 3, respectively. With increasing the amount of the coating, the adsorption of plasma proteins such as albumin, globulin

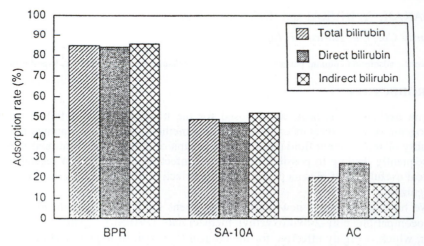

Figure 1. Bilirubin adsorption rate of anion-exchange resins and activated carbon (batchwise experiment). BPR: porous type anion-exchange resin. SA-10A: gel type (non-porous) anion-exchange resin. AC: activated carbon.

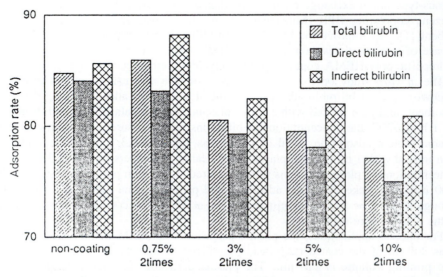

Figure 2. Effect of PHEMA coating on bilirubin adsorption. PHEMA coating conditions: concentration of PHEMA solution (%) and number of coatings (times).

and fibrinogen was reduced, while the adsorption rate of bilirubin tended to gradually decrease. In the *in vitro* column perfusion study, the optimally coated adsorbent showed an excellent adsorption performance for bilirubin and bile acid. The removal rate of total bilirubin was 65% as is seen in Fig. 4. Both direct and indirect bilirubin were adsorbed in the same way. The safety of the coated adsorbent was confirmed by various biological toxicity tests.

In the clinical evaluation, totally 72 plasma perfusion treatments were performed for 14 patients with hyperbilirubinemia. The average volume of plasma treated by each plasma perfusion was 3700 ml. The average removal rates of total bilirubin, direct

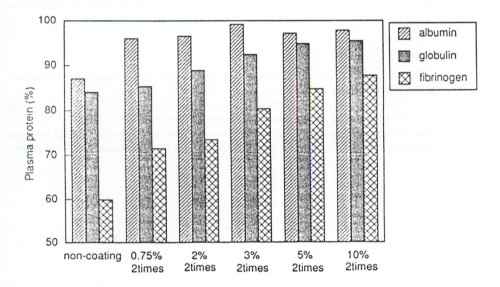

Figure 3. Effect of PHEMA coating on plasma protein levels. PHEMA coating conditions: concentration of PHEMA solution (%) and number of coatings (times).

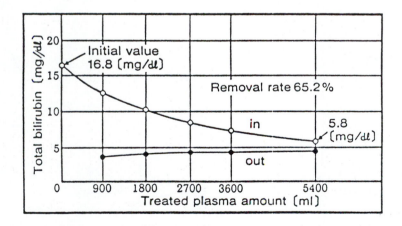

Figure 4. Adsorption performance of total bilirubin (column perfusion).

bilirubin and indirect bilirubin were 35.5, 38.0 and 36.1%, respectively. The bilirubin adsorption capacity of this column was estimated to be more than 5 l of treated plasma volume. No adverse effects were observed during the treatments.

CONCLUSIONS

The new porous type anion-exchange resin showed excellent adsorption performance for bilirubin compared with the gel type (non-porous) ones. The poly-HEMA coating reduced the plasma protein adsorption as well as the release of micro-particles from the adsorbent. The adsorption column exhibited a highly increased adsorption capacity of 5 l and removal rate of 65% *in vitro*. The effectiveness and usefulness of Medisorba BL has been demonstrated in the clinical treatment of hyperbilirubinemia.

REFERENCES

1. T. Watanabe, O. Otsubo, N. Iwadate *et al.* Development of porous type anion exchange resin for purpose of removal of bilirubin. *Jpn. J. Artif. Organs*, **14**, 236–239 (1985).
2. Y. Suzuki, T. Morita, H. Hasegawa *et al.* Clinical performance of an artificial liver support system in severe liver failure: evaluation of four systems. *Ther. Plasmapheresis*, **9**, 77–80 (1991).
3. K. Kabutan, F. Kosaka, S. Mizobuchi *et al.* Comparison of an anion-exchange resin with an uncoated powdered charcoal column in treatment by plasma perfusion. *Ther. Plasmapheresis*, **9**, 335–338 (1991).

Therapeutic Plasmapheresis (XII), pp. 215-218
T. Agishi *et al.* (Eds)
© VSP 1993

Plasma Exchange for 16 Postoperative Liver Failure Patients: A Clinical and Histological Study

Y. ASANUMA, K. KOYAMA, H. NANJO, S. MIYAGATA[1] and K. SAITO[2]

Departments of Surgery, [1]Urology and [2]Pathology, Akita University, Akita, Japan

Key words: plasma exchange; postoperative liver failure; liver cirrhosis; hepatectomy; liver regeneration.

INTRODUCTION

In 7 years, 16 cases of postoperative liver failure were treated with plasma exchange (PE) and five survived. Among the 11 cases who died, seven underwent autopsy. Using these autopsied liver specimens, the significance of PE in cases of postoperative liver failure has been examined.

MATERIALS AND METHODS

The 16 cases are summarized in Table 1. The preceding operations were abdominal surgery in 10 and cardiovascular surgery in six. Autopsy was carried out in seven cases (cases 2, 3, 4, 7, 9, 12 and 16) and their liver specimens were analyzed histologically.

RESULTS

Causes of postoperative liver failure
Postoperative liver failure in the five patients who suffered from HCC on liver cirrhosis resulted from excessive operative insult during hepatectomy (cases 1–5). In cases 6, the short hepatic vein was damaged during surgery, resulting in the loss of 14 860 ml of blood. The patient's blood pressure was below 80 mm Hg for 3 h 20 min, and such hepatic circulatory disturbance was believed to be the cause of the liver failure. Case 7 suffered from fulminant hepatitis induced by halothane or antibiotics. Case 8 suffered from secondary biliary cirrhosis due to postoperative bile duct stricture that occurred after right hepatic lobectomy. Plasma exchange was performed to improve hyperbilirubinemia and mental disturbance. Two patients (cases 9 and 10) developed diffuse peritonitis as a result of anastomotic leakage and peritonitis was believed to be the cause of the hepatic failure. The main cause of liver failure in six patients (cases 11–16) was believed to be a disturbance of hepatic circulation resulting from excessive operative insult. The amount of blood loss ranged from 2430 to 7315 ml and the length of low blood pressure ranged from 0 to 5 h 30 min.

Table 1.
Cases with postoperative liver failure

Case			Disease	Associated chronic liver disease	Operation	Blood loss (ml)	Op time	BP< 80 mmHg time	Initial T.B. (mg/dl)	OP–PE days	Times of PE	Outcome	Liver weight at autopsy (g)
1.	55	M	HCC	+	hepatic resection	3015	5 h 50 min	0	26.4	23	6	alive	—
2.	55	M	HCC	+	hepatic resection	1838	6 h 35 min	0	33.5	27	6	dead	930
3.	75	M	HCC	+	hepatic resection	1696	5 h 35 min	0	6.8	9	9	dead	800
4.	72	F	HCC	+	hepatic resection	3077	7 h	0	13.8	12	6	dead	1400
5.	54	M	HCC	+	hepatic resection	11194	14 h 45 min	30 min	19.8	7	2	dead	—
6.	50	M	HCC	–	hepatic resection	14860	16 h 40 min	3 h 20 min	13.6	10	4	alive	—
7.	63	M	gastric cancer	–	gastrectomy	160	2 h 30 min	0	7.5	16	6	dead	735
8.	50	M	liver injury	–	hepatic resection	2330	6 h 50 min	0	15.3	350	116	dead	—
9.	26	M	gastric cancer	–	gastrectomy	889	4 h 30 min	0	8.7	149	13	dead	1650
10.	48	M	colon laceration SMV rupture	–	colectomy hemostasis	1920	4 h 30 min	4h 35 min	15.0	47	2	alive	—
11.	57	F	Budd–Chiari syndrome	+	IVC–RA bypass	2430	7 h 20 min	0	4.4	8	5	alive	—
12.	55	M	aortic regurgitation	+	re AVR	7315	14 h 50 min	1 h	27.5	14	6	dead	1800
13.	29	M	aneurysma dissecans	–	bypass	4168	9 h 30 min	1 h 30 min	13.2	16	5	alive	—
14.	55	F	combined valvular disease	+	re MVR, TVR	5200	13 h 30 min	6 h	32.6	18	5	dead	—
15.	44	F	combined valvular disease	+	MVR, AVR	6553	7 h 15 min	2 h 30 min	55.2	20	10	dead	—
16.	65	M	arch aneurysm	–	arch reconstruction	4700	16 h 10 min	5 h 30 min	11.1	39	18	dead	2080

Histological examinations of the liver

Histological findings of the liver at the operation and autopsy were comparatively shown in Table 2. Of case 2, moderate mononuclear cell infiltration and P-P bridging fibrosis were found in the portal area of the non-cancerous part of the liver obtained during surgery, indicating chronic active hepatitis. Of the autopsied liver specimen, prominent expansion of the portal area and pseudoductular proliferation and fibrosis of the surrounding area were observed. The parenchyma/interstitium ratio was decreased from 86 to 65%, indicating prominent postoperative liver cell necrosis. Cases 3 and 4 show the similar decrease of liver cell volume at autopsy. Of case 7, the autopsied liver weighed only 735 g and showed extensive hepatic necrosis histologically. Of case 12, enlargement of portal area and pseudoductular proliferation were observed; however, liver cell necrosis was not seen and the parenchyma/interstitium ratio was as much as 75%.

Table 2.
Histologic findings of seven autopsied cases

Case	2		3		4		7	9	12	16
	op	Sek	op	Sek	op	Sek	Sek	Sek	Sek	Sek
Hepatic lesion	CAH	CAH IHCS	CAH	CAH IHCS	LC	LC IHCS	*	IHCS	IHCS	IHCS
Parenchyma/ interstitium	86%	65%	90%	77%	79%	45%	13%	75%	75%	60%
Liver cell necrosis	±	++	±	+	−	+++	++++	+	±	+++
Fatty degeneration	−	−	−	−	−	−	−	+++	−	+++
Cholestasis	−	++	−	++	−	++	±	+	++	+++
Pseudoductule	−	+	−	+	−	++	±	+	++	++

CAH, chronic active hepatitis; IHCS, intrahepatic cholestasis; LC, liver cirrhosis; Sek, autopsy,
*fulminant hepatitis, drug-induced.

DISCUSSION

Babior [1] divided the postoperative liver failure into two categories. In the 'hepatitis' category, liver necrosis progressed quickly, with many of the patients dying within 3–5 days. In the 'vascular' category, liver necrosis developed slow and long after cardiovascular surgery, or shock due to cardiac failure, sepsis or hemorrhage. The structure of the liver was in relatively good shape. Sherlock [2] stated with regard to 'vascular' liver necrosis that jaundice occurred in 20 percent of heart surgery cases in which a pump-oxygenator was used and that the prognosis is particularly bad in patients over 50 years of age. Of the 16 patients examined in this study, one was placed in the 'hepatitis' category (case 7) and 7 in the 'vascular' category (cases 6 and 11–16). Five of the patients (cases 1–5) suffered from liver failure due to deterioration of a pre-existing liver disorder by excessive operative insult.

Judging from the present study, it is believed that operative insult should be lessened in cases of liver cirrhosis, as the liver regeneration cannot be expected during plasma exchange (cases 2–5). Conversely, plasma exchange is efficacious in cases with normal liver (case 6). Plasma exchange is believed to be useful in cases of fulminant hepatitis as long as regeneration is possible, but ineffective in our patient (case 7) with almost total effacement of hepatocytes. Plasma exchange is useful in cases of hepatic failure induced by peritonitis accompanying anastomotic leakage with no pre-existing liver disorders (case 10). Patients with 'vascular' liver necrosis could be saved by temporarily supporting the liver with plasma exchange while the cardiac failure is being treated effectively (cases 11–16).

REFERENCES

1. B. M. Babior and C. S. Davidson. Postoperative liver necrosis. *N. Engl. J. Med.*, **276**, 645–652 (1967).
2. D. S. Sherlock. The hepatic artery and hepatic veins: the liver in circulatory failure. In: *Diseases of the Liver and Biliary System,* 7th edn., pp. 182–198, Blackwell Scientific Publications, Oxford (1985).

Therapeutic Plasmapheresis (XII), pp. 219-222
T. Agishi *et al.* (Eds)
© VSP 1993

A Case with Alcoholic Fulminant Hepatitis-induced Acute Hepatic and Renal Failures, and Obtained Lifesaving by using Plasma Exchange, Plasma Adsorption, Hemofiltration and Hemodialysis

K. OTSUBO, S. UEDA, Y. TAKIGAWA, K. AOYAGI, M. TSUJI,
Y. TERASAKI, R. KUSABA, I. TAKAHASHI, H. NOZAKI and T. INAO

Sangenjaya Hospital, 1-21-5, Sangenjaya Setagaya-ku, Tokyo, Japan

Key words: alcoholic fulminant hepatitis; hepatic coma; alcoholic rhabdomyolysis; acute renal failure; plasma exchange.

INTRODUCTION

In recent years, increasing tendency of death due to acute alcoholism has been a social problem. This time, we report a case (a 21 year old male) with hemorrhage of the digestive tract, hemorrhagic spots of the skin, and hepatic coma which reached grade III–IV because of alcoholic fulminant hepatitis after massive drinking, and complicated with acute renal failure because of rhabdomyolysis due to the acute alcoholic myopathy. We achieved lifesaving by using plasma exchange (PE), plasma adsorption (PA), hemofiltration (HF) and hemodialysis (HD). From the results, it was considered that active extensive treatment of this disease is very important.

CASE REPORT

This case is a 21 year old male employee. Chief complaints were abdominal pain, hematemesis, melena and fever. Familial history revealed no specific findings. Past history of illness showed a habitual heavy drinker (drinking of 2 l of beer, 700 ml of low-class distilled spirits or half bottle of whisky per day).

Present history of illness

This patient drunk a massive amount of alcohol for 2 consecutive days. The patient was admitted to our hospital because of upper abdominal pain, hematemesis, melena, palpitation and fever.

Findings on admission

The findings such as almost clear consciousness, facial pallor, edematous state, body temperature of 38.6 °C, regular pulse rate of 135/min, blood pressure of 150/80 mmHg, conjunctival injection of eyelids, jaundice of conjunctiva bulvi, palpation of the 4th finger breadths, hepatic mass, tenderness, abdominal distention and rigidity, subcutaneous hemorrhagic spots, and decrease of bowel sound were observed. The subcutaneous hemorrhagic spots in extremities and edema in the pretibial region were observed.

General test and clinical course on admission

As shown in Fig. 1, rapid deterioration of the consciousness level and exacerbation of the hepatic coma progressed into grade II, III and IV were observed. Laboratory studies showed high levels such as 215 of GOT, 40 of GPT, 695 of γ-GTP, 5.3 mg/dl of total bilirubin, 3.0 mg/dl of direct bilirubin and 109 mg/dl of ammonia. Anemia of 9.0 g/dl of hemoglobin and 26.1% of hematocrit were also observed. The remarkable decrease of the platelet 1.4×10^4 was observed. The decrease of fibrinogen 93 mg/dl and remarkable reduction of prothrombin activity 25% were observed. The decreases such as cholinesterase 1493 mU/ml and hepaplastin test 39% were observed.

Glucagon–insulin therapy, drip infusion of aminoleban and prednisolone therapy were carried out, and in addition to these therapies, therapy by combined use of PA, HF, PE and HD was performed as shown in Fig. 1; 7.8 l of the isolated plasma went through the adsorbent, N-350 (a product of Asahi Medical Co., Ltd). PE using 50 units of fresh frozen plasma was carried out on the 4th and 8th hospital days. Coma grade was improved from IV to II.

As shown for renal functions in Fig. 2, normal levels of BUN 16.2 mg/dl and creatinine 1.1 mg/dl were observed, but BUN 75.9 mg/dl and creatinine 5.1 mg/dl elevated on the 7th hospital day. The decrease of the urinary output 1500–2000 ml/day was not observed. An abnormally high level of myoglobin in the blood 1400 mg/dl was observed, and CPK elevated to 1328 mU/ml. Acute renal failure due to rhabdomyolysis

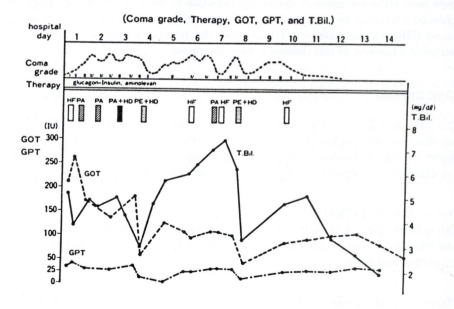

Figure 1. Clinical course of the alcoholic fulminant hepatitis.

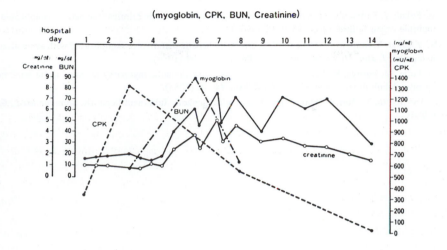

Figure 2. Acute renal failuer due to alcoholic rhabdomyolysis.

was considered because elevation of myoglobin in the blood was observed, and abdominal pain, myalgia of extremities and muscle weakness of extremities were complained of. Renal failure was improved by HF and HD.

DISCUSSION

The therapeutic combined use of PE, PA, HF and HD was useful in alcoholic fulminant hepatitis induced acute hepatic and renal failures. The early diagnosis of liver failure and early treatment including perfusion of the blood were necessary for improving the survival rate because the survival rate in patients with alcoholic fulminant hepatitis who revealed multiple organ failure (MOF) is extremely low. The case within 2 months until death by liver failure after development of the ascites or jaundice is defined as an alcoholic fulminant hepatitis, and many death cases by advancement of the acute hepatic failure due to the complications of MOF with ascites, jaundice and encephlopathy have been reported. A case (a habitual drinker) represented by us was complicated by MOFs including renal failure by acute alcoholic hepatitis and alcoholic myositis due to massive drinking. It was considered that not only conservative therapies but also early perfusion of the blood are effective for the improvement of clinical findings, and improvement and regeneration of destroyed hepatic cells from viewpoints of the impaired function of the reticulo-endothelial system, and participation of endotoxemia and immunological mechanisms.

CONCLUSION

This patient, with multiple organ failures such as hepatic failure, renal failure, hemorrhage of the digestive tract and disseminated intravascular coagulation (DIC), was saved by active therapy using PA, HF, PE and HD.

REFERENCES

1. M. Fukui, T. Furukawa, M. Kurosawa *et al.* A case with alcoholic fulminant hepatitis complicated with multiple organ failure. *Liver*, **95**, 1507 (1987).

2. N. Yoshida, Y. Sumino, Y. Ueno *et al.* A case with hepatic disturbance complicated with acute alcoholic myopathy. *J. Jpn. Digestive Organ Ass.*, **86**, 1701–1704 (1989).

3. M. Fujie, M. Furuya, H. Yanagisawa *et al.* A case with alcoholic myopathy revealed acute renal failure by myoglobulinuria. *J. Jpn. Intern. Med. Ass.*, **74**, 78 (1985).

4. S. Yamamoto, T. Hori, N. Ohgi *et al.* A case with alcoholic fulminant hepatitis. *Shimane Med.*, **6**, 122 (1986).

Therapeutic Plasmapheresis (XII), pp. 223-227
T. Agishi *et al.* (Eds)
© VSP 1993

Clinical Study of Continuous Hemofiltration in Hepatic Failure — Mainly Improvement of Hepatic Encephalopathy

S. MORIISHI, Y. MIYOSHI, S. NAKAYAMA and Y. SUMIDA

Department of Internal Medicine and Surgery, Saisei Foundation Hiroshima Hospital, Japan

Key words: continuous hemofiltration; plasma exchange; multiple organ failure; hepatic failure; hepatic encephalopathy.

INTRODUCTION

Plasma exchange or bilirubin absorption has been generally used for treatment of hepatic failure, while its life-saving rate is still low. We attempted continuous hemofiltration (CHF) in addition to these therapeutic methods and studied improvement of hepatic encephalopathy due to removal of substances with low-to-middle molecular weights in blood.

MATERIAL AND METHODS

CHF or continuous hemodia-filtration (CHDF) was carried out in 12 cases with hepatic failure including multiple organ failure (MOF). The single dose more than 6000 ml of Subload or Sorita for HF was administered by using PS or PAN membrane. This dose was administered in cases using PE concomitantly for a long term (Table 1).

RESULTS

CHF was extremely useful because improvement of the consciousness level was observed in 11 of 12 cases (Table 1, Fig. 1) Fischer's ratio was remarkably improved before and after CHF (Figs 1 and 2). In particularly, aromatic amino acid and ammonia were markedly normalized (Figs 1, 2 and 3).

The comparison of the electroencephalogram (EEG) is shown in the Fig. 4. The improvement of the EEG was clearly observed. The variation of the EEG from delta wave (δ) to theta wave (θ) is mainly observed. However, the normal EEG cannot be observed by the theta wave.

Moreover, all cases showing metabolic acidosis and hypoxia were also improved.

Table 1.

Patients with liver failure treated by CHF and other extracorporeal blood purification therapy

Diagnosis		No. of cases (survivor)	No. of treatments
LC		2(1)	13 (5 CHF, 3 PE, 5 PP)
PBC		1(0)	3 (CHF only)
HCC	(hepatic resection)	2(1)	34 (7 CHF, 23 PE, 2 PP, 2 HD)
	others	1(1)	3 (CHF only)
Adenocarcinoma of CBD (pancreatico-duodenectomy)		2(1)	10 (9 CHF, 1 PP)
MOF	septic shock	2(1)	13 (10 CHF, 3 HD)
	others	2(0)	5 (CHF only)
Total		12(5)	81 (42 CHF, 26 PE, 8 PP, 5HD)

CHF, continuous hemofiltration; PE, plasma exchange; PP, plasma perfusion; HD, hemodialysis.

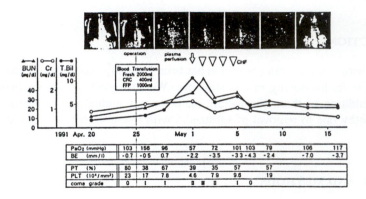

Figure 1. The clinical course of a 77 years old man with adenocarcinoma of common bile duct who developed MOF, evidenced by grade III coma and hypoxia, after pancreatico-duodenectomy. The patient survived following 4 days of CHF and 1 session of plasma perfusion.

The number of patients and the survival rate which were carried out CHF and plasmapheresis except for CHF in our hospital are shown in Table 1. The survival rate was approximately 42%.

The pulmonary edema or ARDS was remarkably improved by using CHF, and arterial oxygen (PaO$_2$) was also normalized.

DISCUSSION

Elevations of the conscious level and Fischer's rate, and improvement of the rate of ketone body by using CHF were observed because the condition of hypoxia might be improved.

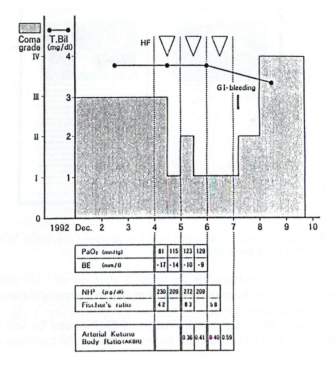

Figure 2. The clinical course of a 59 years old woman with PBC who developed liver failure. The patient died 6 days after three sessions of hemofiltration (HF) because of hepatic coma.

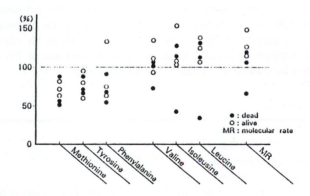

Figure 3. Change of plasma amino acid level (Met, AAA, BCAA, MR) before and after CHF therapy.

The progress of aromatic amino acids (AAA) and branched-chain amino acids (BCAA) before and after the use of CHF are shown in Fig. 2. The decreasing tendency of AAA and elevating tendency of BCAA are observed after use of CHF. The elevating tendency of rate of molecular weight in these acids, so-called Fischer's rate, is observed.

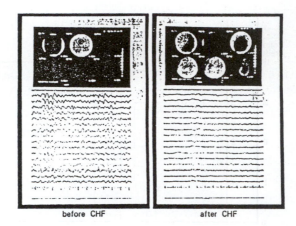

before CHF   after CHF

Figure 4. EEG findings of 54 years old man with HCC who developed liver failure, evidenced by grade III coma. EEG findings improved due to CHF.

The influence due to amino acids for revision after use of CHF may be considered because glucagon–insulin therapy and revision of the amino acids are simultaneously carried out at hepatic failure.

The contradiction for technical application of CHF cannot be felt because plasma exchange (PE) with high level technique has been used for the treatment of the fulminant hepatitis.

CONCLUSIONS

The early improvement of hepatic failure was necessiated because this disease is considered to be a preparatory state of MOF. Various toxic substances with low to high molecular weights occur in hepatic encephalopathy, while removal of substances less than middle molecular weight using CHF was useful as an adjuvant therapy of the metabolism, supporting hepatic function by combined use of PE even though hepatic failure cannot be completely treated by this removal.

Table 2.

General indications
    (1) overhydration
    (2) hyperkalemia
Special indications
    (1) impaired pulmonary diffusion complicated by circulatory failure
    (2) hyper natremia
    (3) multiple organ failure (MOF)
    (4) liver failure or hepatic coma
Questionable indications
    (1) intoxications through poisons or drugs
    (2) severe hyperkalencia or unbalance of mineral due to hemolysis or
        extensive tissue damage

The modification of the indication for CAVH which was proposed by Krammer *et al.* in 1988 [1] is shown in Table 2. The indication for CAVH is varied to CHF and CHDF, but its content is considered to be almost same.

The general indication for renal functional failure and circulatory kinetics is occasionally problematical. This time, encephalopathy and MOF associated with hepatic failure were particularly indicated.

REFERENCE

1. P. Krammer. Intensive care potential of continuous arteriovenous hemofiltration. *Trans. Am. Soc. Artif. Intern. Organs*, **38**, 28–33 (1982).

Therapeutic Plasmapheresis (XII), pp. 229-233
T. Agishi *et al.* (Eds)
© VSP 1993

The Indication of Plasmapheresis Application for Patients with Hepatic Failure

J. MEGURO, N. KAMII, K. ONODERA, M. TAKAHASHI,
H. WITMANOWSKI, K. KUKITA, M. YONEKAWA and A. KAWAMURA

Department of Surgery, Sapporo Hokuyu Hospital,
Artificial Organ and Transplantation Hospital, Sapporo, Japan

Key words: acute hepatic failure; plasma exchange; cryofiltration; bilirubin adsorption.

INTRODUCTION

We have been treating patients with acute hepatic failure by applying various kinds of plasmapheresis. The purpose of treatment is to support them over a period of severe hepatic damage until hepatocytes may regenerate. The state and the cause of acute hepatic failure are important factors for selecting the method of plasmapheresis, such as plasma exchange (PE) [1], cryofiltration (CRYO) [2] and bilirubin adsorption (BA).

MATERIALS AND METHODS

From January 1985 to December 1991, we treated 44 patients with acute hepatic failure, 19 patients with fulminant hepatic failure, 13 with acute on chronic liver diseases, five with post-operative hepatic failure, three with drug-induced hepatic failure and four with other hepatic failure were treated with plasmapheresis (Table 1). PE was performed 183 times. CRYO was performed 95 times and BA was performed 6 times.

Table 1.

Disease	Number	Plasmapheresis			Survival rate
		PE	CRYO	BA	
Fulminant hepatic failure	19	107	51	2	7/19 (36.8%)
Liver cirrhosis	13	56	30	0	0/13 (0%)
Post-operative hepatic failure	5	0	7	4	0/5 (0%)
Drug induced hepatic failure	3	9	6	0	1/3 (33.3%)
Others	4	11	1	0	3/4 (75.0%)
Total	44	183	95	6	11/44 (25.0%)

RESULTS

The survival rate of the patients with fulminant hepatic failure is 36.8%. The overall survival rate is 25%.

PE

The purpose of PE is to remove coma substances, to remove toxic substances and to supply indispensable proteins, such as albumin and coagulation factors. The indication of PE is for the patient with hepatic coma and for the patient with drug-induced hepatic failure.

Eighteen of 19 patients with fulminant hepatic failure were treated with PE. The rate of consciousness improvement was 66.7%. The survival rate was 33.3%. Eleven of 13 patients with liver cirrhosis as acute on chronic hepatic failure received PE. Among 11 patients, only three cases awoke from deep coma and none survived. The total rate of consciousness improvement cases and survivors were 50 and 21.9%, respectively (Table 2).

Table 2.

Disease	Number	Improvement of consciousness	Survival rate
Fulminant hepatic failure	18	12/18 (66.7%)	6/18 (33.3%)
Liver cirrhosis	11	3/11 (27.3%)	0/11 (0%)
Drug	2	1/2 (50.0%)	1/2 (50.0%)
Others	1	0/1 (0%)	0/1 (0%)
Total	32	16/32 (50.0%)	7/32 (21.9%)

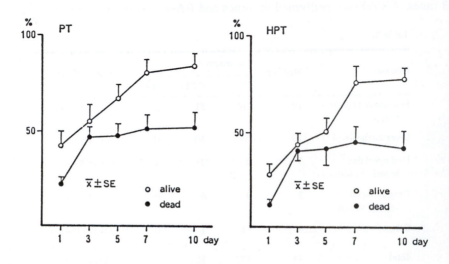

Figure 1.

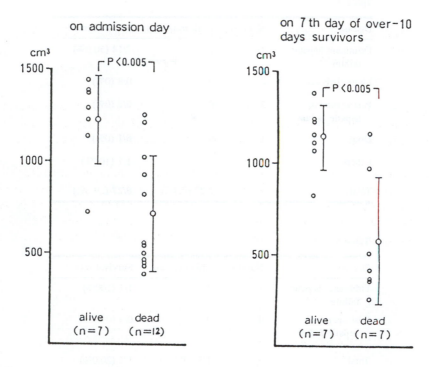

Figure 2.

The activity of PT and HPT of survivors of fulminant hepatic failure on admission day were $42.7 \pm 7.8\%$ and $28.6 \pm 4.6\%$, respectively. The activity of fatal cases on admission day were 21.2 ± 3.2 and $11.6 \pm 2.5\%$, respectively. The difference of PT and HPT between survivors and non-survivors was significant on the 10th day (Fig. 1).

As the indicator of the prognosis of the patients with fulminant hepatic failure, the liver volume calculated by CT is very useful [3]. The values for survivors and non-survivors on admission day were 1221.6 ± 242.0 and $713.5 \pm 315.5 \text{cm}^3$, respectively. On the 7th day, the liver volume between survivors and non-survivors was significant (Fig. 2).

CRYO

Cryofiltration was applied to 27 cases with slight disturbance of consciousness and/or hyperbilirubinemia after the improvement of consciousness [1]. Only two patients with fulminant hepatic failure had a good response (Table 3).

BA

Bilirubin adsorption was performed for one patient with fulminant hepatic failure and four cases with post-operative hepatic failure. In these five cases, only one patient with fulminant hepatic failure survived using BA (Table 4). The indication of BA is to remove the danger of complications due to hyperbilirubinemia.

Table 3.

Disease	Number	High responder	Survival rate
Fulminant hepatic failure	14	2	7/14 (50.0%)
Liver cirrhosis	8	0	0/8 (0%)
Post-operative hepatic failure	3	0	0/3 (0%)
Drug	1	0	0/1 (0%)
Others	1	0	1/1 (100%)
Total	27	2/27 (7.4%)	8/27 (29.6%)

Table 4.

Disease	Number	Effective case	Survival rate
Fulminant hepatic failure	1	1	1/1 (100%)
Post-operative hepatic failure	4	0	0/4 (0%)
Total	5	1/5 (20.0%)	1/5 (20.0%)

Table 5.

Plasma exchange	($n = 20$)	$67.4 \pm 7.6\%$
Cryofiltration	($n = 24$)	$22.9 \pm 10.7\%$
Bilirubin adsorption	($n = 5$)	$40.7 \pm 11.1\%$

We tried to calculate the removal rate of serum bilirubin compared with two other methods. The processed plasma volume of each procedure was 4 l. PE was the most effective method for the removal of serum bilirubin. However, for only the reduction of serum bilirubin, level, BA was useful from the point of view of economics and side-effect problems (Table 5).

DISCUSSION

Figure 3 shows the role and indication of each plasmapheresis. PE should be applied only in case of coma. CRYO is useful for some patients after the improvement of consciousness as a method of immunomodulation. It is difficult for patients of post-operative hepatic failure with infection and patients with liver cirrhosis to survive.

The beneficial effects of PE have been evident in acute hepatic failure [1]. On the other hand, PE has some demerits, such as high-cost, viral infection and anaphylaxis [1].

Role & Indication of Plasmapheresis

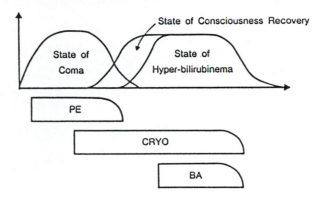

Figure 3.

CRYO has no notable side-effects. These treatments should be tried in the proper state of the clinical course on hepatic failure, in which patients may have the possibility of recovery.

REFERENCES

1. M. Yonekawa, J. Meguro, K. Kukita *et al.* Positive and negative effects of plasma exchange. *Artif. Organs*, **14** (Suppl. 2), 185–187 (1990).
2. Y. Nosé, P. S. Malchesky, J. W. Smith and R. S. Krakauer. *Plasmapheresis: Therapeutic Applications and New Techniques*. Raven Press, New York (1983).
3. K. Kukita, A. Kawamura, T. Ariyama *et al.* Rationality of plasma exchange therapy based on periodic liver CT volume calculation in patients with fulminant hepatitis. In: *Apheresis*, pp. 237–238, Alan R. Liss, New York (1990).

Role & Indication of Plasmaphoresis

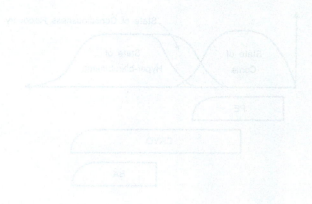

Figure 1.

CRYO has no notable side-effects. These treatments should be tried at the patient state of the clinical course on hepatic failure, in which patients may have the possibility of recovery.

REFERENCES

1. J. M. Yonekawa, J. Megami, K. Kakita et al. Positive and negative effects of plasma exchange, *New Digest*, 14 (Suppl 3), 165–167 (1990).
2. K. Ness, Z. S. Malchesky, J. W. Smith and R. S. Kolff (Eds), *Plasmapheresis: Therapeutic Applications and new Techniques*, Raven Press, New York (1980).
3. K. Kajita, A. Kawamura, T. Aoyama et al. Effectiveness of plasma exchange therapy based on periodic hepatCT volume calculation in patients with fulminant hepatitis, in *Apheresis*, pp. 157–175, Alan R. Liss, New York (1990).

6
Neurological Diseases

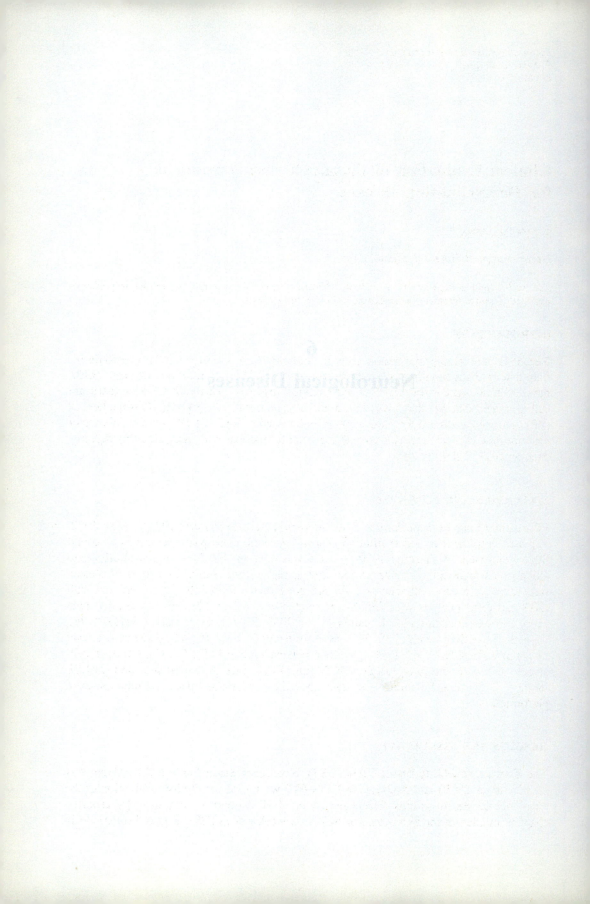

6

Neurological Diseases

Therapeutic Plasmapheresis (XII), pp. 237-238
T. Agishi *et al.* (Eds)
© VSP 1993

Clinical Evaluation of Plasmapheresis Treatment for Demyelinating Disease

S. HOSOKAWA

Utano National Hospital, Kyoto, Japan

Key words: Guillain–Barré syndrome; multiple sclerosis; chronic inflammatory demyelinating polyradiculo-neuropathy; double filtration plasmapheresis; demyelinating diseases.

INTRODUCTION

Recently, demyelinating diseases such as Guillain–Barré syndrome (GBS), chronic inflammatory demyelinating polyradiculoneuropathy (CIDP) or multiple sclerosis (MS), have been thought to be types of autoimmune diseases. Demyelinating diseases are cell-mediated diseases and have abnormalities in humoral factors [1–3]. Plasmapheresis (PP) has been successfully used to treat patients with GBS, CIDP or MS. This paper describes the clinical evaluation of PP treatment for patients with demyelinating diseases such as GBS, CIDP or MS.

MATERIALS AND METHODS

PP treatment has been performed over the period from September 1984 to May 1992. A plasma separator as a first filter and separator of the plasma component as a second filter were used. A Plasouto 1000 machine was used for PP. Electrolytes solution and albumin solution (25% albumin) were used as replacement fluid. Two liters of plasma were treated in each PP therapy. Twenty six patients with MS, seven patients with GBS and three patients with CIDP were treated with PP. In MS, PP was usually done every 2 weeks for 6 months. In patients with CIDP, PP was done every 2 weeks during 3 years. In patients with GBS, PP was done every 2 days. PP was performed a total of 5 times for GBS. IgG, IgM, IgA, total plasma protein (TP), C_3, C_4, CH_{50}, T cell, B cell, NK cell activities, OKT_3, OKT_4 and OKT_8 were measured pre- and post-PP therapy. CBC, liver function, renal function and a general laboratory examination were performed.

RESULTS AND DISCUSSION

The Kurtzke Disability Status Scale (DSS), Functional Status Scale (FSS), Upper Extremity Index (UEI) and Ambulation Index (AI) were used for clinical evaluation of the treatment of MS in general. The Japan National MS Research Committee [4] reported that the incidence and symptoms of MS were weakness in 22% or gait disturbance in

24% at onset, and motor paresis in 68.4% or ataxia in 42.8% during the course of MS. In eight of 26 patients with MS, PP therapy was not effective. We did not find any kind of subjective or objective improvement.

In 18 of 26 patients with MS, subjective improvements were found. However, 18 patients with MS gradually worsened within 2–3 years. PP therapy may possibly improve the electrophysiological findings in nerves that have not yet progressed to demyelination or axonal degeneration followed by muscle denervation in patients with GBS [5]. In seven patients with GBS, all seven patients improved with PP treatment (see Table 1.)

Table 1.
The change of functional grade in GBS with PP therapy (GBS study Group [5])

	Case						
	1	2	3	4	5	6	7
Grade	$3 \rightarrow 2$	$4 \rightarrow 2$	$4 \rightarrow 2$	$5 \rightarrow 3$	$3 \rightarrow 2$	$4 \rightarrow 2$	$3 \rightarrow 2$
Duration (days)	7	14	14	16	8	10	5

The GBS study group [5] reported that PP therapy was effective for GBS. In CIDP, chronic inflammatory demyelination may be the result of a balance between demyelination and remyelination. Macromolecular proteins may contribute to inhibit nerve remyelination because persistent conduction blocks have been found in patients with CIDP. The removal of macromolecular solutes by PP therapy might be beneficial for neurological abnormalities in CIDP patients. In three patients with CIDP, consecutive improvements of grip strength and a general striking improvement were observed during maintenance PP treatment. A recovery of proximal muscle weakness was found. PP therapy is effective for patients with CIDP.

None of the patients with demyelinating diseases such as MS, GBS or CIDP had any side effects with PP therapy.

CONCLUSION

(1) PP is a very effective and safe therapy for patients with GBS or CIDP.

(2) In patients with MS, subjective improvements were observed following PP therapy.

REFERENCES

1. S. D. Cook and D. C. Duwling. The role of autoantibody and immune complexes in the pathogenesis of Guillaine–Barré syndrome. *Ann. Neurol.,* **9,** (Suppl.), 70–79 (1981).
2. M. C. Dalakas and W. K. Engel. Chronic relapsing (dysimmune) polyneuropathy: pathogenesis and treatment. *Ann. Neurol.,* **9,** 134–145 (1981).
3. B. O. Khatri, M. P. McQuillen, G. J. Harrington *et al.* Chronic progressive multiple sclerosis: double blind controlled study of plasmapheresis in patients takings immunosuppresive drugs. *Neurology,* **35,** 312–319 (1985).
4. Y. Kuroiwa. Multiple sclerosis in Japan. In: *Multiple Sclerosis in Asia,* Japan Medical Research Foundation (Ed.), pp. 109–127, University of Tokyo Press (1976).
5. The Guillain–Barré Syndrome Study Group. Plasmapheresis and acute Guillan–Barré syndrome. *Neurology,* **35,** 1096–1104 (1985).
6. R. A. Lewis, A. J. Sumer, M. J. Brown *et al.* Multifocal demyelinating neuropathy with persistent conduction block. *Neurology,* **32,** 958–964 (1982).

Therapeutic Plasmapheresis (XII), pp. 239-242
T. Agishi *et al.* (Eds)
© VSP 1993

Immunoadsorption with Phenylalanine-immobilized Polyvinyl Alcohol versus Plasma Exchange — A Controlled Pilot Study in Multiple Sclerosis

E. SCHMITT, K. von APPEN, E. BEHM, G. KUNDT, K. LAKNER, H. MEYER-RIENECKER, M. PALM, D. SEHLAND and H. KLINKMANN

Departments of Internal Medicine and Neurology, University of Rostock, Germany

Key words: plasmasorption; PVA–phenylalanine; plasma exchange; multiple sclerosis; controlled study.

Despite tremendous efforts there is no sufficient treatment available today for MS. Immunosuppressive and immunomodulatory therapies failed to exhibit significant results. Immunopathogenesis and the poor results of traditional therapies are the reasons why plasmapheresis (PE) has been attempted in MS since 1982. Several teams reported encouraging results with PE [1–3]. Later on Weiner *et al.* [4] found a significant benefit of PE in acute attacks of MS in a controlled trial. When we started to design our protocol we learned that Shibuya [5] had been successfully treating MS by the use of phenylalanine immobilized polyvinyl alcohol (PVA–Ph). Since the etiology of MS is unknown and since there are reasons to believe that immune and inflammatory processes play an important role in MS, we decided to run a double-blind controlled trial.

Thirty patients with clinically definite MS which were either chronically progressive or in an acute exacerbation were included in the study. They were randomly allocated into groups, based on three parameters: (i) sex, (ii) age at onset of the disease (below 30 years or older) and (iii) mode of activity (chronic progression or acute beat). Before entering the study patients gave their informed consent. The ethics committee agreed upon the protocol which comprised the following three groups:

(i) *Group P.* Patients were treated with prednisolone only: 60 mg i.v. per day over 1 week. Then the dose was reduced to 30 mg per day orally which was administered over 4 weeks.

(ii) *Group PE.* The same steroid therapy as in (i). Four plasma exchange treatments were performed within 1 week. The exchange volume was 50 ml/kg body weight at each session using 5% albumin in Ringer's as a substitute.

(iii) *Group IA.* The same steroid regimen as in (i) and (ii). Within 1 week we performed four plasmasorption treatments making use of the Plasmaflo HP-05 and the immunosorbent column PH-350 (containing PVA–Ph) both from Asahi Medical Co., Tokyo, Japan. The plasma volume processed through the column was also 50 ml/kg body weight at each session.

Neurologic examination was carried out before the treatment, after 2 and 12 weeks, and after 1 year. The degree of impairment in the functional systems (FS) was measured according to Kurtzke. Disability was measured by means of the expanded disability status scale (EDSS) also after Kurtzke. Neurologists and patients were blinded as to what kind of extracorporeal treatment was applied. Thirty patients had entered the study, 11 males and 19 females. Sixteen had acute exacerbation and 14 suffered from the chronic progressive form.

When looking firstly at the EDSS results, one can see that after 2 weeks there is a poor or even no effect in the P group. A marked improvement, however, is obtained after 2 and 12 weeks in the PE and in the IA groups. A more pronounced effect is achieved in FS. It is demonstrated that prednisolone alone provides nearly none or only a questionable effect. Mainly in the IA group and less in the PE group, there is a remarkable improvement after 2 weeks which remains over a period of at least 3 months. Generally, the best results are obtained in the acute patients by application of PVA–Ph. After 1 year we found deterioration in all groups (Fig. 1). No side effects were observed in the IA and the P groups. Two of the PE patients developed weakness for a few days and one had to be operated on for a gastric ulcer due to steroids.

In trying to explain (nearly) similar effects in the extracorporeal treatments we analyzed the immunoglobulins and complement behaviour. In Fig. 2 we can see in the upper part that PE reduces immunoglobulins A, G and M as well as fibrinogen by about 75%. In the case of IA there is only a slight decrease of these proteins, by about 15–20%. Therefore the change in the immunoglobulin content cannot be responsible for the therapeutic effect. Turning to a consideration of the hemolytic activity of both the classical and alternate pathways, we found them to be significantly reduced by PE and also by IA. In Fig. 3 the CH_{50} levels of the classical and alternate pathways during the treatments are depicted. One can see a reduction of complement activity by both the IA and PE therapy by about 75% at each session. We would like to speculate that behind this complement reduction we can find the reason for the beneficial effect of both

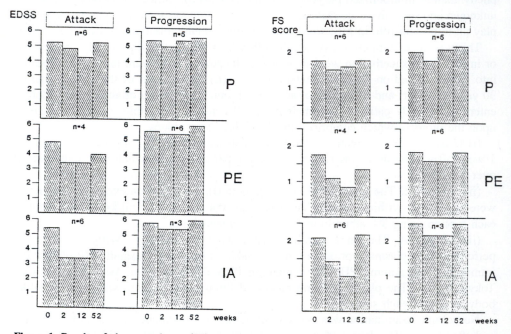

Figure 1. Results of plasma exchange (PE) and immunoadsorption (IA) in MS patients with acute attack or chronic progression.

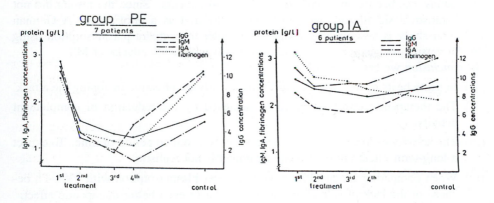

Figure 2. Changes of immunoglobulins and fibrinogen (samples taken before treatments).

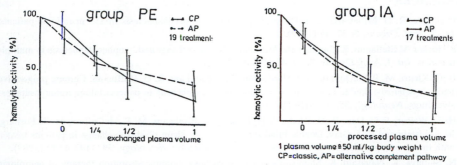

Figure 3. Changes of complement activity in the classic (CP) and alternate pathways (AP) during the procedure.

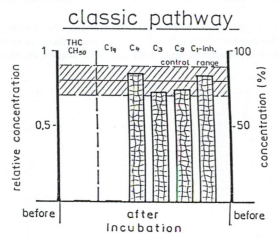

Figure 4. PVA–Ph *in vitro* adsorption of complement factors. C1q binding causes CH_{50} reduction.

extracorporeal treatments. The high capability of PVA–Ph to adsorb C1q is regarded as being responsible for the reduction of complement activity in the IA patients (Fig. 4).

The study has been completed after enroling 30 patients. Since the results did not exhibit statistical significance we had to finish the trial as a pilot study. A German multicenter study is now under preparation in order to compare plasmasorption using PVA–Ph versus prednisolone in around 60 patients with acute attacks of MS.

In *conclusion* we can state that:

(i) In acute beats of MS, the IA and PE treatments are effective in coping the attack.

(ii) The therapeutic effect seems to be achieved by the reduction of complement activity.

(iii) The activity of MS can be influenced for only a limited period of time. To expect a long-term effect after a 1 week treatment is not realistic.

(iv) When comparing IA and PE we would prefer plasmasorption with PVA–Ph because of the lack of side effects and a similar or even better therapeutic effect.

REFERENCES

1. P. C. Dau, R. G. Miller and E. H. Denys. Experience with plasmapheresis in 153 neurologic patients. *Int. J. Artif. Organs*, **5**, 37–46 (1982).

2. P. Höcker, V. Stellamor, K. Summer and M. Mann. Plasma exchange and lymphocytapheresis in multiple sclerosis. *Int. J. Artif. Organs*, **7**, 39–42 (1984).

3. B. O. Khatri, M. P. McQuillen, G. J. Harrington, D. Schmoll and R. G. Hoffmann. Chronic progressive multiple sclerosis: double blind controlled study of plasmapheresis in patients taking immunosuppressive drugs. *Neurology*, **35**, 312–319 (1985).

4. H. L. Weiner, P. C. Dau, B. O. Khatri, J. H. Petajan, G. Birnbaum, M. P. McQuillen, M. T. Fosburg, M. Feldstein and E. J. Orav. Double blind study of true vs. sham plasma exchange in patients treated with immunosuppression for acute attacks of multiple sclerosis. *Neurology*, **39**, 1143–1149 (1989).

5. N. Shibuya, K. Nagasato, K. Shibuyama and H. Kanazawa. Immunoadsorption therapy in neurologic disorders: myasthenia gravis, multiple sclerosis and Guillain–Barré-syndrome. In: *Proc. First Int. Congr. of the World Apheresis Association*, T. Oda, Y. Shiokawa and N. Inou (Eds), pp. 122–128, ISAO Press, Cleveland (1987).

6. M. Palm, E. Behm, E. Schmitt, F. Buddenhagen, B. Hitzschke, M. Kracht, G. Kundt, H. Meyer-Rienecker and H. Klinkmann. Immunoadsorption and plasma exchange in multiple sclerosis: complement and plasma protein behaviour. *Biomat. Artif. Cells Artif. Organs*, **19**, 283–296 (1991).

Therapeutic Plasmapheresis (XII), pp. 243-245
T. Agishi *et al.* (Eds)
© VSP 1993

Treatment of Guillain–Barré Syndrome with Plasma Exchange

J. M. KUTNER, A. MENDRONE Jr, A. M. SAKASHITA, M. A. MOTA,
P. E. DORLHIAC-LLACER and D. A. F. CHAMONE

*Fundação Pró-Sangue Hemocentro de São Paulo and Hematology Department,
University of São Paulo, São Paulo, Brazil*

Key words: Guillain–Barré syndrome; plasma exchange; polyneuropathy; demyelination; respiratory failure.

INTRODUCTION

Guillain–Barré syndrome (GBS), or acute inflammatory demyelinating polyneuropathy, is characterized by peripheral, bilateral, symmetric and progressive neurological impairment. Cerebrospinal fluid (CSF) shows increased albumin levels and no cellular reaction (albuminocytological dissociation). It can be seen in all age groups with a 2:1 preponderance of male patients. The incidence is reported to be 1.7 per 100 000 person-years [1].

Two features are required for the diagnosis: progressive motor weakness and areflexia. Other symptoms such as sensory loss, relative symmetry and cranial nerve involvement strongly support the diagnosis [2]. GBS may progress to respiratory failure and, despite advances in intensive care, mortality remains at 2–3% and long-term morbidity is significant [3].

Although the pathogenesis of GBS has not been elucidated, prevailing opinion is that the syndrome is the consequence of an immune-mediated process [4]. Both humoral and cellular immune mechanisms are thought to be involved [5].

The outcome in untreated patients is unpredictable. A small percentage have very little recovery at all, others undergo a gradual recovery, and may be left with residual symptoms [6]. The median time to recover from severe disease (confined to bed or requiring assisted ventilation) to mild disease (able to walk without support) is reported to be approximately 86 days [3, 6].

Plasma exchange (PE) is now the accepted therapy for GBS [7], although there are reports that do not support this affirmation [8]. In this work we describe the results obtained with a group of seven patients treated with PE and compare them with the results of the current literature.

MATERIALS AND METHODS

Between March 1990 and April 1991, seven patients with GBS (five males, two females), mean age of 28 years (range 10–69), were treated only with automated PE,
using a continuous flow blood separator (Vivacell BT-798, Dideco, Italy). On each
procedure, 1 plasma volume was exchanged for 5% albumin solution.

Patients were assessed according to the following disability scale: grade 0 = healthy;
1 = minor symptoms; 2 = able to walk 5 m without support; 3 = able to walk 5 m
with support; 4 = confined to bed or wheelchair; 5 = requiring assisted ventilation;
6 = dead [6].

The first three PEs were performed daily on consecutive days, and than 2 or 3 times
a week until grade 2 could be reached or, if no improvement was observed, a maximum
exchange of 300 ml/kg (total).

At the moment of the first procedure, five patients presented on grade 4 and two on
grade 5. The mean interval from the disease onset to the first PE was 11 days (range
4–16; median 11). None of the patients received any other specific treatment besides
PE.

RESULTS

The total volume exchanged varied from 4300 to 32 200 ml (mean 16 800 ml), in
3–40 days (mean 10; median 28). Six of the seven patients improved. From the day
of the first PE, the time interval for these six patients to reach grade 3 varied from 1
to 20 days (mean 10; median 12), and grade 2 varied from 3 to 33 days (mean 14,
median 12.5), and to discharge from hospital, from 4 to 37 days (mean 18; median 18).

Only one patient, a 69 year old male who was grade 5 at presentation, did not
improve.

There were no complications related to the therapy.

DISCUSSION AND CONCLUSIONS

The prognosis for GBS is usually good, but a proportion of the patients have a fatal
outcome during the acute illness, while others retain significant residual disability. Effective treatment is needed to reduce the mortality, maximum functional deficit, risk of
residual disability and length of hospital stay.

Controlled studies have not shown that steroids have a beneficial effect on GBS [8].

Since the first report of successful PE in GBS by Brettle in 1978 [9], several reports
have been published favoring its use early in the course of severe GBS [6]. The
rationale for using PE is the existence of a humoral factor that may reproduce the
electrophysiological and histological patterns of demyelination in animal studies [10].

The results observed in this study agree with current literature, since six of the seven
patients studied improved significantly with PE. Of interest is the shorter period of time
(median 12.5 days) necessary to reach grade 2, while other series show from 48 to
55 days (median) for the same outcome [3, 6]. Although this study has a small number
of patients, one of the possible reasons for the better outcome verified might be the
intensive program of PE used at the beginning of therapy.

The only patient who did not improve after PE had two bad prognostic factors,
according to MacKhann *et al.* [3]: his age group and grade at presentation.

Acknowledgments
Supported in part by a grant from Fundação Banco do Brasil.

REFERENCES

1. M. Alter. The epidemiology of Guillain–Barré syndrome. *Ann. Neurol.*, **17**, (Suppl.), S7–S12 (1990).

2. A. K. Asbury and D. R. Cornblath. Assessment of current diagnostic criteria for Guillain–Barré syndrome. *Ann. Neurol.*, **27**, (Suppl.), S21–S24 (1990).

3. G. M. MacKhann, J. W. Griffin, D. R. Cornblath *et al*. Plasmapheresis and Guillain–Barré syndrome: analysis of prognostic factors and the effect of plasmapheresis. *Ann. Neurol.*, **23**, 347–353 (1988).

4. D. E. MacFarlin. Immunological parameters in Guillain–Barré syndrome. *Ann. Neurol.*, **27**, (Suppl.), S25–S29 (1990).

5. L. Svennerholm and P. Fredman. Antibody detection in Guillain–Barré syndrome. *Ann. Neurol.*, **27**, (Suppl.), S36–S40 (1990).

6. J. Tharakan, R. E. Ferner, R. A. C. Hughes *et al*. Plasma exchange for Guillain–Barré syndrome. *J. Royal Soc. Med.*, **82**, 458–461 (1989).

7. G. M. McKhann. Guillain-Barré syndrome: clinical and therapeutic observations. *Ann. Neurol.*, **27**, (Suppl.), S13–S16 (1990).

8. R. J. Greenwood, R. A. C. Hughes, A. N. Bowden *et al*. Controlled trial of plasma exchange in acute inflammatory polyradiculoneuropathy. *Lancet*, **1**, 877–879 (1984).

9. R. P. Brettle, M. Gross, N. J. Legg *et al*. Treatment of acute polyneuropathy by plasma exchange. *Lancet*, **2**, 1100 (1978).

10. French Cooperative Group on Plasma Exchange in Guillain–Barré Syndrome. Efficiency of plasma exchange in Guillain–Barré syndrome: role of replacement fluids. *Ann. Neurol.*, **22**, 753–761 (1987).

Therapeutic Plasmapheresis (XII), pp. 247-252
T. Agishi *et al.* (Eds)
© VSP 1993

Beneficial Effect of Double Filtration Plasmapheresis to Patients with Guillain–Barré Syndrome

N. TAKAGI, H. ODA, Y. TAKEDA, S. YAMAGUCHI, M. YABANA,
S. TANAKA, M. MINAMIZAWA, H. SATSUTA, T. TAKIZAWA, T. IWAMOTO,
M. ISHII, H. TODA,[1] T. TAKAHASHI,[1] Y. SUZUKI[1] and O. HASEGAWA[1]

*Second Department of Internal Medicine and [1]Department of Neurology,
Yokohama City University, School of Medicine, Yokohama 236, Japan*

Key words: double filtration plasmapheresis; Guillain–Barré syndrome.

INTRODUCTION

With the progress in therapeutic plasmapheresis and the spread of its indications, the benefit of plasmapheresis has been reported on neuro-muscular diseases. We experienced two cases of patients with Guillain–Barré syndrome (GBS) respiratory deterioration classified as grade 4 that recovered immediately after performing the double filtration plasmapheresis (DFPP) therapy. In this study, we report two cases and show the beneficial effect of DFPP on GBS.

CASE 1

A 74 year old female was a patient and complained of weakness in her bilateral arms and legs and dysphagia. Her family and past histories were not mentioned this time. On October 12, 1991, she had fever at 37.5 °C and felt weakness of her arms and legs; in addition, she had difficulty in walking.

On October 15, she was not able to walk completely and entered a local hospital. She underwent treatment with 60 mg prednisolone per day, but her numbness progressed and she could not move her fingers. On October 22, she had dysphagia and difficulty in breathing, and was transferred to Yokohama City University Hospital in order to undergo therapy in the intensive care unit (ICU) room.

In her present status, her height was 154 cm, body weight was 41.6 kg and her consciousness was clear. Her blood pressure was 130/70 mmHg and her heart rate was regular at 120 per minute. Her cervical, thoracic and abdominal status were normal physically, but neurologically remarkable numbness of her bilateral arms and legs was recognized and we could not measure her grasping power.

Table 1 shows her clinical data after admission. Her urine, blood and blood chemistry were each within normal limits, and also her liquor properties were normal on October 29. Her vital capacity was 1.2 l and the per cent vital capacity (%VC) was 55%. These values showed deterioration in respiratory function.

Table 1.

Clinical data of case 1 after admission

Urine	
glucose	(–)
protein	(–)
sediments	normal
Blood chemistry	
T-P	6.4 g/dl
Alb	3.6 g/dl
BUN	2.3 mg/dl
Cr	0.5 mg/dl
Na	134 mEq/l
K	4.0 mEq/l
Cl	93 mEq/l
CPK	46 mU/ml
CK-MB	9 mU/ml
aldolase	2.3 mU/ml
T-ch	191 mg/dl
T-G	73 mg/dl
Blood	
WBC	6600 /mm^3
RBC	414 × 10^4/mm^3
Hb	12.3 g/dl
Hct	38.4 %
PLT	22 × 10^4/mm^3
Liquor	
cell count	0/3
glucose	87 mg/dl
protein	35 mg/dl
Respiratory function test	
VC	1.20 l
%VC	55%

Figure 1 demonstrates her progress in our hospital. Immediately after admission, she was inserted with an intratracheal tube in the ICU. She breathed spontaneously, but was assisted with an respirator. On the same day, she underwent DFPP therapy, and also underwent DFPP therapy on October 23 and 25. With DFPP therapy, a total of three times, we prescribed 1000 mg of methylprednisolone to her for 3 days from October 23. Thereafter, the dose of prednisolone was decreased from 60 mg per day at the rate of 10 mg every 2 days. On October 26, her motor nerve conduction velocity (NCV) improved and increased to 20–30% over that at admission. Because her %VC increased to 75%, the intratracheal tube was removed on November 2 and she was discharged from the ICU on November 5. She was transferred from our hospital to another hospital in order to undergo rehabilitation therapy on November 30.

Figure 2 demonstrates the improvement in the NCV of her median nerve. The NCV of the median nerve deteriorated at a speed of 32.2 m/s and its amplitude fell at admission. On November 8, the NCV of the median nerve recovered to a speed of 45.5 m/s and its amplitude recovered.

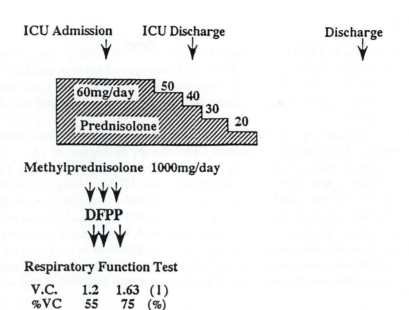

Figure 1. Clinical progress of case 1.

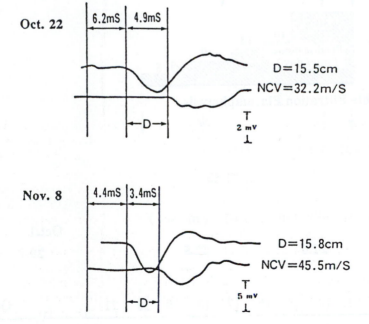

Figure 2. Actual measurements of NCV before and after the DFPP therapy.

CASE 2

A 6 year old boy had a fever at the end of August, 1991. At the beginning of September, he vomitted and complained of weakness and arthralgia of his legs and lumbago. He was admitted into a local hospital on September 6 and diagnosed as GBS from liquor examination data. However, after admission, his symptoms progressed and he could not sit up in bed.

As he complained of a hoarse voice and showed bulbar palsy, he was transferred to our hospital and immediately underwent DFPP therapy on September 13.

In his present status at admission, his height was 116 cm, body weight 19 kg and his consciousness was clear. His blood pressure was 120/80 mmHg and his heart rate was regular at 110 per minute. His cevical, thoracic and abdominal status were normal physically, but neurologically remarkable numbness of his extremities was recognized.

Table 2 shows clinical data at admission. His urine, blood, blood chemistry and immunological examination were within normal limits. However in his liquor on September 11, the protein concentration showed a high value at 370 mg/dl, but the cell number was normal. These results demonstrated proteinocytogenic dissociation that was typical of GBS.

Figure 3 shows his progress in our hospital. On September 13, immediately after admission, he underwent DFPP therapy at first and a total of four times. He was in ICU from September 14 to 19 and he was discharged from ICU because his respiratory function improved from 58.3 to 91% on %VC examination.

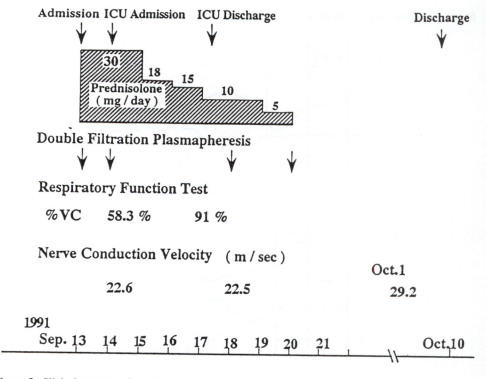

Figure 3. Clinical progress of case 2.

Table 2.
Clinical data of case 2 after admission

Urine			
Gl	(–)		
protein	(–)		
sediments			
RBC	(–)		
WBC	(–)		
Blood chemistry			
T-P	6.8 g/dl		
Alb	4.3 g/dl		
BUN	10 mg/dl		
Cr	0.4 mg/dl		
Na	140 mEq/l		
K	4.1 mEq/l		
Cl	100 mEq/l		
CPK	15 mU/ml		
CK-MB	18 mU/ml		
aldolase	3.2 mU/ml		
GOT	24 mU/dl		
GPT	11 mU/dl		
LDH	266 mU/dl		
T-ch	39 mg/dl		
T-G	26 mg/dl		
Blood			
WBC	8500 /mm^3		
RBC	435 × 10^4 /mm^3		
Hb	12.1 g/dl		
Hct	36.5%		
PLT	34.8 × 10^4 /mm^3		
Immunological examination			
IgG	1060 mg/dl		
IgA	149 mg/dl		
IgM	367 mg/dl		
C3	94 mg/dl		
C4	18 mg/dl		
CH50	12.8 mg/dl		
ANA	(–)		
ADA	(–) < 1.0 IU/ml		
OKT4/8	0.83		
Liquor	September 11	September 17	September 27
cell count	4/3	140/3	25/3
glucose	–	72	67 mg/dl
protein	370	139	8 mg/dl

Prednisolone treatment was started from dose of 30 mg per day on September 13 and rapidly reduced. On September 20, prednisolone was stopped and pulse therapy of methylprednisolone was not needed.

Although his NCV did not improve to normal levels, he was discharged from our hospital on October 10 because he was able to walk by himself.

DISCUSSION

The benefit of plasmapheresis therapy for GBS was recognized by several reports [1–4]. However, their method of plasmapheresis was a simple plasma exchange [1, 2] or immunoadsorbent therapy [3, 4].

The selectivity of an immunoadsorbent column for the pathogenic factor of GBS was not confirmed. Therefore, we tried and performed non-selective therapy of DFPP on the two cases reported. In our two cases, one patient was aged and another case was a child. They were classified as GBS grade 4 with bulbar palsy including respiratory deterioration and had a high risk on extracorporeal circulation. However, they improved remarkably in comparison with other reported cases. At this point, it was suggested that DFPP therapy performed at the time of the early phase of GBS was beneficial and useful.

SUMMARY

(i) We reported two cases of GBS with respiratory deterioration which recovered by DFPP.

(ii) It is suggested that DFPP is beneficial for GBS and should be performed in the early phase of GBS.

REFERENCES

1. Guillain–Barré Syndrome Study Group. Plasmapheresis and acute Guillain–Barré syndrome. *Neurology*, 35, 1096–1104 (1985).
2. J. C. Raphael. French controlled trial-plasma exchange therapy in Guillain–Barré syndrome. Presented at the *6th Ann. Apheresis Symp.*, Chicago, IL (1984).
3. J. D. Pollard. A critical review of therapies in acute and chronic demyelinating polyneuropethies. *Muscle Nerve*, 10, 269–287 (1987).
4. P. J. Dyck. Inflammatory and dysimmune neuropathy. *Curr. Opinion Neurol. Neurosurg.*, 2, 705–707 (1989).

Therapeutic Plasmapheresis (XII), pp. 253-256
T. Agishi *et al.* (Eds)
© VSP 1993

A New Immunoadsorbent for Guillain–Barré Syndrome

H. KANAZAWA, I. TOMITA, A. SUENAGA, H. GOTO and N. SHIBUYA

Department of Neurology, Kawatana National Hospital, Nagasaki, Japan

Key words: immunoadsorbent; autoantibodies; Guillain–Barré syndrome; experimental allergic neuritis; synthetic peptides.

INTRODUCTION

The synthetic peptide consisting of amino acid residues 66–78 of P2 protein (SP66-78) has been reported to induce experimental allergic neuritis (EAN) and cellular hypersensitivity in patients with Guillain–Barré syndrome (GBS) [1]. In addition, SP66-78 is known to stimulate the P2 specific T cell line that mediates EAN [2]. Antibodies to SP66-78 were detected in 73% of patients with GBS. The values of the antibodies decreased in parallel with clinical improvement. We made a new immunoadsorbent-fixed SP66-78 as ligand (SP66-78=PVA). SP66-78=PVA adsorbed more than 90% of antibodies against SP66-78 without loss of other plasma components [3]. Therefore we have treated an EAN model with SP66-78=PVA.

MATERIALS AND METHODS

Induction of EAN
Healthy female rabbits (body weight 2.0 kg) were immunized with two kinds of synthetic peptide (SP66-78 and SP59-78). The inoculum was prepared by mixing each synthetic peptide (1 mg/ml in saline) and complete Freund's adjuvant. Each rabbit received a single subcutaneous multiportal inoculation on the back and the foot pad. Rabbits were periodically weighed and examined, and a clinical score assigned according to the classification. Tibial motor conduction velocity (MCV) was measured. Blood samples were collected at the same time that MCV was measured.

Measurement of antibodies
Antibodies against SP66-78 or SP59-78 were measured by ELISA.

Extracorporeal circulation
Plasma perfusion was performed with SP66-78=PVA on-line with a plasma separator APO2H. One plasma volume (30 ml/kg) was treated in each plasma perfusion.

RESULTS

Five of 10 immunized rabbits showed clinical signs of EAN with a decline of MCV. All five EAN rabbits were induced by SP59-78. Antibodies to SP59-78 were detected in seven of eight rabbits injected with SP59-78. The antibodies were not detected in the rabbit in which EAN did not occur (Table 1, no. 5). Antibodies to SP59-78 were detected in rabbits immunized with SP66-78 (Table 1, no. 2 and 4). IgG class antibodies to SP59-78 were detected in all EAN rabbits, but were found in only two of five rabbits in which EAN was not observed. MCV gradually decreased in EAN rabbits. On the other hand, MCV did not change during 4 weeks in rabbits in which EAN did not occur (Fig. 1). Immunoperfusion therapy with SP66-78=PVA induced recovery from the weakness in EAN rabbits with an improvement of MCV and a decline of anti-SP66-78 antibodies (Fig. 2). A total of four EAN rabbits were treated by extracorporeal circulation with SP66-78=PVA. MCV increased significantly after treatment in all. The mean value of MCV before treatment was 87.4 ± 5.5 m/s and that after treatment was 100.4 ± 4.1 m/s. A decrease of the values of anti-SP66-78 antibodies was observed in all, the reduction rate of γ-gl class antibodies was $42.6 \pm 28.5\%$ and that of IgG class was $36.7 \pm 6.5\%$. There was a significant correlation between the values of antibodies to SP66-78 and SP59-78 ($r = 0.67$, $P < 0.002$). The values of antibodies to SP59-78 were inhibited by SP66-78.

Table 1.
Antibodies to synthetic peptide in EAN

Rabbit			Antibodies to synthetic peptide			
No.	Ag	EAN	SP59-78		SP66-78	
			γ-gl class	IgG class	γ-gl class	IgG class
Exp. 1 1 (JWR)	SP59-78	+	0.49	0.35	0.21	0.30
3 (NZWR)	SP59-78	+	0.57	0.52	0.23	0.31
6 (JWR)	SP59-78	+	0.53	0.35	0.18	0.36
2 (JWR)	SP66-78	−	0.46	0.48	0.21	0.31
4 (NZWR)	SP66-78	−	0.48	0.17	0.30	0.32
5 (JWR)	SP59-78	−	0.10	0.18	0.12	0.29
			(0.13 ± 0.03)	(0.16 ± 0.02)	(0.15 ± 0.03)	(0.16 ± 0.03)
Exp. 2 7 (JWR)	SP59-78	+	1.25	0.41	0.55	0.75
10 (JWR)	SP59-78	+	0.41	0.21	0.64	0.61
8 (JWR)	SP59-78	−	0.90	0.40	0.62	1.10
9 (JWR)	SP59-78	−	0.25	0.07	0.32	0.32
			(0.07 ± 0.01)	(0.09 ± 0.03)	(0.22 ± 0.04)	(0.08 ± 0.03)

Values in parentheses indicate ELISA titers in control

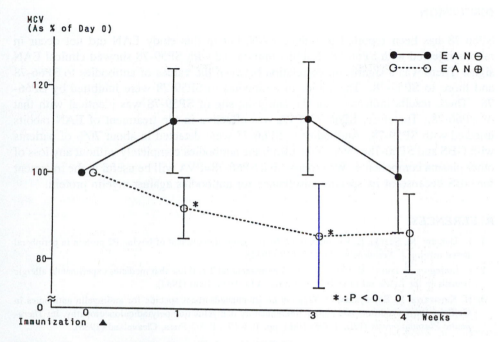

Figure 1. Changes of MCV after immunization with SP59-78.

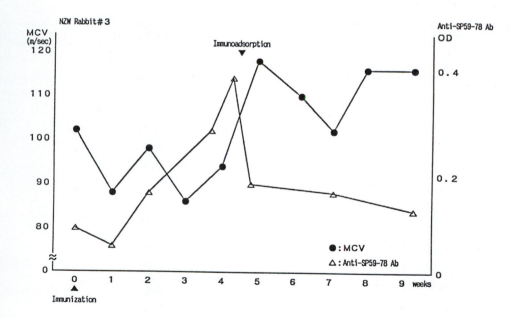

Figure 2. Effects of immunoadsorption on MCV and anti-SP59-78 Ab in an EAN rabbit.

DISCUSSION

SP66-78 has been reported to induce EAN, but in this study EAN did not occur in rabbits injected with SP66-78. Rabbits immunized with SP59-78 showed clinical EAN signs. There was a significant correlation between the values of antibodies to SP66-78 and those to SP59-78. The values of antibodies to SP59-78 were inhibited by SP66-78. These results indicated that the antigenic site of SP59-78 was identical with that of SP66-78. Therefore, SP66-78=PVA was effective in the treatment of EAN rabbits injected with SP59-78. Antibodies to SP66-78 were detected in about 70% of patients with GBS and SP66-78=PVA could adsorb the antibodies completely without any loss of other plasma components. We propose that SP66-78=PVA will be useful in the treatment for GBS because of its specific adsorbance for antibodies against myelin protein.

REFERENCES

1. K. Uemura, M. Suzuki, K. Kitamura et al. Neuritogenic determinant of bovine P2 protein in peripheral nerve myelin. J. Neurochem., **39**, 895–898 (1982).

2. C. Linington, S. Izumo, K. Uemura et al. A permanent rat T cell line that mediates experimental allergic neuritis in the Lewis rat in vitro. J. Immunol., **133**, 1946–1950 (1984).

3. H. Kanazawa, K. Shibayama, G. Takeo et al. Immunoadsorbent specific for antimyelin antibodies in Guillain–Barré syndrome and chronic inflammatory demyelinating polyradiculoneuropathy. In: Therapeutic Plasmapheresis (VII), T. Oda (Ed.), pp. 103–107, ISAO Press, Cleaveland (1988).

Therapeutic Plasmapheresis (XII), pp. 257-259
T. Agishi *et al.* (Eds)
© VSP 1993

Plasmapheresis for Guillain–Barré Syndrome in Japan

A. SUENAGA, H. KANAZAWA, I. TOMITA, H. GOTO and N. SHIBUYA

Kawatana National Hospital, Nagasaki, Japan

Key words: Guillain–Barré syndrome; chronic inflammatory demyelinating polyradiculoneuropathy; plasmapheresis.

INTRODUCTION

Plasmapheresis (PP) has been reported to be efficacious in Guillain–Barré syndrome (GBS) and chronic inflammatory demyelinating polyradiculoneuropathy (CIDP) [1–3].

Although many uncontrolled reports suggested that PP for GBS is useful in Japan, no one knows the actual conditions of PP. Therefore we designed a nationwide questionnaire survey to investigate how PP is applied and evaluated for the treatment of GBS and CIDP in Japan.

MATERIALS AND METHODS

We sent a questionnaire to 374 hospitals and asked clinical data of patients treated with PP between January 1989 and September 1990. Items covered are age, sex, severity due to Hughes' functional grading scale, duration of illness before PP, methods of PP, frequency of PP, time to improve one and two grades, judgement on usefulness, replacement fluids, additional treatments and complications.

RESULTS

Replies were obtained from 157 hospitals. It was found that PP was done at 65 of 157 hospitals on 163 patients [109 patients with GBS, 10 patients with Fisher syndrome and 44 patients with CIDP (Table 1)]. PP for GBS and CIDP was carried out on patients whose severity scores were 4.2 ± 1.0 (mean $\pm$ SD, $n = 109$) and 3.0 ± 1.0 ($n = 44$), respectively. The frequency of PP was 4.3 times for GBS and 11.2 times for CIDP. PP was performed on 11.4 days from the onset of motor deficits in GBS and 500 days in CIDP.

Plasma separation was performed with a membrane separator in 91.4% and with a centrifugation in 8.6% of cases. Immunoadsorption therapy was used in 20.7% of PP treatments.

Replacement fluids were used in treatments with a simple plasma exchange, such as a centrifugation and a single filtration, but not with immunoadsorption.

Albumin products were used in the main and fresh frozen plasma was used in only 10%.

Table 1.
PP performed in Japan between January 1989 and September 1990 (mean ± SD)

	GBS	Fisher	CIDP
No. of patients	109	10	44
Age	39.0 ± 17.9	50.6 ± 10.1	41.5 ± 17.9
Functional Scale	4.2 ± 1.0	3.6 ± 1.2	3.0 ± 1.3
Duration of illness (days)	11.4 ± 11.9	16.4 ± 9.9	501.8 ± 789.1
No. of times of PP	4.3 ± 2.2	4.0 ± 2.5	11.2 ± 18.4

In GBS, PP was employed alone in 35% of the cases and 60% of patients were administered corticosteroids together with PP. In CIDP, corticosteroids and immuno-suppressive drugs were given in about 80% of patients. In about 1000 procedures, side effects occurred in 4.4%; 17 hypotensive reactions and nine inflammatory reactions.

The mean time to recover one functional grade was 28.0 days in GBS, 15.2 days in Fisher syndrome and 20.3 days in CIDP (Table 2). If the efficiency of PP is assessed to be useful by means of the finding of improvement by one functional grade at 4 weeks after PP, it has been shown that PP has a beneficial effect in 64% of GBS, in 90% of Fisher syndrome and in 49% of CIDP. With respects to the duration of illness before PP, methods of PP, the severity of the disease and additional treatments, no significant correlation with efficiency of PP was found statistically.

Table 2.
Time to improve one and two grades on the functional grading scale and effect of PP

	Time to improve (days, mean ± SD)		Effect (%)	
	1 grade	2 grade	+	−
GBS	28.0 ± 34.8	53.6 ± 61.8	70 (64.2)	39 (35.8)
Fisher	15.2 ± 15.1	38.0 ± 29.2	9 (90.0)	1 (10.0)
CIDP	20.3 ± 28.8	69.5 ± 89.2	21 (48.8)	22 (51.2)

The efficiency of PP is assessed to be useful by means of the finding of improvement by one functional grade at 4 weeks after PP.

DISCUSSION

It was found that PP is evaluated to be valuable for the treatment of GBS, Fisher syndrome and CIDP in Japan. In the present study, 64% of GBS patients showed a beneficial effect from PP, which was similar to those identified in previous trials: 52% in the North American trial [1] and 67% in the French trial [2]. With regard to the median time to recover one grade after PP in GBS, it was documented to be 54 days in the North American trial, 70 days in the French trial and 69 days in the Dutch trial [3], in contrast to 28 days in this study. It is also indicated that PP was efficacious if begun early; however, our results showed no significant difference between the effect of PP and the duration of illness. It is difficult to explain the differences between our results and conclusions previously reported. Since this study was a questionnaire survey but not a controlled study based on a common protocol, no comparison can be made simply with respect to the results.

CONCLUSION

PP was applied to 163 patients with inflammatory neuropathy between January 1989 and September 1990 in Japan, and has been evaluated to be efficacious.

REFERENCES

1. The Guillain–Barré Syndrome Study Group. Plasmapheresis and acute Guillain–Barré syndrome. *Neurology*, **35**, 1096–1104 (1985).
2. French Cooperative Group on Plasma Exchange and Guillain–Barré Syndrome. Efficiency of plasma exchange in Guillain–Barré syndrome: role of replacement fluids. *Ann. Neurol.*, **22**, 753–761 (1987).
3. F. G. A. van der Meche *et al.* A randomized trial comparing intravenous immunoglobulin and plasma exchange in Guillain–Barré syndrome. *N. Eng. J. Med.*, **17**, 1123–1129 (1992).

Therapeutic Plasmapheresis (XII), pp. 261-263
T. Agishi *et al.* (Eds)
© VSP 1993

Apheresis in Chronic Inflammatory Demyelinating Polyneuritis

W. F. HAUPT, E. GIBBELS and H. BORBERG[1]

Departments of Neurology and [1]Haemapheresis,
University of Cologne, Germany

Key words: CIDP; immunotherapy; plasma exchange; clinical course.

INTRODUCTION

Idiopathic polyneuritis is an inflammatory disease of unknown etiology leading to discontinuous demyelination of peripheral nerves; an autoimmune pathogenesis seems probable. The disease occurs in two major variants of which the more common form is acute idiopathic polyneuritis, the Guillain–Barré syndrome. The less frequent form is chronic inflammatory demyelinating polyneuritis (CIDP). For both variants diagnostic criteria have been published so that both forms can be clearly distinguished from each other.

However, for CIDP there seem to be a number of subtypes which differ in their clinical course and also in their response to various treatment regimes. With reference to the classification propagated by Dyck [1] and co-workers we propose the following slightly modified definitions, published by Gibbels and Hann [2]:

  (i) Progressive: steadily progressive course.

 (ii) Stepwise progressive: multiple monophasic courses with incomplete remissions and subsequent progression, interval < 1 year.

(iii) Monophasic: monophasic course with progression beyond the 4th week.

(iv) Remitting: monophasic courses with or without defect and subsequent recurrence, interval > 1 year.

The hallmark of the diagnosis of CIDP is that of 'pattern recognition' including clinical findings, electrophysiologic data, CSF values, laboratory tests and on occasion nerve biopsy findings as recently stated by the Ad Hoc Committee of the American Academy of Neurology AIDS Task Force [3]. The most common treatment is steroids usually combined with azathioprin. This regimen seems to be reasonably effective in the majority of cases [1, 4]. However, a number of patients do not respond satisfactorily and can deteriorate to severe clinical conditions leading to respiratory failure and complete paralysis. Especially in the more severe cases, treatment by apheresis has been implemented with sometimes astonishing results [5]. To date, some 50 cases of treatment of CIDP by apheresis have been published. Due to the low incidence of the disease, the reports contain only a few cases each with a maximum of 15 cases in the series of

Dyck *et al.* [6]. These small numbers make evaluation of results extremely difficult, and, so far, only one controlled treatment trial has been documented by Dyck *et al.* [6].

Our own experience is based on the observation of nine patients followed for more than 5 years [7] and another 10 patients with a follow up of less than 5 years. All patients fulfilled the criteria of CIDP and all 19 were treated by plasma exchange.

METHODS

Plasma exchange treatment was performed by removing 100–150% of the plasma volume in three consecutive sessions and another 75–100% in further sessions and replacement with 5% human albumine. Plasma separation was performed with continuous flow blood cell separators, usually in peripheral veno-venous technique. Anticoagulation was performed with preinjection of 2500 IU heparin followed by citrate. In cases of fibrinogen depletion, fresh frozen plasma was substituted.

RESULTS

In the long-term group, we encountered three remitting and six progressive courses. The maximum MRC (Medical Research Council) score of paresis ranged from 3 (unable to walk) to 0 (total paralysis and artificial respiration). The minimal NCV (Nerve conduction velocity) values ranged from 4 to 31 m/s. The plasma exchange treatments showed good results in the three remitting and one progressive case, and moderate results in three progressive cases. In two cases, both progressive, we saw no improvement following treatment. The results of the plasma exchange treatment show that between four and 16 sessions were performed during the first series and that five patients were subjected to further series of plasma exchange. Furthermore, there was no apparent correlation between the severity of clinical findings, NCV data, number of plasma exchange sessions or series and response to treatment. The remitting cases all responded whereas the progressive cases showed a favorable response in half of the cases.

In the 10 cases with a follow up of less than 5 years we encountered six remitting, one progressive, and two monophasic courses. The distribution of the MRC scales was similar to that of the long-term group (1–4, but no grade 0) and the range of the minimal NCV also values between 0 and 47 m/s. Of the six remitting cases, one responded well, three moderately, but two showed no response. The three monophasic courses all showed a moderate response, and, as in the long-term group, the progressive case did not respond. The number of plasma exchanges ranged from two to 16, 3 patients received two series. Here again, the treatment results could not be attributed to the clinical subtype, severity of disease, NCV values, or number of treatments. In four cases (three progressive, one remitting) we performed nerve biopsies in an attempt to correlate clinical and histological findings. The endoneural areas, number of myelinated fibers per sq mm as well as signs of inflammation, de- and re-myelination and onion bulb formation varied widely and without any discernable pattern [8]. The development of NCV values over the course in cases of CIDP with and without plasma exchange treatment also showed no pattern [9].

CONCLUSION

Plasma exchange treatment of CIDP is well-documented in a limited number of cases, mainly due to the low incidence of the disease. The standard treatment with cortisone and azathioprine seems to be successful in less severe cases. It seems that mainly the severe cases are referred to plasma exchange treatment as a last resort which probably causes a negative selection of the patients. Also, the variable courses and response to treatment may reflect the fact that remitting and progressive CIDP are not subtypes of the same disease but actually different entities with variable response to plasma exchange and other treatments. The knowledge of CIDP and its treatment is still quite limited at best and may be improved by uniform documentation and multicenter treatment trials.

REFERENCES

1. P. J. Dyck, A. C. Lais, M. Ohta *et al.* Chronic inflammatory polyradiculoneuropathy. *Mayo Clin. Proc.*, **50**, 621–637 (1975).
2. E. Gibbels and P. Hann. Rezidivierende und chronische Polyneuritiden. In: *Metabolische und entzündliche Polyneuropathien*, Springer, Berlin (1984).
3. D. R. Cornblath, A. K. Asbury, J. W. Albers *et al.* Research criteria for diagnosis of chronic inflammatory demyelinating polyneuropathy (CIDP). *Neurology*, **41**, 617–618 (1991).
4. M. C. Dalakas and W. K. Engel. Chronic relapsing (dysimmune) polyneuropathy: pathogenesis and treatment. *Ann. Neurol.*, **9** (Suppl.), 134–145 (1981).
5. K. V. Toyka, R. Augspach, H. Wiethölter *et al.* Plasma exchange in chronic inflammatory polyneuropathy: evidence suggestive of a pathogenic humoral factor. *Muscle Nerve*, **5**, 479–484 (1982).
6. P. J. Dyck, J. Daube, P. O'Brien *et al.* Plasma exchange in chronic inflammatory demyelinating polyradiculopathy. *New Engl. J. Med.*, **314**, 461–465 (1986).
7. E. Gibbels, K. V. Toyka, H. Borberg *et al.* Plasmaaustauschbehandlung bei chronischen Polyneuritiden vom Typ Guillain–Barré. *Nervenarzt*, **57**, 129–139 (1986).
8. E. Gibbels and M. Kentenich. Umyelinated fibers in sural nerve biopsies of chronic inflammatory demyelinating polyneuropathy. *Acta Neuopathol.*, **80**, 439–447 (1990).
9. W. F. Haupt, E. Gibbels and P. Hann. Chronische Polyneuritis vom Typ Guillain–Barré: Bedeutung der Langzeitverläufe elektroneurographischer Parameter. *Nervenarzt*, **59**, 274–277 (1988).

Therapeutic Plasmapheresis (XII), pp. 265-267
T. Agishi *et al*. (Eds)
© VSP 1993

Beneficial Effect of Plasma Exchange in Fisher Syndrome

K. OTA, Y. SHIMIZU, M. EJIMA, H. TANAKA and S. MARUYAMA

Department of Neurology, Neurological Institute, Tokyo Women's Medical College, Tokyo, Japan

Key words: plasma exchange; plasmapheresis; Fisher syndrome; Guillain–Barré syndrome; ganglioside.

INTRODUCTION

Since Fisher [1] described three patients presenting with external ophthalmoplegia, sever ataxia and loss of tendon reflexes as an unusual variant of acute idiopathic polyneuritis, Fisher syndrome has been thought as a related disease of Guillain–Barré syndrome. This disease is, in general practice, treated with steroids. However, in recent years several reports of a patient with Fisher syndrome undergoing plasma exchange (PEX) were described. We carried out PEX on a series of multiple patients with Fisher syndrome and compared it with steroid therapy with respect mainly to the response of symptoms and duration of illness.

A TYPICAL CASE OF FISHER SYNDROME TREATED BY PEX

The patient was a 42 year old male who developed a cough and fever while traveling. He was admitted 5 days later because of blephaloptosis, diplopia and staggering gait. Neurological examination revealed ophtalmoplegia, absence of deep tendon reflexes and ataxia. Examination of spinal fluid showed albinocytological dissociation. As a result, the diagnosis of Fisher syndrome was made. The symptoms worsened after admission and PEX was performed on the second hospital day. Immediately following the first session of PEX there was an improvement in ophthalmoplegia as well as subjective symptoms such as diplopia. The patient received a total of five sessions on PEX until the 14th hospital day, when ataxia resolved. By the 45th hospital day the patient had only a slight disturbance of abduction and he was discharged from the hospital. The levels of anti-glycolipid antibodies (Ab) in the serum were determined. The only antiglycolipid Ab that was presented was anti-GQ1b Ab. Serial measurements of anti-GQ1b Ab titer were determined. A week after admission anti-GQ1b Ab titer and serum IgG levels decreased suddenly following PEX. However, the following week the levels rose again, presumably due to a rebound increase of IgG after its sudden decrease. Interestingly, during the 5th week of hospitalization anti-GQ1b Ab titers were noted to be low despite an increase in total IgG.

MULTIPLE CASE STUDY

A retrospective study was conducted on 14 patients with Fisher syndrome in our hospital. By modality, this series consisted of four PEX patients, five steroid therapy, three combined PEX and steroid therapy, and two untreated patients. The effect of treatment was evaluated according to the following criteria. (i) The time interval from the onset of Fisher syndrome to the improvement of symptoms was considered the duration of illness. (ii) The time interval from the start of treatment to the disappearance of ocular movements was considered the period of ocular movement recovery. (iii) The patients were considered positive for an early effect when their ocular movements improved within 48 h of the start of treatment and were considered negative when the ocular movements showed no response within the same period of time.

RESULTS

The average duration of illness in patients with Fisher syndrome who were treated with PEX or steroid or had no treatment was 1.4 ± 0.4, 2.5 ± 0.5 or 2.0 ± 0.7 months, respectively. There was no statistically significant difference between each treatment in duration of illness, possibly because of the limited numbers of patients in the respective groups, but it tended to be reduced to a greater extent in the PEX group than in the steroid and the untreated groups. The patient in the PEX group who initially had complete or incomplete ophthalmoplegia recovered over an average of 1 month. The steroid treatment group had all incomplete ophthalmoplegia, recovered over a period of 2 months. As for the early therapeutic effect, the ocular movements improved in all PEX patients within 48 h of the start of treatment, while the rate of effectiveness was 60% for the steroid group. Spinal fluid and blood levels of IgG and albumin were determined in both the acute and recovery phase to calculate IgG index which reflects intrathecal IgG synthesis. Three of eight patients showed an increase in the IgG index, but there was no significant correlation between the change in IgG index and each modality or the effect of treatment.

DISCUSSION

The utility of PEX or plasmapheresis in Fisher syndrome was first reported in 1981 by Littlewood [2] who found it to be very beneficial in a patient presenting with respiratory paralysis. Other investigators have also performed PEX in patients with Fisher syndrome; they all noted that PEX induced improvement in disease status. In our series PEX induced an excellent response with a rapid improvement of ophthalmoplegia and a marked reduction in the duration of illness. Patients with Fisher syndrome are generally said to carry a favorable prognosis. However, some may develop severe complications such as respiratory paralysis. Therefore, PEX may have a good chance to benefit patients with Fisher syndrome if performed in the acute phase of disease activity. In recent years attempts have been made to determine anti-glycolipid Ab in patients with certain neurological diseases including polyneuritis. In 1992 Chiba and associates determined serum levels of anti-glycolipid Ab in multiple patients with Fisher syndrome. They found elevated levels of anti-GQ1b Ab in all of them and postulated that anti-GQ1b Ab is a possible factor related with Fisher syndrome. In the case we discussed the clinical symptoms closely correlated with changes in anti-GQ1b Ab titer. In addition, PEX tended to be more beneficial than steroid in the 14 cases we reviewed. These findings suggest that PEX could benefit patients with Fisher syndrome in cases where a humoral factor such as anti-GQ1b Ab might be eliminated.

CONCLUSION

(i) The effect of PEX was studied in patients with Fisher syndrome.

(ii) Unlike in the group of patients receiving steroid therapy alone, ophthalmoplegia improvement in the group of PEX patients early after the start of treatment and the whole course of Fisher syndrome was reduced. The results of this study suggest that PEX is worthwhile being tried on patients with Fisher syndrome.

(iii) In patients with Fisher syndrome in whom serum level of anti-GQ1b antibody were determined, serum values showed changes consistent with the course of symptoms and the therapeutic effect of PEX.

Acknowledgments
We thank Drs A. Chiba and S. Kusunoki, Department of Neurology, Tokyo University, for determining anti-GQ1b antibody in our patient with Fisher syndrome.

REFERENCES

1. M. Fisher. An unusual variant of acute idiopathic polyneuritis (syndrome of ophthalmoplegia, ataxia and arefrexia). *N. Engl. J. Med.*, **255**, 57–65 (1956).

2. R. Littlewood and S. Bajada. Successful plasmapheresis in the Miller–Fisher syndrome. *Br. Med. J.*, **282**, 778 (1981).

3. A. H. Ropper. Three patients with Fisher's syndrome and normal MRI. *Neurology*, **36**, 1630–1631 (1988).

4. R. Neshige, Y. Kuroda, K. Oda *et al.* Suppression of acute exacerbation of Fisher's syndrome by plasmapheresis. *Neurolog. Ther.*, **3**, 31–34 (1986).

5. H. Matsumoto, K. Yonezawa, N. Kobayashi *et al.* A case of Fisher's syndrome successfully treated by plasma exchange. *Intern. Med.*, **56**, 1189–1192 (1984).

6. A. Chiba, S. Kusunoki, T. Shimizu *et al.* Serum IgG antibody to ganglioside GQ1b is a possible marker of Miller–Fisher syndrome. *Amm. Neurol.*, **31**, 677–679 (1992).

Therapeutic Plasmapheresis (XII), pp. 269-272
T. Agishi *et al.* (Eds)
© VSP 1993

Treatment of Multiple Sclerosis with Lymphocytapheresis using a Leukocyte Adsorptive Column

T. SATO, Y. ISHIGAKI, T. KOMIYA, H. MIWA, J. YOKOTA and H. TSUDA[1]

Departments of Neurology and [1]Internal Medicine, Juntendo University, Tokyo, Japan

Key words: lymphocytapheresis; multiple sclerosis; T cell.

INTRODUCTION

Multiple sclerosis (MS) is an autoimmune disorder of the central nervous system that affects as many 3.9% per 100 000 Japanese. The main symptoms are visual, motor, sensory and urinary disturbances. Although intravenous pulsed methylpredonine therapy followed by oral prednisolone therapy is used to treat MS, some patients still fail to respond to treatment. Three recent double blind studies were carried out on the efficacy of plasmapheresis and immunosuppressive drug therapy in MS. These studies suggest that plasmapheresis, when rendered adequately and in conjunction with immunosuppressive drugs, may benefit MS patients who are in the active state of the disease [1]. However, some MS patients do not respond to treatment by plasmapheresis. Several attempts have been made to treat MS patients using lymphocytapheresis and improvements were noted in some patients [2, 3]. However, one study reported no clear evidence of improvement [4]. Lymphocytapheresis in these reports [2–4] was carried out by the centrifugation method. Recently, we reported preliminary results on a new method of lymphocytapheresis using a lymphocyte and leukocyte adsorption column to treat MS patients in the active state [5]. The method is both simple and safe. A detailed clinical study on the effects of lymphocytapheresis in MS will be reported in a later paper.

PATIENTS AND METHODS

Patients
Twenty-four patients with MS and four with retrobulbar neuritis were treated with lymphocytapheresis using the new method. The clinical status of these patients was as follows: one MS patient and two retrobulbar neuritis patients had acute onset of the disease; 20 MS and two retrobulbar neuritis patients were in the active state of exacerbation; three MS patients with progressive forms were in the active phase of the disease. Although all patients received intravenous pulsed methylpredonine therapy followed by oral high-dose prednisolone therapy, their clinical symptoms did not improve. Clinical symptoms were evaluated according Kurtzke's expanded disability status scale (EDSS) [6]. Prior to treatment with lymphocytapheresis, their EDSS grades varied from 3.0 to 8.5.

Lymphocytapheresis

Lymphocytapheresis was carried out using a 'Cellsorba' lymphocyte adsorption column (Asahi Medical Co., Tokyo). The column employs non-woven fabric made of polyester fibers. About 3000 ml of whole blood was treated with the anticoagulant nafamostat mesilate and passed though the column.

One course of lymphocytapheresis lasted 60 min during which 3000 ml of whole blood was treated and about 9×10^9 lymphocytes were removed. Each patient received 1–15 lymphocytapheresis treatments (average: three treatments) carried out 7–8 days apart.

Lymphocyte subsets

Peripheral lymphocyte subsets were determined before and after limphocytapheresis using monoclonal antibodies [7].

RESULTS

Eight of the 24 patients who underwent lymphocytapheresis therapy showed marked to moderate improvement. These patients ranged in age from 20 to 46 years, with onsets of the disease ranging from 2 weeks to 11 years (Table 1). EDSS grades varied from 4.0 to 8.5 before lymphocytapheresis. Within 4–12 h after therapy each of the eight patients showed EDSS grade improvements of 2 or more steps. Sensory disturbances and weakness of the extremities, pyramidal tract signs and visual disturbances responded well to treatment.

Table 1.

Eight MS cases showing improvement after lymphocytapheresis

No.	Case	Age/sex	Symptoms improvement	EDSS Before	After
1	K.Y.	22/M	s, p	4.0	0
2	N.Y.	20/F	v, s, p	7.5	4.0
3	K.M.	21/F	v, s, p	6.0	4.0
4	Y.K.	24/F	v, s	5.0	0
5	M.S.	39/F	s, p, r	8.0	5.0
6	H.K.	34/M	c, b, s, p	4.0	2.0
7	F.R.	46/F	c, b, s, p	7.0	4.0
8	K.H.	26/F	s, p	8.5	6.0

c: cerebrum, v: opt. N, b: brain stem, s: sensory, p: motor, r: urinary incontinence.

We examined the visual evoked potentials in two patients (nos 2 and 4) with visual disturbances who underwent lymphocytapheresis. Although no response to visual evoked potential was noted before therapy, obvious recovery of evoked potentials was recorded after the second course of lymphocytapheresis. Evoked potentials improved before visual acuity improved. Two other patients (nos 5 and 8), who were unable to walk without assistance before lymphocytapheresis, were able to walk independently after several treatments.

Based on the degree of improvement in EDSS scores, the patients were divided into three groups (Table 2). In group 1, marked to moderate improvement in EDSS scores of two or more steps were observed in eight patients. In group 2, slight improvement in EDSS scores of one step was observed in seven patients with MS and two with retrobulbar neuritis. In group 3, nine patients with MS and two with retrobulbar neuritis failed to demonstrate any objective clinical improvement. The results indicate that MS patients who underwent lymphocytapheresis within 30 days after the onset of the acute phase of the disease were able to respond to therapy.

Although about 50% of all lymphocytes were removed by lymphocytapheresis, Ta1-positive activated T cells were removed more efficiently. None of the patients experienced any side effects following lymphocytapheresis.

Table 2.
Lymphocytapheresis in multiple sclerosis and retrobulbar neuritis

Improvement	No.	F/M	Duration of the disease (year)	Duration before LCP		Relapse after 1 year
				≤ 30 days	> 30 days	
Group 1. ++	8	6/2	5.3 ± 4.2 (0.1–9)	7 (36.8%)	1 (11.1%)	3
Group 2. ++	8	4/4	1.9 ± 2.11 (0.2–7)	6 (31.6%)	3 (33.3%)	4
Group 3. −	9	4/5	5.1 ± 6.0 (0.1–20)	6 (31.6%)	5 (55.6%)	3
Total	28	15/13		19	9	

DISCUSSION

Although lymphocytapheresis was carried out in open rather than blind trials, obvious objective improvements were noted immediately after therapy. In addition, visual evoked potentials showed rapid recovery after therapy. It is commonly known that MS patients in the acute state of exacerbation often demonstrate spontaneous remission over the natural course of the disease. However, the efficacy of lymphocytapheresis was clearly apparent in MS patients who did not respond to treatment with high-dose steroids. Immunological study on the T cell subsets in lymphocytapheresis demonstrated that Ta1-positive T cells were removed at a higher rate than other lymphocyte subsets [7]. It has been reported that MS patients in the active state had an increased number of Ta1-positive activated T cells in both peripheral blood and cerebrospinal fluid [8]. Treatment efficacy seems to be correlated with the removal of certain pathologically-activated lymphocytes, in particular, Ta1-positive T cells.

Lymphocytapheresis using a lymphocyte adsorption column is a relatively simple procedure. Since neither hemolysis nor serious complications were noted in this method, the procedure is considered to be extremely safe.

In conclusion, lymphocytapheresis employing a lymphocyte adsorption column is effective in treating MS patients who do not respond to intravenous pulsed methylpredonine therapy.

Acknowledgments

This study was supported in part by grants provided by the Japanese Ministry of Health and Welfare and the Tokyo Metropolitan Bureau of Health.

REFERENCES

1. B. O. Khatri. Plasmapheresis and immunosuppressive drug therapy in multiple sclerosis. In: *Proc. 4th Int. Congr. of the World Apheresis Association*, Sapporo, Japan (1992).

2. P. Hocker, V. Stellamor, K. Summer and M. Mann. Plasma exchange and lymphocytapheresis in multiple sclerosis. *Int. J. Artif. Organs*, **7**, 39–42 (1984).

3. E. Maida, P. Hocker and E. Mann. Long-term lymphocytapheresis therapy in multiple sclerosis. *Eur. Neurol.*, **25**, 225–232 (1986).

4. S. L. Hauser, M. Fosfurg, S. V. Kevy and H. L. Weiner. Lymphocytapheresis in chronic progressive multiple sclerosis: Immunologic and clinical effects. *Neurology*, **34**, 922–939 (1984).

5. Y. Ishigaki, T. Sato, S. Ikebe, T. Komiya and H. Tsuda. Effects of lymphocytapheresis with a immunoadsorptive column on 4 patients with multiple sclerosis. In: *Therapeutic Plasmapheresis VIII*, T. Oda (Ed.), pp. 114–117, Schattauer, Stuttgartt (1989).

6. J. F. Kurtzke. Rating neurologic impairment in multiple sclerosis: an expanded disability status scale (EDSS). *Neurology*, **33**, 1444–1452 (1983).

7. K. Matsuda, Y. Ishigaki, T. Komiya, Y. Furukawa, H. Tsuda and T. Sato. Lymphocytapheresis in multiple sclerosis: immunologic and clinical effects. In: *Proc. 4th Int. Congr. of the World Apheresis Association*, Sapporo, Japan (1992).

8. D. A. Hafler, D. A. Fox, M. E. Manning *et al. In vivo* activated T lymphocytes in the peripheral blood and cerebrospinal fluid of patients with multiple sclerosis. *N. Engl. J. Med.*, **312**, 1405–1411 (1985).

Therapeutic Plasmapheresis (XII), pp. 273-275
T. Agishi *et al.* (Eds)
© VSP 1993

Improvement of AChR Na$^+$ Influx after IM-T Plasmapheresis in Myasthenia Gravis

T. YAMAMOTO, H. HIRAWAKE and T. SATO

Juntendo University, Department of Neurology, Tokyo, Japan

Key words: myasthenia gravis; anti-acetylcholine receptor antibody; acetylcholine receptor Na$^+$ influx; IM-T column; α-bungarotoxin binding.

TE671 cell line is derived from human rhabdomyosarcoma, which produces human nicotinic acetylcholine receptors (AChR). Lang *et al.* [1] reported that seropositive myasthenia gravis (MG) plasmas reduced Na$^+$ influx through AChR channels (AChR Na$^+$ influx) in these cells, and the inhibition correlated weakly with anti-AChR antibody (Ab) titers and the presence of antibodies directed against the α-bungarotoxin (BuTx) binding sites. Yamamoto *et al.* [2] investigated similar effects of seronegative MG plasma on AChR Na$^+$ influx.

These results suggest that AChR Na$^+$ influx could be a useful tool to estimate AChR function. Plasmapheresis using an IM-T column is known to remove anti-AChR Ab more effectively than double membrane filtration. In some patients, however, clinical improvement cannot be obtained after IM-T column plasmapheresis in spite of the significant reduction in anti-AChR Ab titer.

The purpose of this study is, therefore, to estimate the amount of AChR Na$^+$ influx using plasma before and after IM-T plasmapheresis, thus finding a possible cause of the non-effective cases.

MATERIALS AND METHODS

Plasma was obtained from six patients with MG who had undergone therapeutic plasma exchange using an IM-T column.

MG was diagnosed by a positive response to intravenous edrophonium and/or electrophysiological evidence of disordered neuromuscular transmission. Healthy human plasma was used as the standard control preparation.

The anti-AChR antibody assay was performed using human AChR as the antigen as previously described [1, 3].

TE671 cells ($1-2 \times 10^6$) were cultured in 60 mm Petri dishes for 1–2 days before use [1].

AChR Na$^+$ influx was determined at room temperature by first washing the cells in phosphate-buffered saline solution (PBS) with 1 mM calcium chloride (PBSC) and adding 10^{-3} M carbachol in HEPES–Locke buffer containing ^{22}Na$^+$ at a final concentration of 0.06μCi/ml. After incubation for 1–3 min, the cells were washed rapidly in PBSC three times, extracted with 1% Triton X-100 and counted.

To study the effects of plasma on carbachol-induced Na$^+$ influx, the TE671 cells were preincubated for 2 h at room temperature. In each experiment, triplicate dishes were run with and without carbachol. Carbachol-induced influx was calculated by subtraction of the basal influx, and in each experiment it was expressed as a percentage of that under standard conditions carried out in parallel.

To assess the effect of plasma on the number of α-BuTx binding site, triplicate dishes were treated with MG or pooled control plasma before applying [^{125}I]α-BuTx (1×10^{-8} M) for 2 h at room temperature. Counts per minute (c.p.m.) bound to MG plasma-treated cells are expressed as a percentage of c.p.m. bound to control plasma-treated cells.

RESULTS (FIGS 1 AND 2)

Clinical improvement
One of six MG patients (Pt 1) did not show any clinical improvement after IM-T plasmapheresis, while five patients showed moderate improvement.

Reduction of anti-AChR Ab
Between 59.4 and 76.96% of anti-AChR Ab was removed by IM-T plasmapheresis (6000–9000 ml/3 days).

Improvement of AChR Na$^+$ influx
The amount of AChR Na$^+$ influx before and after IM-T plasmapheresis were 16 to 167% and 27 to 236% of control, respectively. Improvement of AChR Na influx, ranging from 0 to 69% was expressed by subtracting the values before IM-T plasmapheresis from those after pheresis. AChR Na influx in Pt 1 was revealed to be much (167%) more than controls even before IM-T plasmapheresis.

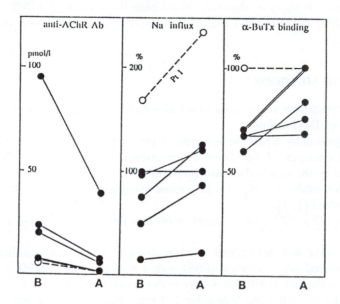

Figure 1. Effect of IM-T column plasmapheresis on MG patients.

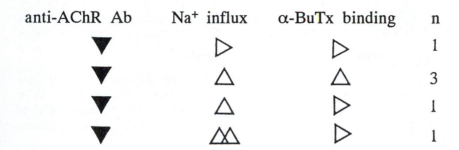

anti-AChR Ab	Na⁺ influx	α-BuTx binding	n
▼	▷	▷	1
▼	△	△	3
▼	△	▷	1
▼	△△	▷	1

Figure 2. Changes of parameters after IM-T column plasmapheresis.

[^{125}I]α-BuTx binding
[^{125}I]α-BuTx binding before and after IM-T plasmapheresis was found to be 59.0 to 100% and 67.6 to 100% ($n = 17$) of control, respectively. Increased values of [^{125}I]α-BuTx binding were 0 to 30.8%. Pt 1 showed 100% binding even before IM-T plasmapheresis.

DISCUSSION

In five patients who showed clinical improvement after IM-T plasmapheresis, anti-AChR Ab was significantly reduced and the number of α-BuTx binding sites was variously increased. These facts suggest that both binding and blocking antibodies were effectively bound to the IM-T column.

On the other hand, one patient (Pt 1) who showed no clinical improvement was revealed to have a different pattern of these three parameters. Although Pt 1 had a significant clinical manifestation, he did not have blocking antibodies and the amount of Na⁺ influx was much more than the control even before IM-T plasmapheresis. This patient may have some factor which keeps AChR Na⁺ channels continuously open.

IM-T column plasmapheresis is found to be effective for MG patients. However, MG patients who have no blocking antibodies or who show high amounts of Na⁺ influx, even before IM-T plasmapheresis, do not seem to be good candidates for IM-T column plasmapheresis.

REFERENCES

1. B. Lang, G. Richardson, J. Rees *et al.* Plasma from myasthenia gravis patients reduces acetylcholine receptor agonist-induced Na⁺ influx into TE671 cell line. *J. Neuroimmunol.*, **19**, 141–148 (1988).

2. T. Yamamoto, A. Vincent, A. Thomas *et al.* Seronegative myasthenia gravis: A plasma factor inhibiting agonist-induced acetylcholine receptor function copurifies with IgM. *Ann. Neurol.*, **30**, 550–557 (1991).

3. A. Vincent and J. Newsom-Davis. Acetylcholine receptor antibody as a diagnostic test for myasthenia gravis: results in 153 validated cases and 2967 diagnostic assays. *J. Neurol. Neurosurg. Psychiatr.*, **48**, 1246–1252 (1986).

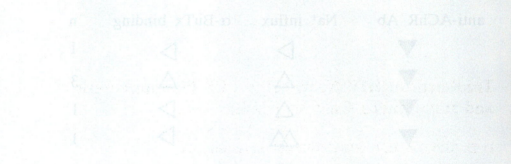

anti-AChR Ab	Na+ influx	α-BuTx binding	n

Figure 2. Changes of parameters after IM-T column plasmapheresis.

[125I]α-BuTx binding

[125I]α-BuTx binding before and after IM-T plasmapheresis was found to be 61% to 100% and 91% to 109% (n = 17) of control, respectively. Increased values of [125I]α-BuTx binding were 0 to 20.8%. Pt 1 showed 100% binding even before IM-T plasmapheresis.

DISCUSSION

In five patients who showed clinical improvement after IM-T plasmapheresis, anti-AChR Ab was significantly reduced and the number of α-BuTx binding sites was variously increased. These facts suggest that both blocking and blocking antibodies were effectively bound to the IM-T column.

On the other hand, one patient (Pt 1) who showed no clinical improvement was revealed to have a different pattern of these three parameters. Although Pt 1 had a significant clinical manifestation, he did not have blocking antibodies and the amount of Na+ influx was much more than the control even before IM-T plasmapheresis. This patient may have some factor which keeps AChR Na+ channels continuously open. IM-T column plasmapheresis is found to be effective for MG patients. However, MG patients who have no blocking antibodies or who show large amounts of Na+ influx, even before IM-T plasmapheresis, do not seem to be good candidates for IM-T column plasmapheresis.

REFERENCES

1. R. Lasek, G. Richardson: Ligne prick fluence [non-specific fascin] activity uptake acetylcholine receptor gated ion, influx into TnnH cell line, J. Neurophysiol., 14: 141-148 (1996).
2. T. Yamamoto, A. Vincent, A. Ciulla et al: Seronegative myasthenia gravis. Antibodies [non inhibiting agonist-induced acetylcholine receptor function] repetitive with IgM anti-titers, 30: 550-557 (1991).
3. G. Vernet and J. Newson-Davis: Acetylcholine receptor antibody: (1) Its detection and its correlation with disease severity in [1] validated method and 2201 diagnostic assays, Clinical Neurol., Neurosurg. Psychiatry, 43: 1246-1252 (1980).

Therapeutic Plasmapheresis (XII), pp. 277-282
T. Agishi *et al.* (Eds)
© VSP 1993

Treatment of HIV Neuropathy with Plasmapheresis and Intravenous Gammaglobulin

D. D. KIPROV, R. B. STRICKER and R. G. MILLER

*Divisions of Immunotherapy and Neurology, Department of Medicine,
California Pacific Medical Center, San Francisco, CA*

Key words: HIV; neuropathy; plasmapheresis; gammaglobulin; AIDS.

INTRODUCTION

Patients with human immunodeficiency virus (HIV) infection may present with a variety of clinical syndromes that resemble autoimmune diseases [1]. These syndromes include immune thrombocytopenic purpura (ITP), polymyositis, autoimmune hemolytic anemia and inflammatory demyelinating polyneuropathy [2–5]. HIV-related demyelinating polyneuropathy may occur as an acute illness clinically resembling Guillain–Barré syndrome, or it may have a more chronic course [6–11]. Autoantibodies against peripheral nerve antigens have been identified in patients with HIV-associated polyneuropathy [4, 12].

Plasmapheresis and intravenous gammaglobulin (IVIg) have been used to treat HIV-negative patients with acute and chronic inflammatory demyelinating polyneuropathy [13, 14]. In this report, we describe the use of these treatment modalities in patients with HIV-related polyneuropathy.

METHODS

Patients
Between 1982 and 1992, 27 patients with HIV-related peripheral neuropathy were seen in the Division of Immunotherapy at California Pacific Medical Center. The clinical characteristics of these patients are shown in Table 1. Patients ranged in age from 24 to 69 years, and all were homosexual men. Twenty-four subjects had AIDS-related complex (ARC), while three had overt AIDS as defined by the CDC criteria [15]. The $CD4^+$ T-cell counts varied widely in these patients from 10 to 1200 cells/μl. The mean $CD4^+$ T-cell count was 640 cells/μl and patients often had disproportionately high $CD4^+$ T-cell numbers, as previously noted in HIV-related neuropathy [4]. Associated conditions are listed in Table 1. Three patients had ITP, while one patient had cryoglobulinemia. All patients seen after 1986 were treated with zidovudine (AZT). Patients with AZT-induced myopathy were excluded from the study.

All patients underwent nerve conduction studies and electromyographic (EMG) testing, as previously described [6]. Response to the treatment regimens was assessed by follow-up physical examination and nerve conduction studies.

Table 1.
Clinical characteristics of study subjects

Number of patients	27
Age	24–69
Sex	All male
HIV status	24 ARC
	3 AIDS
CD4+ T-cell counts	10–1200 cells/μl
Mean CD4+ T-cell count	640 cells/μl
Associated conditions	
immune thrombocytopenic purpura	3
cryoglobulinemia	1
anticardiolipin antibody	20
Karposi's sarcoma	1
Medications	
AZT	12
Trimethoprim/Sulfa	10
Pentamidine	11

Treatment regimens

Plasmapheresis and corticosteroids were used to treat 15 patients with HIV-induced peripheral neuropathy. Between 1982 and 1987, plasmapheresis was performed using the IBM 2997 cell separator. Subsequently, plasma exchange was performed using the Cobe Spectra cell separator and more recently the Fresenius AS104 cell separator. A single-volume plasma exchange was performed during each treatment using 5% albumin replacement. Treatments were done three times a week for 3 weeks and then discontinued. Corticosteroids were given concomitantly in the form of prednisone 1 mg/kg daily. The dose was tapered to 10 mg daily and patients were maintained on this dose indefinitely. Patients were evaluated for neurologic improvement or relapse at biweekly intervals. Antiretroviral therapy (when given) was continued throughout the course of plasmapheresis treatment and subsequent follow-up.

Beginning in 1990, 12 patients with HIV-related neuropathy were treated with a combination regimen of plasmapheresis and IVIg. A single-volume plasma exchange was performed using 5% albumin replacement, followed immediately by IVIg 0.1–0.2 g/kg. This regimen was administered twice weekly for 3 weeks and then tapered to monthly maintenance. Six patients received prednisone 10 mg daily, while the other six received no corticosteroid treatment. Patients were evaluated for neurologic improvement on a biweekly basis, and antiretroviral therapy was continued during combination plasmapheresis/IVIg treatment. The IVIg preparation used was exclusively Gamimune-N (Cutter-Miles Biologicals, Westport, CT).

Lymphocyte subsets

Lymphocyte subsets were analyzed using two-color flow cytometry, as previously described [16]. Subsets that were analyzed included helper/inducer T-cells (CD4+), suppressor/cytotoxic T-cells (CD8$^+$), stimulated suppressor cells (CD8$^+$DR$^+$) and a subset of (CD8$^+$) T-cells defined by the CD38 monoclonal antibody (CD8$^+$CD38$^+$). This subset has previously been shown to correlate with HIV disease activity [17].

RESULTS

The results of treatment with plasmapheresis and corticosteroids are shown in Table 2. The initial response rate in this group was 80% (12/15). However, all but two patients relapsed within 1 months when plasmapheresis was withdrawn. Plasma exchange was reinstituted in five patients. All responded to the second course but then relapsed when the treatment was withdrawn again. An increase in steroid dose failed to control relapses in these patients.

Table 2.
Outcome of treatment protocols for HIV neuropathy

Treatment regimen	Number of patients	Initial response (%)	Persistent response (%)
Plasmapheresis + Corticosteroids	15	12 (80)	2 (13)
Plasmapheresis + IVIg	12	10 (83)	8 (67)

Treatment results with the combined use of plasmapheresis and IVIg are shown in Table 2. Ten of 12 patients responded to this treatment regimen. In contrast to plasmapheresis and corticosteroids use, combined plasma exchange and IVIg with monthly maintenance resulted in sustained remissions (greater than 6 months) in 8/10 patients. The two patients who failed to respond initially to plasmapheresis and IVIg were receiving corticosteroids, while the two patients who subsequently relapsed were not taking corticosteroids. EMG and nerve conduction studies demonstrated significant electrophysiologic improvement in the patients who responded to the combination regimen (data not shown).

There were no side effects related to the plasmapheresis treatments. In contrast, significant side effects were associated with corticosteroid administration. Bone necrosis developed in three patients and two required hip replacement. Although some patients experienced an increase in oral thrush, major infections did not occur with the dose of corticosteroids used in the study. Gastrointestinal bleeding was not seen in any of the study subjects. Reactions to the IVIg preparation included mild headache that was related to the rate of infusion and was easily controlled. There were no major adverse reactions to the brand of IVIg used in the study.

Lymphocyte subset analysis revealed a striking correlation between an increased CD8$^+$CD38$^+$ T-cell level and exacerbation of polyneuropathy (Fig. 1). The CD8$^+$CD38$^+$ T-cell number decreased following treatment with plasmapheresis and IVIg. This decrease in CD8$^+$CD38$^+$ T-cells correlated with improvement of neuropathic symptoms in the patients studied. Significant changes in other T-cell subsets were not observed.

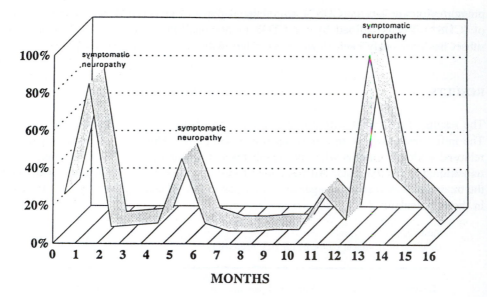

Figure 1. Association between neurologic disease and CD8+CD38+ T-cells in a representative patient.

DISCUSSION

Inflammatory demyelinating polyneuropathy is an autoimmune neurologic disorder that affects up to 10% of patients with HIV infection [5, 9]. The neuropathy may be crippling in individuals with significant weakness and sensory deficits, and it may follow an acute or chronic course. Recently an autoantibody directed against a peripheral nerve antigen has been described in this disorder [12]. The autoimmune nature of the neuropathy has prompted the use of immunosuppressive or cytotoxic agents to control neurologic damage. However, these treatments confer an additional risk of immunosuppression in patients with HIV disease. Thus alternative treatment modalities for polyneuropathy in these patients is essential.

Plasmapheresis has been used to treat various autoimmune disorders in HIV-negative patients [18]. Plasma exchange removes circulating autoantibodies and immune complexes, and it also modulates cellular immune function [19]. Removal of autoantibodies is accompanied by rebound antibody production that requires concomitant immuno-suppression. In HIV-negative patients with acute and chronic demyelinating polyneu-ropathy, plasmapheresis has provided an effective means of controlling the neurologic disease over long periods of time [13].

The first phase of our study demonstrated that plasmapheresis is effective in revers-ing most cases of HIV-related polyneuropathy. Unfortunately, relapse occurred when plasmapheresis was withdrawn and in spite of the use of immunosuppressive therapy with corticosteroids. In addition significant morbidity was associated with corticosteroid use. Thus a more effective form of immunosuppression was required.

IVIg has immunomodulatory properties similar to plasmapheresis [20, 21]. IVIg may down regulate immunostimulatory CD4+ T-cells and decrease autoantibody production by means of negative feedback [21]. These properties prompted the combined use of plasmapheresis with low-dose IVIg in patients with HIV-related polyneuropathy. The combined treatment had a sustained effect on the neuropathy in most patients. In addition, the side-effects of corticosteroids were minimized or avoided with this combination regimen. Baseline immunologic parameters did not change with the combination treatment. However, suppressor/cytotoxic T-cells bearing the CD38 marker increased with disease activity and decreased following treatment with plasmapheresis and IVIg. The implications of these T-cell changes are currently under investigation.

CONCLUSION

Treatment with plasmapheresis plus corticosteroids induces a significant but transient improvement in HIV-related polyneuropathy, and corticosteroid-induced side-effects may be significant. In contrast, combined treatment with plasma exchange plus IVIg leads to sustained remission in many patients with this HIV-related disorder. The combination regimen also avoids the adverse effects of corticosteroids. Further studies with combined plasmapheresis in IVIg in HIV-induced neuropathy are warranted.

SUMMARY

Inflammatory demyelinating polyneuropathy is an autoimmune disease that affects patients with human immunodeficiency virus (HIV) infection. We compared two protocols for the treatment of HIV-related polyneuropathy. In the first protocol, plasmapheresis combined with corticosteroids induced a remission in 80% of patients, but these patients quickly relapsed when plasmapheresis was withdrawn. In addition, significant side-effects were associated with corticosteroid use. In the second protocol, plasmapheresis was combined with low-dose intravenous gammaglobulin (IVIg). This regimen induced remission in 83% of patients and two-thirds had a sustained response to the combination therapy. Side effects related to plasmapheresis and IVIg were minimal. The combination of plasmapheresis and IVIg is a potent immunomodulatory therapy for patients with HIV-related peripheral neuropathy.

Acknowledgments
The authors thank Drs Dale Bredesen and Yuen So for helpful discussion. We also thank Regina Penton, Dulce MacLeod, Sheila Smith, Janet Smith, Lisa Farwood, Janet Leiva, Michelle Sours and Cecilio Dumlao of the Plasmapheresis Unit of California Pacific Medical Center for patient care and sample processing. We are grateful to Mary O'Loughlin for expert technical assistance. Supported by Grants 89-023 and 90-041 from California Pacific Medical Center.

REFERENCES

1. W. J. W. Morrow, D. A. Isenberg, R. E. Sobol, R. B. Stricker and T. Kieber-Emmons. AIDS virus infection and autoimmunity: a perspective of the clinical, immunological, and molecular origins of the autoallergic pathologics associated with HIV disease. *Clin. Immunol. Immunopathol.*, **58**, 163–180 (1991).
2. R. B. Stricker. Hemostatic abnormalities in HIV disease. *Hematol. Oncol. Clin. North Am.*, **5**, 249–265 (1991).
3. M. C. Dalakas and G. H. Pezeshkpour. Neuromuscular diseases associated with human immunodeficiency virus infection. *Ann. Neurol.*, **23** (Suppl. 1), S38–S48 (1988).

4. D. D. Kiprov, W. Pfaeffl, G. Parry, R. Lippert, W. Lange and R. G. Miller. Antibody-mediated peripheral neuropathies associated with ARC and AIDS: successful treatment with plasmapheresis. *J. Clin. Apheresis*, **4**, 3–7 (1988).

5. R. G. Miller, J. P. Gareth, W. Pfaeffl, W. Lange, R. Lippert and D. D. Kiprov. The spectrum of peripheral neuropathy associated with ARC and AIDS. *Muscle Nerve*, **11**, 857–863 (1988).

6. R. G. Miller, G. Parry, W. Lang *et al.* AIDS-related inflammatory polyradiculoneuropathy: prediction of response to plasma exchange with electrophysiologic testing. *Muscle Nerve*, **8**, 626–630 (1985).

7. Y. T. So, D. M. Holtzman, D. I. Abrams *et al.* Peripheral neuropathy associated with acquired immunodeficiency virus infections. *Arch. Neurol.*, **45**, 1084–1088 (1988).

8. D. Eidelberg, A. Sotrel, H. Vogel *et al.* Progressive polyradiculopathy in acquired immune deficiency syndrome. *Neurology*, **36**, 912–916 (1986).

9. R. B. Levy, D. E. Bredesen and M. L. Rosenblum. Neurologic manifestations of the acquired immunodeficiency syndrome (AIDS): experience at UCSF and review of the literature. *J. Neurosurg.*, **62**, 475–495 (1985).

10. W. I. Lipkin, G. Parry, D. D. Kiprov *et al.* Inflammatory neuropathy in homosexual men with lymphadenopathy. *Neurology*, **35**, 1479–1483 (1985).

11. D. R. Cornblath, J. C. McArthur, P. G. E. Kennedy *et al.* Inflammatory demyelinating peripheral neuropathies associated with HTLV-III infection. *Ann. Neurol.*, **21**, 32–40 (1987).

12. R. B. Stricker, D. E. Bredesen, P. D. Neyman, M. A. Wesley and S. K. Hahawar. Autoimmunity in the pathogenesis of HIV-related peripheral neuropathy. In: *Fifth Int. Conf. AIDS*, Montreal, Canada (1989) (Abstract).

13. G. M. McKhann, J. W. Griffin, D. R. Cornblath, E. D. Mellits, R. S. Fisher, S. A. Quaskey *et al.* Plasmapheresis and Guillain–Barré syndrome: analysis of prognostic factors and the effect of plasmapheresis. *Ann. Neurol.*, **23**, 347–353 (1988).

14. F. G. A. Van Der Meche, P. I. M. Schmitz and the Dutch Guillain–Barré Study Group. A randomized trial comparing intravenous immunoglobulin and plasma exchange in Guillain–Barré syndrome. *N. Engl. J. Med.*, **326**, 1123–1129 (1992).

15. Centers for Disease Control. Revision of the CDC surveillance case definition for acquired immunodeficiency syndrome. *MMWR*, **36** (Suppl. 1s), 3–15 (1987).

16. D. D. Kiprov, D. F. Busch, D. M. Simpsom *et al.* Antilymphocyte serum factors in patients with acquired immunodeficiency syndrome. In: *Acquired Immune Deficiency Syndrome*, M. S. Gottlieb and J. S. Groopman (Eds), pp. 299–308, Alan R. Liss, New York (1984).

17. R. S. Stricker, J. V. Giorgi, C. Dumlao and D. D. Kiprov. Significance of CD8$^+$CD38$^+$ T-cells in HIV infection. In: *Seventh Int. Conf. AIDS*, Florence, Italy (1991) (Abstract).

18. K. H. Shumak and G. A. Rock. Therapeutic plasma exchange. *N. Engl. J. Med.*, **310**, 762–771 (1984).

19. D. D. Kiprov, P. C. Dau and P. Morand. The effect of plasmapheresis and drug immunosuppression on T-cell subsets as defined by monoclonal antibodies. *J. Clin. Apheresis*, **2**, 57–63 (1983).

20. S. V. Kaveri, G. Dietrich, V. Hurez and M. D. Kazatchkine. Intravenous immunoglobulins (IVIg) in the treatment of autoimmune diseases. *Clin. Exp. Immunol.*, **86**, 192–198 (1991).

21. M. G. Macey and A. C. Newland. CD4 and CD8 subpopulation changes during high dose intravenous immunoglobulin treatment. *Br. J. Haematol.*, **76**, 513–520 (1990).

7
Rheumatoid Arthritis

Therapeutic Plasmapheresis (XII), pp. 285-288
T. Agishi *et al*. (Eds)
© VSP 1993

Results of Plasmapheresis Treatment in 12 Patients with Rheumatoid Arthritis — Long-term Treatment Cases

H. OGAWA, A. SAITO and Y. MATSUMOTO[1]

Department of Internal Medicine, Shinseikai Dai-ichi Hospital 1–3–2, Tamamizu-cho, Mizuho-ku, Nagoya, Aichi, Japan
[1]*Second Department of Internal Medicine, Nagoya City Univerity, School of Medicine, Nagoya, Japan*

Key words: rheumatoid arthritis; plasmapheresis; long-term treatment cases.

INTRODUCTION

Plasmapheresis (PP) is one form of therapy for collagen disease [1, 2]. It aids recovery from the disease by elimination of autoantibodies and immune complex. In the present investigation, we examined 12 patients undergoing PP treatment, mainly those who had been on it for a long time.

SUBJECTS AND METHODS

As shown in Table 1, a total of 12 patients were studied, five with rheumatoid arthritis (RA), seven with malignant rheumatoid arthritis (MRA). The course of RA or MRA

Table 1.
Profile of the 12 patients

Case	M or F	Age at starting PP (years)	Disease	RA stage	Duration of RA or MRA until PP (years)	Duration of PP therapy (months)
1	F	38	RA	4	12	58
2	F	46	MRA	3	3	46
3	M	60	RA	3	8	9
4	M	64	MRA	4	5	71
5	F	54	RA	4	7	48
6	M	44	MRA	4	10	30
7	F	44	MRA	4	21	27
8	F	46	RA	4	1	18
9	F	52	MRA	2	14	6
10	F	58	MRA	4	3	14
11	F	57	RA	3	1	6
12	M	51	MRA	3	5	3

until PP averaged 7.3 ± 5.9 years, and the duration of PP therapy averaged 29.9 ± 22.7 months. PP treatment was used for (i) cases of vasculitis and accompanying symptoms, and (ii) cases refractory to conventional drugs or unable to be treated because of their side-effects. PP treatment was given 1–4 times per month, but usually 4 times a months. Target symptoms were polyarthritis, neuropathy and vasculitis.

Two PP methods were used, double filtration (DF) and salt–amino acid coprecipitation (SAC) plasmapheresis [3], with treated plasma volume at 2.5 1.

For DFPP, 100 ml of 25% albumin as supplementary solution was employed, while no supplementary solution was employed for SAP plasmapheresis.

Hand gripping force was examined for each cases, and serum levels of CRP, albumin, IgG, IgM and RAHA were also examined.

RESULTS

Figure 1 shows the right hand gripping force over the course of therapy. An examination was made of 10 cases treated by PP for more than 1 year. The level at 12 months $(n = 10)$ into PP treatment was 78.6 ± 46.6 mmHg, whereas the level before PP was 61.6 ± 46.3 mmHg, reflecting a significantly higher level than pretreatment values $(P < 0.01)$. The level at 24 months $(n = 6)$ was 99.0 ± 60.9 mmHg, whereas the level before PP was 79.7 ± 52.2 mmHg, reflecting no significant difference.

The gripping force of the left hand at 12 months $(n = 10)$ was 68.0 ± 45.0 mmHg, whereas the pretreatment value was 60.2 ± 52.3 mmHg, reflecting no significant difference.

Figure 2 shows the level of CRP during PP therapy. The level of CRP at 12 months $(n = 11)$ was 4.6 ± 4.2 mg/dl, whereas the pretreatment level was 7.0 ± 4.4 mg/dl. The

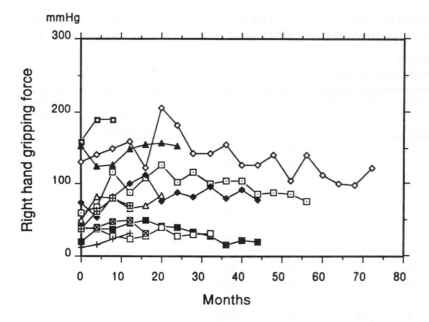

Figure 1. The right hand gripping force over course of PP therapy.

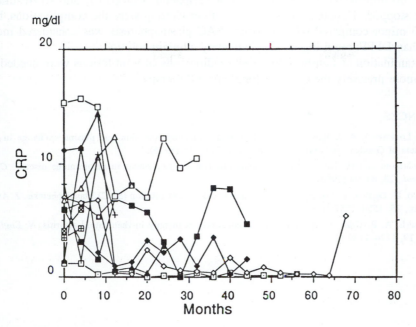

Figure 2. The level of CRP over the course of PP therapy.

levels of CRP at 24 months ($n = 6$) was 3.5 ± 4.4 mg/dl, whereas the pretreatment level was 7.0 ± 5.5 mg/dl. The level of CRP at 12 and 24 months were lower than the pretreatment levels, but no significant difference was found in each period.

Eleven of 12 cases showed RAHA levels beneath the PP pretreatment values.

The plasma IgG and IgM levels tended to decrease during PP treatment, but no significant difference was found in both the IgG level and IgM level.

The reduction rate of the plasma IgG and IgM levels of pre- and post-PP showed no decrease over the initial levels at 1–2 years of PP treatment.

The reasons for stopping PP treatment were as follows: (i) no diminishment of joint pain in one case (no. 11); (ii) no reduction in peripheral neuropathy in one case (no. 12); and (iii) shunt trouble in two cases (nos 8 and 9).

Complications arising in PP treatment were: (i) hepatitis in two cases (two with Type C); (ii) insufficient treated plasma volume in one case due to filter clotting; and (iii) hypotension (one case) and nausea (two cases) during PP treatment.

DISCUSSION

PP is one type of immunotherapy available for the treatment of collagen disease, and is reported to bring about recovery through elimination of autoantibodies and immune complex. However, Dwosh [4] indicated that PP was not an effective form of therapy. In the present study, PP was performed on a total of 12 patients. The focus was especially on patients undergoing PP treatment for over 1 year. Clinical results were obtained with only gripping force and CRP as criteria for evaluation, but there was an evident increase in the former and a clear decrease in the latter. In three patients, however, there was no improvement, for joint pain or peripheral neuropathy, and so treatment had to be stopped. Hypotension, nausea and filter clotting were the complications, but they were minor compared with hepatitis. SAC plasmapheresis was considered more suitable than DFPP, requiring no supplementary albumin solution.

The Examination of Lansbury index and radiographs of joint lesions were needed to evaluate more precisely the effect of long-term PP therapy.

REFERENCES

1. C. M. Lockwood, A. J. Rees and A. J. Rinching. Immunosuppression and plasma exchange in the treatment of Goodpasture's syndrome. *Lancet*, **1**, 711–715 (1976).

2. H. Hashimoto and H. Thuda. Plasmapheresis and lymphocytepheresis in autoimmune disease. *Clin. Immunol.*, **20**, 84–94 (1988).

3. A. Saito, H. Ogawa, T. Takagi *et al.* Salt–Amino acid–Coprecipitation (SAC) Plasmapheresis. *J. Artif. Organs.*, **15**, 1554–1557 (1986).

4. Il. Dowsh, A. R. Giles, P. M. Ford *et al.* Plasmapheresis therapy in rheumatoid arthritis. *N. Engl. J. Med.*, **19**, 1124–1129 (1983).

Therapeutic Plasmapheresis (XII), pp. 289-291
T. Agishi *et al.* (Eds)
© VSP 1993

Therapeutic Effects of Lymphocytapheresis on Rheumatoid Arthritis

T. NIWA, N. KATO,[1] H. ASADA,[1] Y. EMOTO, T. MIYAZAKI, H. MORITA, S. NAKAI and K. MAEDA

Department of Internal Medicine, Nagoya University Branch Hospital, Nagoya, Japan
[1]Yamaguchi Hospital, Aichi, Japan

Key words: lymphocytapheresis; rheumatoid arthritis; leukapheresis filter; immunomodulation; interleukin.

INTRODUCTION

Removal of lymphocytes has been used as an alternative of plasmapheresis [1] for the treatment of rheumatoid arthritis. Lymphocytapheresis has been performed by thoracic duct drainage [2] or centrifuge methods [3]. However, these methods of lymphocytapheresis are not widely used for the routine treatment. A cylindrical leukapheresis filter with polyester fiber fabric has been recently developed to remove leukocytes from blood in extracorporeal circulation [4]. To determine the therapeutic effect of lymphocytapheresis, patients with rheumatoid arthritis were treated by the lymphocytapheresis with the filter.

PATIENTS AND METHODS

Two patients with rheumatoid arthritis were treated by lymphocytapheresis. Case 1 (S.Y.) was a 65 year old, male patient. He had complained of shoulder, elbow, hand, hip and knee joint pain since 7 years ago. He visited our hospital 5 years ago. A non-steroidal anti-inflammatory drug (indomethacin) had been given for the treatment of joint pain. Data before lymphocytapheresis were as follows: BP 121/76 mmHg, TP 7.0 g/dl, Alb 2.3 g/dl, T-chol 158 mg/dl, BUN 23 mg/dl, s-cr 1.7 mg/dl, UA 6.5 mg/dl, CRP 25.3 mg/dl, RAHA 10 240, WBC 10 900/mm^3, RBC 3 370 000/mm^3, Ht 25.5%, Hb 8.1 g/dl, platelet 730 000/mm^3, IgG 5120 mg/dl, IgA 510 mg/dl, IgM 336 mg/dl, C_3 119.4 mg/dl, C_4 38.6 mg/dl.

Case 2 (A.M.) was a 60 year old, female patient. She had complained of morning stiffness and joint pain for 1 year. Steroids had been given for the treatment of rheumatoid arthritis. Data before lymphocytapheresis were as follows: BP 116/74 mmHg, TP 6.1 g/dl, Alb 3.0 g/dl, T-chol 161 mg/dl, BUN 13 mg/dl, s-cr 0.8 mg/dl, UA 5.0 mg/dl, CRP 18.8 mg/dl, RAHA 2560, WBC 9 600/mm^3, RBC 3 070 000/mm^3, Ht 25.6%, Hb 7.2 g/dl, platelet 422 000/mm^3, IgG 1235 mg/dl, IgA 197 mg/dl, IgM 209 mg/dl, C_3 79 mg/dl, C_4 17 mg/dl.

The patients with rheumatoid arthritis were treated three times by lymphocytapheresis. Access to the circulation was achieved by cannulating an internal shut in the forearm or femoral vein. A cylindrical leukapheresis filter (Cellsorba) was perfused with a total blood volume of 2400–2500 ml at a flow rate of 40 ml/min. Nafamostat mesilate was used as an anticoagulant at a dose of 50 mg/h. Using the filter, 97% of the leukocytes ($1.2-1.8 \times 10^{10}$ cells), 100% of the lymphocytes ($2.0-4.0 \times 10^9$ cells), 99% of the platelets and 1% of the erythrocytes that entered the filter were removed.

RESULTS AND DISCUSSION

Using the filter, 97.3 ± 0.5 (SE)% of the leukocytes ($1.2-1.8 \times 10^{10}$ cells), 100% of the lymphocytes ($2.0-4.0 \times 10^9$ cells), $99.0 \pm 0.4\%$ of the platelets ($5.3-9.6 \times 10^{11}$ platelets) and $0.9 \pm 0.7\%$ of the erythrocytes that entered the filter were removed. At the end of lymphocytapheresis, the circulating leukocytes, lymphocytes and platelets decreased to 60.0 ± 12.5, 49.1 ± 2.8 and $55.9 \pm 3.8\%$, respectively, of the number before lymphocytapheresis, while the number of erythrocytes maintained $91.8 \pm 0.8\%$.

Table 1 shows the effects of lymphocytapheresis on activities of rheumatoid arthritis. By lymphocytapheresis, both patients clinically improved as demonstrated by the decrease in Lansbury index. The duration of morning stiffness and erythrocyte sedimentation rate (ESR) decreased in both patients. Grip strength increased in case 2. However, the clinical improvement in our patients was not so remarkable as that observed in the previous report [4] in which patients were more often (9 times) treated by lymphocytapheresis. Long-term, frequent lymphocytapheresis treatment may cause more marked clinical improvement in patients with rheumatoid arthritis.

Table 2 shows the effects of lymphocytapheresis on immunological tests in case 1. Lymphocytapheresis showed immunomodulative effects such as a decrease in plasma levels of IL-2, IL-6 and CRP, and improved proliferative response to PHA, ConA and PWM. The proliferative responses of lymphocytes to lectins are usually suppressed in rheumatoid arthritis as a result of the increased number of monocytes. The removal of monocytes by lymphocytapheresis may have improved the proliferative response of lymphocytes. Lymphokines such as IL-1, IL-6 and TNF are thought to be involved in the progression of arthritis. Plasma levels of IL-6 were increased in case 1 before lymphocytapheresis and decreased after lymphocytapheresis. Since monocytes are the main source of IL-6 in human peripheral blood, the removal of monocytes by lymphocytapheresis may have caused the decrease in plasma IL-6. Il-6 induces liver acute-phase protein synthesis such as CRP. The decrease in CRP may be due to the decrease in the plasma IL-6 level.

Table 1.

Effects of lymphocytapheresis on activities of rheumatoid arthritis

	Case 1		Case 2	
	before	after	before	after
Lansbury index	86	75	79	74
Morning stiffness (min)	180	120	60	45
ESR (mm/h)	117	108	103	100
Grip strength	40	40	40	57
(R+L)/2 (mmHg)				

Table 2.

Effects of lymphocytapheresis (LCP) on immunological tests (case 1)

	Before	After third LCP
IL-1β (pg/ml)	< 15.6	< 15.6
IL-2 (IU/ml)	2.9	< 1.0
IL-6 (pg/ml)	182	42.6
CRP (mg/dl)	25.3	20.6
Proliferative response of lymphocytes		
PHA	5	204
ConA	42	74
PWM	20	82

CONCLUSIONS

Two patients with rheumatoid arthritis were treated by lymphocytapheresis with cylindrical leukapheresis filters. Access to the circulation was achieved by cannulating an internal shunt in forearm or femoral vein. The filter was perfused with total blood volume of 2400–2500 ml at a flow rate of 40 ml/min. Nafamostat mesilate was used as an anticoagulant at a dose of 50 mg/h. By the filter, 97% of the leukocytes (1.6×10^{10} cells), 100% of the lymphocytes (3.4×10^{9} cells), 99% of the platelets (7.7×10^{11} platelets) and 1% of the erythrocytes that entered the filter were removed. The patients clinically improved as demonstrated by the decrease in Lansbury index. Lymphocytapheresis with the filter showed immunomodulative effects such as a decrease in plasma levels of IL-2 and IL-6, and improved proliferative response to PHA, ConA and PWM.

REFERENCES

1. I. A. Jaffe. Comparison of the effects of plasmapheresis and penicillamine on the levels of circulating rheumatoid factor. *Ann. Rheum. Dis.*, **22**, 71–76 (1963).

2. T. Ueo, S. Tanaka, Y. Tominaga *et al.* The effect of thoracic duct drainage on lymphocyte dynamics and clinical symptoms in patients with rheumatoid arthritis. *Arthritis Rheum.*, **22**, 1405–1412 (1979).

3. J. Karsh, D. G. Wright, J. H. Klippel *et al.* Lymphocyte depletion by continuous flow cell centrifugation in rheumatoid arthritis. *Arthritis Rheum.*, **22**, 1055–1059 (1979).

4. T. Kondoh, Y. Hidaka, H. Katoh *et al.* Evaluation of a filtration lymphocytapheresis (LCP) device for use in the treatment of patients with rheumatoid arthritis. *Artif. Organs*, **15**, 180–188 (1991).

8
Hyperviscosity

Therapeutic Plasmapheresis (XII), pp. 295-297
T. Agishi *et al.* (Eds)
© VSP 1993

Efficacy of Plasmapheresis on Multiple Myeloma with Renal Insufficiency

K. TSUNEMI, M. HIDA, Y. TAKEBAYASHI, J. WATANABE, K. TANAKA, T. IIDA, S. HIRAGA and T. SATOH

Tokai University Hospital, Kidney Center, Kanagawa, Japan

Key words: plasmapheresis; multiple myeloma; renal failure.

INTRODUCTION

Renal insufficiency occurs in over 50% of multiple myeloma (MM) patients at the time of diagnosis. In recent years, plasmapheresis in conjunction with chemotherapy has been performed on MM patients with renal insufficiency, and the favorable effect of recovery of renal function has been reported.

PATIENTS AND METHODS

Patients

From 1983 to 1991 eight patients with acute renal failure (ARF) caused by MM were referred to our kidney center and one patient with chronic renal failure (CRF) and MM admitted to our center. They included seven males and two females who were 56–74 years old. All patients were either followed up to death or up to December 1991.

The diagnosis of MM was established by standard hematologic criteria. Myeloma was staged using the Durie and Salmon classification (1975). ARF was defined as previous findings of normal or near normal serum-creatinine (S-Cr) and normal kidney size. All patients were treated with hemodialysis (HD). Some clinical and laboratory data of the patients are summarized in Table 1.

Treatment protocol (Table 2)

Plasma exchange (PE) was performed in all nine patients. DFPP (double filtration plasmapheresis) was performed to Ig myelomas with a plasma separator of PVA or OP-05 and we used EVAL4A, 3A, or 2A as a plasma filter. The treated plasma volume was 3000 ml per treatment, replaced by albumin added lactate Ringer solution.

Total PE was performed to light chain myelomas with a plasma separator of EVAL2A, PVA or OP-05. The treated plasma volume was 3000 ml per treatment, replaced by fresh frozen plasma or albumin added lactate Ringer solution.

RESULTS

HD was required in all patients. Three patients, cases 7, 8 and 9, recovered renal function after PE, evaluated as a fall in serum creatinine level and suspension of HD,

Table 1.
Clinical and laboratory data, therapy and follow up

Case	Age	Sex	Type	BJP	S-Cr (mg/dl)	T-P (g/dl)	Hb (g/dl)	Alb (g/dl)	MOF number	Stage	Med.	HD	PE frequency	Outcome (month)
1	65	M	IgG λ	+	3.6	13.4	8.9	2.3	4	III B	P, M	I	2	*D* < 1
2	55	M	IgG λ	+	14.6	13.8	7.4	2.0	4	III B	P, M, V, C	I	4	D 5
3	70	M	IgG κ	+	5.6	6.5	7.5	2.2	5	III B	P, M, C, INF	I	2	D 42
4	56	M	BJP λ	+	13.8	9.2	6.9	3.5	1	III B	INF	M	3	D 3
5	65	F	BJP κ	+	4.6	5.3	6.4	2.7	5	III B	INF	I	1	D 3
6	58	M	IgA κ	+	12.7	6.8	10.1	2.7	2	III B	P, V, C	M	7	D 5
7	74	F	BJP κ	+	7.3	4.5	5.8	3.6	0	III B	P, M, INF	S	1	A 36
8	65	M	IgG κ	+	3.2	13.8	7.3	3.1	1	III B	P, M, INF	S	20	D 7
9	63	M	IgA λ	+	4.9	8.0	9.2	3.6	0	III B	P, V, C, INF	S	3	D 4

MOF, multiple organ failure; Med., medication; P, prednisolone; M, melpharan; V, vincristine; C, cyclo-phosphamide; INF, α-interferon; I, intermittent; M, maintenance; S, suspension; D, dead; A, alive.

Table 2.
Plasma exchange methods

	Target monoclonal serum type	Plasma separator	Plasma filter	Treated plasma volume (ml)	Replaced solution
DFPP	IgG, IgA	PVA, OP-05	EVAL4A, 3A, 2A	3000	4–5%, 7%. 8%, 10% Alb. Lactate Ringer
Total PE	BJP	EVAL2A, PVA, OP-05	none	3000	3% Alb. Lactate Ringer, FFP

who were defined as responders. Non-responders, i.e. cases 1, 2, 3, 4, 5 and 6, required continued dialysis and their frequency of HD did not decreased.

Statistical analysis was performed using the unpaired t-test for evaluation of the significance of the differences between the two groups, i.e. responders and non-responders.

We found no significant differences in diuresis, S-Cr, total protein (T-P), Hb, Ca, the intervals from diagnosis to ARF and ARF to PE, and the frequency of PE and HD between the two groups. However, there were significant differences between the two groups in serum albumin value and the numbers of organ failure.

DISCUSSION

We performed plasmapheresis on nine MM patients with renal insufficiency for the past 8 years, and investigated the efficacy of the treatment for the recovery of renal function, retrospectively. Pozzi *et al.* [2] reported that the most important clinical prognostic factors were T-P, S-Cr and myeloma type. However, in our study, the albumin value

Table 3.
Comparison between responder and non-responder patients

Parameters	Responders (nos 7, 8, 9)	Non-responders (nos 1, 2, 3, 4, 5, 6)	P
Age (years)	67.3 ± 5.9	61.5 ± 6.0	NS
Male/female	2/1	5/1	
Light chain/Ig Myeloma	1/2	2/4	
κ/λ	2/1	3/3	
Diuresis (ml/D)	656.7 ± 573.3	608.3 ± 261.6	NS
S-Cr (mg/dl)	5.13 ± 2.06	9.15 ± 5.06	NS
T-P (g/dl)	8.76 ± 4.70	9.17 ± 3.66	NS
Hb (g/dl)	7.43 ± 1.70	7.86 ± 1.38	NS
Ca (mEq/l)	5.03 ± 1.01	6.26 ± 1.18	NS
Alb (g/dl)	3.43 ± 0.28	2.56 ± 0.53	$P < 0.05$
Interval (months) (MM→ARF)	0 ± 0	9.8 ± 17.8	NS
Interval (days) (ARF→PE)	17.7 ± 7.23	13.8 ± 6.71	NS
PE (frequency)	8.0 ± 10.4	3.16 ± 2.13	NS
HD (frequency)	4.0 ± 1.0	17.4 ± 30.6	NS
MOF (number)	0.33 ± 0.57	3.5 ± 1.64	$P < 0.05$

and the numbers of organ failures at the time of starting HD and PE were significant statistically. Judging from several factors such as transferin, urinary protein, energy intake, etc., we concluded that patients nutritive condition could be evaluated with the serum albumin value at the initiation of HD and PE. It was suggested that the increase in the number of organ failures meant progression and deterioration of the primary disease.

It seems important to start timely HD and PE for the treatment of renal insufficiency due to MM before the general condition becomes worse.

REFERENCES

1. P. Zucchelli, S. Pasquali, L. Cagnoli and G. Ferrari. Controlled plasma exchange trial in acute renal failure due to multiple myeloma. *Kidney Int.*, **33**, 1175–1180 (1988).
2. C. Pozzi, S. Pasquali, U. Donini *et al.* Prognostic factors and effectiveness of treatment in acute renal failure due to multiple myeloma: a review of 50 cases. *Clin. Neph.*, **28**, 1–9 (1987).
3. S. Pasquali, L. Cagnoli, C. Rovinetti *et al.* Plasma exchange therapy in rapidly progressive renal failure due to multiple myeloma. *Int. J. Artif. Organs*, **8**, (Suppl. 2), 27–30 (1985).
4. M. Kajtna-Koselj, J. Drinovec, S. Kaplan *et al.* Plasma exchange in myeloma renal failure. *Apheresis*, **1**, 271–273 (1990).

Therapeutic Plasmapheresis (XII), pp. 299-304
T. Agishi *et al.* (Eds)
© VSP 1993

Hemorheological Properties Changed by Therapeutic Plasmapheresis: Patients with Waldenström's Macroglobulinaemia

G. PARDEMANN, I. PAWLOW,[1] G. MATTHES,[1]
M. PAULITSCHKE and D. LERCHE

Humboldt University Berlin (Charité), Institute of Medical Physics, Biophysics and
[1]*Institute of Transfusiology and Transplantation, Germany*

Key words: Waldenström's macroglobulinaemia; therapeutic plasmapheresis; cascade filtration; proteinshifts; hemorheological properties.

INTRODUCTION

There has been considerable interest to improve the treatment of patients with Waldenström's macroglobulinaemia by chemotherapy and therapeutical plasmapheresis (PPH). It seems to be useful to measure protein shifts in plasma due to PPH by physical methods and to evaluate changes of the blood properties using hemorheological methods [1–5]. The goal of these measurements is also to optimize the therapy so as to estimate the effectiveness of blood purification for personal therapy planning. The rapidly increased plasmaviscosity in patients with macroglobulinaemia is the base of complex hemorheological, biochemical and pathophysiogical processes [3]. Our preliminary results show that a temporary improved flowability of blood can be achieved after PPH.

MATERIAL AND METHODS

Five ambulant patients with monoclonal increased IgM were treated by PPH. Blood samples were taken before and after PPH (anticoagulant heparin).

We used two methods for *blood purification*: (i) in cases with high IgM levels mainly partially PPH (Hemonetics PCS Ultralite with discontinuous flow) to remove 20% of the plasma volume on three following days in common without substitution (3 RV 20) and (ii) a cell separator with continuous flow (Dideco Vivacell BT 798, Italy) connected with a cascade filter (Dideco-Albusave BT 902) for selective IgM removal (CF).

Plasma measurements: plasmaviscosity (PV), using a capillary viscosimeter (25°C); density (D), using as high precision method a fluid-filled vibrating U-tube (25°C), Firma Paar, Graz; Colloid osmotic pressure (COP), using a membrane osmometer from the Institute of Laboratory Diagnostic (Dresden) (37°C, pH7.4). Biochemical routine methods: Total Protein Content (TPC), Albumin (A), serum- and immuno-electrophoresis.

Hemorheological measurements: blood viscosity (BV), using Low Shear Viscosimetry-System LS 40 of Mettler/Toledo, Switzerland (25°C); Aggregometer (Hct=0.45; 25°C), an infrared backscattering technique, and Filtrometer (cellulose filters, 25°C, Hct=0.60), both Institute of Medical Physics (Berlin), reviewed in [1].

RESULTS

Experimental data were evaluated in relation to parameters determined from plasma donors (Table 1).

Table 1.
Normal values of measured quantities

quantity		mean value	SD	N
D	g cm^{-3}	1.0247	±0.00120	40
PV	mPas	1.618	±0.069	40
COP	kPa	3.84	±0.33	30
TPC	g l^{-1}	75.90	±3.70	30
A	g l^{-1}	47.60	±2.60	30
FI (filtration index)		11.60	±2.20	22
AI (aggregation index)		0.65	±0.07	22

Figure 1 shows long-term monitoring of PPH by physical methods (PV, COP, D). The density depends linearly on TPC. It should be noted that the lower borderline of the oncotic pressure does not exceed at the end of the last PPH.

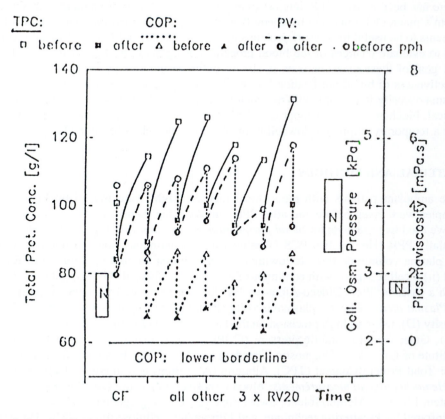

Figure 1. Protein shifts due to PPH monitored by physical measurements (PV, COP, D) patient: G. F., M. Waldenström CF: 2.10.90 3 RV 20: 22–24.5.91; 24–26.6; 29–31.7.92; 29.10–1.11; 4.3–6.3.92; 27.4–29.4.92.

Using the results of all biochemical measurements we found a non-linear relationship between IgM concentration and measured PV, presented in Fig. 2 and expressed by an exponential function.

We can see from Fig. 3 that the COP is remarkable influenced by high levels of the paraproteins (IgG plasmocytom, IgM: M. Waldenström). Globulins in plasma of patients with high IgM levels produce about 40–50% of COP. The effect of albumin concentration on COP is estimated by means of the virial equation, given in Fig. 3 with an experimentally determined virial coefficient for albumin: $B_A = 0.84 \, \text{m}^3 \, \text{mol}^{-1}$.

As the result of the aggregometer measurements we obtained a positive linear correlation between the AI and PV: $AI = -0.523 \, PV + 1.429$ for PV<2.8 mPas. If the PV is higher than 2.8 mPas, it is necessary to use diluted suspension media (plasma: PBS) in order to estimate the RBC aggregation loss by blood purification.

We used filtrometer measurements to characterize RBC deformability. As a rule, we measured clearly increased FIs compared with the normal group (11.6 ± 2.2) and significantly decreased FI of blood after PPH.

The apparent blood viscosity (BV), depending on shear rates ($0.01–100 \, \text{s}^{-1}$), is shown in Fig. 4 for blood samples before and after PPH. The BV in low shear rates is diminished by PPH due to reduced RBC–RBC interactions. There exist difficulties in patients with high IgM concentrations when trying to measure blood viscosities exactly that are caused by rapid sedimentation of the cell aggregates in the viscosimeter gap.

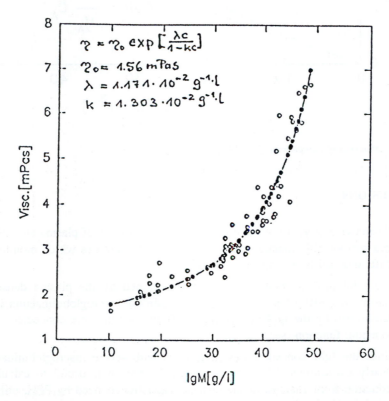

Figure 2. Plasmaviscosity as a function of the IgM concentration (patients with M. Waldenström).

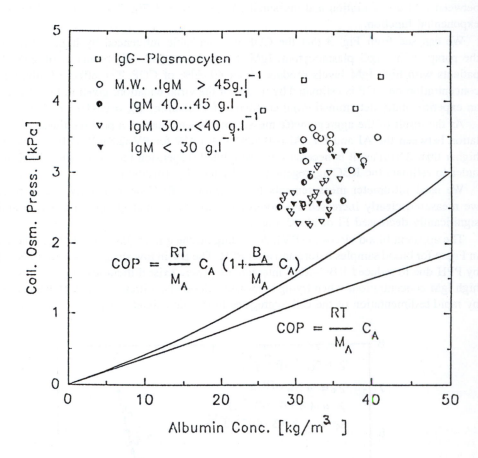

Figure 3. Influences of paraproteins (IgG, IgM) on COP.

CONCLUSIONS

(i) Plasma viscosity, colloid osmotic pressure and density of plasma are quickly and in a reproducible manner measurable physical quantities which monitor protein shifts induced by therapeutical PPH.

(ii) The total protein content is exactly determined by the plasma density. The plasma viscosity of patients with Waldenströms macroglobulinaemia is mainly determined by the IgM concentration. Both quantities are connected by an exponential function (see Fig. 2).

(iii) Since the IgM concentrations in patients with severe macroglobulinaemia are clearly overestimated by immunoelectrophoresis, it is useful to calculate IgM reduction from changes of the plasma viscosities induced by PPH, utilizing the exponential equation.

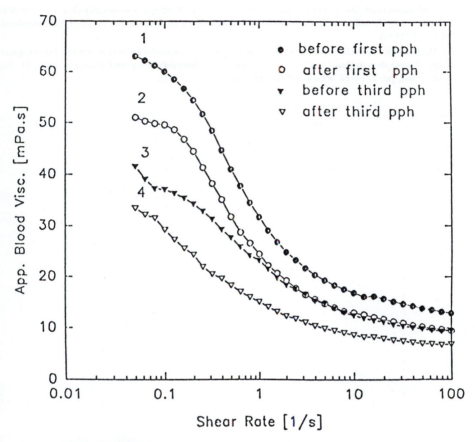

Figure 4. Influences of PPH (3RV20) on apparent blood viscosity, depending on shear rate (patient G. F., M. Waldenström) 1: PV=7.44 mPas, Hct=0.29; 2: PV=5.57 mPas, Hct=0.28; 3: PV=4.98 mPas, Hct=0.31; 4: PV=3.94 mPas, Hct=0.28.

(iv) Monoclonal increased immunoglobulins (IgM, IgG) in human plasma contribute remarkably to the oncotic pressure. Therefore, the virial coefficient (B_{IgM}) of the pentamer ($M = 900 \, \text{kg mol}^{-1}$) was estimated to about $50 \, \text{m}^3 \, \text{mol}^{-1}$ (see Fig. 3).

(v) If PV>3 mPas measurements of hemorheological quantities (apparent blood viscosity, aggregation parameters) are connected with measuring technical problems. Presently the improved flow ability of blood after plasmapheresis can be estimated only quantitatively.

REFERENCES

1. D. Lerche *et al.* Flow properties of blood and hemorheological methods of quantification. In: *Phisical Characterization of Biological Cells*, W. Schütt *et al.* (Eds), pp. 189–214, Berlin Verl. Gesundheit (1991).

2. T. Somer. Rheology of paraproteinaemias and the plasma hyperviscosity syndrome. *Baillieres Clin. Haematol.*, **1**, 695–723 (1987).

3. F. Stoltz, M. Donner and A. Larcan. Introduction to hemorheology: theoretical aspects and hyperviscosity syndrome. *Int. Angiol.*, **6**, 119–132 (1987).

4. G. Pardemann *et al.* Die Überwachung der therapeutischen Plasmapherese mit physikalischen Meßverfahren — eine Grundlage zu ihrer mathematischen Modellierung. *Biomed. Techn.*, **35** (Ergänzungsband), 316–317 (1990).

5. M. Paulitschke *et al.* Untersuchungen zu Änderungen der Plasmaviskosität und -dichte der therapeutischen Plasmapherese. In: *Aktuelles aus der klinischen Mikrozirkulation und Hämorheologie*, H. Jung *et al.* (Eds), pp. 181–186, Blackwell Wissenschaft, Berlin (1992).

Therapeutic Plasmapheresis (XII), pp. 305-308
T. Agishi *et al.* (Eds)
© VSP 1993

Effect of Plasmapheresis for Hyperviscosity Syndrome in a Patient with Sjögren's Syndrome Associated with Macroglobulinemia

T. NAKABAYASHI, A. SAGAWA, N. OGURA, T. ATSUMI, K. OHNISHI, A. FUJISAKU and S. NAKAGAWA

The Second Department of Internal Medicine, Hokkaido University School of Medicine, Sapporo, Japan

Key words: hyperviscosity syndrome; Sjögren's syndrome; plasmapheresis; Sephacryl S-300 gel chromatography; immune complexes.

INTRODUCTION

Hyperviscosity syndrome is a rare but severe disorder that accompanies monoclonal and occasionally polyclonal paraproteinemias [1]. Large molecular compounds with a high intrinsic viscosity are especially prone to cause hyperviscosity.

We studied the effect of plasmapheresis on a case with Sjögren's syndrome with hyperviscosity symptom whose serum had monoclonal IgM, positive rheumatoid factor (RF) and anti-SS-A antibody. Plasmapheresis relieved her symptoms related with hyperviscosity syndrome. We discuss the elimination of immune complexes were probably composed of RF and IgG, some of which had anti-SS-A activity, by plasmapheresis.

CASE REPORT

A 69 year old woman was admitted to our hospital on June 11, 1985, for evaluation of elevated IgM in her serum. The patient had been suffering for 5 years, from bilateral parotid gland enlargement and dry mouth, since April, 1984. Sialography and biopsy of the parotid gland were performed and then she was diagnosed as Sjögren's syndrome. Physical examination on admission showed bilateral parotid enlargement and lymph node enlargement in the right axilla. The laboratory studies revealed that hemoglobin level was 6.8 g/dl, hematocrit value was 20.1% and white blood cell count was 5200/μl. The total protein level was 7.0 g/dl with gamma fraction, 42.7%. Protein electrophoresis of her serum showed a monoclonal peak existed in the slow gamma region, which was identified as an IgM(kappa). The concentration of IgM was increased, 3075 mg/dl, but IgG and IgA were within normal limits. Serum immunoelectrophoresis showed normal IgG and IgA precipitin arcs. The IgM and light chain kappa arcs showed M bow. A Bence–Jones protein of kappa-type was detected in a 50-fold concentrated specimen of urine. Cryogelglobulin was detected in her serum at room temperature. Immunological findings revealed high tittered RF activity, positive antinuclear antibody and anti-SSA antibody.

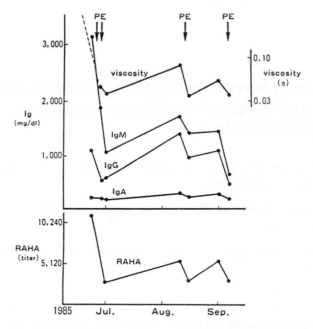

Figure 1. Changes in the viscosity, the levels of immunoglobulins (Ig) and RAHA titer of her serum during the course.

On the 10th hospital day, the patient developed transient confusion and sudden onset of bilateral visual disturbance. Funduscopic examination demonstrated retinal bleeding and dilated veins, confirming the diagnosis of hyperviscosity syndrome. Plasmapheresis was applied and her serum was replaced with lactated Ringer's solution, ACD solution and albumin in a total volume of 2000 ml by Haemonetics model S-30. After pheresis, the electrophoresis of her serum showed that the monoclonal component in the slow gamma region was markedly reduced.

Figure 1 illustrates changes of serum viscosity, immunoglobulin levels and RAHA titer during the course of plasmapheresis. After pheresis, her serum viscosity decreased, associated with reduction of the concentration of IgM and IgG and titer of RAHA, while the concentration of IgA was unchanged. Her symptoms related to hyperviscosity improved during the whole course of this study.

MATERIALS, METHODS AND RESULTS

The components which might be responsible for hyperviscosity were studied.

For starters, analysis with ultracentrifugation of her serum showed some macromolecular peaks in 0.05 M tris buffered saline (TBS), pH 8.0. But after treatment of the serum with 0.1 M acetate buffer, pH 4.1, these macromolecular peaks disappeared (data not shown).

Next, her serum was fractionated by gel filtration. The chromatographic elution pattern of her serum protein from Sephacryl S-300 gel are shown in the upper panels in Fig. 2. The five main peaks in 0.05 M TBS, pH 8.0 (Fig. 2A), were shifted to three

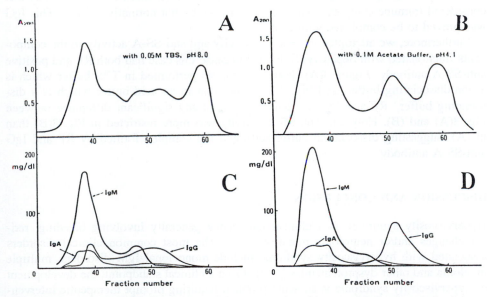

Figure 2. The elution profile of her serum and the concentration of immunoglobulins in each fraction.

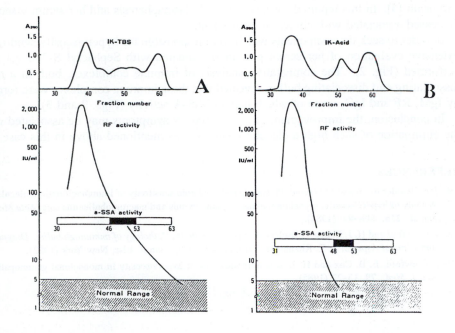

Figure 3. The elution profile of her serum and RF activity and anti-SS-A activity in each fraction.

peaks in 0.1 M acetate buffer, pH 4.1 (Fig. 2B). The lower panels of Fig. 2 show the concentration of immunoglobulins measured by laser nephelometry in the above eluted fractions. We have two peaks of IgG (fractions 39 and 51) in Fig. 2(C), while we have only one peak of IgG in Fig. 2(D). The first peak of IgG (fraction 39) in Fig. 2(C) was considered immune complex because IgG alone would not normally existed. This IgG was proved to be complexed with IgM.

Furthermore, we attempted to seek RF activity and anti-SS-A activity in the components fractionated with Sephacryl S-300 gel because this case had both RF and positive anti-SS-A antibody. Figure 3(A) shows an analysis performed in TBS buffer which is a non-dissociating buffer, and Fig. 3(B) shows that in an acid buffer which is a dissociating buffer. RF activity was detected without any significant difference between Fig. 3(A) and (B). However, anti-SS-A activity was more restricted in Fig. 3(B) than in (A), suggesting dissociating buffer separated the complex formed by RF and IgG anti-SS-A antibody.

DISCUSSION AND CONCLUSION

Hyperviscosity syndrome is a clinical emergency generally involving bleeding, retinal changes and/or neurologic manifestations. The most common clinical disorders associated with hyperviscosity syndrome include monoclonal IgM disorders, multiple myeloma and other dysproteinemias [1, 2]. From a clinical standpoint, the development of hyperviscosity syndrome is an acute problem requiring prompt therapeutic intervention such as plasmapheresis. Although the initial signs and symptoms are reversible with early treatment, delay in therapy leads to permanent visual loss, stroke, bleeding and death [3]. In this reported case, we applied plasmapheresis and her serum viscosity decreased associated with clinical improvement.

In order to seek the components which were responsible for hyperviscosity syndrome, extensive evaluation of her serum protein fractionated with Sephacryl S-300 gel was performed (Fig. 2). The comparative analysis of immune complexes, both in a non-dissociating and dissociating buffer, revealed that these immune complexes were formed by IgM, RF and IgG, some of which had anti-SS-A activity (Figs 2 and 3).

In conclusion, the improvement of hyperviscosity symptoms may be associated with the elimination of such high molecular complexes as mentioned above in this case.

REFERENCES

1. J. G. Waldenström and U. Raiend. Plasmapheresis and cold sensitivity of immunoglobulin molecules. I. A study of hyperviscosity, cryoglobulinemia, euglobulinemia and macroglobulinemia sera. *Acta Medica Scand.*, **216**, 449–466 (1984).
2. J. Crawford and H. J. Cohen. Disorders of hyperviscosity. In: *Pathology of immunoglobulins: Diagnostic and Clinical Aspects*, S. E. Ritzumann (Ed.), pp. 237–259, Alan R. Liss, New York (1982).
3. J. Crawford, E. B. Cox and H. J. Cohen. Evaluations of hyperviscosity in monoclonal gammopathies. *Am. J. Med.*, **79**, 13–22 (1985).

Therapeutic Plasmapheresis (XII), pp. 309-313
T. Agishi *et al.* (Eds)
© VSP 1993

Changes in Blood and Plasma Viscosity Accompanying Plasmapheresis on Patients with Rheumatoid Arthritis

K. YAMAJI, Y. KANAI, T. KAWANISHI, M. TOUMYO, S. FUJITA,
M. YOKOYAMA, H. TSUDA, H. HASHIMOTO and S.-I. HIROSE

*Division of Rheumatology, Department of Internal Medicine, Juntendo University,
Tokyo, Japan*

Key words: plasmapheresis; viscosity; rheumatoid arthritis.

INTRODUCTION

Recently, there have been many reports that suggested the availability of plasmapheresis (PP) to rheumatoid arthritis (RA) patients, but many of these reports were based on investigations of immunological changes. In the present study, we measured blood and plasma viscosity before and after PP and investigated changes in viscosity and association with RA activity and clinical symptoms.

SUBJECTS AND METHODS

The subjects were 18 patients, who were diagnosed according to the criteria of the American Rheumatism Association. We divided them into two groups, A and B, according to their ESR levels. Group A patients consisted of nine persons, whose erythrocyte sedimentation rate (ESR) level was 50 mm/h and higher. Group B patients consisted of nine persons, whose ESR level was under 50 mm/h (Table 1).

Table 1.
Patient profile of RA patients

	Cases	Male:Female	Age (mean)
Group A (ESR≥50 mm/h)	9	3:6	47–73 (60.0)
Group B (ESR<50 mm/h)	9	2:7	42–61 (50.8)

We performed PP on the 18 patients using double filtration and employed a second filter that had a 0.02 μm pore size. We measured the blood viscosity using a cone-plate type viscometer manufactured by Brookfield Inc. on sample of whole blood and corrected blood using autoplasma to 35% Ht. We used a shear rate of five steps with centipoise (cP) as the unit. Plasma viscosity was measured by the capillary viscometer of Isogai's method and these data are shown as viscosity relative to distilled water.

RESULTS

We investigated these results and clinical symptoms before and after PP, comparing the findings in Group A with those of Group B. The values of blood viscosity of whole blood in Group B were slightly higher than those of Group A, but the difference was not significant. We thought that these results may have been affected by differences in Ht and so on (Fig. 1).

The values of blood viscosity of corrected blood in Group A were slightly higher than those of Group B (Fig. 2).

Plasma viscosity is shown in Table 2: Group A values were significantly higher than those of Group B.

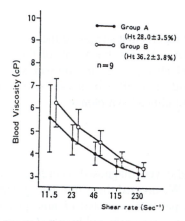

Figure 1. Blood viscosity of RA patients: whole blood.

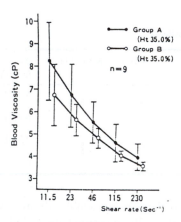

Figure 2. Blood viscosity of RA patients: corrected blood.

Table 2.
Plasma viscosity of RA patients

Group A	1.994 ± 0.143	
Group B	1.751 ± 0.058	P < 0.01

Table 3.
Lansbury index

Group A	78.96 ± 21.54	
Group B	38.63 ± 13.90	P < 0.01

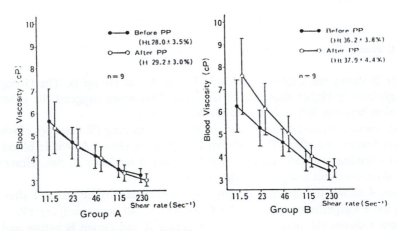

Figure 3. Whole blood viscosity of RA patients (cP).

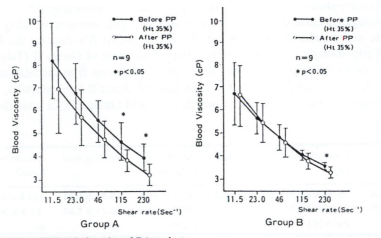

Figure 4. Corrected blood viscosity of RA patients.

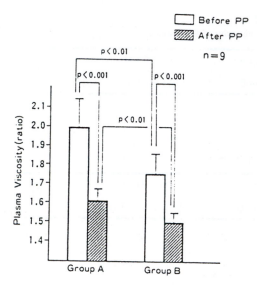

Figure 5. Plasma viscosity of RA patients.

Table 3 shows the Lansbury index in Group A and Group B. The Group A value was significantly higher than that of Group B. This result suggests the existence of a correlation between RA activity and plasma viscosity.

Next, we investigated changes in viscosity accompanying PP. Changes of whole blood viscosity before and after PP are shown in Fig. 3. In Group A, whole blood viscosity showed a tendency to fall and in Group B showed a tendency to rise. However, these results do not exhibit a significant difference.

Figure 4 shows the changes in corrected blood viscosity before and after PP. Both groups have a significant tendency for the values to fall accompanying PP.

Figure 5 shows the plasma viscosity in Group A and Group B before and after PP. Group A's plasma viscosity was higher than that of Group B, both before and after PP. Plasma viscosity showed a significant tendency to fall accompanying PP.

We investigated Lansbury index, morning stiffness, grip strength, walking time and joint score, and compared Group A with Group B. Group A's data for the Lansbury index and grip strength were significantly poorer than those of Group B (Table 4).

Table 5 shows the difference between Group A and Group B in the laboratory data. Group A's data were significantly higher than those of Group B for γ-globulin, IgG, IgA and Fibrinogen. Group A's data were lower than those of Group B's for total-cholesterol.

Table 4.

	Lansbury index (%)	Morning stiffness (min)	Grip strength (mmHg)	Walking time (s)	Joint score (point)
Group A	75.96 ± 21.54	88.9 ± 104.3	78.1 ± 33.0	18.83 ± 6.15	113.3 ± 56.3
Group B	38.63 ± 13.90	28.9 ± 50.2	146.3 ± 63.4	14.24 ± 1.83	81.4 ± 38.0
	$P < 0.001$	ns	$P < 0.05$	ns	ns

Table 5.

	ESR (mm/h)	γ-globulin (g/dl)	IgG (mg/dl)	IgA (mg/dl)	IgM (mg/dl)	T-CHO (mg/dl)	Fibrinogen (mg/dl)
Group A	77.7	1.559	1928.0	473.3	174.2	174.7	439.6
	±22.4	±0.365	±354.4	±186.8	±107.3	±20.8	±121.1
Group B	25.6	0.978	1212.3	265.1	102.4	213.8	322.4
	±9.9	±0.178	±298.0	±80.4	±31.4	±29.9	±79.0
	$P < 0.01$	$P < 0.01$	$P < 0.01$	$P < 0.05$	ns	$P < 0.01$	$P < 0.05$

Table 6.

	Grip strength (mmHg)		Walking time (s)		Joint score (point)	
	before PP	after PP	before PP	after PP	before PP	after PP
Group A	78.1±33.0	129.3±79.9	18.83±6.15	15.00±2.00	113.3±56.3	89.5±18.5
Group B	146.3±63.4	172.7±35.5	14.24±1.83	13.00±1.50	81.4±38.0	72.5±21.5

This time we investigated changes in the clinical symptoms before and after PP, in both Group A and Group B for grip strength, walking time and joint score. These data show tendency for improvement accompanying PP (Table 6).

DISCUSSION AND CONCLUSION

We measured the blood and plasma viscosity before and after PP, and investigated the changes of viscosity and relevancy to RA activity and clinical symptoms. Plasma viscosity is related to RA activity. In addition, plasma viscosity, clinical symptoms and RA activity show a tendency to improve accompanying PP. Our findings indicate that plasma viscosity is related to RA activity, and that plasma viscosity clinical symptoms and RA activity show a tendency to improve accompanying PP.

Because of these results, we believe that plasma viscosity can serve as a therapeutic indicator for PP in RA patients.

REFERENCES

1. M. Harreby, B. Danneskiold-Samoe, J. Kjer and M. Lauritzen. Viscosity of plasma in patients with rheumatoid arthritis. *Ann. Rheum. Dis.*, **46**, 601–604 (1987).
2. M. E. Pickup, J. S. Dixon, C. Hallett, H. A. Bird and V. Wright. Plasma viscosity — a new appraisal of its use as index of disease activity in rheumatoid arthritis. *Ann. Rheum. Dis.*, **40**, 272–275 (1981).
3. R. M. Pope, M. Mannik, B. C. Gilliland and D. C. Teller. The hyper viscosity syndrome in rheumatoid arthritis due to intermediate complexes formed by selfassociation of IgG-rheumatoid factors. *Arthritis Rheum.*, **18** No. 2 (1975).
4. R. M. Hutchinson and R. D. Eastham. A comparison of the erythrocyte sedimentation rate and plasma viscosity in detecting changes in plasma proteins. *J. Clin. Pathol.*, **30**, 345–349 (1977).
5. R. A. Crockson and A. P. Crockson. Relationship of the erythrocyte sedimentation rate to viscosity and plasma proteins in rheumatoid arthritis. *Ann. Rheum. Dis.*, **33**, 53 (1974).

9
Transplantation–relevant Apheresis

Therapeutic Plasmapheresis (XII), pp. 317-319
T. Agishi *et al.* (Eds)
© VSP 1993

Peripheral Blood Stem Cell Collection with the Excel

M. VALBONESI, P. CARLIER, G. LERCARI, G. FLORIO and G. GIANNINI

Immunohematology Services, San Martino Hospital, Genova, Italy

Key words: peripheral blood stem cell collection; mononuclear cell.

INTRODUCTION

Progenitor stem cells are found in both marrow and peripheral blood which can be collected by apheresis. It is most effective to collect the peripheral blood stem cells (PBSCs) during the rise in white count that follows induction chemotherapy. PBSCs have been shown to be capable of restoring hematopoiesis after induction chemotherapy in patients suffering from hematological malignancies or solid tumors. This is of peculiar interest in patients at risk for anesthesia or with hypocellular or infiltrated bone marrow. More frequently, acute leukemia, melanoma, chronic myelogenous leukemia (CML) in blastic crisis, lymphoma, as well as breast, lung and ovarian Cancers are treated and long-term disease-free cases have been recorded. Several apheresis instruments and methods have been employed for PBSC collection [1], both of the DFC and CFC type, with progressive interest in automated CFC techniques [2, 3].

In this study we report on the efficacy of the Dideco-Excel (Dideco Srl, Mirandola, Modena, Italy) in collecting mononuclear cells (MNC) to be used for autologous PBSC transplantation.

THE PRINCIPLE OF PBSC COLLECTION

The separation of MNC from red blood cells (RBC) occurs in a PVC belt which during separation phase assumes a double stage configuration. In the primary chamber the buffy coat (BC) is separated from packed red blood cells (PRBC) and progressively accumulated in the upper position of the primary chamber.

Plasma is continuously separated and it flows freely from the primary to the secondary separation chamber. The BC, which contains the MNC, is maintained in a fixed position by the action of a CCD sensor which acts upon the PRBC reinfusion pump. The BC is in a very unstable position and it tends to escape the sensor control (continuous spillover). When this occurs the PRBC pump is activated and the precarious equilibrium of the BC is obtained.

The BC that escapes from the primary chamber is brought out of the belt by the action of a specific peristaltic pump whose velocity may be adjusted according to the operator's decisions.

The program which operates the collection of MNC can be modified by the operator in such as way that MNC collection is continuous, as described, or discontinuous.

With this second option, which is recommended for very low white blood cell (WBC) counts, a prefixed amount of blood (50–500 ml) is collected from the patient to allow the formation of the BC which at the end of the collection is discontinuously collected (discontinuous spillover). This is obtained by automatically halting the PRBC pump and inactivating the CCD sensor feedback for a prefixed and programmable volume in order to allow the BC to invade the secondary separation chamber.

The belt which is used for PBSC is the usual for PLT apheresis. The ACD-A to blood ratio is 1/15, the blood flow rate (BFR) is from 5 to 70 ml/min and the centrifuge speed is 1800 r.p.m. At this centrifugation speed 400 g are determined at the primary to secondary chamber passage and 600 g at the collection port.

PATIENTS AND RESULTS

Ten procedures have been carried out in patients undergoing PBSC collection because of CML in blastic crisis (five), NHL (three) and breast cancer (two). Six were male and four were female; their mean body weight (BW) was of 56 kg. The precollection hematological values (Technicon H 6000; Technicon Corp., Tarrytown, NY) are summarized in Table 1.

Table 1.
Preliminary study of PBSC collection with the Excel and comparison with the results obtained in the same patients when the AS 104 apparatus was used

	Dideco Excel		Fresenius AS 104
No. of procedures		10	
M/F ratio		6/4	
Mean body weight (kg)		56	
Mean HCT%		26,7	
WBC precount/μl	470		455
MNC precount/μl	410		424
PLT precount $\times 10^3 \mu$l	31		28
WBC yield $\times 10^9$	1,9		2,57
MNC %	84		90
PLT contamination $\times 10^{11}$	2,8		2,3
HCT % in the product	11		8
Volume of blood processed (l)	10		10
Mean blood flow rate (ml/min)	41		44
Procedure time (min)	243		227

The yields in terms WBC, MNC, RBC, PLT, as well as the volume of the product are summarized in the same table, where they are compared with the results obtained in the same patients employing the Fresenius AS 104 apparatus in a crossover study.

DISCUSSION

PBSC collection is becoming one of the main tasks for apheresis units. As to our most recent experience, in the last 6 months over 150 procedures have been carried out using the CS 3000+ or the Fresenius AS 104 CF separators.

Excel is the very latest third generation automated CF apparatus that Dideco has presented for high speed and efficiency platelet collection and therapeutic procedures. The machine has several pieces of new technologies which seem to justify its introduction in the international market if PBSC is performed adequately.

This study gives very preliminary answers to the question of the adequacy of Excel to this task. In fact, our results indicate that even with the presently used prototype, PBSC collection is possible even if it must be recognized that this result represents approximately 76% of those obtained in comparable patients by the use of the Fresenius AS 104 apparatus. Refinements of the procedure and ameliorations of the results are necessary for this machine that, in terms of other apheresis procedures, has shown its competitivity.

REFERENCES

1. H. C. Schouten, A. Kessinger, D. Smith *et al.* Counterflow centrifugation apheresis for the collection of autologous peripheral blood stem cells from patients with malignancies: a comparison with a standard centrifugation apheresis procedure. *J. Clin. Apheresis*, **5**, 140 (1990).
2. D. Padley, R. G. Strauss, M. Wieland *et al.* Concurrent comparison of the cobe spectra and fenwal CS3000 for the collection of peripheral blood mononuclear cells for autologous peripheral stem cell transplantation. *J. Clin. Apheresis*, **6**, 77 (1991).
3. A. Iacone, A. Dragani, A. M. Quaglietta *et al.* Collection of blood-derived hemopoietic stem cells with a CS 3000 blood cell separator. *Bone Marrow Transplant.*, **5**, (Suppl. 1), 70 (1990).

Therapeutic Plasmapheresis (XII), pp. 321-323
T. Agishi *et al.* (Eds)
© VSP 1993

Plasma Exchange for Reduction of Anti-A/Anti-B Levels Before Bone Marrow Transplantation

A. MENDRONE Jr, J. M. KUTNER, M. A. MOTA,
A. M. SAKASHITA, M. C. ZAGO, A. M. ARRIFANO,
P. E. DORLHIAC-LLACER and D. A. F. CHAMONE

*Fundação Pró-Sangue Hemocentro de São Paulo and Hematology Department,
University of São Paulo, São Paulo, Brazil*

Key words: ABO incompatibility; bone marrow transplantation; plasma exchange; hemolysis; isoagglutinins.

INTRODUCTION

Major ABO incompatibility in bone marrow transplantation has been reported to occur in 15–20% of HLA identical donor recipient pairs [1–3]. Marrow engraftment,
incidence of rejection, incidence and severity of graft versus host disease (GVHD),
and patient survival have all been shown to be unrelated to this incompatibility [1–5].
However, infusion of ABO incompatible marrow can cause serious acute hemolysis in
recipients with high levels of anti-A and anti-B. To avoid this complication, the approach can be either to remove red blood cells (RBC) from the marrow product (by
gravity sedimentation after addition of hydroxyethyl starch or dextran amidotrizoate,
or using cell separator equipment), or to reduce the patient's isoagglutinin levels [by
infusion of ABO incompatible RBC or A/B substances, extracorporeal immunoabsorb-
tion of anti-A/anti-B or plasma exchange (PE)] [2, 6]. When plasma exchange is the
chosen method, it is useful to be able to predict the efficiency of the procedure on a
given patient. We devised this study in order to investigate how efficient the reduction
of anti-A/anti-B levels after plasma exchange would be in our institution.

MATERIALS AND METHODS

Thirty-nine PEs were performed in 12 nonbone marrow transplant patients (one cryoglobulinemia; one myasthenia gravis; three systemic lupus erythematosus; two ITP; one
acute renal transplant rejection; three Guillain–Barré syndrome; one chronic polyradicu-
loneuritis). The equivalent to 1 plasma volume (individually calculated) was exchanged
for 5% albumin solution during each procedure, using a continuous flow blood separator
(Vivacell BT-798, Dideco, Italy) and ACD-A as anticoagulant.

During every procedure, anti-A and/or anti-B levels were determined pre- and post-PE.
IgM detection was performed by saline agglutination of type-specific cells at room
temperature and at 37 °C. IgG titers were determined by indirect Coombs' test after
inactivation of IgM by means of the 2-mercaptoethanol technique.

Twenty-one samples were analyzed for IgM anti-A, 39 for IgM anti-B (total = 60), 18 for IgG anti-A and 24 for IgG anti-B (total = 42).

Statistical analysis was performed using the chi-square method.

RESULTS

The results obtained are described in Table 1.

Table 1.
Alterations of anti-A/anti-B isoagglutinins after plasma exchange

	Titer	IgM	IgG
Reduction of	1 titer	38 (63%)	7 (17%)
	2 titers	7 (12%)	7 (17%)
	3 titers	3 (5%)	1 (2%)
Elevation		0	5 (12%)
No alteration		12 (20%)	22 (52%)
Total		60	42

Every patient who had previous IgM levels of more than 1/16 had a reduction of at least 1 titer (data not shown).

For the 22 procedures where no IgG alteration could be detected, the levels of this isoagglutinin ranged from 1/2 to 1/16.

No other correlations could be made between preprocedure titers and degree of reduction, independent from the levels of these titers.

DISCUSSION

Not every bone marrow transplantation center uses plasma exchange to prevent acute hemolysis after the infusion of ABO incompatible marrow. For the ones who still do, the data obtained is helpful in scheduling the number of procedures necessary to reach the desired level of isoagglutinins. The level considered to be safe is 1/16 [2].

From our data it can be verified that 80% of the procedures resulted in a reduction of 1 or more titers of IgM; however, for IgG, this reduction could be reached in only 36%, while in 52% no alteration was observed ($P < 0.0005$). This can be explained by the fact that IgM is predominantly intravascular and only about 45% of IgG is in this compartment.

Of interest is the rebound verified by the elevation of IgG levels in five procedures (all of just 1 titer).

CONCLUSIONS

We can conclude that with the exchange of 1 plasma volume by 5% albumin solution, IgM titers (anti-A and/or anti-B) are expected to be reduced by at least 1 titer in 80% of the procedures. For IgG, titer reductions can be expected in only 36% of the procedures, being aware of the fact a titer elevation is a possible outcome.

Acknowledgments
Supported in part by a grant from Fundação Banco do Brasil.

REFERENCES

1. W. I. Bensinger, C. D. Buckner. R. A. Clift *et al.* Plasma exchange and plasma modification for the removal of anti-red cell antibodies prior to ABO-incompatible marrow transplant. *J. Clin. Apheresis*, **3**, 174–177 (1987).

2. L. D. Petz. Immunohematologic problems asociated with bone marrow transplantation. *Transf. Med. Rev.*, **1**, 85–100 (1987).

3. B. Haustein, H. Achenbach, A. Weißflog *et al.* Plasma exchange for removal of anti-A and anti-B group antibodies in ABO major-incompatible bone marrow transplantation. *Folia Haematol.*, **3–4**, 463–467 (1989).

4. P. I. Warkentin, J. M. Hilden, J. H. Kersey *et al.* Transplantation of major ABO-incompatible bone marrow depleted of red cells by hydroxyethyl starch. *Vox. Sang*, **48**, 89–104 (1985).

5. R. P. Gale, S. Feig, W. Ho *et al.* ABO blood group system and bone marrow transplantation. *Blood*, **50**, 185–194 (1977).

6. A. Müller, J. Hermann, D. Fuchs *et al.* Transplantation of major ABO-incompatible bone marrow: removal of red cells by dextrane sedimentation. *Folia Haematol.*, **3–4**, 475–479 (1989).

Therapeutic Plasmapheresis (XII), pp. 325-327
T. Agishi *et al.* (Eds)
© VSP 1993

Experience with Peripheral Blood Stem Cell Collection for Autografts in Children with Active Cancer

Y. TAKAUE, T. WATANABE, T. ABE, S. SAITO, T. SHIMIZU, J. SATO, T. SUZUE, A. HIRAO, Y. KAWANO and Y. KURODA

Department of Pediatrics, University Hospital of Tokushima, Tokushima, Japan

Key words: blood hematopoietic stem cells; children; cancer; leukemia; lymphoma.

INTRODUCTION

Few guidelines for collecting peripheral blood stem cells (PBSC) have been published for use with pediatric patients and the impact of PBSC autografts (PBSCT) on the clinical management of childhood cancer has not yet been understood. Problems associated with the apheresis procedure in small children include access to blood, tolerance of an extracorporeal circulation and postapheresis cytopenia. Identification of the optimal conditions for effectively and safely harvesting PBSC from children needs accumulation of new information. This report, concerning a larger number of children, updates our experience on mobilization, collection and utilization of PBSC to gather further information about the PBSCT program in pediatric patients.

COLLECTION RESULT OF BLOOD STEM CELLS

Eighty-two children with various types of cancer were referred for the harvest of PBSC for autografts. Because of refractory disease or deteriorating liver dysfunction, 13 patients were subsequently removed from the study, thus leaving us 69 patients (40 boys and 29 girls; 7 months to 17 years with a median of 8 years), including 22 children aged 4 years or less. The mean body weight was 29 kg (range 7–70 kg). Diagnoses included ALL, 40; AML, 12; non-Hodgkin's lymphoma (NHL), 7; solid tumors, 10. Informed consent to participate in the study was obtained from the guardians. Details of the collection procedure and the hematopoietic progenitor assay have been previously published [1–3]. Harvest was repeated to the point where cell yield decreased and no more clinical benefits were suggested by apheresis.

A total of 295 aphereses were performed by a CS 3000 cell separator during bone marrow recovery after chemotherapy and when the monocyte ($> 10\%$) and platelet ($> 150 \times 10^9$/l) counts were rising rapidly. The mean number of procedures per patient was 3.6 ± 1.4 (range 1–10). The volume of blood/kg of patients' body weight (bw) processed in each apheresis ranged from 67 to 429 ml (mean $\pm$ SD, 193 ± 79 ml). Although profound thrombocytopenia occurred in all cases, generally the morbidity related to PBSC harvest was small. A threshold of $\geqslant 3 \times 10^5$ colony-forming unit-granulocyte-macrophage (CFU-GM)/kg bw were collected in 35 of 69 children (51%) by a mean of 3.1 (range 1–5) aphereses and $\geqslant 1 \times 10^5$ CFU-GM/kg in 52 children (78%) with a low incidence of serious morbidity.

FACTORS PREDICTING PROGENITOR YIELDS BY APHERESIS

By univariate analysis, both patient age ($r = -0.470$, $P < 0.01$) and duration of preapheresis chemotherapy ($r = -0.334$, $P < 0.01$) had an impact on total number of CFU-GM yields, but when multivariate analysis was performed, age of the patients was the only significant predictor of CFU-GM yield ($P = 0.009$). Thus, PBSC harvest can be done more effectively in younger children than in their older counterparts or adult patients and they are better candidates for PBSC collection. When apheresis or chemotherapy was repeated, the progenitor yields decreased rapidly. Hence, to obtain sufficient stem/progenitor cells for autografts, the collection protocol must be installed early in the chemotherapy. Detailed data will be published in a separate paper [4]. We also confirmed that blood progenitors can be frozen by an alternative uncontrolled procedure without losing their clonogenic viability.

HEMATOPOIETIC RECONSTITUTION AFTER PBSCT

Whether blood stem cells can permanently restore hematopoiesis after marrow-ablative therapy used to be a major concern, but this has proved not to be a major issue as survival of autologous stem cells is almost universal, even after high-dose chemoirradiation. We have so far performed 48 PBSCT, successful and rapid hematopoietic engraftment was achieved in patients who received $> 3 \times 10^5$ CFU-GM/kg [5]. On the other hand, no association was seen between the number of burst-forming units for erythroid (BFU-E) infused and the speed of hematopoietic recovery. We suggest that early recovery of myelopoiesis is correlate with the infused dose of CD34$^+$ cells, which represent very immature human progenitor cells, possibly including some of the stem cell population, and the minimum requirement of blood CD34$^+$ cells resulting in a successful and rapid engraftment is 1.0×10^7/kg.

All patients showed a transient decrease in the number of once recovered granulocytes and platelets 3–7 weeks after transplantation without jeopardizing their clinical course. This is in accordance with most of the published reports on adult patients. In a patient who received a small number of CFU-GM (2.2×10^4/kg), incomplete platelet recovery was observed despite complete granulocyte recovery; this is the major limiting factor for PBSC autografting.

SERUM CYTOKINE KINETICS STUDY AFTER PBSCT

The current strategy to enhance hematopoietic engraftment after BMT is the use of recombinant cytokine. However, most clinical trials of granulocyte-CSF (G-CSF) or granulocyte-macrophage-CSF (GM-CSF) in recipients of autologous or allogeneic BMT have been done without considering *in vivo* production of those CSFs in recipients. Widespread use of cytokine is costly. Improved understanding of the endogenous production of cytokines will lead to better selection of patients.

In our study endogenous production of G-CSF, GM-CSF, interleukin-3 (IL-3), and interleukin-6 (IL-6) was investigated in 10 children who underwent a total of 12 courses of PBSCT by measuring their serum levels using immunoassay kits. We found a marked and sustained increase of serum G-CSF level in the early course of PBSCT, which reached the therapeutic range when injected. On the other hand, increase in the IL-6 levels was not remarkable, and for GM-CSF this was transient and insignificant. IL-3 was not detected.

Measurement of plasma cytokine levels would not always evaluate the *in vivo* productive kinetics of cytokines or their actual role in hematopoiesis, and the contribution of endogenously secreted cytokines to the early hematopoietic recovery after PBSCT needs to be clarified. However, it is very probable that infused monocytes are activated to become the main source of the dramatic rise in G-CSF levels during the critical early engraftment period and such endogenously secreted cytokines provide sufficient stimulation on hematopoietic engraftment without an exogenous supply.

COMMENTS

In a large number of children with active cancers we found that collection of PBSC is a safe and practical procedure with a low incidence of serious morbidity. Our program is also the first to examine therapeutic efficacy of PBSCT for the treatment of childhood cancer and clinical data have been published elsewhere [6]. Although the number of patients is too small and the follow-up period is too short, the preliminary data justify the incorporation of PBSCT in the design of salvage protocols for patients with early or multiple relapse from ALL.

The focus on PBSCT is now moving in another area important for the use of CSFs. Trials have been performed to increase the efficiency of harvesting blood progenitors by the administration of CSFs in patients with malaised hematopoiesis. In children, G-CSF induces an increase in the number of circulating stem/progenitor cells harvested by apheresis and this permits a more rapid recovery of hematopoiesis [5]. Future clinical trials of G-CSF with patients undergoing PBSCT should be focused on this strategy.

REFERENCES

1. Y. Takaue, T. Watanabe, K. Kawano *et al.* Isolation and storage of peripheral blood hematopoietic stem cells for the autotransplantation in cancer children. *Blood*, **74**, 1245–1251 (1989).
2. Y. Takaue, Y. Kawano, C. L. Reading *et al.* Effects of recombinant human G-CSF, GM-CSF and IL-3 on the growth of purified human peripheral blood progenitors. *Blood*, **76**, 330–335 (1990).
3. Y. Takaue. Peripheral blood stem cell autografts in children with acute lymphoblastic leukemia and lymphoma: updated experience. *Leuk. Lymphoma*, **3**, 241–256 (1991).
4. Y. Takaue, T. Watanabe, T. Abe *et al.* Experience with peripheral blood stem cell collection for autografts in children with active cancer. *Bone Marrow Transplant.*, **10**, 241–248 (1992).
5. Y. Kawano, Y. Takaue, T. Watanabe *et al.* Effects of progenitor cell dose and preleukapheresis use of human recombinant granulocyte colony-stimulating factor on the recovery of hematopoiesis after blood stem cell autografting in children. *Exp. Hematol.*, **21**, 103–108 (1993).
6. Y. Takaue, Y. Hoshi, T. Abe *et al.* Treatment of childhood acute leukemias and lymphoma with high-dose chemotherapy and peripheral blood stem cell autografts. In: *Autologous Bone Marrow Transplantation V*, K. A. Dicke, J. O. Armitage and M. J. Dicke-Evinger (Eds), pp. 811–821, University of Nebraska Medical Center Press, Omaha (1991).

Therapeutic Plasmapheresis (XII), pp. 329-332
T. Agishi *et al*. (Eds)
© VSP 1993

Preliminary Analysis of a Modified Method of Photopheresis in the Treatment of Cardiac Transplant Rejection

J. ROBINSON, E. HUBBELL, M. R. COSTANZO-NORDIN,
G. WINTERS and R. PIFARRE

Loyola University of Chicago, Foster G. McGaw Hospital Medical Center, Maywood, USA

Key words: photopheresis; cardiac transplant rejection.

INTRODUCTION

In spite of the continuing introduction of new immunosuppressive strategies, the incidence and significance of cardiac allograft rejection remains a formidable problem. The most recent novel immunosuppressive therapies, such as monoclonal antibodies, have proven useful in rescue situations only and an old agent such as methotrexate, has proved to be effective in the treatment of stubborn or recalcitrant rejection [1], but has the potentially serious side-effect of infection in the face of drug induced leucopenia. The well known deleterious effects of corticosteroids (CS) on both a short and long-term basis also promote continued exploration of new and safer steroid-free strategies for treating allograft rejection. Experimental observations of the immunomodulating effects of UV light on mononuclear effector cells (MNC) prompted us to evaluate photopheresis (PHO) in the treatment of patients with moderate rejection (MRE) without associated hemodynamic compromise. This discrete stage of rejection was selected in order to allow us to assess both the safety of PHO in the transplant setting and, as a pilot effort, compare its efficacy in comparison to the use of conventional CS pulse therapy [2].

In an effort to collect a maximum number of circulating potential allograft reactive precursor cells for immunomodulation by UV-A and psoralen, we modified the conventional method of PHO. MNC were collected from psoralen pre-medicated cardiac transplant patients (CTP) using the Cobe Spectra® blood cell separator. A minimum of two times the patient's whole blood volume was processed. The resulting relatively large yield of MNC in all but one instance precluded a second day of therapy. The collected MNC were exposed to UV-A in standard fashion on the Therakos UVAR® system. The advantages in terms of efficiency of cell collection, necessity for single instead of dual treatment sessions, and cost have been presented elsewhere [3].

MATERIALS AND METHODS

Nine CTP were treated with the modified method of photopheresis after documentation of moderate rejection (ISHT grades 2 and 3) on routine endomyocardial biopsies (EMB). No patient at the time of study had hemodynamic compromise. Gender distribution of this patient sample was five female/four male with an age range from 28 to 64. The period of time from allotransplantation to the first treatment with PHO ranged from 15 to 2003 days. The CTP sample size and highly variable time of entry into PHO after transplantation precluded meaningful statistical analysis of the demographics and clinical identifiers of these patients; however, the percentage of females within the sample study group is markedly higher than our overall CT population. A minimum of 5×10^9 MNC were collected as described above. If this number of cells could not be collected on the first day of treatment, the MNC pheresis and UV-A exposure was repeated within 24 h. Mean hematocrit of the pheresis product was 2.44.

RESULTS

There were 14 episodes of moderate rejection (MRE) in these nine CT patients that required 19 treatments with PHO. Thirteen MRE were completely reversed with PHO. Eight of the 13 MRE reversed with one PHO session while the remaining five of 13 reversed after two sequential PHO 7 days apart (Tables 1–3). The average number of MNC treated/MRE was 8.9×10^9 and only one PHO failed to exceed the target of 5×10^9 8-Mop treated MNC required for UV-A exposure; in the latter case PHO was repeated 24 h later and the target cell population was attained. There were no hemodynamic side-effects associated with MNC collection. There were no serious infections associated with the treatment, nor was the incidence of any infection different than in our non-PHO treated transplant population.

Table 1.
Clinical course of CTP treated with PHO

Patient no.	Age	Sex	Days to rejection	Resolution with PHO	Subsequent rejection
3	53	M	16	yes	no
5	60	F	17	no	
			26	yes	no
7	50	F	8	yes[a]	no[b]
8	20	M	43	no	
			50	yes	no

[a] Required two spectra collections 24 h apart.
[b] Died of post-transplant lymphoma.

One patient failed to respond to PHO and was subsequently treated with methotrexate. The time to improvement of the EMB was 8.8 days with complete resolution by 30.0 days. Immunophenotypic analysis of EMB infiltrates revealed no substantial change in CD4, CD8, IL-2 or granzyme A$^+$ cells from pre-PHO EMB (Table 4) but there was a substantial reduction in total infiltrating cells in the allografts and a suggestive reduction of B cells and total T cells. Endomyocardial biopsy appearance of several CTP after

Table 2.
Clinical course of CTP treated with PHO

Patient no.	Age	Sex	Days to rejection	Resolution with PHO	Subsequent rejection	RX
2	64	M	15	no		
			22	yes	yes	PHO
			147	yes	no	
4	38	F	17	yes	yes	PHO
			184	yes	yes	CS[a]
6	28	F	568	no		
			578	yes	yes	PHO
			731	yes	yes	CS

[a] Corticosteroids.

Table 3.
Clinical course of CTP treated with PHO

Patient no.	Age	Sex	Days to rejection	Resolution with PHO	Subsequent rejection	RX
1	59	M	2003	yes	yes	PHO
			2195	yes	yes	PHO
			2365	yes	no	
9	29	F	63	no		
			70	no	yes	MTX[a]

[a] Methotrexate.

Table 4.
Cell immunophenotypes in endomyocardial biopsies before and after treatment of rejection by photopheresis

	Total Leukocytes	Total T cells	CD4	CD8	B cells	IL-2	GRZ-A
Pre-PHO[a]	126 ± 52	57 ± 34	19 ± 13	24 ± 22	16 ± 13	2.5 ± 3.0	20 ± 22
Post-PHO	88 ± 73	36 ± 28	23 ± 29	27 ± 38	6 ± 6	1.9 ± 2.9	18 ± 26

[a] Photopheresis by modified method.

photopheresis was substantially different than that found in the EMB after conventional CS treatment. There was a unique and striking persistence of T cell infiltrates without myonecrosis in several EMB. Two patients also developed a giant cell reaction or broad band infiltrates with normal intravening tissue. These histologic findings confounded the interpretation of the PHO biopsies.

DISCUSSION

This 'pilot trial' of PHO in the treatment of MRE reveals that PHO is associated with not only prevention of progression of MRE to more serious forms of rejection, but also its ultimate reversal, although the temporal course of reversal appears to be different in some patients in that cellular infiltrates persist apparently without cytotoxic potential. The use of modified PHO also appears safe. There are several possible mitigating factors, however that preclude significant conclusions being made from this study. First, there is increasing awareness within the cardiac transplant community that there are certain forms of MRE that may not require any treatment. Unfortunately, this subset of MRE patients has no unique identifiers to-date and thus it is possible that one or more patients in our trial with PHO were within that subset. Second, the treatment course was short and the optimal number of MNC to be treated with UV-A and the number and frequency of PHO remains unknown. Conversely, it appears clear that MRE, at least in some patients, does respond to PHO. Photopheresis in two patients with more aggressive resistant rejection has recently been reported to be effective [4].

The use of UV light in the treatment of transplant rejection is an attractive form of therapy. There is a substantial body of experimental evidence that UV-B irradiation is a potent immunomodulator in the allograft setting. The effects of UV-B appear to be mediated through its ability of impairing the homing of T cells and antigen presenting cells to high endothelial venules, possible alteration or damage to T cell receptors and accessory T cell molecules and finally inhibition of effective antigen presentation by antigen presenting cells [5, 6]. Whether UV-A light and psoralen has some of the same immunomodulatory effects as UV-B remains to be proven; in fact, it is currently not even certain whether psoralen is required as an adjuvant molecule to potentiate the UV-A effects of conventional photopheresis when used for therapies other than the treatment of cutaneous T cell leukemia. We believe that PHO is a potential therapeutic modality for the treatment of transplant rejection; but more importantly, if used early after allograft placement, it may have substantial promise is a tolerance inducer. Hopefully a large multicenter trial can be mounted to test this hypothesis in cardiac and lung transplantation.

REFERENCES

1. M. R. Costanzo-Nordin, B. B. Grusk, M. A. Silver *et al.* Reversal of recalcitrant cardiac allograft rejection with methotrexate. *Transplant. Proc.*, **20**, 3 (1988).

2. M. R. Costanzo-Nordin, E. Hubbell, J. O'Sullivan *et al.* Successful treatment of heart transplant rejection with photopheresis. *Transplantation*, **53**, 808–815 (1992).

3. E. A. Hubbell and J. A. Robinson. A potentially more efficient method of photopheresis. In: *Abstract (Oral); American Society for Apheresis, 12th Annual Meeting*, New Orleans, LA (991).

4. M. Wieland, M. J. Randels, R. G. Strauss *et al.* Promising therapy for intractable cardiac allograft rejection. In: *Abstract (Oral); American Society for Apheresis, 13th Annual Meeting*, Chicago, IL (1992).

5. M. Mitchell, M. Kripke and S. Ullrich. Suppression of the elicatation of the immune response to alloantigen by ultraviolet radiation. *Transplantation*, **47**, 1008–1013 (1989).

6. J. Simon, R. Tifelaar, P. Bergstresser *et al.* Ultraviolet B radiation converts langerhans cells from immunogenic to tolerrogenic antigen-presenting cells. *Transplantation*, **146**, 485–491 (1991).

Therapeutic Plasmapheresis (XII), pp. 333-336
T. Agishi *et al.* (Eds)
© VSP 1993

Harvesting of Peripheral Blood Stem Cells by Haemapheresis in Children with Solid Tumors

A. LANDOLFO, A. ANGIONI, G. DEB,[1] A. JENKNER,[1] R. COZZA,[1] L. DE SIO,[1] C. DOMINICI,[2] P. BALLONI and A. DONFRANCESCO[1]

Blood Bank and [1]Department of Pediatric Oncology, Ospedale Pediatrico 'Bambino Gesu', Rome, Italy
[2]Department of Pediatrics, University 'La Sapienza', Rome, Italy

Key words: peripheral blood stem cells; apheresis; autografting; solid tumors; low weight children.

INTRODUCTION

Autologous bone marrow transplantation (ABMT) allows for a significant increase in drug dosage and a higher cure rate in those tumors in which a steep dose–response curve has been demonstrated [1]. However, patients who present with a high anesthesiologic risk, serious pelvic malformations, marrow metastases, or who have undergone pelvic or craniospinal radiotherapy are excluded from this treatment. For these patients peripheral blood stem cell (PBSC) reinfusion may represent the ideal method of rescue after marrow-ablative chemo/radiotherapy [2]. The increase in PBSC number observed shortly after administering myelosuppressive chemotherapy and/or hematopoietic growth factors allows for a more efficient harvest, with a cell yield suitable for clinical use [3]. Many childhood tumors may be amenable to high-dose chemotherapy and PBSC reinfusion. However, few studies have been carried out [4, 5]. We report on a technique of PBSC collection in children that can be easily performed and appears to have overcome the problems related to low weight, vascular access and anticoagulant side effects, making apheresis a reliable and safe procedure in children.

PATIENTS AND METHODS

From April 1989 to April 1992, PBSC were collected from 14 patients (12 males and two females) with solid tumors: five neuroblastomas (NB), three medulloblastomas (MB), two Ewing's sarcomas (ES), one Hodgkin's disease (HD), one primitive neuroectodermal tumor (PNET), one ependymoma (EP) and one hepatoblastoma (HB). Patient age ranged from 22 months to 18 years (median 8 years), weight ranged from 10 to 60 kg (median 24.5 kg). All patients had relapsed or resistant disease at the time of collection. Informed consent was obtained from the patients and/or parents in accordance with institutional guidelines.

Following two courses of chemotherapy, leukaphereses were performed by means of a Baxter CS-3000 Plus continuous flow cell separator (Fenwal, Deerfield, IL) using the

1-special program for mononuclear cell collection. The cell separator was first primed with normal saline. This was replaced with a mixture of irradiated leukocyte-poor packed red blood cells (PRBC), fresh frozen plasma and 5% albumin solution, adjusted to the same hematocrit of the patient or to a higher one in case of anemia. The priming was stopped as soon as 400 ml of this mixture, which equals the extracorporeal volume, had been processed. Venous access was obtained in eleven patients by means of a double lumen central venous catheter (Quinton), in two patients by a percutaneous subclavian catheter (15G Secalon Hydrocath, Viggo) according to Seldinger's technique and in one patient by a 18G cannula inserted into the antecubital fossa veins of both arms. Patients under 25 kg of weight were heparinized (1 U/ml) to reduce the ACD-anticoagulant load to a ratio of 1:30, in order to prevent citrate toxicity. Blood pressure, heart rate and activated clotting time were continuously monitored during the whole procedure; serum electrolytes were checked before and after apheresis. PBSC harvesting was started at the moment of the steepest increase during the recovery from the nadir of white blood cells (WBC) and platelets (PLT), i.e. when WBC were $\geqslant 1500/\mu l$ and PLT $\geqslant 80\,000/\mu l$; it was continued on alternate days until the WBC counts reached $3000/\mu l$. For each procedure, which lasted about 2.5 h, a blood volume equal to two times the patient's volume was processed. Detection of tumor cell infiltration in patients with neuroectodermal tumors (NB, MB, ES, PNET) by means of indirect immunofluorescence employing a panel of monoclonal antibodies was performed in both bone marrow and PBSC collections in seven patients, in PBSC collections only in two patients and in bone marrow only in two patients. The panel of monoclonal antibodies was kindly provided by Dr J. T. Kemshead, Imperial Cancer Research Fund, Bristol, UK.

RESULTS

A total of 50 PBSC collections were performed, with an average of 3.6 collections per patient (range 1–9). A median of 0.73×10^8 (range 0.37–1.82) mononuclear cells/kg patient weight were harvested during each procedure. No side-effects were observed during the procedure besides chills and fever in one patient. Bone marrow infiltration was detected by means of the employed panel of monoclonal antibodies in four of nine patients (three NB and one ES); tumor cells could also be detected in one of nine PBSC collections (one NB).

Two patients (one MB, one ES) underwent autografting with both bone marrow and PBSC. Engraftment (defined as $\geqslant 1000$ WBC count and $\geqslant 50\,000$ platelet count) was observed on day 25 (MB) and day 105 (ES). Two patients (one ES, one NB) were grafted with PBSC only. Engraftment was observed on day 22 (ES) and day 25 (NB). Four patients (one MB, one HD, one NB, one PNET) underwent high-dose chemotherapy with PBSC rescue. Recovery (defined as $\geqslant 1000$ WBC count and $\geqslant 50\,000$ platelet count) was observed on day 13 (HD) and day 25 (MB); the other two patients are too early to evaluate. The patient with tumor cell infiltration in the PBSC collection did not perform autografting.

DISCUSSION

The harvesting of PBSC in small children is limited because of several technical problems [6]. Venous access is critical in order to obtain adequate blood flow rates, a minimum of 20 ml/min with a constant blood flow being necessary to obtain a good recovery and a high mononuclear cell yield. Double lumen central venous catheters are needed in children requiring chronic chemotherapy, while for short-term collections percutaneous catheters are also satisfactory. The use of a continuous-flow cell separator primed with PRBC and albumin solution is necessary to prevent hypovolemia in small infants. No more than 15% of the patient's blood volume, estimated at 80 ml/kg body weight, should be in the extracorporeal circulation. Citrate toxicity related to ACD overload is a common side-effect in pediatric apheresis. Symptoms include pallor, bradycardia, hypotension and acute abdominal pain with or without vomiting [7]. Employing both heparin and ACD enables us to reduce ACD dosage, thus lowering the risk of ACD toxicity. Since this technique may result in a low ACD concentration in the collection bag, we added 20 ml of ACD directly to the bag. Careful monitoring of the activated clotting time before, during and after collection is used to adjust the dose of heparin.

Table 1.
PBSC collection in children with solid tumors: results

Diagnosis	Age/sex	Weight (kg)	Apheresis no.	MNC $\times 10^8$/ kg (Mean + SEM)	Involvement	
					BM	PBSC
1. MB	5/M	15	9	1.04 + 0.11	no	—
2. MB	13/M	50	3	0.40 + 0.06	no	no
3. NB	2/M	11	5	0.96 + 0.13	yes	no
4. NB	8/M	25	3	0.37 + 0.12	yes	no
5. HD	18/M	46	3	1.10 + 0.25	—	—
6. ES	10/M	27	8	0.87 + 0.08	yes	no
7. PNET	14/M	50	3	1.03 + 0.10	—	no
8. NB	1/F	10	1	0.82	no	—
9. ES	13/M	37	2	0.58 + 0.09	—	no
10. MB	8/M	20	3	0.39 + 0.11	no	no
11. HB	6/F	18	4	1.82 + 0.17	—	—
12. NB	2/M	14	2	0.66 + 0.09	yes	yes
13. EP	13/M	60	1	0.62	—	—
14. NB	5/M	24	3	0.38 + 0.10	no	no

CONCLUSIONS

In conclusion, this study indicates that PBSC harvesting in children and toddlers can be a safe and practical clinical procedure. The feasibility of PBSC autografting is again confirmed and the advantage obtained by PBSC rescue in terms of reduced transfusional requirements and increased dose-intensity seems also promising.

REFERENCES

1. E. D. Thomas. Marrow transplantation for malignant disease. *J. Clin. Oncol.*, **1**, 517–531 (1983).
2. A. Kessinger, J. O. Armitage, J. D. Landmark *et al.* Autologous peripheral hematopoietic stem cell transplantation restores hematopoietic function following marrow ablative therapy. *Blood*, **71**, 723–727 (1988).
3. C. M. Richman, R. S. Weiner and R. A. Yankee. Increase in circulating stem cells following chemotherapy in man. *Blood*, **47**, 1031–1039 (1976).
4. L. C. Lasky, B. Bostrom, J. Smith *et al.* Clinical collection and use of peripheral blood stem cells on pediatric patients. *Transplantation*, **47**, 613–616 (1989).
5. T. Watanabe, Y. Takaue, Y. Kawano *et al.* Peripheral blood stem cell autotransplantation in treatment of chilhood cancer. *Bone Marrow Transplant.*, **4**, 261–265 (1989).
6. D. O. Kasprisin. Techniques, indications and toxicity of therapeutic hemapheresis in children. *J. Clin. Apheresis*, **5**, 21–24 (1989).
7. S. V. Kevy and M. Fosburg. Therapeutic apheresis in childhood. *J. Clin. Apheresis*, **5**, 87–90 (1990).

Therapeutic Plasmapheresis (XII), pp. 337-340
T. Agishi *et al.* (Eds)
© VSP 1993

A Peripheral Blood Stem Cell Collection Program in a Regional Blood Center

H. KIYOKAWA, C. TSURU, K. MURAKAMI, N. UEDA, M. OHYAMA, Y. IRITA, S. YAMAMOTO, K. TOKUNAGA, H. SHIRAKI and Y. MAEDA

Fukuoka Red Cross Blood Center, Fukuoka, Japan

Key words: peripheral blood stem cell collection; mobile PBSC collection program; rHuG-CSF; blood cell separator; leukapheresis.

INTRODUCTION

Growth in the selective collection of blood components and in the application of innovative therapeutic techniques has been making a revolution in transfusion medicine. Recently, hospitals have begun to collect new therapeutic components from patients. Autotransfusion using peripheral blood stem cells (PBSC) has been successfully applied to the treatment of malignancies. Fukuoka Red Cross Blood Center has initiated a mobile PBSC collection program to the Fukuoka community since 1990.

MATERIALS AND METHOD

In the Fukuoka region, there are 3.5 million people and 25 hospitals which have more than 300 beds. We have 60 blood cell separators and 50 registered nurses to collect single donor platelets which cover more than 90% of total platelet collection including

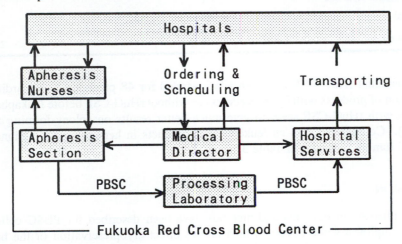

Figure 1. Administration of the PBSC collection program.

random donor platelets. In the special services for hospitals, there are four clinical programs (therapeutic plasmapheresis, intraoperative autologous plateletpheresis and autologous blood collection) including PBSC collection. We have provided a mobile PBSC collection program to four hospitals in the Fukuoka region since 1990 (Fig. 1). This program includes collection and cryopreservation of PBSC.

RESULTS

PBSC collection in 12 cases of hematopoietic malignancies and 13 cases of solid tumors has been carried out on the Cobe Spectra during July 1990 to April 1922 (Table 1). About 20 days before starting leukapheresis, chemotherapy was done in all patients. The 25 patients experienced 75 Cobe Spectra procedures. The processed volume was 6782 ml in whole blood on average and the yield of MNC was 3.0×10^9. The number of CFU-GM and CFU-C were 14.8×10^5 (2.6×10^4/kg) and 192.8×10^5, respectively.

Table 1.
PBSC collections (31 July 1990–30 April 1992)

Diagnosis	No. of patients	No. of cases		Clinical course		
		collection	transplantation	alive	death	unknown
Hematological malignancies						
ALL	1	1	1			1
ANLL	9	9	4	1	2	1
non-Hodgkin's lymphoma	2	2	1	1		
total	12	12	6	2	2	2
Solid tumors						
breast cancer	7	8	7	5	2	
ethmoid sinus cancer	1	2	1		1	
metastatic lymph node cancer	1	2	2		1	
lung cancer	3	3	2	1	1	
malignant thymoma	1	1				
total	13	16	12	6	5	
Grand total	25	28	18	8	7	2

Supplemental rHuG-CSF had been administrated for 48 procedures. Regarding the comparison of products with (27 procedures) or without rHuG-CSF before leukapheresis, the cases with rHuG-CSF seem to give much better results on colony-forming assays (Table 2). Comparable data on leukapheresis products in hematological malignancies and solid tumors is shown in Table 3.

DISCUSSION

Several apheresis instruments and methods have been described for PBSC collection [1]. We employ a Cobe Spectra which allows direct cryopreservation of the harvest without further manipulation to reduce red cell contamination.

Table 2.
Comparison of products with or without rHuG-CSF before leukapheresis

rHuG-CSF	Processed blood volume (ml)	Leukapheresis products				
		total NC[a] ($\times10^9$)	total MNC[b] ($\times10^9$)	recovery[c] (%)	CFU-C (1×10^5)	CFU-GM (1×10^5)
−	6805±1889 [26]	5.4±2.9 [24]	3.2±2.2 [24]	48±25 [21]	54±33 [9]	6.7±5.2 [9]
+	6497±2015 [+]	7.6±4.9 [36]	2.8±1.8 [46]	56±26 [38]	254±268 [24]	18.6±18.1 [24]

[ ], Number of leukapheresis.
[a] Nucleated cell.
[b] Mononuclear cell.
[c] $\text{Recovery(\%)} = \dfrac{\text{Total MNC count in apheresis product}}{\text{MNC count(/ml) in patient before leukapheresis} \times \text{Processed blood volume (ml)}} \times 100.$

Table 3.
Comparison of leukapheresis products in malignancies

Diagnosis	Processed blood volume (ml)	Leukapheresis products				
		total NC ($\times10^9$)	total MNC ($\times10^9$)	recovery (%)	CFU-C (1×10^5)	CFU-GM (1×10^5)
Hematological malignancies						
ALL	9237±166 [3]	1.2±0.5 [3]	0.8±0.4 [3]	16±3 [3]	ND[a]	ND[a]
ANLL	7298±1683 [23]	7.1±4.0 [23]	3.5±2.3 [21]	57±26 [21]	52±55 [7]	7.1±7.1 [10]
non-Hodgkin's lymphoma	9336±1350 [4]	6.6±3.1 [4]	4.1±2.4 [4]	35±11 [4]	61±21 [4]	5.4±2.1 [4]
Solid tumors						
breast cancer	5412±1083 [23]	5.7±3.1 [23]	2.3±1.5 [23]	60±25 [19]	196±218 [8]	19±18 [8]
ethmoid sinus cancer	5650±594 [6]	9.5±2.2 [6]	3.8±2.1 [5]	61±9 [3]	ND	ND
metastatic lymph node cancer	5400±534 [6]	2.3±0.8 [6]	1.8±0.4 [5]	70±32 [4]	16.2 [1]	0.2 [1]
lung cancer	6839±3296 [6]	12.6±5.5 [7]	4.2±1.1 [6]	40±2 [4]	501±263 [3]	25±19 [7]
malignant thymoma	8017±1427 [3]	9.3±4.6 [3]	3.8±1.1 [3]	37 [1]	241±204 [3]	28±16 [3]

[ ], Number of leukapheresis.
[a] Not done.

The timing and extent of PBSC rebound is difficult to predict, and depends upon several factors including the amount of chemotherapy and the mobilizing agent. We currently use a recovering peripheral blood leukocyte count of $1 \times 10^3/\mu l$ as a surrogate marker to initiate leukapheresis and carry out three procedures over subsequent days.

The use of recombinant growth factors appears both to facilitate the harvesting of hematopoietic stem cells from peripheral blood and hasten engraftment after transplantation.

CONCLUSIONS

The operator's direct responsibilities are to provide adequate cell yields and to work as a beneficial member of the bone marrow transplant team. The final success of the program depends on the smooth operation of the procedure between the blood center and the hospitals. Results of our blood center, providing a mobile PBSC collection, have been gratifying to all involved.

REFERENCE

1. D. Padley, R. G. Strauss, M. Wieland and M. J. Randels. Concurrent comparison of the Cobe Spectra and Fenwal CS3000 for the collection of peripheral blood mononuclear cells for autologous peripheral stem cell transplantation. *J. Clin. Apheresis*, **6**, 77–80 (1991).

Therapeutic Plasmapheresis (XII), pp. 341-344
T. Agishi *et al.* (Eds)
© VSP 1993

Thoracic Duct Drainage Pretreatment in Living Related Kidney Transplantation

Y. ONO, S. OHSHIMA,[1] T. KINUKAWA,[1] O. MATSUURA,[1] N. TAKEUCHI,[1] R. HATTORI,[1] K. TANAKA,[1] S. YAMADA, O. KAMIHIRA and O. KURIKI[1]

Department of Urology, Komaki Shimin Hospital, Komaki, Japan
[1]*Department of Urology, Shakai Hoken Chukyo Hospital, Nagoya, Japan*

Key words: thoracic duct drainage; pretreatment; living related transplantation; kidney.

INTRODUCTION

The beneficial effect of preoperative lymphocyte depletion through thoracic duct drainage (TDD) on graft survival has been reported in HLA one-haploidentical living related kidney transplantation [1, 2]. Complete success was achieved for the first and second years in transplant patients treated even under conventional immunosuppressive therapy. However, some transplant patients lost their graft from immunological events in the third and forth years. To minimize graft loss, TDD pretreatment and low-dose cyclosporin (CsA) and steroid immunosuppressive treatment have been used in HLA one-haploidentical kidney transplant patients since July 1986. Moreover, it was extended to high-risk transplant patients receiving secondary grafts, HLA non-haploidentical grafts and ABO incompatible grafts. In this paper, we present our results to evaluate the significance of TDD pretreatment in the CsA era.

MATERIALS

One hundred and thirty four patients with end-stage renal disease entered into our living related transplant program between July 1980 and December 1991. Seventy nine patients were treated with lymphocyte depletion through TDD preoperatively. Seventy three received primary grafts and four received secondary grafts from HLA one-haploidentical donors. Of the four patients, one was transplanted an ABO incompatible (A → O) graft. Two received primary grafts from HLA non-haploidentical siblings. Of 73 patients, 16 were treated with high-dose steroid and azathioprine therapy between July 1980 and January 1985, 28 with low-dose steroid and azathioprine therapy between March 1983 and June 1986, and 29 with low-dose CsA and steroid therapy between August 1986 and June 1990. Of six high-risk patients, one was treated with high-dose steroid and azathioprine therapy and five with low-dose CsA and steroid therapy. Details of patients' characteristics in each group are shown in Tables 1 and 2.

Table 1.

Posttransplant immunosuppression	High-dose steroid + AZ	Low-dose steroid + AZ	Low-dose steroid + Low-dose CsA
No. of patients	16	28	29
Sex (male/female)	16/0	20/8	19/10
Age (mean±SD)(years)	32±6	29±9	26±7
Original disease			
glomerulonephritis	15	25	21
nephrotic syn.	1	0	2
pyelonephritis	0	1	3
others	0	2	3
TDD pretreatment			
duration (days)	35±5	36±4	33±6
removed cells (×10⁹)	118±43	132±37	107±37

Table 2.

	Age	Sex	Original disease	TDD duration (days)	No. of removed cells (×10⁹)	No. of Tx	Donor	Histocompatibility	Graft survival (months)	Recent S-Cr (mg/dl)
LD 57	23	M	CGN	41	65	2	parent	one-haploidentical	lost in 29	
KLD 7	37	M	CGN	35	81	2	parent	one-haploidentical	29	1.4
LD167	28	M	CGN	30	43	2	parent	one-haploidentical	17	1.2
KLD11	32	M	CGN	41	86	2	parent	one-haploidentical	8	1.8
								A → O		
LD153	34	M	CGN	44	134	1	sibling	non-haploidentical	37	1.4
LD163	35	M	CGN	30	133	1	sibling	non-haploidentical	21	1.2

METHODS

TDD pretreatment

TDD was established as described by Starzl *et al.* [3]. A 5–7 Fr. Swan-Ganz double lumen catheter was placed into the duct after cutting off the balloon. Postoperatively, heparinized saline was infused through one lumen to prevent clotting of the lymph and the lymph was collected through the other lumen into a plastic bag. The drained lymph was frozen and thawed three times to destroy lymphocytes. The lymphocyte-free lymph was infused to maintain the level of serum protein in the patients. TDD was maintained for 4–5 weeks before transplantation. TDD was closed on the day of transplant.

Posttransplant immunosuppressive treatment

The first 17 patients were treated with the high-dose steroid regimen, which began at a dosage of 200–250 mg prednisolone for 3 days. The dose then was reduced progressively from 2 mg/kg to 50 mg at 30 days and to 30 mg at 60 days. The second 28 patients were treated with the low-dose steroid regimen, which began at a dosage of 200–250 mg for 3 days and was then reduced abruptly to 30 mg at 3 days and 25 mg at 30 days postoperatively. Azathioprine was also given at a dosage of 3 mg/kg from 4 days before transplantation and at a dosage of 1–3 mg/kg after transplantation in both groups. The third 34 patients were treated with the low-dose CsA and steroid regimen. CsA was started at a dosage of 6 mg/kg, maintained for 4 weeks. Then the dose was reduced to 4–5 mg/kg as an initial maintenance dose. One gram methylprednisolone was given intravenously on the day of transplant. Prednisolone was started at the dose of 20 mg/day, which was maintained for 4 weeks. Then the dose was reduced to 15 mg/day. Any rejection crisis was treated with 1 g methylprednisolone and increased dosage of prednisolone (200–250 mg) followed by progressively reduced doses.

RESULTS

Seventy-three patients received primary grafts from HLA one-haploidentical living related donors

TDD pretreatment. TDD pretreatment was performed for 35 ± 5 days (mean $\pm$ SD) in the first 16 patients, 36 ± 4 days in the second 28 patients and 33 ± 6 days in the third 29 patients. The total number of removed cells in each group was $118 \pm 43 \times 10^9$ (mean $\pm$ SD), $132 \pm 37 \times 10^9$ and $107 \pm 37 \times 10^9$, respectively.

Graft survival. Graft survival was 94% at 1–2 years, 88% at 3 years, and 63% at 4–10 years in TDD plus the high-dose steroid and azathioprine treated patients; 96% at 1–2 years, 89% at 3 years, 86% at 4–5 years, 75% at 6 years, 71% at 7 years, 64% at 8 years and 56% at 9–10 years in TDD plus the low-dose steroid and azathioprine treated patients; and 97% at 1 year, 87% at 2 years, 83% at 3 years, 76% at 4–5 years in TDD plus the low-dose CsA and steroid treated patients. There are no statistically significant differences in the three groups.

Patient survival. Patient survival was 94% at 1–3 years, 88% at 4–6 years and 84% at 7–10 years in TDD plus the high-dose steroid and azathioprine treated patients; 100% at 1–2 years, 96% at 3–5 years, 93% at 6 years, 88% at 7–8 years and 79% at 9–10 years in TDD plus the low-dose steroid and azathioprine treated patients. In TDD plus the low-dose CsA and steroid treated patients it was 97% at 1–5 years.

Six high-risk patients

Outcome of six high-risk patients in shown in Table 2. Of four patients receiving secondary grafts, two had well-functioning grafts for 17 and 29 months, and one lost in 29 months. One patient transplanted an ABO incompatible (A → O) kidney had a well-functioning graft for 8 months. Two patients receiving kidneys from HLA one-haploidentical sibling also had well-functioning grafts for 21 and 37 months.

DISCUSSION

In conventional immunosuppressive therapy consisting of steroid and azathioprine, lymphocyte depletion through TDD had been reported to have beneficial effects on graft survival in cadaveric kidney transplantation by some authors [3, 4]. The results of the first 16 patients treated with the high-dose steroid and azathioprine therapy indicated that TDD pretreatment could have beneficial effects on the first 2 years of graft survival in HLA one-haploidentical living related kidney transplantation [1, 2]. Moreover, it was indicated from the second 28 transplant patients that the combination of TDD pretreatment and the low-dose steroid and azathioprine therapy might have long-term (over 5 years) beneficial effects on graft survival. This paradoxical phenomena between the high-dose steroid group and the low-dose steroid group has been reported elsewhere [5]. Our results strongly support that TDD pretreatment has beneficial effects on graft survival in steroid and azathioprine treated patients, especially those receiving HLA one-haploidentical grafts. In the CsA era, graft survival was also improved in HLA one-haploidentical living related kidney transplant patients. It was 91% at 1 year, 83% at 2 years and 72% at 5 years even in the recipients without any pretreatment [6]. These figures were very similar with those of our third 29 patients treated with TDD pretreatment and low-dose CsA and steroid therapy. These findings indicate that TDD pretreatment is not necessary in CsA treated HLA one-haploidentical living related kidney transplant patients. In the high-risk transplant patients receiving secondary grafts, ABO incompatible grafts and HLA non-haploidentical grafts, the outcome has been accepted to be poor. Then, in the CsA era, the results for transplant patients receiving HLA non-haploidentical living related graft greatly improved and their 5 years graft survival reached 82% [6]. However, the outcome of transplant patients receiving secondary grafts and ABO incompatible grafts is still poor. In our CsA treated high-risk patients, all had well-functioning grafts for 8–37 months. These results indicate that TDD pretreatment might have beneficial effects on graft survival in high-risk patients receiving secondary grafts and ABO incompatible grafts under CsA immunosuppressive therapy.

REFERENCES

1. S. Ohshima, Y. Ono, T. Kinukawa, O. Matsuura, N. Takeuchi and R. Hattori. The beneficial effects of thoracic duct drainage in HLA-1 haplotype identical kidney transplantation. *J. Urol.*, **138**, 33 (1987).
2. Y. Ono, S. Ohshima, T. Kinukawa, O. Matsuura and S. Hirabayashi. MLR suppression and MLR-suppressor activity induced by thoracic duct drainage prior to transplantation. *Transplant. Proc.*, **19**, 1985 (1987).
3. T. E. Starzl, R. Weil, III, L. J. Koep, R. T. McCalmon, Jr P. I. Terasaki, Y. Iwaki, G. P. J. Schroter, J. J. Franks, V. Subryan and C. G. Halgrimson. Thoracic duct fistula and renal transplantation. *Ann. Surg.*, **190**, 474 (1979).
4. H. K. Johnson, G. D. Niblack, M. B. Tallent and R. E. Richie. Immunological preparation for cadaver renal transplant by thoracic duct drainage. *Transplant. Proc.*, **9**, 1499 (1977).
5. T. Kinukawa, S. Ohshima, Y. Ono, O. Matsuura, N. Takeuchi, R. Hattori, S. Hasegawa, S. Sugiyama and K. Tsuzuki. Paradoxical effects of acute rejection in long-term kidney allografts after pretreatment with thoracic duct drainage. *Transplant. Proc.*, **21**, 2192 (1989).
6. The Japan society for transplantation, annual report of kidney transplantation 1990. *Jpn. J. Transplant.* **26**, 494 (1991).

Therapeutic Plasmapheresis (XII), pp. 345-347
T. Agishi *et al.* (Eds)
© VSP 1993

Effect of Plasmapheresis on ABO-Incompatible Kidney Transplantation

K. UCHIDA, T. SHINDO, T. TAMAI, M. ICHIKAWA, T. KONDO,
M. MANNAMI,[1] Y. KIMURA,[2] S. YUASA[3] and H. MATSUO[3]

Departments of Medicine and [1]*Urology, Uwajima City Hospital, Uwajima, Japan*
[2]*Kimura Medical Office, Uwajima, Japan*
[3]*The Second Department of Internal Medicine, Kagawa Medical School,*
Kagawa, Japan

Key words: living donor kidney transplantation; ABO-incompatibility; immunoadsorption; double filtration plasmapheresis.

INTRODUCTION

Living donor kidney transplantation offers several advantages, including no distressing waiting time, immediate functioning of the transplant, better long-term graft and patient survival, over cadaver transplantation. However, many recipients are still being denied the benefit of living donor kidney transplantation because of ABO-incompatibility of the potential donor. Recently, successful ABO-incompatible living donor kidney transplantation has been performed by removal of patient's isoagglutinins with plasmapheresis and splenectomy in combination [1–3]. We report herein the experience of nine living donor kidney transplantations between ABO-incompatible donors and recipients.

PATIENTS AND METHODS

From February 1990 to October 1991, nine splenectomized patients received ABO-incompatible living donor kidney transplants in Uwajima City Hospital. The donor–recipient ABO incompatibilities were A to 0 in three cases, B to A in two cases and B to 0 in four cases. Six patients received double filtration plasmapheresis (DFPP) 23 times and four patients immunoadsorption 10 times. Table 1 summarizes the clinical profile of each case. The DFPP apparatus used in this study was a KM-8500 (Kuraray Medical Co., Osaka, Japan). Plasmacure^{TM} (Kuraray) was used as plasma separator and Evaflux^{TM} (Kuraray) was used as second filter. Biosynsorb^{TM} (Kuraray), which can adsorb and remove of anti-A and anti-B blood group antibodies from biological media [4, 5], was used as an adsorbent column for immunoadsorption therapy. The quantity of plasma disposition at DFPP was 1860–9000 ml, and the average quantity was 4529.2 ml. Each immunoadsorption therapy treated 6000–8950 ml of plasma.

Table 1.

ABO-incompatible living donor kidney transplantation: recipient relationships and preoperative data

Reci-pient No.	Date of transplant	ABO-incompatibility	DFPP	Immuno-adsorption	Titer anti-ABO (IgG)	
					before PP	after PP
1	02/28/90	B to 0	0	4 (31 350 ml)	1/128	1/1
2	07/04/90	B to A	4 (12 260 ml)	2 (15 680 ml)	1/8	1/4
3	04/25/90	B to 0	0	3 (23 930 ml)	1/16	1/1
4	11/28/90	A to 0	6 (23 000 ml)	0	1/128	1/16
5	02/06/91	A to 0	5 (20 000 ml)	0	1/256	1/16
6	04/17/91	A to 0	5 (44 000 ml)	0	1/1024	1/16
7	05/14/91	B to 0	1 (5000 ml)	0	1/1	1/1
8	06/11/91	B to 0	2 (7500 ml)	0	1/16	1/16
9	08/28/91	B to A	0	1 (6000 ml)	1/1	1/1

RESULTS

Total Ig anti-A and/or anti-B titer decreased to $1:16$ after either DFPP or immunoadsorption therapy in all patients.

In case no. 3, Ig anti-B titer elevated to $1:256$ on the ninth day following transplant, and renal function deteriorated rapidly. DFPP (three times) and immunoadsorption therapy (two times) were performed, but improvement of renal function was not observed. Nephrectomy was carried out on the 15th day. The other patients did not receive acute vascular rejection. In cases no. 7 and no. 9, chronic rejection occurred and the function of the transplanted kidneys deteriorated. These two patients had induced hemodialysis therapy. Case no. 9 received ABO-compatible living donor kidney transplantation thereafter. However, pneumonia had developed and he died of untreatable infection. In cases no. 1, 2, 4, 5, 6 and 8, transplanted kidneys have evaded acute and chronic rejection, and are now functioning.

DISCUSSION

Long-term results of ABO-incompatible living donor kidney transplantation in Uwajama City Hospital have not yet been obtained. We have a few cases (nine cases) of ABO-incompatible kidney transplantation. However, we found favorable results in comparison with ABO-compatible living donor kidney transplantation at present for escaping acute vascular rejection. It is generally believed that ABO-incompatibility is a major barrier to living kidney transplantation and often causes accelerated or hyperacute rejection. Our results suggest that plasmapheresis and splenectomy may be useful procedures for ABO-incompatible living donor kidney transplantation.

REFERENCES

1. G. P. J. Alexandre, J. P. Squifflet, M. De Bruyere *et al.* Splenectomy as a prerequisite for successful human ABO-incompatible renal transplantation. *Transplant. Proc.*, **17**, 138–143 (1985).
2. G. P. J. Alexandre, J. P. Squifflet, M. De Bruyere *et al.* Present experience in a series of 26 ABO-incompatible living donor renal allografts. *Transplant. Proc.*, **19**, 4538–4542 (1987).

3. A. D. Bannett, R. F. McAlack, R. Raja *et al.* Experience with known ABO-mismatched renal transplant. *Transplant. Proc.*, **19**, 4543–4546 (1987).

4. W. I. Bensinger, D. A. Baker, C. D. Buckner *et al.* Immunoadsorption for removal of A and B blood-group antibodies. *N. Engl. J. Med.*, **304**, 160–162 (1981).

5. R. Raja, A. D. Bannett, R. Coruana *et al.* Removal of antibodies with immunoadsorption from an ABO-incompatible recipient prior to renal transplant. *Trans. Am. Soc. Artif. Intern. Organs*, **32**, 102–103 (1986).

Therapeutic Plasmapheresis (XII), pp. 349-351
T. Agishi *et al.* (Eds)
© VSP 1993

Plasma Treatment Prior to ABO-Incompatible Kidney Transplantation

T. YAGISAWA, K. TAKAHASHI, T. AGISHI, T. TAKAHASHI and K. OTA

Kidney Center, Tokyo Women's Medical College, Tokyo, Japan

Key words: ABO blood type incompatible kidney transplantation; immunoadsorption; Biosynsorb; double filtration plasmapheresis; deoxyspergualin.

INTRODUCTION

Hyperacute rejection caused by the ABO antigen–antibody reaction is a major problem in kidney transplantation across the ABO barrier. However, some plasma treatment technologies [1] made possible the removal of anti-A and/or B antibodies to prevent the rejection. In this paper, we report the results of ABO-incompatible kidney transplantation with extracorporeal plasma treatment.

MATERIALS AND METHODS

Removal of anti-A and anti-B antibodies

We first applied immunoadsorption with Biosynsorb, produced by Chembiomed Ltd and supplied by Kawasumi Laboratories Inc., to remove the antibodies. The adsorbent is composed of silica beads embedded with blood type A or B antigen-expressing-trisaccharides. Adsorbent (80 g) was placed in a column; 3500–7000ml of plasma produced by membrane plasmaseparation was led to the column per each time and the antibodies were adsorbed. A series of one to four immunoadsorptions was carried out according to the antibody titer level to allow the titers to be reduced by 8 times. If it was difficult to reduce the antibody titers by immunoadsorption or anaphylactoid reactions were observed during immunoadsorption, then the antibodies were removed by double filtration plasmapheresis.

Immunosuppression

Five drugs (cyclosporin, azathioprine, steroid, anti-lymphocyte globulin and a new immunosuppressant, deoxyspergualin [2]) were initially used. Thereafter, treatment with three drugs (cyclosporin, azathioprine, steroid) was continued.

In addition, splenectomy was performed simultaneously at the time of transplantation.

Patients

A total of 35 patients were treated with this protocol of plasma treatment and received kidney grafts from ABO-incompatible living donors. Mean age was 34.6 ± 14.3 years. Twenty-one were male and 14 were female. Two cases were second grafts. Twenty-four patients received grafts from their mothers or fathers. Eight received grafts from their wives or husbands.

As for the blood type, 13 cases were A_1 type donors to O type recipients. 10 cases were B donors to O recipients. The mean mismatch number of HLA-A, B, OR was 2.4 ± 1.4. The mean one-way MLC SI was 24.2 ± 19.1.

RESULTS

Preoperative removal of the antibodies

The total volume of treated plasma was $22\,011 \pm 5033$ ml for anti-A antibody, $23\,924 \pm 6289$ ml for anti-B antibody in immunoadsorption.

Concerning anti-A antibody, the titers were reduced 4.9 ± 5.0 times in immunoglobulin G and 2.7 ± 1.7 times in immunoglobulin M. Concerning anti-B antibody, similarly, the titers were reduced 2.8 ± 3.5 times in IgG and 2.4 ± 3.2 times in IgM.

Patient and graft survival rates

The 1 year survival rate of patients was 87% and the 1 year survival rate of grafts was 80%. The 2–2.5 year survival rates of patients and grafts were equal to 1 year rates.

Rejection episodes

In 14 out of 35 patients (40%), rejection did not occur. Hyperacute rejection occurred once in one patient and accelerated acute rejection occurred once in four patients. Acute rejection occurred once in nine patients, twice in four patients, 3 times in one patient and 4 times in two patients. Three patients lost their grafts due to acute rejection.

Causes of graft loss and death

Seven out of 35 patients lost their grafts. Four patients out of seven died. Two out of four died of malignant B dell lymphoma and cerebral hemorrhage with functioning grafts. The remaining two patients died of ischemic colitis with DIC and cerebral hemorrhage after graft loss. Graft loss caused by rejection occurred in only three patients.

Complications

Cytomegalovirus infection occurred in four patients. Leukopenia was observed in three patients. The fatal complications were cerebral hemorrhage and malignant B cell lymphoma.

Antibody titers after transplantation

Immunoadsorption was required twice in only one patient for the elevation of the titers, postoperatively. The mean titers of anti-A and anti-B antibodies were maintained at below 8 times dilution after transplantation.

DISCUSSION AND CONCLUSIONS

Until now, kidney transplantation across the ABO barrier contraindicated, because of an occurrence of hyperacute rejection caused by the ABO antigen–antibody reaction.

In this trial, we performed ABO-incompatible kidney transplantation after removal of anti-A and/or anti-B antibodies by mainly immunoadsorption [1] and used a new immunosuppressive regimen [2] after transplantation.

Our trial showed that ABO-incompatible transplantation using immunoadsorption (or double filtration plasmapheresis) and our immunosuppressive regimen brought about clinically acceptable results.

REFERENCES

1. T. Agishi, K. Takahashi, T. Yagisawa *et al.* Immunoadsorption of anti-A or anti-B antibody for successful kidney transplantation between ABO incompatible pairs and its limitation. *ASAIO Trans.*, **37**, M496–498 (1991).
2. K. Takahashi, K. Tanabe, S. Oba *et al.* Prophylactic use of a new immunosuppressive agent, deoxyspergualin, in patients with kidney transplantation from ABO-incompatible or performed antibody-positive donors. *Transplant. Proc.*, **23**, 1078–1082 (1991).

Therapeutic Plasmapheresis (XII), pp. 353-355
T. Agishi *et al.* (Eds)
© VSP 1993

Induction of Immunosuppression in Renal Transplant Recipients by Lymphocytapheresis

A. TAJIMA, N. MORIYAMA, T. KITAMURA, T. UEKI and Y. ASO

Department of Urology, Faculty of Medicine, The University of Tokyo, Tokyo, Japan

Key words: renal transplantation; lymphocytapheresis; immunosuppression.

INTRODUCTION

It has been well known that various types of lymphocytes play an important role in the occurrence of acute rejection in the grafted kidney. Therefore, removal of lymphocytes may prevent the occurrence of acute rejection.

Using blood cell separators (IBM 2997 and Haemonetics V50 Pheresis System), we have carried out removal of lymphocytes, lymphocytapheresis (LA), as a pretransplant immunosuppressive treatment from 1981, and have obtained excellent graft survival [1, 2]. In this paper, the immunosuppressive state caused by LA pretreatment is presented.

PATIENTS AND METHODS

Sixty-six patients who received grafts from HLA one-haploidentical living related donors (LRD) have undergone LA as a pretransplant immunosuppression.

Between 6 and 8 l of whole blood was processed at the time of LA that resulted in the collection of approximately 200 g of lymphatic fluid in 60–120 min. Usually, 1–10 billion peripheral lymphocytes were removed in one process [3]. Fifteen repeated processes of LA were the goal of pretreatment for each patient. As post-transplant immunosuppression, cyclosporine and steroids were administered.

To evaluate the immunosuppressive state induced by LA, differences in peripheral lymphocytes, lymph nodes (LN) and the values of mixed lymphocytes reaction stimulation indices (MLR SI) before and after pretreatment with LA were examined; the numbers of peripheral lymphocytes and T cell subsets of peripheral lymphocytes (the ratio of OKT4/8 cells and the numbers of OKT10 cells) were studied. Inguinal LN biopsies done before LA were compared histologically with pelvic LN obtained during the transplant operation.

RESULTS

Complications
No serious complications attributable to LA were observed.

Graft survival

The graft survival rates at 1 year and 2 year in our cases were 96% and 94%, respectively; 93% and 87% in LRD registration cases of the Japan Transplantation Society (1986–1990).

Changes of peripheral lymphocytes

Repeated LA decreased significantly the number of recipient lymphocytes (1436 ± 637 to 780 ± 309/mm^3). The OKT4/8 ratio significantly dropped, whereas the number of OKT10 cells was elevated.

MLR SI

High MLR responders were converted to low ones.

LN

Biopsy of LN after LA showed distinct atrophy.

DISCUSSION

The effectiveness of LA was anticipated in renal transplantation, since thoracic duct drainage and antilymphocyte globulin (ALG) have already been shown to improve graft survival. Thoracic duct drainage, however, necessitates a complicated and time-consuming procedure, and cannulation into the thoracic duct may evoke infection. Similarly, ALG sometimes causes an allergic reaction.

This study shows that LA can be effectively and safely performed. The efficacy of LA in clinical organ transplantation has been reported by Kurland [4] and Iwatsuki [5]. Their clinical trials, however, were done in only a small number of cases, without basic analysis.

Our results of immunological and histological investigations point strongly to the immunosuppressive potential of LA. It is interesting that the number of OKT10 cells was elevated after LA, because OKT10 cells, immature lymphocytes, may have favorable effects on graft acceptance.

SUMMARY

Using blood cell separators, we have carried out removal of lymphocytes, lymphocytapheresis (LA), as a pretransplant immunosuppressive treatment from 1981, and have obtained excellent graft survival. The immunosuppressive state caused by LA pretreatment in 66 patients who received grafts from HLA one-haploidentical living related donors is presented.

Between 6 and 8 l of whole blood was processed at the time of LA, that resulted in removal of 10^9 to 10^{10} peripheral lymphocytes in 60–120 min. This procedure was repeated 15 times, and repeated LA decreased significantly the number of recipients' peripheral lymphocytes. In addition, the following data were obtained after the LA pretreatment: (i) biopsy of lymph nodes after LA showed distinct atrophy, (ii) high MLR responders were converted to low ones and (iii) the OKT4/8 ratio of peripheral lymphocytes significantly dropped, whereas the number of OKT10 cells was elevated. These results suggest that an immunosuppressive effect was induced by LA. LA was safely carried out without any complications.

REFERENCES

1. A. Tajima *et al.* Lymphocytapheresis as pretransplant immunosuppression. *Transplant. Proc.*, **21**, 1722–1725 (1989).

2. A. Tajima *et al.* Lymphocytapheresis by the V50 pheresis system: Pretreatment of kidney transplantation recipients. In: *Therapeutic Plasmapheresis (IX)*, N. Koga *et al.* (Eds), pp. 523–526, ICAOT Press, Cleveland (1991).

3. A. Tajima *et al.* Apheresis as an immunosuppressive method in renal transplantation — an evaluation of lymphocytapheresis and plasmapheresis. In: *Therapeutic Plasmapheresis (V)*, T. Oda (Ed.), pp. 417–419, Schattauer, New York (1986).

4. J. Kurland *et al.* Treatment of renal allograft rejection by exchange plasma–lymphocytapheresis. *Transfusion*, **20**, 337–340 (1979).

5. S. Iwatsuki *et al.* Lymphapheresis in organ transplantation: preliminary report. In: *Cytapheresis and Plasma Exchange: Clinical Indication*, W. R. Vogler (Ed.), p. 219, Alan R. Liss, New York (1982).

Therapeutic Plasmapheresis (XII), pp. 357-361
T. Agishi *et al.* (Eds)
© VSP 1993

Prolongation of Cardiac Xenograft Survival by Double Filtration Plasmapheresis and *ex vivo* Xenoantibody Adsorption

M. SHINKAI, M. KIMIKAWA, H. SUGA, T. AGISHI, Y. HAYASAKA,
S. TERAOKA, K. OTA, K. ICHINOHE,[1] H. NAKAJIMA[1] and M. ABE[1]

The Third Department of Surgery, Kidney Center, Tokyo Women's Medical College, Tokyo, Japan
[1]*Kawasumi Chemical Laboratory Inc., Japan*

Key words: double filtration plasmapheresis; *ex vivo* antibody adsorption; xenotransplantation.

INTRODUCTION

Hyperacute xenograft rejection is associated with preformed xenogeneic antibodies in discordant species [1]. We have utilized double filtration plasmapheresis (DFPP) and *ex vivo* xenoantibody adsorption (EXA) to deplete these antibodies, and evaluated the effects on xenograft survival [2].

MATERIALS AND METHODS

Swine–canine heart transplant combinations were used and they were divided into four experimental groups of cardiac transplantation according to the methods of preoperative immunomodulation (Group 1: no immunomodulation; group 2: DFPP alone; group 3: EXA using donor spleen subsequent to DFPP; group 4: EXA using donor liver subsequent to DFPP).

Donor operation

Under general anesthesia the heart was excised after infusion of cardioplegic solution into the ascending aorta. Splenectomy or hepatectomy was performed before heart excision in groups 3 and 4 to utilize these organs for EXA.

Recipient operation

Following preoperative DFPP and/or EXA, splenectomy was performed through a midline laparotomy [3] and the swine heart was transplanted heterotopically onto the cervical vessels of the dog.

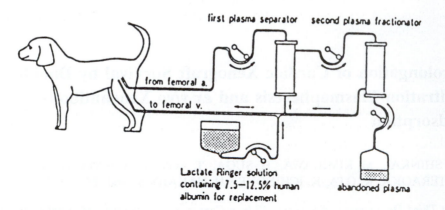

Figure 1. Circuit diagram of DFPP.

Plasmapheresis
Canine blood was obtained from the femoral artery and the plasma was continuously separated by KPS-015 (Kawasumi Chemical Laboratory Inc.); the fraction of large molecules, such as immunoglobulin, was selectively replaced with 7.5–12.5% solution of human albumin using EVAFLUX 2A (Kawasumi Chemical Laboratory Inc.), see Fig. 1.

Ex vivo antibody adsorption
The plasma separated by KPS-015 was perfused *ex vivo* through the isolated donor spleen or liver for 1–3 h to further eliminate donor-specific canine antibodies and then returned into the recipient femoral vein, see Fig. 2.

Immunosuppression
   Group 2. Cyclosporin and azathioprin were administered orally at a dose of 15 and 5 mg/kg/day, respectively, on day −2, −1 and the day of transplantation and methyl-prednisolone (25 mg/kg) was administered i.v. during operation. Gabexate mesilate (FOY) was also infused at a dose of 100 mg/kg.

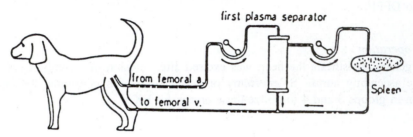

Figure 2. Circuit diagram of EXA.

Groups 3 and 4. Cyclosporin (5 mg/kg/day), 15-deoxyspergualin (DSG) (10 mg/kg/day) and methylprednisolone (25 mg/kg) were administered i.v. on the day of transplantation. FOY (100 mg/kg) or nafamostat mesilate (FUT) (20 mg/kg) was infused as anti-coagulation therapy.

RESULTS

Swine hearts transplanted into the untreated dogs (group 1) were rejected within 15 min. In contrast, cardiac grafts in groups 2, 3 and 4 had a mean survival of 98 ± 42, 217 ± 146 and 225 ± 74 min, respectively (Table 1).

Table 1.
Effects of DFPP and EXA on swine cardiac graft survival

Group	n	Graft survival (min)	Mean ± SD (min)
No. treatment	3	5, 7, 15	9 ± 5
DFPP	6	60, 60, 70, 110, 120, 165	98 ± 42
DFPP+splenic perfusion	13	60, 75, 120, 120, 125, 170, 180, 205, 240, 330 360, 240, 600	217 ± 146
DFPP+hepatic perfusion	4	120, 240, 270, 270	225 ± 74

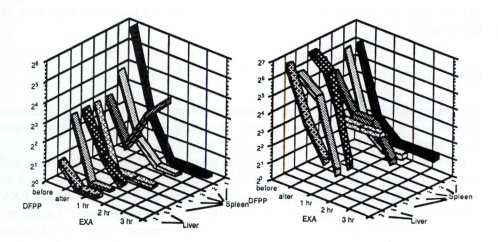

Figure 3. Effect of DFPP and EXA on serum levels of anti-swine hemagglutinating antibodies (left) and lymphocytotoxic antibodies (right).

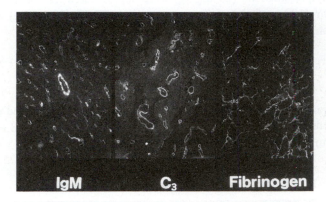

Figure 4. Deposition of IgM, C3 and fibrinogen on vascular endothelium of the cardiac grafts in group 4 (pretreated with DFPP and EXA).

Serum levels of IgG and IgM were remarkably decreased after DFPP and these depletion rates (comparing pre-DFPP to post-DFPP titers) were 85.5 and 93.3%, respectively. EXA, on the other hand, had little influence on IgG and IgM levels.

The amount of xenoantibody removal by *ex vivo* organ perfusion was evaluated by anti-swine hemagglutination and lymphocytotoxicity. Hemagglutinating antibodies were efficiently removed by DFPP except for one case and were hardly detectable by the first 1 h during *ex vivo* antibody adsorption. Lymphocytotoxic antibodies were also reduced significantly by DFPP and EXA with their depletion rate of 95.3% (Fig. 3).

The histological picture of rejection of the hearts transplanted after DFPP and EXA showed interstitial edema, intramuscular hemorrhage and microthrombosis in capillaries in moderate fashion. The immunohistological study revealed deposition of canine IgM and C3 along the vascular endothelium but no evidence for significant deposition of IgG (Fig. 4).

DISCUSSION

A major obstacle to success in discordant xenotransplantation is the presence of xenoantibodies which initiate hyperacute rejection. This study reveals the effect of depletion of xenoantibodies by DFPP and EXA on graft survival.

DFPP and EXA effectively removed the majority, not all, of xenoantibodies and allowed for a significant prolongation of swine graft survival. But small amounts of antibodies, as was shown in lymphocytotoxicity, remained following DFPP and EXA and immunohistological staining demonstrated the deposition of IgM and C3 along endothelial surfaces, suggesting that residual xenoantibodies, especially IgM, could induce hyperacute rejection in less pronouncing fashion than the controlled [4]. More effective methods to eliminate xenoantibodies or interrupt the deposition of antibodies and complements would be needed for success in xenotransplantation.

REFERENCES

1. R. J. Fishel, J. L. Bolman III, J. S. Najarian *et al.* Removal of IgM anti-endothelial antibodies results in prolonged cardiac xenograft survival. *Transplant. Proc.*, **22**, 1077 (1990).

2. T. Agishi, K. Kaneko, Y. Hasuo *et al.* Double filtration plasmapheresis. *Trans. Am. Soc. Artif. Intern. Organs*, **26**, 406 (1980).

3. G. P. J. Alexandre, P. Gianello *et al.* Plasmapheresis and splenectomy in experimental renal xenotransplantation. In: *Xenograft 25*, pp. 259–266, Elsevier, Amsterdam (1989).

4. J. L. Platt, R. J. Fischel *et al.* Immunopathology of hyperacute xenograft rejection in a swine-to-primate model. *Transplantation*, **52**, 214–220 (1991).

Therapeutic Plasmapheresis (XII), pp. 363-365
T. Agishi *et al.* (Eds)
© VSP 1993

Processing of Bone Marrow with the CS-3000 Plus using the Small Volume Collection Chamber

A. WAGNER, P. HÖCKER and K. GERHARTL

Clinical Institute of Blood Serology and Transfusion Medicine,
Department of Transfusion Medicine, University Hospital Vienna, Vienna, Austria

Key words: bone marrow processing; cell separator; small volume collection chamber.

INTRODUCTION

Bone marrow (BM) harvesting for either autologous or allogenic transplantation usually results in a vast amount of a BM peripheral blood mixture containing plasma, culture medium, anticoagulant, red cells, granulocytes as well as mononuclear cells (MNCs) containing the hematopoietic cell population. It may also be of concern that several plasma factors are activated during the harvesting process. Thus several procedures have been developed to reduce the volume and to remove undesirable cells like red cells, granulocytes and platelets to achieve a relatively small volume of MNC concentrates. Recently a method has been described using the Baxter CS-3000 Plus Cell Separator with a special program for BM processing using by the A-35 chamber [1]. We have modified the technique by replacing the A-35 chamber by the small volume collection chamber (SVCC). Instead of human albumin 5%, we took a mixture of hydroxyethyl starch and saline which results in a small volume end product enriched with MNCs and preserved red cells for retransfusion leach to the donor.

MATERIALS AND METHODS

BM from 32 donors (26 autologous and six allogenic) were harvested by multiple punctions from the posterior iliac chrest into a tissue culture medium containing conservans free heparin. BM were then centrifuged at 2858 g for 30 min and the fat supernatant was removed. A mixture of 2/3 saline and 1/3 HES 6% (plasmasterile R Fresenius) was used to prime the Fenwal, CS-3000 Plus Baxter after setting up with the standard open collection kit and the SVCC. A special program was provided from the manufacture based on an established program for lymphapheresis. Except the connection from the red cell return with a dialysis needle all other connections between the BM bag, red cell bag and inlet line were done by the sterile connecting device Haemonetics R.

After removing the fat rich supernatant, also in a closed bag system, the BM was adjusted to a hematocrit (HCT) of 25% with the HES/saline mixture also used for priming. Then the BM was connected to the inlet line and the red cell retransfusion bag and the procedure was started with a flow of 25 ml/min. The baseline detector was set when the color of the plasma line turn to light yellow (usually after 150–170 ml plasma was processed). The red cells were collected in a bag containing HES/saline mixture. After BM was processed once, the red cells were adjusted again to 25% HCT, transferred to the BM bag and processed again with the same settings. This was done in the last 16 BMTs, the first 16 BMTs were processed without adjusting the red cells. When the second run was finished, the bag with the BM concentrate was removed and the red cells were collected by gravity from the separation chamber to the retransfusion bag.

Cell counts were performed with an electronic cell counter CC-780 (Sysmex). The percentage of MNCs and granulocytes was determined microscopically from a stained smear. As MNCs, lymphocytes, monocytes, promyelocytes and myeloblasts were counted and CD34 positive cells were determined by FACS analysis as percentage of MNCs gained after density separation, CFU-GM and BFUe were assayed in a methylcellulose system as described elsewhere.

Total CFU-GMs were calculated by the formula

$$\text{mean number of colonies/plate} \times \text{total MNCs} \times 10^{-5}.$$

The recovery was calculated by dividing the number of CFU-GM of the centrifuged fat depleted BM. Engraftment was defined when a white cell count above $10^9/l$ was achieved.

RESULTS

The results of BM processing with and without HCT adjustment before the second run are shown in Table 1. There was an overall reduction in volume of about 95% with a similar reduction in red cells. This provides an excellent tolerance in ABO-incompatible donor recipient pairs with rapid engraftment. The loss of CFU-GM cells and in MNCs was minimal. This procedure presents more consistent results.

Table 1.
Results of BM processing with the Fenwall CS-3000 Plus and the SVCC

	BM post fat removal	BM concentrated
Volume (ml)	I 1065 (738–1326)	93 (51–210)
	II 1101 (850–1440)	66 (50–92)
NC ($\times 10^8$)	I 161.4 (60.4–247)	80.7 (20.4–155.3)
	II 147.5 (109.5–321.2)	89.4 (46.3–298.4)
MNC ($\times 10^8$)	I 25.6 (6.3–46.7)	22.5 (3.97–58.6)
	II 34.3 (18.1–60.8)	32.4 (19.1–58.9)
CFU-GM ($\times 10^4$)	I 204.8 (69.9–383.6)	200.9 (72.6–417.6)
	II 261.8 (56.1–896.9)	230.3 (34.2–684.9)
Seg. + Band ($\times 10^8$)	I 87.5 (16.6–131.8)	36.6 (3.6–82.4)
	II 98.1 (61.3–151.4)	26.8 (6.9–68.1)
Plts ($\times 10^{11}$)	I 2.0 (0.6–3.47)	0.5 (0.07–1.1)
	II 1.7 (0.5–3.1)	0.6 (0.1–1.4)
Red cells	I 334 (211–418)	
	II 335 (227–416)	

I, without; II, with adjusting HCT to 25% before the second run.

PATIENTS OUTCOME (TABLE 2)

In comparison to the conventional method there was minimal discomfort for the recipient due to the low volume in both the allogenic as well as in the autologous setting. Engraftment was not delayed but slightly enhanced in allogenic BMT. It can be speculated that this may be due to the removal of granulocytes, platelets and substances in the supernatant which may possibly inhibit or compete with the seeding of the transfused heamatopoietic cells. One additional advantage for the donor is the fact that no blood donation prior to BM harvest is necessary because the packed red cells are retransfused.

Table 2.
Engraftment

	Days	WBC 1000/μl	Plts-Tx independ.
Allogenic BM (6)	14	(10–21)	10 (6–15)
Autologous BM (7)	17	(12–19)	17 (7–28)

CONCLUSION

There are several advantages of BM processing considering both allogenic and autologous BMT

Allogenic BMT
- Minimal discomfort for the recipient due to the low volume.
- Retransfusion of red cells to the donor (no previous blood donation necessary).
- Excellent tolerance in ABO mismatched donor/recipient pairs.
- Rapid engraftment (withdrawal of toxic or activated substances).

Autologous BMT
- Small volume for further purging procedures.
- Small volume minimizing DMSO toxicity.
- Good engraftment (with or without growth factor).

We recommend this procedure for allogenic as well as for autologous BM harvesting and processing.

REFERENCE

1. E. M. Areman *et al.* Automated processing of human bone marrow can result in a population of mononuclear cells capable of achieving engraftment following transplantation. *Transfusion*, **31**, 724–730 (1991).

Therapeutic Plasmapheresis (XII), pp. 367-369
T. Agishi *et al.* (Eds)
© VSP 1993

Harvesting and Transfusion of Peripheral Blood Stem Cells without and with Autologous Bone Marrow

P. HÖCKER, A. WAGNER, K. GERHARTL, C. PETERS,
W. LINKESCH and W. HINTERBERGER

Bloodbank and Haematological Department, University Hospital,
St Anna Children's Hospital, Vienna, Austria

Key words: PBSC apheresis; small volume collection chamber; autologous bone marrow transplantation.

INTRODUCTION

Autologous bone marrow transplantation (ABMT) has become a widely used therapeutic tool for the treatment of certain malignant diseases like malignant lymphomas or solid tumors. An alternative approach is the collection of peripheral blood stem cells (PBSC). To harvest a sufficient number of PBSC it is common to induce a profound myelosuppression and to perform PBSC apheresis during the recovery phase, when increased levels of circulating PBSC can be expected [1]. This effect can be enhanced by simultaneous application of haematopoietic growth factors, thus allowing the harvesting of large amounts of PBSC necessary for a rapid and complete engraftment [2]. However, both methods as well as ABM harvest and PBSC collection can be of limited efficacy when the patient is heavily pretreated with cytotoxic chemotherapy resulting in low yields of bone marrow haematopoietic cells or circulating PBSC, which may result in delayed or incomplete engraftment. We have therefore tried to collect ABM and PBSC without priming from such patients and to retransfuse both ABM and PBSC simultaneously to shorten the period of myeloaplasia. We compared this group of patients to patients who received only PBSC after myeloablative therapy.

MATERIAL AND METHODS

PBSC collections were performed from 32 patients after myelosuppressive therapy in the recovery phase. PBSC harvest was started when the WBC count was above $1.0 \times 10^9/l$ and the platelet count exceeded $80 \times 10^9/l$ with clear evidence of a rapid increase. PBSC was done on consecutive days with the target to collect at least 3.0×10^8 mononuclear cells per kg body weight. When platelet recovery or WBC increase was delayed, two or three additional cytaphereses were performed. The stem cell concentrates were frozen after adding DMSO as cryoprotectant.

To collect PBSC, first, a cell separator type Haemonetics 30® was used. But most of PBSC aphereses were performed with the Fenwal CS-3000® cell separator. When the small volume collection chamber became available this was used, resulting in small concentrate volumes with relatively low red cell and platelet contamination and decreased DMSO load, thus minimizing side-effects during retransfusion.

BM harvest was performed in 24 patients for autologous purposes by multiple punctions of the posterior iliac chrest. Usually, 10 ml/kg body weight was collected during a session. BM was then concentrated by spinning it and removing the supernatant. Afterwards the cryoprotectant was added and the BM was frozen. PBSC collection was performed immediately before conditioning the patient with high dose myeloablative therapy prior to BM retransfusion without a specific priming procedure. Usually two to three PBSC collections were performed and the stem cell concentrates were processed as described above.

Evaluation of CFU-GM was done by a CFU-GM assays in a methycellulose system as described elsewhere [3].

RESULTS

The results of the PBSC collections done after myelosuppressive therapy are shown in Table 1 and those with no conditioning of the patients in Table 2. The results of the timed collections were far better than the yields obtained from the patients without priming, but it may be of interest that no correlation was found between the number of MNCs collected and the CFU-GM yield ($r = 0.35$) in the group of primed patients but a relatively fair correlation was found in the group of patients without priming between MNCs collected and CFU-GM harvested.

Table 1.
Results of PBSC collections after myelosuppressive therapy during the recovery phase (the mean value of the total yields harvested from each patient is shown).

	No. of ph.	MNC ($\times 10^8$/kg)	CFU-GM ($\times 10^4$/kg)
Mean	6.4	3.32	3.82
Range	2–14	1.5–7.36	0.83–14.3

Table 2.
Results of PBSC collections without myelosuppressive therapy during the recovery phase (the mean value of the total yields harvested from each patient is shown).

	No. of ph.	MNC ($\times 10^8$/kg)	CFU-GM ($\times 10^4$/kg)
Mean	3.1	1.93	0.78
Range	2–7	1.1–4.16	0.09–2.73

The results of ABM harvesting together with the yields of the PBSC collections from these patients are shown in Table 3.

Due to the heavy pretreatment prior to BM harvesting, the CFU-GM yield was rather poor and with the PBSC added the total number of CFU-GM did not exceed the number of PBSC collected by phereses only after appropriate timing.

Retransfusion of either PBSC or BM plus PBSC was performed after myeloablative therapy by bed side thawing and rapid infusion. Engraftment was started when the WBC

Table 3.
Results of BM harvesting together with the CFU-GM yield of the PBSC collection in those patients who underwent ABM harvest

	CFU-GM ($\times 10^4$/kg)	
	PBSC	ABM
Mean	0.78	1.18
Range	0.09–2.73	0.06–1.72
Total	1.98	
	0.86–3.11	

Table 4.
Engraftment after reinfusion of PBSC only and after reinfusion of ABM + PBSC. Numbers indicate days (median and range).

	PBSC only	PBSC + ABM
WBC > 1 $\times 10^9$/l	19 (8–135)	14 (10–38)
Plts 20 $\times 10^9$/l	28 (8–219)	21 (11–129)

count was above 1×10^9/l for three consecutive days. Sufficient thrombopoiesis was established when the platelet count remained above 20×10^9/l without further platelet transfusions (Table 4).

There was a more rapid engraftment after the reinfusion of ABM plus PBSC despite the low number of CFU-GM compared with the data obtained after reinfusion of PBSC only. This may indicate a superior quality of progenitor cells from the BM but may also demonstrate an additional effect of peripheral stem cells for the engraftment.

Thus we recommend additional PBSC harvesting from patients who are candidates for ABM but have only a small yield of haematopoietic stem cells when BM is harvested.

REFERENCES

1. A. Bell *et al.* Circulating stem cell autografts. *Bone Marrow Transplant.*, **1**, 103–110 (1986).
2. R. Pettengell *et al.* The engraftment capacity of peripheral blood progenitor cells (PBSC) with chemotherapy ± G-CSF. *Int. J. Cell Cloning*, **10**, (Suppl. 1), 59–61 (1992).
3. K. Geißler *et al.* Circulating stem cells in patients with acute leukemia in remission. *Exp. Haematol.*, **13** (Suppl. 17), 50 (1985).

Therapeutic Plasmapheresis (XII), pp. 371-374
T. Agishi *et al.* (Eds)
© VSP 1993

CD8 Positive T Cell Depleted Bone Marrow Transplantation from a Class I MHC-Mismatched Related Donor

M. IMAMURA, S. HASHINO, H. KOBAYASHI, M. KOBAYASHI,
Y. FUJII, M. KASAI, T. HIGA, K. SAKURADA, T. MINAGAWA,
S. HIRANO and T. MIYAZAKI

*The Third Department of Internal Medicine and The Department of Microbiology,
Hokkaido University School of Medicine and The Sapporo Hokuyu Hospital,
Sapporo, Japan*

Key words: CD8; cytokines; graft-versus-host; host-versus-graft; mixed chimerism.

INTRODUCTION

Graft-versus-host disease (GVHD) is one of the major obstacles in allogeneic bone marrow transplantation (BMT) even in the case of human leukocyte antigen (HLA)-matched donor to recipient combinations. Therefore, in the case of HLA-mismatched allogeneic BMT much more severe GVHD occurs. T cell depletion from MHC-mismatched donor bone marrow cells reduced the incidence of severe GVHD but induced frequent engraftment failure and leukemia relapse [1]. On the other hand, Champlin *et al.* [2] reported that selective depletion of CD8 positive T cells was effective for the prevention of GVHD in allogeneic BMT from HLA-matched siblings although it was not performed in HLA-mismatched ones and the incidence of engraftment failure and leukemia relapse has not been ascertained. In this paper, we shall discuss clinical efficacy of CD8 positive T cell depletion in class I MHC-mismatched BMT.

MATERIALS AND METHODS

Case
The patient was a 20 year old male with acute lymphocytic leukemia (L1). He was admitted to our hospital in July, 1989 and achieved complete remission in August, 1989.

HLA typing and mixed lymphocyte reaction (MLR)
HLA typing was carried out by microcytotoxicity assay. MLR was carried out by the method described elsewhere [3].

Preconditioning regimens and GVHD prophylaxis
The patient received cyclophosphamide (60 mg/kg/d × 2) followed by fractionated total body irradiation for a total dose of 1200 cGy in six fractions. Prophylaxis of acute GVHD was performed by continuous infusion of cyclosporin A (3 mg/kg/d) plus short-term methotrexate therapy (15–10 mg/m^2). Prednisolone (40 mg/d) was also administered from day 1 to day 7 followed by a gradual taper.

CD8 positive T cell depletion of donor bone marrow cells
Bone marrow cells were obtained from his younger brother by density gradient centrifugation with Ficoll-Hipaque. Cells were washed with balanced salt solution and suspended in TC 199 medium at a concentration of 10^{10}/ml. The cells were treated with 5 μg of monoclonal anti-CD8 antibody (Nichirei Co., Tokyo, Japan) for 30 min at 4 °C. After washing the cells, they were resuspended in medium followed by addition of baby rabbit complement (Pelfreeze Lab., Brown Deer, WI) in a 1:5 dilution for 1 h at 37 °C. Then, 2.4 × 10^9 cells in 200 ml medium were administered intravenously to the patient. Cytotoxicity of this monoclonal antibody plus complement against donor bone marrow cells was 7.7% while complement alone showed 4.0% cytotoxicity. This procedure eliminated 90% of CD8 positive T cells in the peripheral blood. Colony formations were not inhibited by this procedure. The clinical protocol was approved by the Institutional Review Boards of the Hokkaido University School of Medicine and BMT was performed with the informed consent of the patient and his family.

Measurement of serum cytokine levels
IFN-γ (Centocor Inc., Malvern, PA) and TNF-α (Medgenix Diagnostics, Brussels, Belgium) were measured by RIA kits. IFN-β, IL-6 (Toray Industries Co., Tokyo, Japan), IL-2, M-CSF and GM-CSF (Ohtsuka Pharmaceutical Co., Tokushima, Japan) were measured by ELISA kits.

RESULTS

HLA typing and MLR
HLA of the patient is consisted as A2, 33, B51, 62, C9, DR13, 8.1, w52, DQ1 whereas the HLA of his brother is consisted of A26, 33, B51, 54, C1, DR13, 8.1, w52, DQ1. MLR showed that the host anti-donor reaction is high (SI:11.3) whereas the donor anti-host reaction is low (SI:0.6).

Clinical course after BMT
Although the patient had a mild liver dysfunction, skin eruption and diarrhoea around day 29 showing the presence of grade II acute GVHD, it disappeared 2 weeks later by the treatment of prednisolone (Fig. 1). We used GM-CSF from day 1 to day 28; however, no increase of granulocyte counts was observed. Since hematopoietic recovery was delayed, we subsequently used G-CSF from day 29 to day 54. Then, leukocyte, erythrocyte and platelet counts gradually increased. HLA typing was performed in order to ascertain the engraftment by using antiserum against HLA-A2 or HLA-A26 2 months after BMT. Only 20% of donor-type cells were observed in the peripheral blood and the remaining 80% was of host-type cells. Although donor-type cells were no longer detected 6 months after BMT, no evidence of leukemia recurrence has been documented so far (2.5 years after BMT) and the patient keeps 100% performance status.

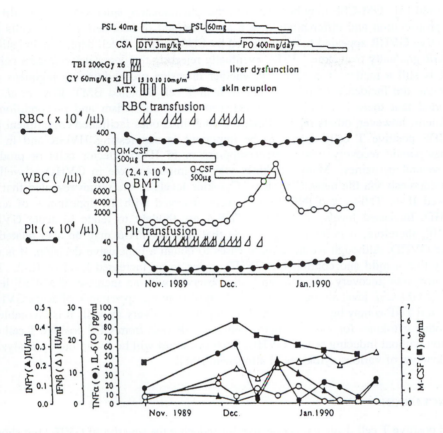

Figure 1. Clinical course and serum cytokine levels in CD8 positive T cell depleted BMT from class I MHC-mismatched donor.

Serum cytokine levels

As shown in Fig. 1, serum IFN-β, TNF-α and IL-6 levels were gradually increased at the time of the appearance of grade II acute GVHD. Prednisolone once inhibited the production of these cytokines, although these cytokine levels showed fluctuating kinetics with a taper of prednisolone. However, IFN-β level gradually increased dissimilar to the kinetics of other cytokines, indicating that this cytokine may be not involved in acute GVHD. M-CSF increased when the hematopoietic recovery occurred; however, increased levels of IL-2 and GM-CSF were not detected (data not shown).

DISCUSSION

When mixed chimerism is established, it lasts for a long time as a stable mixed chimerism without having GVHD or frequent leukemia recurrence [4]. The reason for a rejection of the donor-type cells appears to be due to partial T cell depletion, the presence of strong HVGR, an insufficient preconditioning regimen, the use of cytokines or too few infused cells.

It is interesting to know how the host-derived hematopoietic stem cells survive in spite of receiving a lethal dose of chemoradiotherapy although this phenomenon really occurred [5]. GM-CSF may be related to this phenomenon, since GM-CSF facilitates the proliferation and differentiation of a small amount of host-derived stem cells [6]. Effective GVHR appeared to be weakened by CD8 positive T cell depletion and strong HVGR gradually overcame GVHR, eventually rejecting the donor-derived stem cells.

It is still a matter of controversy whether intensive preconditioning regimens can decrease the incidence of mixed chimerism in T cell depleted BMT. Roy *et al.* [7] reported that there is no correlation between mixed chimerism and preconditioning regimens; however, others reported that the intensified ones facilitated engraftment [8].

CD8 positive T cells appear to be important in suppressing HVGR and in the hematopoietic recovery, via a direct suppression of HVG effector cells or producing several cytokines. Many cytokines play an important role in GVHD as well as hematopoiesis via the network system. Cytokine levels in the serum revealed that increased IL-6, TNF-α and INF-β levels were observed with the appearance of acute GVHD. Increased levels of IL-2 and TNF-α are thought to relate to acute GVHD [9, 10]; therefore, it is interesting to note that IL-6 or IFN-β may be also related to acute GVHD. Although we need more cases to obtain a conclusive decision, it is unlikely that a mild and controllable GVHD is due to an increased level of IL-2. The hematopoietic recovery was concomitantly observed with an increase of M-CSF level but not GM-CSF level although it slightly delayed from the appearance of acute GVHD. IL-6 and TNF-α may be related to the hematopoietic recovery as well. It is favorable to use other cytokines for substituting the deficiency derived from CD8 positive T cell depletion without inducing severe GVHD. Such cytokines will be found out by analyzing the kinetics of various cytokines in allogeneic BMT.

CONCLUSION

CD8 positive T cell depletion is effective for reducing the severity of GVHD but should be carefully used in class I MHC-mismatched BMT, since it readily induces the rejection of donor-type cells.

REFERENCES

1. R. Champlin, W. G. Ho, R. Mitsuyasu *et al. Transplant. Proc.*, **19**, 2616–2619 (1987).
2. R. Champlin, J. Gajewski, S. Feig *et al. Transplant. Proc.*, **21**, 2947–2948 (1989).
3. M. Imamura, H. Fujimoto, S. Hashino *et al. Immunobiology*, **180**, 441–457 (1990).
4. A. Schattenberg, T. Dewitte, M. Salden *et al. Blood*, **73**, 1367–1372 (1989).
5. E. D. Thomas, R. Storb, E. R. Giblett *et al. Exp. Hematol.*, **4**, 97–102 (1976).
6. B. R. Blazar, M. B. Widmer, C. C. B. Soderling *et al. Blood*, **72**, 1146–1154 (1988).
7. D. C. Roy, R. Tantravachi, C. Murray *et al. Blood*, **75**, 296–304 (1990).
8. C. C. B. Soderling, C. S. Song, B. R. Blazar *et al. J. Immunol.*, **135**, 941–946 (1985).
9. E. Holler, H. J. Kolb, A. Moller *et al. Blood*, **75**, 1011–1016 (1990).
10. M. Malkovsky, R. Brenner, S. Hunt *et al. Cell. Immunol.*, **103**, 476–480 (1986).

Therapeutic Plasmapheresis (XII), pp. 375-378
T. Agishi *et al.* (Eds)
© VSP 1993

Efficacy of Cryofiltration in Kidney Transplantation

K. KUKITA, H. KON, N. KAMII, K. ONODERA, M. TAKAHASHI,
H. WITMANOWSKI, J. MEGURO, M. YONEKAWA and A. KAWAMURA

Department of Surgery, Sapporo Hokuyu Hospital, Artificial Organ and Transplantation Hospital, Sapporo, Japan

Key words: cryofiltration; kidney transplantation.

INTRODUCTION

Cryofiltration is a modified double membrane filtration method [1]. We have been applying this technique for the removal of antibodies in many kinds of diseases [2–4]. The purpose of this study is to evaluate the efficacy of cryofiltration in kidney transplantation.

PATIENTS AND METHOD

Cryofiltration was applied in 14 kidney transplantation patients. Six cases were done before transplantation, eight cases were done after transplantation. Five cases were done after donor specific blood transfusion because antilymphocyte antibodies appeared. Anti-T antibodies were detected in three of these cases. Anti-B warm and B cold antibodies were detected in case 2 on the lymphocyte toxicity test with anti-human globulin. Cryofiltration was tried to see whether these antibodies could be removed or not. In two chronic rejection cases cryofiltration was tried to ascertain whether the restart time of hemodialysis could be delayed or not by the reduction of antilymphocyte antibodies (Table 1).

Table 1.
Cases

Time	Cases	Donor	Others
Pre-RTx	5	living	post-DST
	1	cadaver	
Post-RTx	6	living	
	1	cadaver	CHR. REJ
	1	living	CHR. REJ

RTx, renal transplantation; DST, donor specific blood transfusion; CHR. REJ, chronic rejection.

In one cadaveric kidney transplantation case (case 6) cryofiltration was applied as a prophylaxis for rejection to reduce antibodies. The anti-B warm and B cold antibodies were detected after living kidney transplantation within 2 months in six cases. Cryofiltration was performed on these cases (Table 2).

Table 2.
Crossmatch test after DST

Case	LCT			AHG		
	T	Bw	Bc	T	Bw	Bc
1	+	+	+			
2	+	+	+	+	+	+
3	+	+	+	+	+	+
4	−	−	−	−	+	+
5	−	−	−	−	+	+

DST, donor specific blood transfusion.

RESULTS

Table 3 shows the numbers and effects of cryofiltration and the courses of patients sensitized by donor specific blood transfusion. Lymphocyte cytotoxicity was reduced by cryofiltration in cases 1 and 5.

Table 3.
The numbers and effects of cryofiltration and courses (post-DST cases)

Case	Number	Effect	Course
1	1	+	RTx succeeded
2	28	−	observation
3	2	−	observation
4	1	−	RTx succeeded
5	3	+	RTx succeeded

DST, donor specific blood transfusion; RTx, renal transplantation.

Case 1 received donor specific blood transfusions 3 times in October 1988. Anti-T antibodies were not detected after these transfusions. However, in this period he had a gastric ulcer complication and renal transplantation was postponed. A direct crossmatch test was performed twice after the cure of the gastric ulcer. All antibodies appeared in this period and the cryofiltration procedure was performed. The antibodies, except anti-B cold antibodies, disappeared after only one cryofiltration procedure. Renal transplantation was successfully done and no acute rejection episode was observed. The anti-B warm and B cold antibodies were detected in April 1992, but the graft was well functioning.

In case 5, anti-B warm and B cold antibodies were detected at the antilymphocyte cytotoxicity test with anti-human globulin after donor specific blood transfusions twice.

Renal transplantation might have been possible in this period, but we tried cryofiltration 3 times. The cytotoxicity decreased gradually and only anti-B cold antibodies remained after 3 months. No rejection episode was experienced after transplantation.

Lymphocyte cytotoxicity was not reduced in other cases. Kidney transplantation could be done in case 4, but could not be done in cases 2 or 3 because their anti-T antibodies were still positive. In case 6, the evaluation of cryofiltration effect is difficult, but the kidney is functioning normally over 2 years after transplantation.

Table 4 shows the over 50% antilymphocyte antibody reduction ratio and the graft function. The ratio was a poor 5% in case 8 and the graft failed after 1 year and 6 months of transplantation. The ratios were good in other cases and the graft functions were good except case 9.

Table 4.

Over 50% antilymphocyte antibody reduction ratio and graft function

Case	Ratio (no.)	Graft
7	100% (2/2)	6Y functioning
8	5% (1/21)	1Y 6M graft failure → HD
9	100% (1/1)	1Y 3M graft failure → HD
10	100% (1/1)	complication death
11	100% (1/1)	4Y 2M functioning
12	100% (1/1)	2Y functioning

HD, hemodialysis.

Table 5.

Crossmatch test after cryofiltration (cytotoxicity:%:LCT) (case 14)

			'86		'87						'88			
			11	12	2	4	6	8	10	12	2	4	6	8
T cell		pre	—	—	—	—	—	—	—	—	—	—	—	—
		post	—	—	—	—	—	—	—	—	—	—	—	—
B cell	37°C	pre	100	20		80	100	60	100	90	90	60	20	20
		post		20		80	20	40	20	15	90	40	10	10
	4°C	pre	100	70		100	100	100	100	60	90	80	10	10
		post		70		90	20	100	20	10	90	10	10	10

Cryofiltration was tried in two chronic rejection cases. Table 5 shows the cytotoxicity test on case 14. Cryofiltration was started over 2 weeks from July 1986. The anti-B warm and B cold antibodies were reduced after cryofiltration.

Serum creatinine in this case was about 5 mg/dl in July 1986. The elevation of creatinine was not sharp. The value of creatinine reached 10 mg/dl in August 1988 and hemodialysis was re-started (Fig. 1). In one other chronic rejection case, cryofiltration was started somewhat later because his creatinine level reached 8 mg/dl, so after 2 months hemodialysis had to be started.

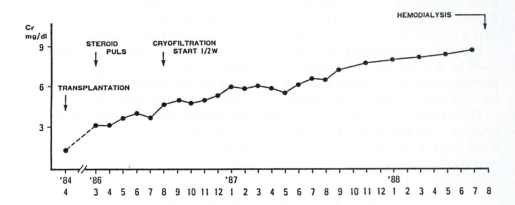

Figure 1. Change of creatinin (case 14).

DISCUSSION AND CONCLUSION

Cryofiltration was applied in 14 patients before or after kidney transplantation. The main purposes are to reduce anti-T, anti-B warm and other antibodies.

We experienced one case whose anti-T lymphocyte cytotoxicity test was changed to negative after cryofiltration and the re-start of hemodialysis was delayed for 2 years and 6 months after rejection episode. It is reported that in cases of chronic renal failure, the duration of hemodialysis was about 10 months [5]. Compared with that it could be said cryofiltration was very effective. In some cases the efficacy of cryofiltration is not clear. In some cases, of course, cryofiltration was not effective because antilymphocyte toxicity could not be reduced.

In conclusion, cryofiltration is effective in some cases, perhaps not high responders or not so highly damaged kidney cases, in the reduction of antilymphocyte antibodies.

REFERENCES

1. Y. Nosé, P. S. Malchesky *et al. Plasmapheresis: Therapeutic Applications and New Techniques.* pp. 1–22. Raven Press, New York (1983).
2. M. Yonekawa, A. Kawamura *et al.* Cryofiltration for treatment of immune complex diseases. In: *Therapeutic Plasmapheresis (VII)*, pp. 167–170, ISAO Press, Cleveland (1988).
3. M. Yonekawa, A. Kawamura *et al.* Therapeutic trials of cryofiltration in patients with acute hepatic failure. In: *Therapeutic Plasmapheresis (VII)*, pp. 404–408, ISAO Press, Cleveland (1988).
4. K. Kukita, J. Meguro *et al.* Therapeutic trials of cryofiltration in patients with myeloma kidney. In: *Therapeutic Plasmapheresis (VIII)*, pp. 56–60, ISAO Press, Cleveland (1990).
5. T. Deguchi, Y. Yuasa *et al.* Clinical evaluation of AST-120 on chronic renal failure cases. *Rinsho Toseki*, 563–568 (1986).

Therapeutic Plasmapheresis (XII), pp. 379-382
T. Agishi *et al.* (Eds)
© VSP 1993

Cytokine Therapy Prior to Bone Marrow Transplantation: the Effects of IL-1, IL-2, TNF and IL-6 on Hematopoietic and Immunologic Recovery

Y. FUJII,[1] M. IMAMURA,[1] S. HASHINO,[1] H. KOBAYASHI,[1] M. HAN,[1]
M. KOBAYASHI,[1] M. KASAI,[2] K. SAKURADA[1] and T. MIYAZAKI[2]

[1]*The 3rd Department of Internal Medicine, Hokkaido University School of Medicine, Sapporo, Japan*
[2]*Sapporo Hokuyu Hospital, Sapporo, Japan*

Key words: IL-1; IL-2; TNF; IL-6; bone marrow transplantation.

INTRODUCTION

Delayed reconstitution of hematopoiesis and retarded recovery of immune functions are among the major complications associated with bone marrow transplantation (BMT) therapy. Cytokines such as interleukin-1 (IL-1), IL-2, tumor necrosis factor (TNF) and IL-6 have an apparent capacity to promote hematopoiesis and immune functions through their direct and/or indirect effects on stromal cells (fibroblasts, endothelial cells and tissue macrophages). The present experiments were conducted to assess stromal cell-mediated effects of these cytokines on the early-stage recovery of hematopoiesis and immune functions in lethally irradiated recipients treated with syngeneic bone marrow cells. For these aims, the cytokines were administered to prospective marrow recipients (BALB/c mice) before total body irradiation (TBI) and syngeneic BMT.

MATERIALS AND METHODS

Mice
BALB/c mice at 10–12 weeks old were used for the experiments, and maintained on laminar air-flow shelves under specific pathogen-free conditions.

Cytokines
rhIL-1β, rhIL-2, rmTNF and rhIL-6 were kindly provided by Ohtsuka Pharmaceutical Co. (Tokyo), Shionogi Pharmaceutical Co. (Tokyo), Asahi Chemical Industry (Tokyo) and Tohre (Tokyo), respectively. Mice were given i.p. injections of rhIL-1β (0.2 μg per injection), rhIL-2 (2×10^4 U per injection), rmTNF (1×10^4 U per injection), rhIL-6 (0.5 μg per injection) or an equal volume (100 μl) of diluent on days -3, -2 and -1 before TBI and BMT (day 0).

Irradiation and BMT

Recipient mice received 6.5 Gy TBI, administered at a dose rate of 25 cGy/min, followed by syngeneic BMT ($5–6 \times 10^6$ BM cells) on day 0.

CFU-GM assay

Bone marrow cells (5×10^4) or spleen cells (1×10^5) in 1 ml IMDM supplemented with 0.9% methylcellulose, 30% FCS, 1% bovine serum albumin and 5% PWM-stimulated mouse spleen conditioned medium were plated into 35-mm Petri dishes. Colony formation was enumerated after 7 days of incubation at 37 °C in a fully humidified atmosphere of 5% CO_2 in air.

Proliferative response

Spleen cells (2.5×10^5) were cultured in 96-well flat bottom plates in a 0.2 ml volume of RPMI 1640 containing 5% FCS, 5×10^5 M 2-ME and sodium pyruvate. The cultures were incubated in a humidified atmosphere of 5% CO_2 in air for 72 h. [^{3}H]thymidine (1 μCi/well) was added for the last 6 h of the culture. The plates were harvested by using an automated multiple sample harvester and the [^{3}H]thymidine incorporated was assessed by liquid scintillation counter.

RESULTS

Enhanced splenic CFU-GM numbers after BMT

Numbers of CFU-GM per femur and spleen were assessed on days 7 and 14 post-BMT. CFU-GM numbers per spleen were remarkably increased on day 7 whether or not the mice were given injections of IL-1, IL-2, TNF or IL-6, with approximately 30 times the normal level. However, on day 14, greater numbers of CFU-GM per spleen were maintained in the mice given injections of the cytokines compared with the control mice (Table 1).

Table 1.
Numbers of CFU-GM/spleen 14 days after BMT

Cytokine therapy	CFU-GM/spleen ($\times 10^3$)
rhIL-1	39.7 ± 2.3^a
rhIL-2	52.3 ± 15.7^a
rmTNF	48.6 ± 6.4^a
rhIL-6	51.0 ± 11.9^a
Control	29.9 ± 5.1
Normal	1.3 ± 0.8

[a] Significantly different from the control value ($P < 0.05$).

Recovery of CFU-GM in femur was comparable between the control mice and the mice given injections of the cytokines, with approximately 25% of normal level on day 7 and a full recovery on day 14 post-BMT (data not shown). Recovery of peripheral blood cells was comparable between the cytokine-injected mice and the control mice (data not shown).

Enhanced response to mitogens

Proliferative responses of spleen cells to PWM, LPS and PHA were assessed at various times after BMT. In the cytokine-injected mice, splenic responses to PWM and LPS were significantly greater on day 28 (Table 2) and those to PHA were significantly greater on day 42 than in the control mice (data not shown).

Table 2.
Proliferative responses of spleen cells 28 days after BMT

Cytokine therapy	% of normal values	
	PWM	LPS
rhIL-1	103.9 ± 16.3^a	110.8 ± 9.0^b
rhIL-2	131.7 ± 17.2^a	83.3 ± 8.5^b
mmTNF	127.8 ± 24.8^a	92.0 ± 5.6^b
rhIL-6	68.9 ± 9.1^a	79.2 ± 6.5^b
Control	26.6 ± 11.8	57.9 ± 6.5

[a,b] Significantly different from the control value ($P < 0.05$).

DISCUSSION

The present studies were conducted to assess effects of IL-1, IL-2, TNF and IL-6 administered in prospective recipients of bone marrow cells on their hematopoietic and immunologic recovery after BMT. IL-1, IL-2, TNF and IL-6 have been reported to stimulate stromal cells to produce CSF and cytokines. The stromal cells are thought to be resistant to 6.5 Gy irradiation [1]. Thus, the present studies are thought to assess an indirect *in vivo* effect of these cytokines that is mediated by stimulation of stromal cell functions.

The present studies showed that numbers of CFU-GM per spleen and responses to PWN, LPS and PHA were greater in the mice given injections of one of these cytokines than in the control mice. Administrations of IL-1 and TNF prior to TBI in the absence of BMT have been reported to exert radioprotective effects and thus accelerate the recovery of CFU-GM and peripheral blood WBC numbers in myelosuppressed host [2, 3]. However, administration of IL-2, which is not associated with radioprotective effects [2], exerted effects on splenic CFU-GM numbers and mitogen responses comparable to that of IL-1, TNF and IL-6. This finding suggests that the immunologic and hematopoietic effects of the cytokine therapies are due to stimulation of donor progenitor cells through activated stromal cell functions rather than direct protection by the administered cytokines of recipient progenitor cells against irradiation. In fact, the radioprotective effects of IL-1 in the absence of BMT are ascribed to both a direct effect on hematopoietic stem cells and an induced production of endogenous cytokines such as CSF and IL-6 from stimulated stromal cells [4]. IL-1 administration after sublethal irradiation of mice without BMT was reported to cause suppressed responses of spleen cells to LPS as well as to Con A [5]. In the present study, splenic responses to LPS were enhanced (Table 2). This finding suggests that cytokine administration prior to TBI may have different outcomes whether in the presence or absence of BMT [6].

CONCLUSION

Our data suggest that posttransplant immunologic and hematopoietic effects of administrations of IL-1, IL-2, TNF and IL-6 to prospective recipients of bone marrow cells are mediated through stimulation of recipient stromal cells, and that exogenous administration of these cytokines in prospective marrow recipients could be useful for enhancement of hematopoietic and immunologic reconstitution after BMT.

REFERENCES

1. Y. Imai and I. Nakao. *In vivo* radiosensitivity and recovery pattern of the hematopoietic precursor cells and stem cells in mouse bone marrow. *Exp. Hematol.*, **15**, 890–893 (1987).

2. R. Neta, S. N. Vogel, J. J. Oppenheim *et al.* Cytokines in radioprotection. Comparison of the radioprotective effects of IL-1 to IL-2, GM-CSF and IFNγ. *Lymphokine Res.*, **5**, S105–S110 (1986).

3. R. Neta, J. J. Oppenheim, R. D. Schreiber *et al.* Role of cytokines (interleukin 1, tumor necrosis factor, and transforming growth factor β) in natural and lipopolysaccharide-enhanced radioresistance. *J. Exp. Med.*, **173**, 1177–1182 (1991).

4. R. Neta, S. N. Vogel, J. M. Plocinski *et al. In vivo* modulation with anti-interleukin-1 (IL-1) receptor (p80) antibody 35F5 of the response to IL-1. The relationship of radioprotection, colony-stimulating factor, and IL-6. *Blood*, **76**, 57–62 (1990).

5. P. Morrissey, K. Charrier, L. Bressler *et al.* The influence of IL-1 treatment on the reconstitution of the hematopoietic and immune systems after sublethal radiation. *J. Immunol.*, **140**, 4204–4210 (1988).

6. J. J. Oppenheim, R. Neta, P. Tiberghien *et al.* Interleukin-1 enhances survival of lethally irradiated mice treated with allogeneic bone marrow cells. *Blood*, **74**, 2257–2263 (1989).

Therapeutic Plasmapheresis (XII), pp. 383-387
T. Agishi *et al.* (Eds)
© VSP 1993

Systemic Administration of IL-2 after Autologous Bone Marrow Transplantation

S. HASHINO, M. IMAMURA, S. KOBAYASHI, H. KOBAYASHI, Y. FUJII,
M. KOBAYASHI, S. HIRANO,[1] T. MINAGAWA,[1] M. KASAI,[2]
K. SAKURADA and T. MIYAZAKI

*The 3rd Department of Internal Medicine and [1]Department of Microbiology,
Hokkaido University, School of Medicine and [2]Sapporo Hokuyu Hospital,
Sapporo, Japan*

Key words: IL-2; bone marrow transplantation; IFN-γ, TNF-α.

INTRODUCTION

IL-2 is presently undergoing extensive trials after autologous bone marrow transplantation (ABMT) in various hematological malignancies for elimination of minimal residual disease (MRD) [1–3]. In this study, we started IL-2 therapy just after ABMT, and investigated an antitumor efficacy and side-effects.

Patients and Methods

Two patients with acute myeloblastic leukemia were treated with chemo-radiotherapy and ABMT. Case 1 was a 20 year old female patient with AML (M2) and her conditioning regimen for ABMT consisted of cytosine arabinoside, etoposide and cyclophosphamide. Case 2 was a 26 year old male patient with AML (M3) and his conditioning was cyclophosphamide, etoposide and total body irradiation. IL-2 was started on day 0 and the day when granulocyte counts in peripheral blood reached $500/\mu l$. Case 1 received two courses of a 5-day cycle of IL-2 ($5–50 \times 10^4$ U/day) and case 2 received three courses of a 7-day one ($50–100 \times 10^4$ U/day). IL-2 was administered as an intravenous infusion for 6 h (case 1) or a continuous infusion for the period (case 2). At several times after ABMT, antitumor effects were immunologically investigated by measuring LAK (anti-Daudi) and NK (anti-K562) activities, lymphocyte subpopulations and serum cytokine concentrations (IL-2, IL-6, M–CSF, GM–CSF, IFN-γ and TNF-α).

RESULTS

In both cases, hematological recovery was slightly impaired without graft failure. In case 1, LAK and NK activities of peripheral blood were low even after IL-2 therapy, but both activities were enhanced by *in vitro* IL-2 stimulation (Fig. 1). There was no significant change on lymphocyte subpopulations of peripheral blood and cytokine concentrations in the serum except for a slight increase of IFN-γ (Fig. 2). In case 2, LAK and NK

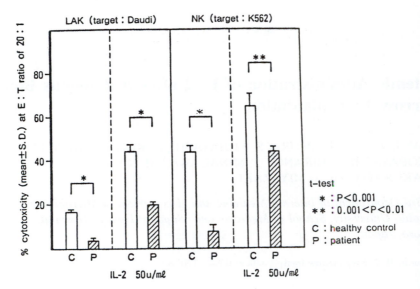

Figure 1. LAK and NK activities (case 1).

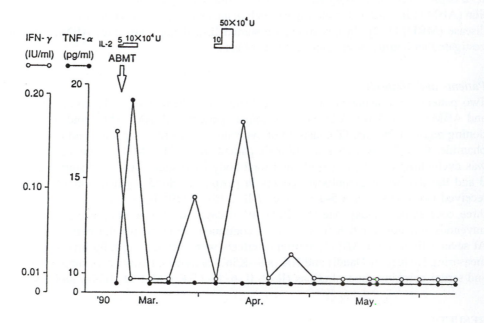

Figure 2. Serum cytokine concentrations (case 1).

activities were enhanced in both peripheral blood (Fig. 3) and bone marrow (data not shown). Percentages of CD11b, CD16 and CD57 positive lymphocytes significantly increased (data not shown), and many large granular lymphocytes appeared on blood smears. Among several cytokines measured, only TNF-α serum level was elevated after

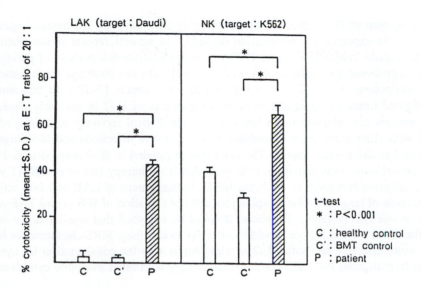

Figure 3. LAK and NK activities (case 2).

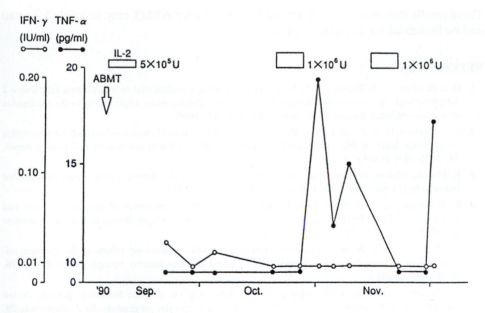

Figure 4. Serum cytokine concentrations (case 2).

IL-2 therapy (Fig. 4). Clinical toxicities involving nausea, mild to moderate fever and general fatigue occurred during IL-2 therapy, but reversed on cessation of the infusions. Case 1 relapsed and died 8 months after ABMT, but case 2 is alive and well 20 months after ABMT and IL-2 therapy.

DISCUSSION

Administration of IL-2 after ABMT or intensive chemotherapy for hematological malignancies is expected for elimination of MRD. In several reports it was mentioned that IL-2 could induce IFN-γ and TNF-α to enhance antitumor activity of patients, but that it suppressed the hematopoetic system [4–6]. On the contrary, the enhancement of hematopoiesis due to IL-2 was reported in some papers [7–10]. In this study we investigated immunological and hematological effects of IL-2 in the early phase after bone marrow transplantation. In two cases hematological recovery was delayed compared with other autologous transplants, but any severe infections and bleedings were not found in the aplastic phase. The cells that responded to IL-2 were detected in the early period after transplantation, indicating that IL-2 therapy just after ABMT will be a very effective treatment to eradicate MRD. Enhancement of LAK and NK activities, the increase of large granular lymphocytes and the elevation of IFN-γ and TNF-α were found in our two patients. Therefore, it could be expected that smaller doses of IL-2 than the doses used in Europe would be effective to eliminate MRD. In future we have to study more effective and safer IL-2 administration after the consideration for cytotoxic effects to malignant cells and combination therapy with other available cytokines.

CONCLUSIONS

These results indicates that IL-2 administration just after ABMT may be safely tolerated and be beneficial for elimination of MRD.

REFERENCES

1. D. J. Gottlieb, M. K. Brenner, H. E. Heslop et al. A phase I clinical trial of recombinant Interleukin-2 following high-dose chemo-radiotherapy for hematological malignancy: applicability to the elimination of minimal residual disease. Br. J. Cancer., 60, 610–615 (1989).

2. D. J. Gottlieb, H. G. Prentice, H. E. Heslop et al. Effects of recombinant Interleukin-2: administration on cytotoxic function following high-dose chemo-radiotherapy for hematological malignancy. Blood, 74, 2335–2342 (1989).

3. R. Foa, G. Meloni, S. Tosti et al. Treatment of acute myeloid leukemia patients with recombinant Interleukin-2; a pilot study. Br. J. Haematol., 77, 491–496 (1991).

4. H. E. Heslop, D. J. Gottlieb, A. C. M. Bianchi et al. In vivo induction of gamma interferon and tumor necrosis factor by Interleukin-2 infusion following intensive chemotherapy or autologous marrow transplantation. Blood, 74, 1374–1380 (1989).

5. D. Blaise, D. Olive, A. M. Stoppa et al. Hematologic and immunologic effects of the systemic administration of recombinant Interleukin-2 after autologous bone marrow transplantation. Blood, 76, 1092–1097 (1990).

6. A. Guarini, F. Sanovia, A. Noverino et al. Thrombocytopenia in acute leukaemia patients treated with Interleukin-2: cytolytic effect of LAK cells on megakaryocytic progenitors. Br. J. Haematol., 79, 451–456 (1991).

7. M. R. Schaafsma, W. E. Fibbe, D. Harst et al. Increased numbers of circulating haematopoietic progenitor cells after treatment with high-dose Interleukin-2 in cancer patients. Br. J. Haematol., 76, 180–185 (1990).

8. E. Tritarelli, E. Rocca, U. Testa et al. Adoptive immunotherapy with high-dose Interleukin-2: Kinetics of circulating progenitors correlate with Interleukin-6, granulocyte colony-stimulating factor level. Blood, 77, 741–749 (1991).

9. H. E. Heslop, A. S. Duncombe, J. E. Reittie *et al.* Interleukin-2 infusion induces haemopoietic growth factors and modifies marrow regeneration after chemotherapy or autologous marrow transplantation. *Br. J. Haematol.*, **77**, 237–244 (1991).

10. S. Hashino, M. Imamura, M. Han *et al.* The effects of Interleukin-2 on immunological and hematological systems of syngeneic bone marrow transplantation in mice. In: *Myelodysplastic Syndrome and Cytokines*, T. Miyaraki *et al.* (Eds), pp. 195–198, Elsevier, Amsterdam (1991).

Therapeutic Plasmapheresis (XII), pp. 389-391
T. Agishi *et al.* (Eds)
© VSP 1993

Removal of Immunoglobulins by Exchange Blood Transfusion Utilizing PHP Solution

H. LIU, T. AGISHI, T. KAWAI, Y. NAKAGAWA, T. TAKAHASHI, Y. HAYASAKA, K. TAKAHASHI, S. TERAOKA, M. NOZAWA and K. OTA

The 3rd Department of Surgery, Tokyo Women's Medical College, Tokyo and Department of Surgery, Meikai University, Japan

Key words: exchange blood transfusion; PHP solution; rat.

INTRODUCTION

Polyethylene glycol conjugate of pyridoxalated human hemoglobin solution (PHP), which has been developed as a blood substitute, is an oxygen carrier that does not contain any solid component and its molecular size is much smaller than that of erythrocytes. Improvements in peripheral circulation and disturbed organs have been reported in past case treated with PHP solution [1–4]. In the present study, we performed total blood exchange transfusion in rat using PHP solution as the replacement solution, and monitored changes in IgG, IgA and IgM to assess the possibility of removing immunologic substances.

MATERIALS AND METHODS

Lewis rats ($n = 8$) weighing 250–350 g were used. Under ether anesthesia, the left external jugular vein and left external femoral artery of the animal were exposed to insert indwelling 24 gauge catheters. At room temperature, blood was removed from the left external femoral artery at the rate of 15–20 ml/h using a blood pump; with the same speed, the PHP solution was injected from the external jugular vein (Figs 1 and 2).

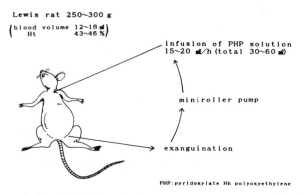

Figure 1. Exchange transfusion with PHP solution for the purpose of removal of immunoglobulins.

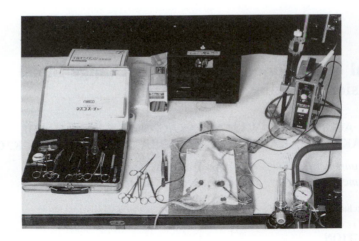

Figure 2.

During the procedure, hematocrit (Ht) was monitored at frequent intervals, the blood exchange was continued until the condition of Ht dropped to 4–5%. Postoperatively, general symptoms, changes in body weight, and level of serum IgG, IgA and IgM concentrations were monitored at specific intervals to evaluate possible effects of total blood exchange on the immunologic system.

RESULTS AND DISCUSSION

After the total blood exchange procedure, body weight decreased temporarily but gradually returned to normal by 3 weeks postoperatively. Blood IgG, IgA and IgM concentrations decreased to less than 10% of the baseline levels, but these returned to normal concurrently with the recovery of body weight (Figs 3 and 4).

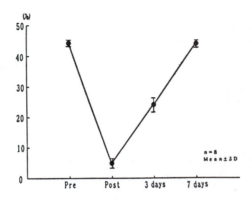

Figure 3. Reduction and recovery in Ht after exchange transfusion with PHP solution.

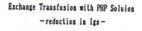

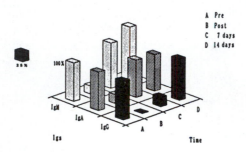

Figure 4. Reduction in Igs after exchange transfusion with PHP solution.

The results suggested that total blood exchange transfusion with PHP solution may be useful in preoperative removal of xenograft antibodies in xenotransplantation.

REFERENCES

1. K. Iwasaki and Y. Iwashita. Preparation and evaluation of hemoglobin polyethylene glycol conjugate (Pyridoxalated polyethylene glycol hemoglobin) as an oxygen-carrying resuscitation fluid. *Artif. Organs*, **10**, 414 (1986).

2. M. Matsushita, A. Yabuki, M. Nasu, T. Horiuchi, J.-F. Chen, J. Goldcamp, S. Murabayashi, H. Harasaki, P. S. Malchesky, Y. Iwashita and Y. Nose. Oxygen transport by a pyridoxalated-hemoglobin polyoxyethylene conjugate. *Trans. Am. Soc. Artif. Intern. Organs*, **33**, 352 (1987).

3. M. Matsushita, A. Yabuki, P. S. Malchesky, H. Harasaki and Y. Nose. *In vivo* evaluation of a pyridoxylated-hemoglobin-polyoxyethylene conjugate. *Biomat. Art. Cells Art. Organs*, **16**, 247 (1988).

4. H. Liu, T. Agishi, T. Kawai *et al.* Removal of immunoglobulins by exchange blood transfusion utilizing PHP solution. *Jpn. J. Artif. Organs*, **21**, 1236–1239 (1992).

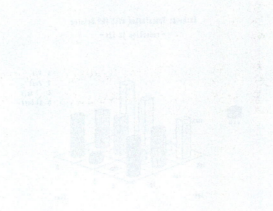

Figure 4. Reduction in IgG after storage based on cold storage.

The results suggested that total blood exchange transfusion with THP solution may be useful in preoperative removal of xenograft antibodies in xenotransplantation.

REFERENCES

1. K. Iwasaki and Y. Iwashita, Preparation and evaluation of hemoglobin-polyethylene glycol conjugate. "Hydroxylated polyethylene glycol hemoglobin (P) as an oxygen carrier for transfusion, *Artif. Organs*, 10, 474 (1986).

2. M. Matsushita, A. Yabuki, M. Piazza, T. Horiuchi, J.P. Chen, J. Golkzateg, S. Hanabusa, H. Isawa, F. S. Malchesky, Y. Iwashita and Y. Nose, Oxygen transport by a cytostabilized hemoglobin polyoxyethylene conjugate, *Trans. Am. Soc. Artif. Intern. Organs*, 34, 292 (1987).

3. M. Matsushita, A. Yabuki, P. S. Malchesky, H. Harasaki and Y. Nose, In vivo evaluation of a pyridoxalated-hemoglobin polyoxyethylene conjugate, *Biomat. Art. Cells Art. Organs*, 16, 247 (1988).

4. H. Ohi, T. Aigah, T. Kurai et al, Removal of immunoglobulin by exchange blood transfusion utilizing THP solution, *Japan J. Artif. Organs*, 21, 1236-1239 (1992).

Therapeutic Plasmapheresis (XII), pp. 393-395
T. Agishi *et al.* (Eds)
© VSP 1993

Cytapheresis Cryopreserved Platelets to Support Autologous Bone Marrow Transplantation (ABMT)

C. Th. SMIT SIBINGA, A. WESTERTERP-MAAS, M. WEGGEMANS,
P. C. DAS, P. O. M. MULDER-DIJKSTRA[1] and N. H. MULDER[1]

*Red Cross Blood Bank Groningen-Drenthe and [1]Division of Clinical Oncology,
University Hospital, Groningen, The Netherlands*

Key words: thrombocytapheresis; platelet freezing; bone marrow transplantation; cryopreservation.

INTRODUCTION

The demand for platelet transfusion has increased considerably in almost all countries. This is partly due to the intensive support necessary to combat thrombocytopenia in oncology and leukemia patients and also due to transplantation and complex surgery. This has certainly provided the impetus to freeze platelets for subsequent clinical use.

Platelets are capable of a variety of functions of which hemostatic plug formation is the main concern in platelet transfusion. Following freezing the cryoinjury of the platelets did not seem to be uniform — half of the platelets were ballooned and de-granulated while the other half seemed to be structurally normal [1]. There are other parameters that are affected by freezing: compared to fresh platelets, aggregation activity is reduced, and so are the ATP and ADP contents. On the other hand, the recovered platelets circulate normally *in vivo* with 45% recovery in a healthy autologous situation [2].

MATERIALS AND METHODS

Platelets were autologously collected from patients who would receive ABMT following chemo-radiotherapy. For functional assessment, three tests were chosen arbitrarily (Table 1). The recovery of platelets following freezing and thawing was about 70–80% in DMSO. Under electronmicroscopy (EM) 50% of the platelets are shown to be damaged. However, the functional parameters for frozen platelets show significant changes in all three tests (Table 1).

RESULTS

Using DMSO-cryopreserved platelets, transfusions were given to patients prophylactically. The initial study has compared *in vitro* functional tests in eight consecutive patients who were treated with ABMT following ablative chemotherapy for solid tumours. From each patient a sample was collected before platelets were harvested by an

Table 1.

Platelet functions (%) following cryopreservation in DMSO

	Before freezing			After thawing		
	mean	(SD)	n	mean	(SD)	n
HSR	62.1	(10.9)	30	20.6	(12.3)	20*
Aggregation	81.2	(12.1)	27	59.7	(12.5)	18*
Clot retraction	66.3	(11.6)	26	49.6	(16.1)	18*

*Significant difference ($P < 0.05$).

Table 2.

In vivo results of DMSO frozen platelets (autologous)[a]

	Autologous (cryopreserved) $n = 5$	Allogeneic (fresh) $n = 5$
Platelets transfused	237 ± 89	362 ± 85
($\times 10^9$)	(123–430)	(278–512)
1 h increment	13.6 ± 6.2	39.6 ± 24
($\times 10^9$/l)	(6–25)	(7–73)
1 h corrected increment	11 ± 6.5	19.8 ± 9.5
($\times 10^9$/l)	(2.2–22.1)	(4.1–30.9)
Predicted recovery	46 ± 25	82 ± 40
%	(8–100)	(17.5–131)

[a] Results are expressed as mean ± SD (range).

apheresis machine, which were subsequently frozen according to our standard method. Following thawing the functional activities of ADP, collagen, ristocetin aggregation tests and hypotonic response show that while 80% platelets were recovered, the *in vitro* functional tests reflected 40% loss of activity following freezing and thawing.

However, when they were transfused to patients there was no correlation between the *in vitro* functional tests, the individual platelet transfusion and the *in vivo* recovery. A comparison is also available between frozen and autologous platelets and fresh (single donor) apheresis derived allogeneic donor platelets in six consecutive patients (Table 2). A similar clinical study [3] comparing fresh versus frozen autologous platelets considered to transfuse 2.5 times as many cryopreserved platelets to achieve a similar number of circulating platelets as produced by transfusion of fresh platelets. On the other hand, it ought to be noted that leukemic patients' own platelets collected and frozen during remission, when given to the patient during thrombocytopenic stage, were as good as frozen HLA-matched platelets derived from normal donors [4]. Comparison of DMSO washed with non-washed platelets in 42 transfusions involving 12 patients indicated no significant difference in the percentage recovery or in corrected platelet increment.

DISCUSSION AND CONCLUSION

Expertise is now available for freezing platelets, although it is relatively costly. It can, however, be justified in selected areas:

(i) Autologously in selected patients such as in oncology. Despite poor recovery advantages are: no-immunization, no GvHD and no potential blood borne infection.

(ii) Another potential area perhaps is to stockpile HLA-typed platelet concentrates for patients with refractory thrombocytopenia.

(iii) Access to frozen platelet panels in the laboratory could expedite platelet serological work and cross matching.

In the future further improvements of frozen platelets in their clinical application are to be expected. Amongst the technical advancements one interesting area is to be noted. The circulating platelets may be further fractionated on the basis of their size and volumes represented by different subpopulations. A recent study [5] has shown that when these fractionated platelets are frozen separately, the larger platelets tend to retain better aggregability than that of the pooled platelet concentrate. Currently, machinery and expertise are available to harvest a selection of separated platelets. Such an approach may further improve the fate of cryopreserved platelets in clinical practise.

REFERENCES

1. H. Baythoon, E. G. D. Tuddenham and R. A. Hutton. Morphological and functional disturbances of platelets induced by cryopreservation. *J. Clin. Pathol.*, **35**, 870–874 (1982).

2. I. Djerassi, S. Farber, A. Roy and J. Cavins. Preparation and *in vivo* circulation of human platelets preserved with combined dimethylsulfoxide and dextrose. *Transfusion*, **6**, 572–576 (1966).

3. A. J. Melargno, R. Carciero, H. Fengold, L. Talarico, L. Weintraub and C. R. Valeri. Cryopreservation of human platelets using 6% dimethylsulfoxide and storage at −80 °C. *Vox Sang*, **49**, 245–258 (1985).

4. C. G. Lazaras, E. A. Kanicki-Green, S. E. Warm, M. Aikanta and R. H. Herzig. Therapeutic effectivenes of frozen platelets concentrate for transfusion. *Blood*, **57**, 243–249 (1981).

5. H. C. van Prooijen, J. H. van Heugten, M. I. Riemens and J. W. N. Akkermann. Differences in the susceptibility of platelets to freezing damage in relation to size. *Transfusion*, **29**, 539–543 (1989).

Therapeutic Plasmapheresis (XII), pp. 397-400
T. Agishi *et al.* (Eds)
© VSP 1993

Simplification of Apheresis Purification Step and Freezing of Bone Marrow Cells for Autologous Transplantation

P. C. DAS, S. WENDEL[1] and C. Th. SMIT SIBINGA

Red Cross Blood Bank Groningen-Drenthe, Groningen, The Netherland
[1]*Blood Blank, Hospital Sirio Libanes, Sao Paulo, Brazil*

Key words: bone marrow transplantation; cryopreservation; cytapheresis; autologous bone marrow.

INTRODUCTION

Autologous Bone Marrow Transplantation (ABMT) is a current supportive therapy of many oncological diseases [1]. The complex procedures have been limited to developed countries. It seems that, with slight modifications of the complex protocols, it is possible to start an ABMT program using equipment usually available in regular blood banks.

MATERIALS AND METHODS

The Dutch Group follows a complex protocol (Table 1) for ABMT. However, in Brazil, with limited resources we could modify the technique using a mechanical freezer (−80 °C) and ordinary plastic bags (Fenwal PL-146).

Experimental materials
- Donor derived blood buffy coat (+ plasma and red cells).
- Waste material from processed bone marrow.

Freezing Materials
- LN2 programmed freezer and mechanical freezer (−80 °C).
- Tubes (Nunc), plastic (PVC) blood bags (Fenwal), kapton/teflon bags (Gambro).

Tests
- Cell counts, morphology and viability by trypan blue.
- Bacteriology.

Clinical Materials
- Patients undergoing ABMT.

RESULTS

To simplify the protocol, the sedimentation process was investigated. Figures 1 and 2 show the effect of length of time on sedimentation. Tables 2 and 3 show the effects of several conditions during freezing and thawing. These experiments led to a simple procedure (Table 1).

Table 1.
Complex and simplified procedures

Complex procedure	Simple procedure
Bone marrow	Bone marrow
Cell separation by apheresis	Sedimentation with HES
Sedimentation (RBC) with HES (6%)	Concentration by centrifugation
Concentration by centrifugation	DMSO
Program controlled freezing with LN$_2$	Freezing in mechanical freezer −80 °C (PVC bag)
Storage in kapton/teflon bags (Gambro) or polystyrene tubes (Nunc)	Storage −80 °C

Table 2.
Comparison of freezing conditions and containers on mononuclear cells (MNC)

Condition	After thawing	
	yield (%)	viability (%)
Tubes: direct freezing at −80 °C	86	74
Tubes: snap freezing	127[a]	43
Tubes: LN$_2$ progress freezer	146[a]	90
Tubes: in −80 °C freezer	85	90
Bag: in −80 °C freezer	88	86
Bag: in −80 °C freezer	122[a]	86
Bag: snap frozen	127[a]	35

[a] Difficulties in counting after thawing.

Table 3.
Effect of reducing the plasma volume of buffy coats during freezing (−80 °C) and thawing

Condition	MNC 10^9/l		After thawing	
	before freezing	after thawing	yield (%)	viability (%)
Bags: standard volume	21.0	9.6	46	88
Bags: reduced volume	19.5	18.7	96	90

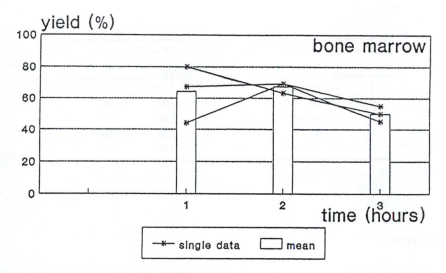

Figure 1. Sedimentation: effect of length of time on cell harvest.

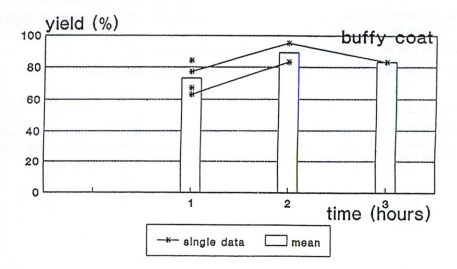

Figure 2. Sedimentation: effect of length of time on cell harvest.

Groningen

A child's (9 year) bone marrow (150 ml) processed by the simplified method yielded 85% of the nucleated cells.

Sao Paulo

Five patients have been transplanted using the modified technique. Four of them showed engraftment within 3 weeks (Table 4). The fifth patient died day 16 due to septicaemia without signs of engraftment.

Table 4.

ABMT on five Brazilian patients

Patient	Sex	Diagnosis	Age	Storage (days)	Infuse	Take (days)
1	M	Ewing	6	45	2.13[a]	12
2	M	HL	31	10	1.27	30
3	M	Melan	42	13	1.01	10
4	F	ALL	7	45	2.54	died[b]
5	F	ALL	12	13	3.80	11

HL, histiocytic lymphoma.
[a] 10^8/kg bw.
[b] no take.

CONCLUSIONS

(i) ABMT is possible in countries with limited resources.

(ii) Ordinary plastic bags can be used instead of kapton/teflon or polystyrene tubes.

(iii) No controlled rate freezer is necessary. The use of a $-80\,^{\circ}$C mechanical freezer seems to be satisfactory.

(iv) BM can be stored for several months in this system.

(v) The simplified method permits handling of children's BM easily.

REFERENCE

1. P. J. Stiff, A. R. Koester, M. K. Weidner, K. Dvorak and R. I. Fisher. Autologous bone marrow transplantation using unfractionated cells cryopreserved in dimethylsulfoxide and hydroxyethyl starch without controlled rate freezing. *Blood*, **70**, 974–978 (1987).

Therapeutic Plasmapheresis (XII), pp. 401-404
T. Agishi *et al.* (Eds)
© VSP 1993

Application of Apheresis to Bone Marrow Transplantation

M. KASAI, T. NAOHARA, N. MASAUJI, M. WATANABE, A. MATSUURA,
J. TANAKA, K. MORII, Y. KIYAMA, M. SAITO, T. HIGA, M. IMAMURA,[1]
K. SAKURADA[1] and T. MIYAZAKI[1]

Department of Internal Medicine, Sapporo Hokuyu Hospital,
Artificial Organ and Transplantation Hospital and
[1]*Third Department of Internal Medicine, Hokkaido University*
School of Medicine, Sapporo, Japan

Key words: bone marrow transplantation; apheresis.

INTRODUCTION

Bone marrow transplantation (BMT) has offered a new therapeutic methodology for hematological malignancies, aplastic anemia, lymphomas, some congenital disorders and some solid tumors.

Apheresis technology has greatly donated to BMT by selecting an adequate method for therapeutic purposes or avoiding the complications in BMT. BMT has some unique aspects in that the patients receive high-dose chemotherapy with or without total body irradiation, resulting in severe bone marrow suppression and bone marrow cells are rescued and graft versus host disease (GVHD) is usually observed in allogeneic BMT.

In these circumstances, cytapheresis can be performed not only for cell component collection from peripheral blood but also for processing bone marrow cells after harvesting. Plasmapheresis could be also performed for hepatic failure including veno-occlusive disease (VOD) of the liver, which is one of the hazardous complications in BMT, and antibody removal including anti-platelet antibody, allo-antibodies and anti-blood group antigen antibodies.

PATIENTS AND METHODS

Allogeneic and autologous BMT patients were entered into the study. Underlying diseases were leukemia, myelodysplastic syndrome, aplastic anemia, lymphoma, germ cell tumor, breast cancer and neuroblastoma. Pretransplant conditioning for hematological malignancies consisted of high dose busulfan (16 mg/kg) and cyclophosphamide (120 mg/kg) [1] or cyclophosphamide plus total body irradiation of 12 Gy. All the patients for allogeneic BMT were prophylactically immunosuppressed with cyclosporine A (CyA) and short-term methotrexate. The regimen for solid tumors differs by the type of tumor.

Cytapheresis was performed to collect the aimed cell component from patients by using CS-3000 (Fenwal, USA) processing 4–8 l of whole blood per cycle. Plasmapheresis

402   *M. Kasai* et al.

including whole plasma exchange, double filtration, cryofiltration and specific adsorption was performed for removing reactive allo-antibodies or specific antibodies and for hepatic failure after BMT by using Plasauto 1000 (Asahi Medical, Japan) processing 4 l of plasma per cycle. For cryofiltration and double filtration, the first plasma separator was AP-05H and the second macromolecule filter was AP-06M (Asahi Medical).

In ABO-incompatible BMT, Biosynsorb column (Kawasumi, Japan) was used to reduce anti-A or -B isoantibodies directed at the ABO antigens.

RESULTS AND DISCUSSION

Applications of apheresis methods to BMT are listed in Table 1. The yields of lymphocytapheresis by one cycle of processing 4 l of peripheral blood by CS-3000 was 8.8×10^9 total cells on average. Lymphocyte depletion by lymphocytapheresis from a BMT patient with GVHD would be an effective treatment in combination with the administration of other immunosuppressants.

Table 1.

Application of apheresis to bone marrow transplantation

Method	Purpose
1. Cytapheresis	
(a) Granulocytapheresis	—— Granulocyte transfusion
(b) Lymphocytapheresis	Lymphocyte transfusion / Immunological control
(c) Platelet pheresis	—— Platelet transfusion
(d) Peripheral blood stem cell (PBSC) collection	—— PBSC transplantation
(e) Bone marrow cell collection	—— Bone marrow cell processing
2. Plasmapheresis	
(a) Whole plasma exchange	Hepatic failure (VOD)
(b) Cryofiltration	Allo-antibody removal
(c) Double filtration	Anti-RBC Ab removal
(d) Immunoadsorption	

Peripheral blood stem cells (PBSC) have recently been used for autologous BMT for leukemia and solid tumors [2]. Peripheral blood cells contain a large number of colony forming unit-granulocyte macrophages (CFU-GM) which can be collected by leukapheresis during the rapid hematological recovery phase after chemotherapy. Although the timing of apheresis and effective mobilization protocols are needed to achieve the good yield of PBSC, our data showed that the CFU-GM number in peripheral blood is about 10–20% of bone marrow cells, detected by colony forming assay in the coincidental comparison of PBSC collection and bone marrow harvest (Fig. 1).

The main purpose of plasmapheresis is antibody removal for successful BMT in order to avoid complications (Table 2). In particular, antiplatelet antibody or anti-HLA antibody is obstacle to the efficacy of platelet transfusion. As the patients undergone BMT have already received many cycles of platelet transfusion before BMT, the platelet

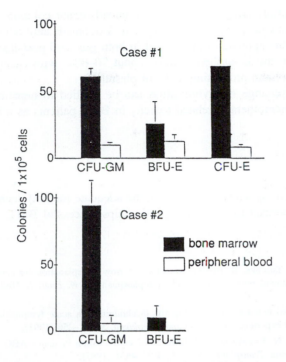

Figure 1. Colony forming ability of bone marrow and peripheral blood.

Table 2.
Purpose of antibody removal

1. Anti-RBC antibody removal in major ABO mismatch BMT
2. Anti-minor blood group antigen antibody removal for avoiding hemolysis
3. Anti-HLA antibody removal
4. Anti-WBC antibody removal
5. Anti-platelet antibody removal

Table 3.
Corrected platelet increment (CPI) before and after cryofiltration

Transfused PC	Before cryofiltration		After cryofiltration	
	1 h	18 h	1 h	18 h
HLA compatible PC	0.60 ± 0.61	0.35 ± 0.64 ($n = 4$)	1.20 ± 0.29	0.83 ± 0.42 ($n = 9$)
random PC	0 ($n = 2$)	0 ($n = 4$)	—	—

CPI = (post-pre) × body surface area × 10^{11}/transfused platelet number.

number in some patients would not increase in spite of HLA compatible platelet transfusion. In such patients, cryofiltration effectively removed allo-antibodies indicating not only the increase of corrected platelet increment (Table 3), but also clinical amerioration of the hemorrhagic tendency. Cryofiltration can also reduce anti-A or -B antibody titer to the half of original titer by processing 4 l of plasma [3].

In ABO incompatible allogeneic BMT, immunoadsorbent columns containing synthetic A or B antigen can specifically remove anti-A or anti-B antibodies and can avoid hemolysis [4]. So this approach can be used in both pre- and post-BMT. The average decline of anti-A or anti-B antibody titer is about 70–80% with each procedure with immunoadsorbent column processing 7–8 l of plasma.

Whole plasma exchange or cryofiltration can be applied to hepatic failure caused by VOD or other chemotherapy related toxicity in BMT patients as a liver supporting therapy.

CONCLUSION

Clinical application of apheresis by selecting the adequate method depending upon the patient's need is beneficial to BMT and greatly helps successful BMT.

REFERENCES

1. G. W. Santos, P. J. Tstschka, R. Brookmeyer *et al.* Marrow transplanation for acute nonlymphocytic leukemia after treatment with busulfan and cyclophosphamide. *N. Engl. J. Med.*, **309**, 1347–1353 (1983).

2. Y. Takaue. Peripheral blood stem cell autografts in children with acute lymphoblastic leukemia and lymphoma: updated experience. *Leukemia and Lymphoma*, **3**, 241–256 (1991).

3. M. Kasai, K. Imai, N. Kobayashi *et al.* Efficacy of cryofiltration in major ABO-incompatible bone marrow transplantation. *Transplant. Proc.*, **19**, 4629–4631 (1987).

4. I. William, W. I. Bensinger, D. A. Baker *et al.* Immunoadsorption for removal of A and B blood-group antibodies. *N. Engl. J. Med.*, **304**, 160–162 (1981).

10
LDL Apheresis

Therapeutic Plasmapheresis (XII), pp. 407-410
T. Agishi *et al.* (Eds)
© VSP 1993

Affinity Chromatography in the Treatment of Lipid Metabolic Disorders

S. POKROVSKY, A. SUSEKOV, I. ADAMOVA,
O. AFANASIEVA and V. KUKHARCHUK

Cardiology Research Center, Moscow 121552, Russia

Key words: apheresis; immunosorbent; low-density lipoprotein; lipoprotein (a); atherosclerosis.

INTRODUCTION

Atherogenic lipoproteins are considered the major risk factor for the development of atherosclerosis and thus cardiovascular diseases. Increased levels of low-density lipoprotein (LDL) in patient plasma are attributed to a genetic deficiency in the specific cell surface LDL receptor protein. These patients suffer from familial hypercholesterolemia (FH) characterized by the development of fatal premature atherosclerosis vascular lesions [1]. For most of homozygous forms of FH and for some heterozygous forms which do not respond to lipid lowering drugs therapy, extracorporeal LDL elimination is an alternative.

The atherogenic role of lipoprotein (a) [Lp(a)] is postulated at present. Its concentration in human plasma is significantly correlated with atherosclerosis plaque formation. Lp(a) has been found in the atheromatous lesions of human aorta and coronary arteries. At present there is practically no diet, drugs and other treatment that can lower increased Lp(a) level [2].

We have developed and used immunosorbents specific for LDL and Lp(a) in extracorporeal procedures for the selective removal of these atherogenic apoB containing particles from human plasma.

MATERIALS AND METHODS

Preparation of immunosorbents

Three types of antibodies were used as ligands for immunosorbent preparation: monospecific sheep polyclonal antibodies (PcAb) to human apoB 100, mouse monoclonal antibodies (McAb) to human apoB 100 and sheep polyclonal antibodies to human Lp(a). Antibodies were covalently linked to Sepharose CL-4B (Pharmacia Fine Chemicals, Sweden) activated by cyanogen bromide. The immunosorbents were tested for specificity and antigen binding capacity by *in vitro* affinity chromatography.

Production of columns

Antibody solution was sterilized before the immobilization procedure. Columns were made in aseptic clean conditions and washed by sterile solutions. After this each column was tested for sterility and pyrogenicity. Two columns of 400 ml (for adult) or 200 ml (for child) volume were assigned for each patient.

Apheresis procedure

The apheresis procedure was performed by continuous flow blood cell separator cen-trifuge (IBM-2997 or Cobe Spectra, USA). The plasma perfusion rate through the col-umn during the procedure was 25–50 ml/min. Anticoagulation was achieved using an infusion of 12 000–20 000 units of heparin solution. The time of one LDL aphere-sis procedure was 2–3.5 h depending on the baseline cholesterol level. Each column worked once per procedure or the first column worked twice and the second once per procedure. The time of the Lp(a) apheresis procedure was 3 h. Each column worked once per procedure.

Patients

A total of 24 patients with homozygous or heterozygous forms of FH were treated by LDL apheresis with Immunoliposorber PcAb or Immunoliposorber McAb since 1984. In all cases diagnosis was confirmed by evaluation of receptor status from fibroblast cultures prior to the initiation of therapy. All patients had a high initial total and LDL cholesterol level resistant to cholesterol lowering diets and hypolipidemic drugs during 3 month therapy. Six patients had xantomas of the tendons or skin. All adult patients had baseline coronary angiography. Stenotic changes were demonstrated in all cases.

Three patients (men) with high Lp(a), normal total cholesterol and normal LDL-chol-esterol levels were treated by Lp(a) apheresis. These patients had coronary vessels disease documented by angiography.

RESULTS

Patients received a total of more than 4000 LDL apheresis procedures with Immunoli-posorber PcAb and Immunoliposorber McAb. The effect of LDL apheresis procedure on plasma total cholesterol (TC) and LDL cholesterol (LDL-C) levels is shown in Table 1.

The volume of plasma treated during each procedure ranged from 1.8 to 4.5 l depend-ing on body weight and the rate of blood flow. Under these conditions TC and LDL-C

Table 1.

Concentration of lipids before and after LDL apheresis with Immunoliposorber PcAb and McAb

Patient no.	Treatment interval (days)	TC (mg/dl) (mean ± SD)		LDL-C (mg/dl) (mean ± SD)	
		before	after	before	after
1	7	528±32	72±9	453±21	33±4
2	7–21	398±15	85±11	324±13	42±6
3	7–10	509±25	216±14	443±17	173±12
4	5	450±19	159±10	398±20	125±9
5	7–14	284±14	123±10	229±15	87±10

Patients 1, 2 and 3 were treated by Immunoliposorber PcAb and patients 4 and 5 by Immunoliposorber McAb. Patients 2 and 4 were treated by 200 ml columns, all others were treated by two columns containing 400 ml of gel.

concentrations reduced dramatically. The high density lipoprotein cholesterol (HDL-C) level remained practically unchanged. No significant decrease in plasma total protein, albumin or electrolyte concentrations were observed. LDL apheresis was generally well tolerated by the patients; side effects were observed in 5% of procedures.

The procedure for the selective removal of Lp(a) with an anti-Lp(a) immunosorbent was applied for the treatment of three patients. The level of Lp(a) during Lp(a) apheresis was lowered by 80%, while other plasma compounds, including LDL, remained practically unchanged. After the treatment a rapid rebound of Lp(a) was observed during the first 3 days. The subsequent daily elevation was rather slow. We now have experience of 18 months of treatment by Lp(a) apheresis.

DISCUSSION

LDL apheresis with immunosorbents is widely and successfully applied at present for the treatment of FH [3, 4]. Our experiments on the synthesis and clinical trials of the immunosorbent with anti-human apoB polyclonal antibodies stimulated further development of high specific sorbents. As a result of intensive *in vitro* testing of monoclonal antibodies to human apoB 100 we succeeded in preparing Immunoliposorber McAb [5]. It has high LDL binding capacity and a longer effective time application.

The results of our clinical trials of Immunoliposorber PcAb and Immunoliposorber McAb can be compared with those of other researchers who applied immunosorbents with polyclonal antibodies [3, 6]. Long-term application of these sorbents (up to 8 years) for the treatment of patients led to amelioration of cardial symptoms, improved myocardial function, complete regression of xanthomas, and prevention of the progression and/or beginning of the regression of stenosis in patients with severe FH.

To test the possibility that patients undergoing long-time treatment by immunosorbents become sensitibilisated we developed immunoassay analysis to show the increase of second human antisheep or antimouse antibody concentrations in patient plasma. The results of analysis of patient plasma collected during 8 years of treatment with Immunoliposorber PcAb show no significant differences between plasma samples.

Since 1991 we have developed a new type of procedure — Lp(a) apheresis. A new sorbent containing polyclonal sheep antibodies against human Lp(a) permits highly specific removal of this atherogenic lipoprotein. At present, Lp(a) apheresis appears to be a unique, effective method for lowering high Lp(a) levels without affecting other plasma lipids and proteins. We hope that Lp(a) apheresis will help us to understand the role of Lp(a) particles in atherosclerotic plaque formation.

CONCLUSION

Affinity chromatography with immunosorbents can be successfully applied in the treatment of different lipid metabolic disorders. Application of immunosorbents, containing polyclonal or monoclonal antibodies against human apoproteins from atherogenic lipoproteins, permits highly specific removal of these lipoproteins. LDL apheresis and Lp(a) apheresis procedures are safe and effective methods for removal of atherogenic lipoproteins from human blood.

REFERENCES

1. J. L. Goldstein and M. S. Brown. Familial hypercholesterolemia. In: *The Metabolic Basis of Inherited Diseases*, J. B. Stanbury, J. B. Wyngaarden, D. S. Fredrickson *et al.* (Eds), p. 622, McGraw-Hill, New York (1983).

2. J. D. Morrisett, J. R. Guyton, J. W. Gaubatz and A. M. Gotto. Lipoprotein (a): structure, metabolism and epidemiology. In: *Plasma Lipoproteins*, A. M. Gotto (Ed.), p. 129, Elsevier, Amsterdam (1987).

3. H. Borberg, A. Gaczkowsky, V. Hombach *et al.* Treatment of familial hypercholesterolemia by means of specific immunoadsorbtion. *J. Clin. Apheresis*, **4**, 59–65 (1988).

4. V. Kukharchuk, G. Konovalov, A. Vedernikov *et al.* Long-term application of three types of sorbents for LDL-apheresis. *Plasma Ther. Transfus. Technol.*, **9**, 45–47 (1988).

5. I. N. Trakht, K. A. Kovaleva, E. V. Janushevskaya *et al.* Investigation of human blood plasma apoB-containing lipoproteins by means of monoclonal antibodies against low density lipoproteins. *Atherosclerosis Rev.*, **17**, 51–66 (1988).

6. S. D. Saal, T. S. Parker, B. R. Gordon *et al.* Removal of low-density lipoproteins in patients by extracorporeal immunoadsorption. *Am. J. Med.*, **80**, 583–588 (1986).

Therapeutic Plasmapheresis (XII), pp. 411-413
T. Agishi *et al.* (Eds)
© VSP 1993

Evaluation of Cholesterol and Lipoprotein (a) Removal by Low Density Lipoprotein Apheresis

S. KOJIMA, M. HARADA–SHIBA, Y. TOYOTA, K. MURAKAMI,
G. KIMURA, M. TSUSHIMA, M. KURAMOCHI, A. YAMAMOTO and T. OMAE

National Cardiovascular Center, Suita, Japan

Key words: low density lipoprotein; lipoprotein (a); plasmapheresis; familial hypercholesterolemia.

INTRODUCTION

Hypercholesterolemia is one of the major risk factors for athelosclerotic cardiovascular disease. Although its pharmacological treatment became convenient due to the development of new antilipidemic drugs, plasmapheresis is indispensable for the treatment of severe hypercholesterolemia, such as homozygous familial hypercholesterolemia (FH). Further, the lowering of serum cholesterol below the normal value is expected to lead to the regression of athelosclerosis which is mainly ascribed to hypercholesterolemia. In order to selectively remove low density lipoprotein (LDL), a column packed with dextran-sulphate (DS) cellulose was devised. LDL apheresis with this column enabled us to decrease serum levels without limitation. It is interesting to know whether the intensive removal of LDL with apheresis using this column causes excessive exclusion of cholesterol as compared with the decrease of the plasma cholesterol reserve. Lipoprotein (a) [Lp(a)], recognized recently as an independent risk factor [1], is also removed with LDL apheresis because it shares apolipoprotein B with LDL that has affinity for DS. The present study is also aimed to investigate the efficacy of LDL apheresis to remove Lp(a).

PATIENTS AND METHODS

Patients consisted of one homozygous and five heterozygous cases of and one case of unknown cause. Four of the patients were men and the remainder were women, all between 16 and 65 years of age. Mean serum cholesterol level of these patients before apheresis was 280 ± 83 mg/dl (mean $\pm$ SD). All these patients were under regular LDL apheresis once a week or every other week. For LDL apheresis, we used a computer-controlled machine equipped with one plasma filter and two DS columns (MA01, Kanegafuchi Chemical Industry, Osaka, Japan). The total treated volume of plasma was 3 000–6 000 ml, and it took 3–4 h for one apheresis session. Hemoglobin, hematocrit and serum concentrations of albumin, total cholesterol, and Lp(a) were measured before and after LDL apheresis. The decrease of intra-vascular reserve for cholesterol and Lp(a) was calculated from serum concentrations and circulating plasma volume before and after apheresis. Blood volume before apheresis was calculated according to the formula of Ogawa *et al.* [2] in Japanese volunteers:

$$BV = 168 \times H^3 + 50 \times W + 444 \text{ (for men)}$$
$$BV = 250 \times H^3 + 63 \times W - 662 \text{ (for women)}$$

where BV is blood volume (ml), H is body height (meter), and W is body weight (kg) before apheresis. Blood volume after apheresis was estimated as follows:

$$BV_a = BV_b \times Hg_b/Hg_a$$

where a is the value after apheresis, b is the value before apheresis and Hg is the hemoglobin concentration. Plasma volume (PV) was determined from blood volume and hematocrit (Ht) using the formula:

$$PV = BV \times (1 - Ht/100)$$

We found good agreement between plasma volume estimated by this method and that directly measured by a dilution technique using indocyanine green dye [3]. The amount of plasma components removed during LDL apheresis was determined by the decrease in plasma reserve. The loss of cholesterol and Lp(a) in the discarded fluid was determined by multiplying these concentrations in the discarded fluid by the discarded volume. Statistical comparison of paired data was undertaken by Student's t-test. The correlation between the two variables was evaluated using Pearson's coefficient of correlation. Values are shown as mean ± SEM.

RESULTS

Serum cholesterol and Lp(a) were decreased by LDL apheresis, respectively, from 280 ± 31 to 103 ± 7 mg/dl and from 23.9 ± 5.9 to 6.6 ± 1.5 mg/dl. The intra-vascular reserve of cholesterol, Lp(a) and albumin decreased, respectively, from 6.65 ± 1.09 to 2.74 ± 0.33 g, from 569 ± 164 to 177 ± 43 mg and from 100.1 ± 7.7 to 94 ± 7.6 g. The decrease in intra-vascular reserve of these plasma components was therefore 3.91 ± 0.77 g, 392 ± 124 mg and 6.09 ± 1.55 g, respectively. On the other hand, the amount of these plasma components removed in the discarded fluid was, respectively, 4.53 ± 0.78 g, 397 ± 124 mg and 7.56 ± 0.80 g. Although the discarded amount of cholesterol was significantly ($P < 0.05$) greater than the decrease in the intra-vascular reserve of cholesterol, there were no significant differences in Lp(a) and albumin between the discarded amount and the decrease in the intra-vascular reserve. There were significant correlations between the discarded amount and the decrease in intra-vascular reserve as for cholesterol ($r = 0.97$, $P < 0.01$) and Lp(a) ($r = 0.97$, $P < 0.01$), indicating that the method for evaluating the balance of these plasma components was appropriate.

DISCUSSION

We evaluated the amount of cholesterol and Lp(a) removed by LDL apheresis and found these plasma components were effectively removed during this treatment. Moreover, the detailed comparison between the decrease in intra-vascular reserve and the removed amount in the discarded fluid disclosed the differences between these two lipids. Although the discarded amount of cholesterol was significantly greater than the decrease in intra-vascular reserve of cholesterol, there were no significant differences between these two values in Lp(a). These findings suggest different metabolism between LDL and Lp(a). The difference between the discarded amount and the decrease in intra-vascular reserve of cholesterol, 0.61 ± 0.22 g, indicates the synthesis of cholesterol and/or extraction of cholesterol from the peripheral tissues. In patients with homozygous FH, Joven *et al.* [4] reported that the production of apolipoprotein B is 13.69 mg/kg/day which corresponds to approximately 1.6 g/day of cholesterol production in patients with 60 kg of body weight. Since the time required for LDL apheresis is about 4 h, the excessive removal of cholesterol over the decrease in intra-vascular cholesterol reserve is about 3.66 g/day. This amount appears to be rather greater as compared with the value of cholesterol production. Since LDL apheresis was done in the morning, this dissociation may be accounted for by the diurnal variation of cholesterol synthesis. Further, the decrease in plasma cholesterol levels during apheresis may activate cholesterol synthesis through the dissolution of a LDL receptor mediated negative feedback mechanism. Finally, the excessive cholesterol removal may be accounted for by cholesterol release from the peripheral tissues. The last assumption will give a rational basis for maintaining of low serum cholesterol by intensive apheresis in order to regress athelosclerosis. In contrast to cholesterol, the decrease in intra-vascular Lp(a) reserve was almost equal to the removed Lp(a) in the discarded fluid. This finding indicates that the metabolism of Lp(a) is retarded as compared with LDL. Although Lp(a) is an independent risk factor of athelosclerosis, the rationality of Lp(a) removal remains unknown.

REFERENCES

1. M. Seed, F. Hoppichler, D. Reaveley *et al.* Relation of serum lipoprotein (a) concentration and apolipoprotein (a) phenotype to coronary heart disease in patients with familial hypercholesterolemia. *N. Engl. J. Med.*, **322**, 1494–1499 (1990).

2. R. Ogawa, T. Fujita and T. Fukuda. Normal value of circulating blood volume in Japanese, Appendix in: *Blood Volume and Extracellular Fluid Volume*, S. N. Albert (Ed.), translated into Japanese by T. Fujta, pp. 252–261, Shinko Koheki Co., Tokyo (1974).

3. B. C. Bradley and J. W. Barr. Determination of blood volume using indocyanine green dye. *Life Sci.*, **7**, 1001–1007 (1968).

4. J. Joven, C. Villabona, E. Vilella *et al.* Abnormalities of lipoprotein metabolism in patients with the nephrotic syndrome. *N. Engl. J. Med.*, **323**, 579–584 (1990).

Therapeutic Plasmapheresis (XII), pp. 415-420
T. Agishi et al. (Eds)
© VSP 1993

Three Years Experience with the Liposorber System in Hypercholesterolemia

R. BAMBAUER, H. E. KELLER and R. SCHIEL

University of Saarland, D-6650 Homburg/Saar, Germany

Key words: liposorber; hypercholesterolemia.

INTRODUCTION

Despite large progress in diagnostics, pharmacokinetics as well as in cardiosurgical possibilities, coronary heart disease still maintains its position at the top of the morbidity and mortality statistics in industrial nations. Cholesterol concentrations exceeding 200 mg/dl involve an increased coronary risk, while the coronary risk of cholesterol values of 200–250 mg/dl is double and even four times as high at 200–300 mg/dl [1]. In addition to familial disposition towards coronary heart disease, risk factors such as smoking, adipositas, diabetes mellitus, stress, reduced high density lipoprotein (HDL), increased LP (a) and fibrinogen concentrations must be mentioned. LP (a) can, in particular, be regarded as a risk factor for coronary heart disease when accompanied by increased low density lipoprotein (a) concentrations [2].

For the most part, severe hypercholesterolemia is caused by a relative or absolute reduction in the liver's capacity to assimilate and/or secrete lipoproteins [3, 4]. Consequently, all therapeutic measures in severe familial dyslipoproteinemia must focus on a drastic reduction of cholesterol. In particular of LDL and LP (a), as well as on a increase in HDL. Since the introduction of HMG-CoA reductase inhibitors, also combined with other drugs, reduction of LDL concentrations by up to 50% of the initial concentration has been achieved; however, this does not always succeed in severe cases [5]. With the introduction of plasmapheresis, specifically the LDL apheresis methods, all forms which were until then therapy-resistant, are now treatable and reductions of LDL can be achieved.

METHODS AND PATIENTS

From early 1989 on, we applied Kaneka's Liposorber system and since 1991 we have been implementing the immunoadsorption system from Baxter. The plasma obtained by a primary separation system is perfused through columns containing cellulose microplates on which dextran sulfate has been immobilized. The dextran sulfate adsorbs from the plasma all cholesterols containing apoplipoprotein-B, such as total cholesterol, LDL, VLDL, triglycerides, Apo B, lipoprotein (a), etc. Adsorption occurs between the Apo B component and dextran sulfate. Immunoadsorption is a reversible binding of antigen–antibodies according to the principle of affinity chromatography. Antibodies against the protein component of human LDL cholesterol (apolipoprotein B-100), obtained from sheep, are equivalently bound to sepharose particles. These are heteroclonal sheep antibodies against apoprotein B. Two columns are necessary as, after the perfusion of 500–800 ml of plasma, their capacity is exhausted and they have to be regenerated. However, in both methods, there is not a 100% selectivity, as fibrinogen is also reduced by approximately 10–20%, probably together with other coagulation factors, such as, for example, Factor VIII. In total 20 patients have been treated with the liposorber system and one female patient with the LDL therasorp immunoadsorption system. Five patients only received treatment for a few sessions. Two of them died. One further patient was lost to follow-up, while one patient improved under therapy and another patient retained high cholesterol values.

Fifteen further patients are still under treatment; ten female and five male patients. The average age is 42 (Table 1). Nineteen patients have a heterozygous and one a homozygous form of hypercholesterolemia. In three patients a severe coronary vascular

Table 1.
Patients with familial hypercholesterolemia (FH) treated with liposorber system from 1989 to 1992

No.	Age (years)	Sex	Diagnosis	LDL apheresis		Course
				n	months	
1	57	f	FH CHD SLE	4	2	improvement
2	58	m	FH Type II b CHD	2	1	?
3	12+	f	FH Type II a	1	1	unchanged
4	51	f	FH, diabetes mellitus, ESRD	2	2	died
5	55	m	FH Type II b ESRD	5	2	died
6	55	m	FH Type II a CHD	35	8	improvement
7	49	m	FH Type II b CHD	24	5	improvement
8	23+	f	FH Type II a CHD	185	36	improvement
9	51	f	FH Type II a CHD (3 ACVB)	104	26	improvement
10	50++	f	FH Type II a CHD (3 ACVB)	96	26	improvement
11	38	m	FH Type II a CHD (3 myoc. infarction)	64	23	improvement
12	59	f	FH Type II b CHD	86	22	improvement
13	57	m	FH Type II b CHD	70	17	improvement
14	56+++	f	FH Type II a CHD	66	17	improvement
15	29+++	f	FH Type II a	60	16	improvement
16	24++	f	FH Type II a	52	13	improvement
17	20	f	FH Type II a (homozygous)	48	11	improvement
18	48	f	FH Type II a	25/24	5/6[a]	improvement
19	53	f	FH Type II b CHD	8	3	improvement
20	38	m	FH Type II b CHD (2 ACVB)	8	3	improvement

CHD: Coronary heart disease, ESRD: end-stage renal failure.

[a] Immuno adsorption with the Therasorb System.

+, ++, +++: mother and daughter.

disease rendered a bypass operation necessary prior to commencement of therapy. The patients were treated for a period ranging from 2 to 36 months. Mostly, we conducted one treatment with an average perfusion volume of 6 l, and subsequently only one treatment per week, respectively, every 2 weeks.

Vascular access was effected via peripheral veins with two needles, the blood flow was between 50 and 120 ml/min, the filtration flux, responsible perfusion flux was between 20 and 50 ml/min. Treatment lasted on average 2.4 h per patient. Anticoagulation was effected using non-fractionated heparin in the case of 17 patients and low molecular heparin in three patients.

RESULTS

The following only relates to the 15 patients who are still under treatment. In these patients, who were treated for between 2 and 36 months, an average reduction of 50% of total cholesterol and LDL was achieved in comparison with pretreatment values. HDL rose by approximately 11% on average in all patients during the treatment period. Triglycerides dropped on average by 42%, whereby it was observed that a greater elimination took place in the patients with greatly increased triglycerides than in the

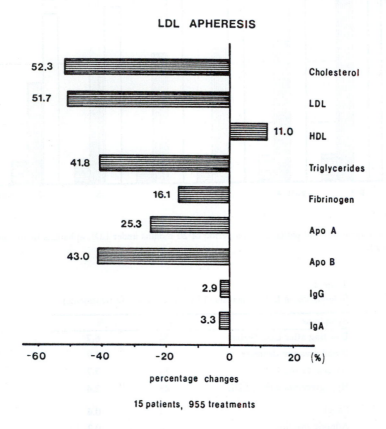

Figure 1. Percentage changes in 15 patients with familial hypercholesterolemia under LDL apheresis ($n = 10 - 100$ treatments/patient).

patients with normal triglycerides. Apoplipoprotein B was reduced by an average of 43%, while apolipoprotein A only dropped by 25%. Fibrinogen was reduced by an average of 16%, while the immunoglobulins only showed a minimal drop of 3%. The remaining parameters, such as hemoglobin, total protein, PTT, etc., hardly changed their status during the period of observation (Fig. 1).

During an observation period of 20 months, the courses of eight patients showed that LDL, in particular, could be reduced to values of approximately 150 mg/dl, while HDL rose minimally (Fig. 2). In the course of treatment an improvement in general well-being and increased performance was experienced by all the patients. Furthermore, a reduction of nitrate medication in the case of most patients with cardiac complaints was observed.

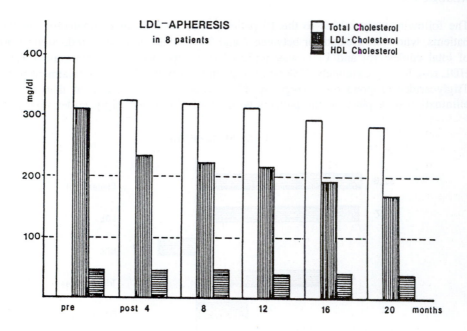

Figure 2. The course of eight patients over a period of 20 months under LDL apheresis treatments (values expressed as x).

Table 2.
Side-effects in LDL apheresis (15 patients, $n = 955$ treatments)

Symptoms	n	%
Bleeding after LDL (veins)	64	6.7
Blood pressure decrease	56	5.9
Nausea during LDL	36	3.7
Hypoglycemia during LDL	23	2.4
Shock	4	0.4
Allergic reaction	2	0.2
Total	185	19.3

Slight side-effects were registered during 185 treatment sessions (19.3%), such as post-treatment bleeding, sickness, drop in blood pressure and hypoglycemia. A positive influence on the bleeding was obtained by reducing the heparin or switching over to low molecular heparin. Serious side-effects, such as, for example, shock symptoms, were observed in four treatments (0.4%) and strong allergic reactions in two LDL aphereses. These side-effects were corrected by immediate discontinuation of treatment and appropriate therapeutic methods (Table 2). Antibodies against dextran sulfate or against sheep LDL antibodies have not been registered up to now, not even in the cases of allergic reactions.

DISCUSSION

Today there is little doubt that severe forms of hypercholesterolemia, in particular given familial disposition, represent a very high coronary risk. Despite a strict diet regimen and the application of cholesterol synthesis blockers, the aim of achieving a sufficient reduction in cholesterol is often not achieved in these patients. In these cases LDL apheresis has proved very effective.

The results, which we were able to collect over a period of 3 years, of 15 patients with familial hypercholesterolemia are very encouraging. Not only the whole cholesterol, but also LDL cholesterol was reduced by over 50%. The other substances containing apoplipoprotein B could also be effectively reduced. Serious side-effects are rare (under 1% during our treatment).

As LDL apheresis is not an emergency indication, all other conservative therapy possibilities must first be exhausted. Furthermore, an exact lipoprotein diagnostic is necessary.

As a result of the still extremely high costs of all these methods, the following indications have been compiled in Germany for LDL apheresis:

(i) Homozygous form of hypercholesterolemia.

(ii) Severe hypercholesterolemia in the case of young patients with coronary heart disease, familial disposition and LDL cholesterol not under 200 mg/dl, despite maximum diet regimen and medication therapy, and cardiovascular deterioration, substantiated cardioangiographically.

(iii) Severe hypercholesterolemia and coronary heart disease with a cardio-angiographically-documented heart disease and LDL cholesterol, not below 135 mg/dl, despite maximum medication therapy.

However, the pre-requisite for all extracorporeal LDL measures is a maximum diet and medication regimen.

REFERENCES

1. R. Ross. Antherosclerosis: a problem of the biology of the arterial wall cells and their interaction with blood components. *Arteriosclerosis*, 1, 291–311 (1981).

2. P. Cremer, D. Nagel, B. Labrot, R. Muche, H. Elster, H. Mann and D. Seidel. Göttinger Risiko-, Inzidenz- und Prävalenzstudie (GRIPS) entwicklung einer diagnostischen strategie zur früherkennung und präventiven behandlung koronargefährdeter. In: *5-Jahres-Ergebnisse einer prospektiven Inzidenzstudie*, Springer, Berlin (1991).

3. V. W. Armstrong, P. Cremer, E. Eberle, A. Manke, F. Schulze, H. Wieland, H. Kreuzer and D. Seidel. The association between serum atherosclerosis. *Atherosclerosis*, 61, 249–257 (1986).

4. M. S. Brown and J. L. Goldstein. A receptor medated pathway for cholesterol homeostasis. *Science*, **232**, 34–37 (1986).

5. J. Thiery, V. Armstrong, T. Bosch, T. Eisenhauer, P. Schuff-Werner, D. Seidel. Maximaltherapie der Hypercholesterinämie bei koronarer Herzerkrankung. *Ther. Umsch.*, **47**, 520–529 (1990).

Therapeutic Plasmapheresis (XII), pp. 421-422
T. Agishi *et al.* (Eds)
© VSP 1993

A Clinical Trial of Low Density Lipoprotein Apheresis on Diabetic Gangrene

H. NAKAHAMA,[1] T. NAKANISHI,[1] O. UYAMA,[1] M. SUGITA,[1]
M. MIYAZAKI,[2] N. IMAI,[2] T. YOKOKAWA,[2] M. OKADA[1] and S. KUBORI[1]

[1]*Fifth Department of Internal Medicine, Hyogo College of Medicine, Nishinomiya, Japan*
[2]*Department of Medicine, Kansai Rosai Hospital, Amagasaki, Japan*

Key words: low density lipoprotein apheresis; diabetic gangrene.

INTRODUCTION

Diabetic gangrene is a serious and debilitating complication of diabetes mellitus which is usually resistant to currently available medications. Recently, low density lipoprotein (LDL) apheresis, which removes serum LDL by repeated extracorporeal adsorption with dextran sulphate cellulose columns, has been reported to be beneficial in improving peripheral circulation in patients with arteriosclerosis obliterans [1].

We studied the efficacy of LDL apheresis on peripheral circulation in two patients with diabetic gangrene of the foot.

PATIENTS AND METHODS

Repeat LDL apheresis was performed in two diabetic patients suffering advanced diabetic gangrene of the foot. The patients (No. 1, 76 year old male; No. 2, 46 year old female) were undergoing hemodialysis therapy for chronic renal failure for 3 months and 6 years, respectively.

The gangrene had resisted conservative treatments. LDL apheresis (Liposorber System, Kaneka Corp., Osaka, Japan) was performed according to routine methods. A total of 3000 ml of plasma, produced over approximately 3 h by a membrane plasma separator, was treated by a single LDL apheresis. LDL apheresis was initiated twice a week for an induction period, then reduced to once a week or every other week. Eight LDL aphereses procedures were performed on each patient.

RESULTS

The average calculated reduction during each treatment was 47.4±3.5% for total cholesterol, 57.3±4.4% for LDL cholesterol and 58.8±4.9% for lipoprotein (a) [Lp(a)]. Blood viscosity was reduced by 6.8–12.2%. No marked changes in hematologic or biochemical data and no serious complications were observed.

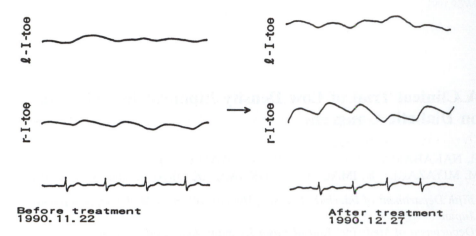

Figure 1. Improvement in amplitude of pulsation in the toes (patient no. 1).

The pulse amplitude on plethysmograms of the toes was increased by 40–50% in patient no. 1. In this patient, thermograms showed a 1.00–1.26 °C increase in the lower extremities temperature. No such favorable changes in plethysmograms or thermograms were observed in patient no. 2.

No clinical signs of improvement in the peripheral circulation were noted in either patients and diabetic gangrene was clinically resistant to LDL apheresis treatment.

DISCUSSION

LDL apheresis mainly removes serum of LDL cholesterol. It has recently been shown to be equally effective in removing Lp(a), which is now considered an important, independent risk factor for such atherosclerotic vascular diseases as ischemic heart disease and stroke. Indeed, a remarkable reduction in lipoprotein (a) by LDL apheresis was observed in our patients.

LDL apheresis was originally developed to prevent the development or recurrence of atherosclerotic cardiovascular diseases. It has recently been recognized to be effective for arteriosclerosis obliterans. The improvement in blood flow to the lower limbs has been attributed to the simultaneous removal of several plasma constituents leading to reduced plasma and total blood viscosity [2].

Our relatively short course (eight procedure) trial of LDL apheresis on diabetic gangrene shows that it is partially effective in improving peripheral circulation. The effect, however, is barely detectable by plethysmograms or thermograms. It is not sufficient for improving either subjective or objective signs of diabetic gangrene.

It remains to be shown whether intensive and long-term LDL apheresis treatment may prove to be beneficial in the treatment of diabetic gangrene.

REFERENCES

1. T. Agishi, Y. Kitano, T. Suzuki *et al.* Improvement of peripheral circulation by low density lipoprotein adsorption. *ASAIO Trans.*, **35**, 349–351 (1989).
2. P. Rubba, A. Iannuzzi, A. Postiglione *et al.* Hemodynamic changes in the peripheral circulation after repeat low density lipoprotein apheresis in familial hypercholesterolemia. *Circulation*, **81**, 610–616 (1990).

Therapeutic Plasmapheresis (XII), pp. 423-424
T. Agishi *et al*. (Eds)
© VSP 1993

Eicosapentanoic Acid Ethyl Ester (EPA-E) Modifies Lipids and Platelet Aggregation in Low Density Lipoproteins Apheresis Patients

H. NAKAHAMA,[1] T. NAKANISHI,[1] O. UYAMA,[1] M. SUGITA,[1]
M. MIYAZAKI,[2] K. INOUE,[2] N. IMAI,[2] T. YOKOKAWA,[2]
M. OKADA[2] and S. KUBORI[1]

[1]*Fifth Department of Internal Medicine, Hyogo College of Medicine,*
 Nishinomiya, Japan
[2]*Department of Medicine, Kansai Rosai Hospital, Amagasaki, Japan*

Key words: EPA-E; LDL apheresis.

INTRODUCTION

Familial hypercholesterolemia (FH) is a hereditary disorder of plasma lipoprotein me-tabolism caused by a defect in the low density lipoprotein (LDL) receptor. The strong predilection for premature development of atherosclerotic cardiovascular disease is often refractory to the conventional lipid-lowering drug regimens. Recently, LDL apheresis, which removes serum of lipoproteins containing apolipoprotein-B (apo-B), has been shown to be extremely effective in the management of these patients [1].

A low incidence of ischemic heart disease among people consuming large quantities of fish has been attributed to increased intake of eicosapentanoic acid, which reduces serum cholesterol, serum triglyceride and platelet aggregation [2]. We assessed the effects of eicosapentanoic acid ethyl ester (EPA-E) on heterozygous FH patients under-going regular LDL apheresis treatment.

PATIENTS AND METHODS

EPA-E 600 mg t.i.d. (EPADEL Capsules 300, Mochida, Japan) was administered to five heterozygous FH patients undergoing LDL apheresis regularly every other week. EPA-E was administered for 20 weeks. No alterations in other lipid-lowering drugs were made during the study period. LDL apheresis was performed using a Liposorber System (Kaneka Corp., Osaka, Japan) according to the routine methods. Between 3000 and 4500 ml of plasma was treated by a single LDL apheresis treatment. The following laboratory parameters were monitored: total cholesterol, triglycerides, phospholipid, β-lipoprotein, HDL-cholesterol, NEFA, LDL-cholesterol, lipoprotein (a), apoproteins A-1, B, E, EPA, arachidonic acid (AA), DHLA, DHA, platelet aggregation (ADP, col-lagen).

RESULTS

A summary of the changes in the major laboratory parameters is shown in Table 1.

After 8 weeks of EPA-E therapy, there was a 119% increase in serum EPA concentration, a 11% reduction in total cholesterol, a 16% reduction in phospholipid, a 10% reduction in LDL cholesterol and a 50% reduction in platelet aggregation to collagen. After 20 weeks of EPA-E therapy, there was a 27% reduction in triglyceride and a 21% reduction in platelet aggregation. No adverse effects were noted.

Table 1.
Changes in major laboratory parameters with EPA-E administration in five FH patients undergoing LDL apheresis

	0 weeks	8 weeks	20 weeks
EPA (μg/ml)	71.7 ± 38.9	157.7 ± 55.9^b	226.5 ± 118.3
EPA/ AA	0.50 ± 0.21	1.17 ± 0.25^b	1.35 ± 0.33^b
T. Chol (mg/dl)	238.0 ± 42.1	212.2 ± 33.6^b	226.0 ± 30.9
TG (mg/dl)	122.2 ± 55.1	100.6 ± 55.2	89.2 ± 46.2
PL (mg/dl)	220.0 ± 43.8	185.0 ± 31.4^a	200.6 ± 23.0
LDL (mgl/dl)	172.5 ± 26.6	155.9 ± 22.3^a	169.8 ± 23.6
Lp(a) (mg/dl)	48.2 ± 19.2	45.6 ± 21.9	44.2 ± 17.0
Platelet aggregation			
collagen 2 μg/ml(%)	61.2 ± 23.2	30.6 ± 14.5^a	35.0 ± 23.2
collagen 5 μg/ml(%)	76.6 ± 14.6	70.4 ± 10.2	60.4 ± 18.3^a

$^a P < 0.05$ vs 0 weeks.
$^b P < 0.01$ vs 0 weeks.

DISCUSSION

It has been reported that the maximal lipid lowering effects was observed after 8 weeks of EPA administration [3]. This period of time is necessary for the incorporation of omega-3 fatty acids into the cell membranes of erythrocytes, platelets, hepatocytes and spleen cells.

According to this observation and considering the relatively mild effect of EPA-E compared with other lipid-lowering drugs and LDL apheresis, we assessed the long-term effects of EPA-E on FH patients undergoing LDL apheresis, which is the most effective method currently available for removing LDL-cholesterol.

The results presented here suggest that adjunct administration of EPA-E produces beneficial effects on lipids and platelet aggregation, and, in turn, reduces cardiovascular mortality in high-risk FH patients undergoing LDL apheresis.

REFERENCES

1. S. Yokoyama, R. Hayashi, M. Satani, *et al.* Selective removal of low density lipoprotein by plasma-pheresis in familial hypercholesterolemia. *Arteriosclerosis*, **5**, 613–622 (1985).
2. J. Dyerberg and H. O. Bang. Haemostatic function and platelet polyunsaturated fatty acids in Eskimos. *Lancet*, **ii**, 433–435 (1979).
3. N. Rolf, W. Tenschert and A. E. Lison. Results of a long-term administration of omega 3-fatty acids in hemodialysis patients with dyslipoproteinaemia. *Nephrol. Dial. Transplant.*, **5**, 797–801 (1990).

Therapeutic Plasmapheresis (XII), pp. 425-427
T. Agishi *et al.* (Eds)
© VSP 1993

Plasmapheresis in the Management of Hyperlipidemia

J. WATANABE, M. HIDA, T. KAKUTA, K. TANAKA, T. IIDA,
S. HIRAGA and T. SATO

*Department of Transplantation 1, Kidney Center, Tokai University Hospital,
Kanagawa, Japan*

Key words: hyperlipidemia; plasmapheresis; double filtration plasmapheresis; LDL-adsorption.

INTRODUCTION

Hypercholesterolemia (HCHO) is invariably accompanied by premature coronary artery disease (CAD) and secondary hyperlipidemia in chronic renal failure is a risk factor for ischemic heart disease or atherosclerosis.

We discuss the use of plasmapheresis (PP) on a patients with HCHO and with hypertriglycemia (HTG).

PATIENTS AND METHODS

We performed PP on six patients. Three patients were male and three were female, the mean age of the patients was 53.8 ± 9.6 years. Three patients had HCHO and two patients had hyperlipidemia due to chronic renal failure (CRF), and the rest were HTG due to CRF. Their complications are shown in Table 1. Two patients had angina pectoris, one patient had myocardial infarction, one patient had both myocardial infarction and angina pectoris. One patient had achiles tendon xanthoma and one patient had paroxysmal atrial tachycardia (Table 1).

Table 1.
Patient profiles

Case no.	Age	Sex	Original desease	Complications
1	52	M	familial hypercholesterolemia	angina pectoris, fatty liver
2	55	F	familial hypercholesterolemia	achilles tendon xanthoma
3	38	M	familial hypercholesterolemia	angina pectoris
4	62	F	hyperlipidemia due to CRF	myocardial infarction
5	48	M	hyperlipidemia due to CRF	myocardial infarction, angina pectoris
6	68	F	hypertriglycemia due to CRF	paroxysmal atrial tachycardia

For treatment of hyperlipidemia, we performed various types of PP. They included double filtration plasmapheresis (DFPP) using EVAL (a copolymer of ethylene and vinyl alcohol)-3A, 4A, 5A and LDL-adsorption using Liposorber. Plasma separators made from cellulose acetate or polyvinyl alcohol or polysulfon were used for continuous separation of the plasma of the patients using two-channel blood and plasma pumps with a Kuraray KM-8500 pressure monitoring system. The blood flow rate was 80–100 ml/min and the plasma flow rate was 20–30 ml/min. Between 2.5 and 3 l of the patient's plasma was treated at each plasmapheresis (Table 2).

Table 2.
Removal rates (%)

	LDL-adsorption	DFPP 3A	DFPP 4A	DFPP 5A
Total cholesterol	52.0 ± 4.6	50.0	61.9 ± 7.9	64.1 ± 9.3
Triglyceride	70.9 ± 11.2	14.9	66.5 ± 15.1	70.5 ± 7.2
β-lipoprotein	62.2 ± 0.9	43.1	57.3 ± 8.6	74.2 ± 5.7
HDL-cholesterol	9.3	18.5	45.3 ± 15.1	24.5 ± 5.5
LDL-cholesterol	58.1	48.7	72.6 ± 2.8	69.9 ± 7.1
Total protein	18.2 ± 2.3	4.2	18.9 ± 8.0	15.9 ± 4.0

RESULTS

Differences of removal rates among each PP are shown in Table 2. As for removal of total cholesterol, β-lipoprotein and LDL-cholesterol, there were no significant difference between each of the methods. However, as for removal of triglycerides, DFPP using EVAL-3A was worse than other methods. On the other hand, as for recovery of HDL-cholesterol, LDL-adsorption was superior to other methods (Table 2). Table 3 shows effects of PP. Reduction of anginal attack was recognized in three patients and suppression of progressive renal failure was recognized in one patient. However, in two patients there were no symptomatical changes. During PP, no significant side-effects were experienced.

Table 3.
Effects of plasmapheresis

Case no.	Age	Sex	Prognosis	Side-effect
1	52	M	reduction of anginal attack	none
2	55	F	no change	none
3	38	M	reduction of anginal attack	none
4	62	F	no change	none
5	48	M	reduction of anginal attack	none
6	68	F	suppression of progressive renal failure	none

DISCUSSION

EVAL-filter, types 3A, 4A and 5A are generally used as a second filter in double filtration system to remove macromolecular substances from the patient's plasma filtrate. Our PP methods using EVAL membranes are most useful for removal of total cholesterol and other substances. However, these methods require albumin as replacement fluid. There need be no replacement fluid in LDL-adsorption. The Liposorber shows better removal of total cholesterol, triglycerides and other substances, and shows better recovery of HDL-cholesterol than DFPP using EVAL membranes.

CONCLUSION

  (i) Four types of hemopurification were performed on patients with hyperlipidemia.
 (ii) The removal rates of total cholesterol, triglycerides and LDL-cholesterol were almost satisfactory.
(iii) LDL-adsorption was superior to DFPP with regard to the recovery rate of HDL-cholesterol and did not require replacement fluid.
 (iv) In four patients, clinical symptoms were improved.
  (v) During PP in the present series, no significant side-effects were experienced.

REFERENCES

1. J. Watanabe, K. Tanaka *et al.* Changes in LDL-cholesterol by double filtration plasmapheresis using new type of Evaflux as the second filter. *ISAO Press*, **313**, 125–127 (1990).
2. P. S. Malchesky, A. Werynski *et al.* Thermofiltration in hypercholesterolemia treatment: analysis of removal and posttreatment cholesterol recovery. *J. Clin. Apheresis*, **5**, 145–150 (1990).
3. B. A. Kottke, A. A. Pineda *et al.* Hypercholesterolemia and atherosclerosis: present and future therapy including LDL-apheresis. *J. Clin. Apheresis*, **4**, 35–46 (1988).
4. S. D. Saal, T. S. Parker *et al.* Removal of low-density lipoproteins by extracorporeal immunoadosorp-tion. *A. J. Med.*, **80**, 583–589 (1986).

Therapeutic Plasmapheresis (XII), pp. 429-433
T. Agishi *et al*. (Eds)
© VSP 1993

Maximal Treatment of Hypercholesterolemia by HELP LDL Apheresis and HMG-CoA Reductase Inhibitors: Long-term Experience in Coronary Artery Disease Patients

J. THIERY, T. H. BOSCH,[1] T. H. EISENHAUER,[2] P. SCHUFF-WERNER,[2] H. J. GURLAND[1] and D. SEIDEL

Institute of Clinical Chemistry, [1]and Department of Nephrology, Medical Clinic I, University Hospital Grosshadern, Munich, Germany
[2]Center Internal Medicine, University of Göttingen, Germany

Key words: HELP; LDL apheresis; HMG-CoA reductase inhibitors; hypercholesterolemia; coronary artery disease.

INTRODUCTION

Plasma LDL-cholesterol is the leading risk factor for premature atherosclerotic vascular disease and the clinical outcome of patients with preexisting coronary lesions. Clinical trials showed that lowering plasma LDL-cholesterol below 100 mg/dl decreases the rate of myocardial infarction and may induce regression in patients with coronary heart disease.

However, in cases with severe hypercholesterolemia and plasma LDL-cholesterol concentrations exceeding 220 mg/dl, LDL can often not be lowered sufficiently by dietary and drug therapy alone.

METHODS

In the last decade several extracorporeal procedures have been developed eliminating LDL from the plasma mechanically. These procedures are collectively referred to as LDL apheresis, but only one system selectively removes the atherogenic lipoproteins LDL and Lp (a) together with plasma fibrinogen, an additional independent risk for coronary artery disease. This apheresis procedure was established in 1982 in collaboration with the B. Braun company (Melsungen, Germany) and is based on the specific precipitation of LDL, Lp (a) and fibrinogen at acid pH in the presence of heparin. Only a limited number of other heparin binding plasma proteins are coprecipitated to various extent. Protective lipoproteins as well as albumin or immunoglobulins are not affected.

This method was designated 'heparin mediated extracorporeal LDL-precipitation' or HELP [1].

The HELP system offers some unique features:

(i) It removes LDL, Lp (a) and fibrinogen with high efficiency.

(ii) It increases HDL on long-term treatment.

(iii) It uses disposable material only and avoids regeneration of any of the used elements.

(iv) It avoids the use of compounds with immunogenic or immunostimulatory activity.

(v) It does not modify or oxidize lipoproteins.

(vi) It does not change plasma concentrations of cell mediators.

(vii) It is a technically safe and well standardized procedure; short- and long-term treatment tolerance are excellent.

RESULTS AND DISCUSSION

Up to now more than 300 patients have been treated in over 100 centers with more than 30 000 single HELP apheresis treatments. Overall treatment tolerance has been very good and no major complications have been observed on long-term apheresis for over 5 years. A typical follow-up kinetic for LDL and Lp (a) under HELP treatment is shown in Fig. 1.

The 33 year old coronary bypass and PTCA-treated patient showed LDL-C levels at baseline above 300 mg/dl and marked Lp (a) elevations above 160 mg/dl. LDL-cholesterol could be lowered by the HMG-CoA reductase inhibitor simvastatin by about

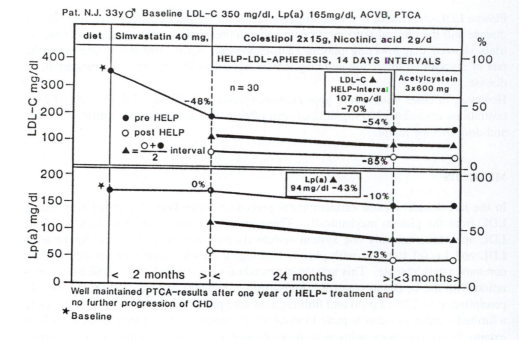

Figure 1. Long-term effects of HELP treatment on LDL and Lp (a). Follow up of LDL and Lp (a) under simvastatin and HELP treatment.

48% to a concentration of 170 mg/dl. No effect on Lp (a) levels was observed. In a combination of maximal drug therapy with regular HELP treatment, we were able to maintain the LDL concentration in the treatment interval at 110 mg/dl. In addition, HELP treatment resulted in a marked decrease of postapheresis Lp (a) concentrations from 160 mg/dl at baseline by more than 70%. The interval Lp (a) levels between two aphereses sessions were maintained around 90 mg/dl, representing a long-term Lp (a) lowering effect of over 40%. An additional treatment with a high dosage of acetylcysteine, which was reported to lower Lp (a), revealed no effect. After 2 years, of treatment, PTCA results were well maintained and no further progression of CAD was observed.

To evaluate the efficiency and safety of the HELP system as well as to demonstrate the effects of this procedure on coronary artery disease (CAD), a clinical multicentre study was initiated in 1988. Fifty one patients with LDL-cholesterol concentrations above 200 mg/dl under diet and drug therapy (without HMG-CoA reductase inhibitors) were treated in 10 centers with weekly HELP LDL apheresis for two years [2]. On long-term treatment preapheresis LDL-cholesterol levels dropped from 287 to 203 mg/dl, representing a 28% decrease, whereas patients with the highest baseline LDL-cholesterol values displayed the greatest percent reduction. The post-apheresis LDL-cholesterol values could be reduced below 80 mg/dl, representing a decrease of more than 60% at each treatment. The mean LDL-cholesterol concentrations between two HELP treatments were maintained around 140 mg/dl, representing a reduction of 50%. In contrast to LDL, mean preapheresis HDL-cholesterol levels rose in the first 12 months by 19%. In addition, plasmafibrinogen was decreased by 46%. First evaluations of the 2 years reangiographs with quantitative determination of stenoses parameters reveal a regression of the CAD 2-fold more than progression in the HELP multicentre study patients; 39% of the patients showed a clear tendency of stenosis regression.

HMG-CoA reductase inhibitors were not available when the HELP multicentre study was started. In the meantime we have investigated and are following the additional efficiency of a combined therapy, using lovastatin, simvastatin or pravastatin together with HELP apheresis in 16 FH patients. They are treated now between 2 and 5 years without any severe adverse effects. The HELP treatment alone reduced the LDL-concentrations by 50% and the combination of the two treatments resulted in a reduction of LDL-cholesterol of up to 70%. HDL-cholesterol rose in each therapeutic regimen, but a significant decrease of Lp (a) and plasma fibrinogen was achieved with the HELP procedure only (Table 1). In all patients angina pectoris, dyspnoe and physical capacity improved remarkably.

A special feature of the HELP treatment is the improvement of rheological factors by eliminating plasma fibrinogen, thus drastically reducing plasma viscosity and erythrocyte aggregation. These rheological findings may be responsible for the impressive improvement of ischemic events in our patients 2–3 months after start of therapy [3]. This unique effect of the HELP procedure is now under further investigation in acute treatment studies of patients suffering from stroke or occlusive peripheral artery disease.

An important therapeutic application of the HELP systems the preventive treatment of patients showing homozygous form of familial hypercholesterolemia. Since 1985 we and our colleagues in Frankfurt are treating an FH patient, born in 1979, with the HELP procedure (Fig. 2). Before start of treatment, LDL-cholesterol concentrations exceeded 800 mg/dl. Under regular HELP apheresis LDL levels in the treatment intervals were

Table 1.

Percentage changes of lipoproteins and plasmafibrinogen by HMG-CoA reductase inhibitors, HELP and combined treatment

HMG-CoA reductase inhibitor		HELP	HELP+HMG-CoA reductase inhibitor
LDL-cholesterol	−38 ± 12	−51 ± 14	−69 ± 12
HDL-cholesterol	+10± 9	+12± 3	+14± 6
Apo B	−30± 9	−46± 2	−53± 8
Apo A1	+13± 4	+9 ± 10	+12± 9
Lp(a)	no change	−45 ± 15	−43± 7
Fibrinogen	no change	−43 ± 12	−44 ± 10

Treatment: 48 months (23–77). Interval values of around 1400 aphereses. n = 16 FH patients.

Pat. Ch.J. ♀, 7y. homozyg. FH Baseline LDL-C 820 mg/dl

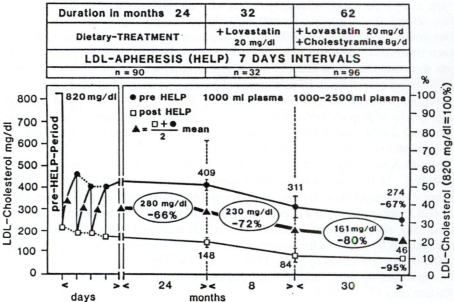

Figure 2. Maximal treatment of follow up of LDL-C in a FH patient under HELP treatment and a combined drug therapy.

maintained at about 280 mg/dl. Under additional drug regimen and by increasing the plasma volume treated the LDL-cholesterol concentrations can now be stabilized at around 160 mg/dl, representing a long-term LDL-lowering effect of 80% [4].

The therapy was excellently tolerated and regression of multiple xanthomata was observed. The girl is well and shows normal growth development. No signs of cardio-vascular symptoms have been noted.

Based on the present experience a German consensus panel has recently recommended guidelines for indication of HELP apheresis and similar extracorporeal procedures [5]. These are as follows:

(i) *Primary prevention of coronary artery disease.* Homozygous form of familial hypercholesterolemia. Severe hypercholesterolemia in young patients (LDL-C under medication >200 mg/dl) with positive family history of CAD and early coronary artery alterations

(ii) *Secondary prevention of coronary artery disease*: Severe CAD and LDL-C under medication >135 mg/dl. Therapeutic goal: LDL-C <110 mg/dl.

REFERENCES

1. V. W. Armstrong, M. Windisch, H. Wieland *et al.* Selective continous extracorporeal elimination of lowdensity lipoproteins with heparin at acid pH. *Trans. Am. Soc. Artif. Intern. Organs,* **29**, 323–327 (1983).

2. D. Seidel, V. W. Armstrong, P. Schuff-Werner for the HELP study group. The HELP–LDL apheresis multicentre study, an angiographically assessed trial on the role of LDL-apheresis in the secondary prevention of coronary heart disease. I. Evaluation of safety and cholesterol-lowering effects during the first 12 months. *Eur. J. Clin. Invest.,* **21**, 375–383 (1992).

3. P. Schuff-Werner, E. Schütz, W. C. Seyde *et al.* Improved haemorheology associated with a reduction in plasma fibrinogen and LDL in patients being treated by heparininduced extracorporeal LDL precipitation (HELP). *Eur. J. Clin. Invest.,* **19**, 30–37 (1989).

4. J. Thiery, A. K. Walli, G. Janning *et al.* Low-density lipoprotein plasmaapheresis with and without lovastatin in the treatment of the homozygous form of familial hypercholesterolemia. *Eur. J. Pediatr.,* **149**, 716–721 (1990).

5. H. Greten, W. Bleifeld, F. U. Beil *et al.* LDL-Apherese: Ein therapeutisches Verfahren bei schwerer Hypercholesterinämie (LDL-apheresis: a therapeutic principle in severe hypercholesterolemia). *Deutsches Ärzteblatt,* **89**, 48–49 (1992).

Therapeutic Plasmapheresis (XII), pp. 435-438
T. Agishi *et al.* (Eds)
© VSP 1993

Simvastatin and LDL Apheresis — A New Treatment of Hypercholesterolemia and Prevention of Coronary Artery Disease After Heart Transplantation

K. WENKE, J. THIERY,[1] N. ARNDTZ, B. MEISER,
D. SEIDEL[1] and B. REICHART

Department of Cardiac Surgery and [1]Institute of Clinical Chemistry,
University Hospital Grosshadern, Munich, Germany

Key words: hypercholesterolemia; heart transplantation; LDL apheresis; coronary artery disease.

INTRODUCTION

Experimental and epidemiological evidence shows that in humans the development of coronary artery disease is very unlikely at plasma LDL-cholesterol concentrations below 110 mg/dl. However, 80% of our heart transplantations show elevated plasma LDL-cholesterol up to pathological concentrations. In long-term follow-up after heart transplantation (HTx), the development of accelerated coronary artery disease remains the major cause of death [1]. The precise pathogenesis of this specific vasculopathy is, however, unknown. Many causative factors may be involved, including elevated serum cholesterol levels after transplantation [2]. In order to minimize the consequences of this postoperative hypercholesterolemia, we initiated a clinical study to prove the beneficial

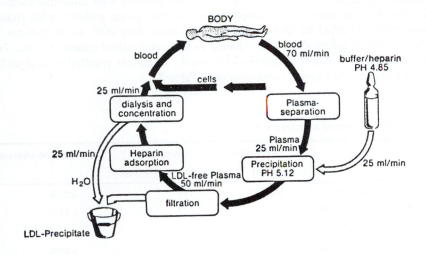

Figure 1. Flow sheet of the HELP procedure.

effects and clinical safety of simvastatin, an inhibitor of cholesterol biosynthesis. For severe hypercholesterolemia we added an extracorporeal LDL elimination procedure, the HELP (heparin mediated extracorporeal LDL-cholesterol precepitation) system (Fig. 1). The overall goal of this trial was to determine whether intensive lipid lowering therapy to less than 110 mg/dl will decrease accelerated coronary disease of the graft within a follow-up time of 4 years.

PATIENTS AND METHODS

After heart-transplantation, patients were randomized either into a treatment group or a control group. Both groups were maintained on a dietary program for the duration of the trial.

Patients in the treatment group received a dose of 5–20 mg of simvastatin once a day. If the LDL-cholesterol exceeded 135 mg/dl on three consecutive visits inspite of simvastatin treatment, additional HELP LDL apheresis was applied. In contrast, the control group received only conventional standard lipid lowering therapy. Until now, 21 patients have been included in the treatment group and 11 patients in the control group. The average age of the patients (30 males and two females) was 45.5 ± 15.5 years. The indication for heart transplantation was either ischemic cardiomyopathy ($n = 13$) or dilatative cardiomyopathy ($n = 19$). All patients received standard triple drug immunosuppression (cyclosporin A, azathioprin, corticosteroids). In each patient, a full clinical chemistry panel as well as measurements of immunological parameters, specific lipids and lipid proteins were obtained regularly. In order to monitor drug therapy and its interaction with cyclosporin A, cyclosporin and simvastatin plasma concentrations were recorded.

RESULTS

Before heart transplantation, patients with diagnosis of ischemic coronary artery disease had significantly higher LDL-cholesterol levels than patients with dilatative cardiomy-opathy. Six months after heart transplantation control group patients with ischemic cardiomyopathy revealed an increase of LDL by more than 20% while patients with dilatative cardiomyopathy showed no change in LDL-cholesterol concentrations. However, in patients with either diagnosis, simvastatin treatment resulted in a significant decrease of plasma cholesterol concentrations (Table 1).

Table 1.
Follow-up of LDL-cholesterol after heart transplantation

		Preoperative (mg/dl)	Postoperative (6 months) (mg/dl)	Δ% LDL-cholesterol
Group A (isch. CMP)	control	145	177	+22%
	simvastatin	170	129	−18%
Group B (dil. CMP)	control	124	121	−2%
	simvastatin	120	87	−28%

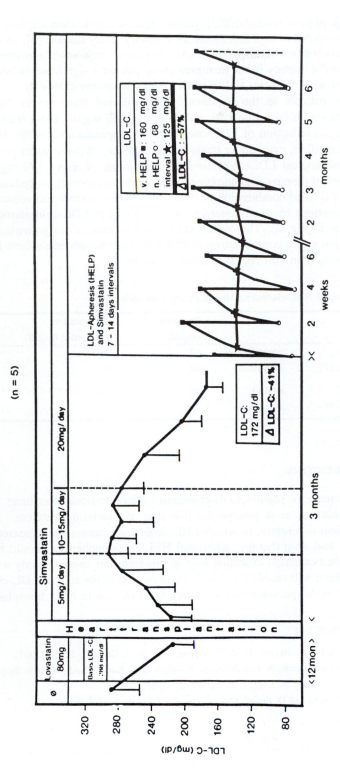

Figure 2. Follow-up of LDL-cholesterol under combined simvastatin and HELP treatment (*n* = 5 patients).

High plasma levels of HDL protect against arteriosclerosis, low HDL plasma levels are considered to be a risk factor for coronary artery disease [3]. In our control patients, HDL-cholesterol levels after heart transplantation were in a normal range. However, simvastatin therapy in the treatment group caused a significant increase of HDL in both, patients with ischemic and dilatative cardiomyopathy (Table 2).

Five patients in the treatment group suffered from severe familial hypercholesterolemia with base line LDL values above 280 mg/dl. Drug treatment resulted in an impressive reduction of LDL-cholesterol by approximately 40%. However, after heart transplantation, even under treatment with 20 mg of simvastatin per day, these patients had pathological LDL-cholesterol concentrations of above 170 mg/dl. In these cases, simvastatin therapy was combined with an extracorporeal procedure to eliminate LDL: HELP [4]. The combination of these two treatment strategies reduced LDL-cholesterol concentrations by approximately 60%, resulting in LDL-cholesterol levels of less than 125 mg/dl (Fig. 2). The overall treatment tolerance of the patients has been extremely good. No major complications or clinically relevant adverse effects have been observed after more than 100 HELP treatment courses.

Table 2.
Follow-up of HDL-cholesterol after heart transplantation

		Preoperative (mg/dl)	Postoperative (6 months) (mg/dl)	Δ% HDL-cholesterol
Group A	control	49	53	+8%
(isch. CMP)	simvastatin	48	61	+27%
Group B	control	56	58	+4%
(dil. CMP)	simvastatin	55	65	+18%

CONCLUSIONS

The increase of plasma LDL-cholesterol concentrations after heart transplantation can be avoided in most patients by low dose simvastatin treatment. In cases of severe hypercholesterolemia, in which LDL-cholesterol cannot be decreased below 135 mg/dl by diet and drug therapy, additional HELP plasmapheresis should be considered. The complete evaluation of annual angiograms from our ongoing study will soon provide results which will enable a rational determination of the role of LDL-cholesterol lowering therapy in the prevention of coronary heart disease in heart transplant patients.

REFERENCES

1. M. Barbir, N. Banner, G. R. Thompson *et al. Int. J. Cardiol.*, **32**, 51 (1991).
2. B. Radovancevic, S. Poludexter, S. Birouljev *et al. Eur. J. Cardiothoracic Surg.*, **4**, 309 (1990).
3. S. M. Grundy. *N. Engl. J. Med.*, **319**, 24 (1988).
4. T. Demant and D. Seidel. *Current Opinion Lipidol.*, **3**, 43 (1992).

Therapeutic Plasmapheresis (XII), pp. 439-441
T. Agishi *et al.* (Eds)
© VSP 1993

Low Density Lipoprotein Apheresis in Atherosclerosis Disease with Hyperlipidemia

S. NAGANUMA, T. AGISHI and K. OTA

Department of Surgery, Kidney Center, Tokyo Women's Medical College, Tokyo, Japan

Key words: low density lipoprotein apheresis; atherosclerosis; hyperlipidemia.

INTRODUCTION

Reports of clinical results of low density lipoprotein (LDL) apheresis have been mostly limited to effects on coronary stenoses and xanthomas. An aim of this paper is to present the effectiveness of LDL apheresis using a sorbent column on clinical improvements of peripheral circulation in atherosclerotic patients with excessively high LDL levels.

MATERIALS AND METHODS

Patients

Indications of LDL apheresis were directed to patients who had (i) clinical signs of poor peripheral circulation such as a cold feeling, decoloration and/or ulcer formation of the extremities or intermittent claudication, which is identified to Fontaine classification grade II or more, (ii) refractoriness to conventional medical and/or surgical treatments, (iii) an excessively high LDL level in spite of drug therapy and (iv) acceptable conditions for extracorporeal circulation and the punctuable peripheral vessels. Table 1 shows the profile of the patients who entered into this clinical trial.

LDL apheresis

LDL apheresis was carried out by adsorption utilizing a Liposorber column (dextran sulfate cellulose beads) installed in a reciprocative double column system (MA-01).

Typically, 4000–4500 ml of plasma, produced by a membrane plasma separator for approximately 3 h in each session, was led into the adsorption system.

The regimen of LDL apheresis was as follows: the apheresis was done twice weekly during the first 2 weeks, intending to normalize a pretreatment LDL level. Once weekly during the next 2 weeks, apheresis was repeated so as to maintain a pretreatment LDL level normal once every other week during 8 weeks; in total 10 times during 3 months in each patient.

Table 1.
Profile of patients treated by LDL apheresis

	Total (28 patients)	Male (22 patients)	Female (6 patients)
Average age (year)	70	71	66
Hyperlipidemia (mg/dl)			
TC	255 ± 43	252 ± 43	265 ± 41
LDLC	158 ± 32	155 ± 32	171 ± 29
Fontaine classification [case (%)]			
I	0	0	0
II	12 (42.9)	8 (36.4)	4 (66.6)
III	11 (39.3)	10 (45.5)	1 (16.7)
IV	5 (17.8)	4 (18.1)	1 (16.7)
Pre-therapy (no.)			
medical	21	17	4
surgical	8	6	2

RESULTS

Clinical symptoms

At 2–3 weeks after initiation of the treatment, improvements in clinical symptoms of the poor peripheral circulation started showing as feelings of warmth or lightness in the lower extremities, walking easier or elongation of the distance until claudication (Table 2).

Laboratory examination

The average reduction rates for 142 treatments, calculated as $[1 - (\text{posttreatment level}/\text{pretreatment level}) \times 100]$ were $64.9 + 18.7\%$ for LDL cholesterol, $47.0 + 20.5\%$ for triglyceride, $50.5 + 11.8\%$ for total cholesterol and $4.3 + 12.5\%$ for high density lipoprotein (HDL), respectively. No marked changes were noticed in hematological data and biochemical analysis.

A pretreatment LDL level became normalized within 2–3 weeks after initiation of the treatment and maintained normal levels during treatment.

Thermogram and plethysmogram

Thermograms showed a 2–4 °C increase in temperature of the lower and upper extremities in 10 of 10 patients. Improvements in plethysmographic findings were observed in 13 of 14 patients (92.9%).

Table 2.
Clinical impact of LDL apheresis in ASO with dyslipidemia

	Total no.	Improve		No change		Worse	
		case no. (%)		case no. (%)		case no. (%)	
Subjective							
coldness	19	17	(89.5)	2	(10.5)	0	
numbness	8	5	(62.5)	2	(37.5)	0	
leg dullness	20	20	(100.0)	0		0	
intermittent claudication	17	14	(82.4)	3	(17.6)	0	
rest pain	18	15	(83.3)	3	(16.7)	0	
Objective							
skin color	8	6	(75.0)	2	(25.0)	0	
pulsation	16	12	(75.0)	4	(25.0)	0	
ulcer/gangrene	5	3	(60.0)	2	(40.0)	0	
Laboratory data							
hypertention	14	7	(50.0)	7	(50.0)	0	
conciousness	10	10	(100.0)	0		0	
plethysmography	6	6	(100.0)	0		0	
thermography	14	13	(92.9)	0		1	(7.1)
AP index	14	11	(78.6)	5	(21.4)	0	

DISCUSSION

We have reported the effectiveness of LDL apheresis on peripheral circulation in arteriosclerosis obliterans (ASO) with hyperlipidemia [1]. Peripheral circulation of ASO patients was clinically improved by LDL apheresis. LDL apheresis could improve the blood viscosity and the deformability of red blood cells, and might reduce atheromatous plaque formation in vessel walls. Subsequent to our own previous successful results of LDL adsorption in the patients with clinical symptoms of poor peripheral circulation, a control study was applied to the same category of patients.

LDL apheresis, i.e. removal of LDL by adsorption, was supposed to be effective in the treatment of peripheral circulation disturbances due to atherosclerotic lesions from both clinical and laboratory points of view.

REFERENCE

1. T. Agishi, Y. Kitano, T. Suzuki and A. Miura. Improvement of peripheral circulation by low density lipoprotein adsorption. *Trans. Am. Soc. Artif. Intern. Organs*, **35**, 349–351 (1989).

Therapeutic Plasmapheresis (XII), pp. 443-445
T. Agishi *et al.* (Eds)
© VSP 1993

Hemorheological Effects of Low Density Lipoprotein Apheresis on Atherosclerosis Disease with Hyperlipidemia

S. NAGANUMA, T. AGISHI and K. OTA

Department of Surgery, Kidney Center, Tokyo Women's Medical College, Tokyo, Japan

Key words: LDL; hemorheology; viscosity; cell deformability.

INTRODUCTION

Low density lipoprotein (LDL) is known to be one of the most important risk factors for the development of coronary and peripheral arteriosclerosis. Although LDL apheresis proved to be effective on regression of arteriosclerosis in a large vessel, the mechanism of improvement of peripheral microcirculation by LDL apheresis has not yet been clarified. The objective of this study was to evaluate the hemorheological effect of LDL apheresis on atherosclerosis disease with hyperlipidemia.

MATERIALS AND METHODS

LDL apheresis

LDL apheresis has been done utilizing two Liposorber columns (Kaneka, Japan) installed in a reciprocative double column system (MA-01). The treated plasma volume was 4000–4500 ml.

The regimen of LDL apheresis was as follows. For an induction period, apheresis was done twice weekly for 2–3 weeks, intending to normalize a pretreatment LDL level. For a maintenance period, apheresis was repeated every other week so as to maintain the pretreatment LDL level.

Patients

Indications of LDL apheresis were directed to patients who had Fontaine II or more degree clinical signs of poor peripheral circulation and an excessively high LDL level in spite of drug therapy. Patients were five males and two females, average 68.7 ± 7.5 year old.

Blood/plasma viscosity

Viscosity was measured using a rotational viscometer (EIECOOL, ECW-6WEN). Measurement was done at 37 °C in a water-bath, and the reading of shear rate at 75 and 150 s was done by a rotary viscometer.

Red blood cell deformability
Red blood cell deformability was estimated by the red blood cell filtration rate using a
5 μm Nuclepore microfilter. The time for 1 ml of red cells passing through the filters
was measured at room temperature. The result was expressed as μl/s as the average of
triplicate measurements.

RESULTS

LDL apheresis by adsorption was effective and safe in removing LDL specifically from
arteriosclerotic and hyperlipidemic patients. The average reduction rate was 64.9% for
LDL-cholesterol, 50.5% for total cholesterol and 4.03% for HDL-cholesterol.
     Figure 1 shows the change of blood and plasma viscosity by LDL apheresis. There
was a significant positive correlation of plasma viscosity and LDL level.
     The deformability of red blood cells was improved significantly by LDL apheresis.
Figure 2 shows the correlation of red blood cell deformability and LDL level, which
has negative correlation. In this study, LDL apheresis reduced plasma viscosity and
probably reflected changes in the rheologic properties of red blood cell deformability.

DISCUSSION

The mechanism of the effect of LDL apheresis on the improvement of peripheral circulation in atherosclerotic patients is thought to be the selective removal of macromolecular

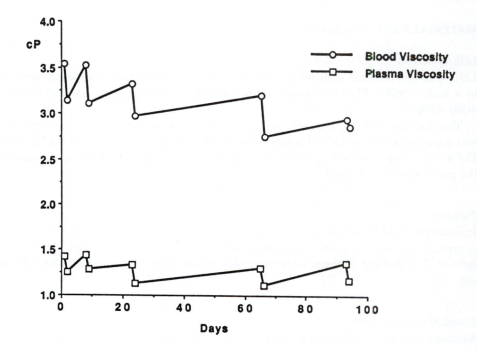

Figure 1. Change of viscosity by LDL apheresis.

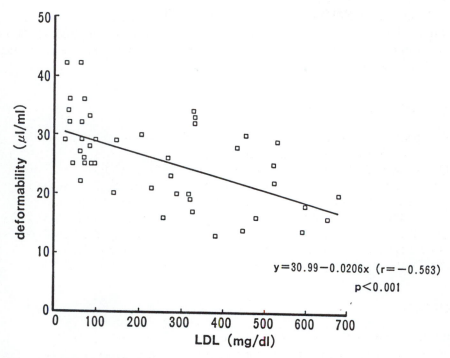

Figure 2. Correlation of red blood cell deformability and LDL level in seven patients.

substances such as LDL, fibrinogen and globulins from blood, thus rapidly producing a desirable decrease in plasma viscosity to improve microcirculation, and, further, to prevent the progression of atherosclerosis in the long-term period.

This course of treatment, which lasted only 3 months, could not produce a regression of atherosclerotic lesions significant enough to improve peripheral circulation. The most likely explanation for the arterial peripheral circulation increase is a reduction of blood viscosity.

After a few apheresis treatments in this study, a significant reduction in blood viscosity was seen in the patients. In addition to blood viscosity, the deformational properties of the red blood cells and the interaction between cells and plasma proteins to form aggregates were improved. In this study, LDL apheresis reduced plasma viscosity and probably reflected changes in the rheologic properties of red blood cell deformability.

REFERENCE

1. P. Rubba, A. Iannuzzi, A. Postiglione *et al.* Hemodynamic changes in the peripheral circulation after repeat low density lipoprotein apheresis in familial hypercholesterolemia. *Circulation*, **81**, 610–616 (1990).

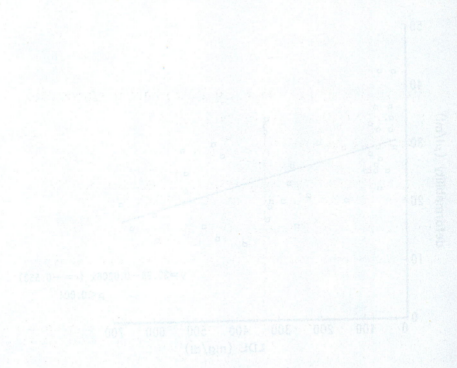

Therapeutic Plasmapheresis (XII), pp. 447-450
T. Agishi *et al.* (Eds)
© VSP 1993

Biocompatibility of Low Density Lipoprotein Apheresis: Contact with Artificial Surfaces Leads to Complement Activation

V. V. KUKHARCHUK, I. F. CHERNIADJEVA, E. T. BOKCHUBAEV,
V. V. SINITZYN, N. I. BACHOV and S. N. POKROVSKY

Cardiology Research Center, Moscow, Russia

Key words: LDL apheresis; anti-apoB immunosorbents; dextran sulfate; heparin sorbent; complement.

INTRODUCTION

In 1981 a therapeutic extracorporeal specific immunoadsorption (SIA) system was introduced for the removal of low density lipoprotein (LDL) from the circulating blood of patients with familial hypercholesterolemia (FH). We reported that coronary stenosis did not progress or regress in FH patients treated with LDL apheresis for 2–5 years and followed with serial coronary angiograms. Columns containing either heparin sepharose or anti-apoB were used.

PATIENTS AND METHODS

Patients with FH (type IIa and IIb) under regular LDL apheresis therapy were studied. Patients were homozygous (3) and heterozygous (15). COBE 2997 or COBE Spectra were used as plasma separators. Heparinized whole blood was separated into fractions as flow circumferentially around the channel. Tubings, single stage channel, sets (input, collection and return) consisted of polyvinyl chloride, acrylonitrile butadiene styrene and nylon.

LDL was removed by passing patient's plasma through columns, contained four types of sorbents: monospecific polyclonal sheep anti-human apoB antibodies (PCAB) and monoclonal mouse anti-human apoB antibodies (MCAB) coupled to Sepharose CL-4B (Moscow, Russia); heparin covalently coupled to Sepharose 4B (Heparin sorbent or HS) (Moscow, Russia) and cellulose beads covalently bound to dextran sulfate (DS) (Kanegafuchi Chemical Industry, Japan) [1].

Samples for testing were drawn at four points: in venous blood of patients before (1) and after (4) the treatment, in plasma separated from the blood cells before (2) and after (3) passage through the column.

The concentration of C3a and/or C3a desarg antigen and C5a and/or C5a desarg antigen was measured according to the method of Chenoweth and Hugli using the radioimmunoassay developed by Amersham. CH50 hemolytic activity measurements were performed in buffer containing calcium and magnesium ions.

RESULTS

The contact between blood and artificial surfaces of the separator and fluid pathway caused anaphylatoxin generation as was measured in points (2) and (1) (Fig. 1). These results are in agreement with the information [2] that activation of complement by polyvinyl chloride may occur during plasma separation when heparin is used as an anticoagulant. The interaction of heparinized blood with the surfaces of the separator caused approximately 30% of CH50 units consumption, assuming initial CH50 units before treatment corresponded to 100% (Fig. 1). So, the pre-column anaphylatoxins level did not remain within the normal range; it was increased, which proves the uninertness of primary separation

Various sorbents had different abilities for adsorption of anaphylatoxins generated by the separator surfaces: PCAB and MCAB did not have this ability. Moreover, contact of patient's plasma with PCAB and MCAB triggers complement activation through the classical or alternative pathways and generation C3a and C5a (Fig. 2). These results are in agreement with data reported by Kadar and Borberg [3].

Columns with PCAB- or MCAB–Sepharose CL-4B decreased CH50 units by 5% the same as column-placebo, containing Sepharose CL-4B (without coupled antibodies). This suggested anti-apoB inertness and also relatively inefficient terminal complement activation compared with C3 convertases and C5 convertase formation.

The level of C3a and/or C3a desarg and C5a and/or C5a desarg in venous blood after SIA is lower than anaphylatoxin levels in post-column plasma (Fig. 3).

Columns with HS have high anticomplementary activity: the anaphylatoxin levels in post-column plasma was very low (Fig. 2) — 22% CH50 consumption by HS suggests complement components adsorption onto the surface of HS.

The anaphylatoxin concentration in post DS-column plasma also decreased suggesting anticomplementary activity of DS and, probably, protein adsorption onto sorbent surface. The latter suggestions are in agreement with 21% CH50 consumption during passing plasma through the DS columns.

DISCUSSION

Anaphylotoxin generation occurs upon interaction between cell-free plasma and sorbent. C3a and C5a in plasma are rapidly transformated into stable desarg derivates. Detection of increased anaphylatoxin levels in venous blood after SIA implies that receptor sites on the neutrophils are saturated. Influence of high C5a desarg concentrations on blood cells of FH patients (after SIA) requires further investigation. Formation of C3 convertases and C5 convertase onto the polymer (but not cell) surface excludes interaction between C3b and C5b with cell receptors.

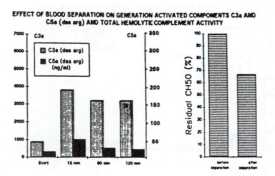

Figure 1.

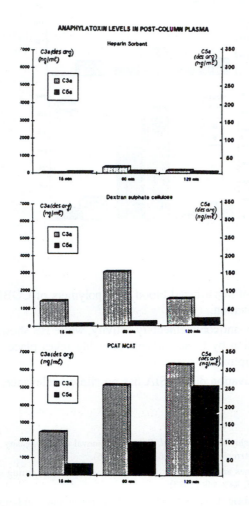

Figure 2.

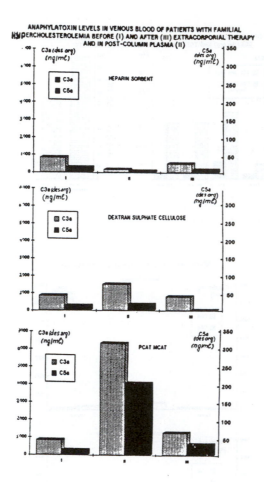

Figure 3.

CONCLUSIONS

(i) The interaction of heparinized blood with polymers of COBE separators causes complement activation.

(ii) HS and DS show anticomplementary activity, while HS shows it more evidently. CH50 consumption by these sorbents probably takes place due to complement component absorption.

(iii) Complement activation during SIA has no clinical relevance.

REFERENCES

1. S. Yokoyama, R. Hayashi, M. Satani *et al.* Selective removal of low density lipoproteins in familial hypercholesterolemia. *Arteriosclerosis*, **5**, 613–622 (1986).

2. B. C. McLeod, A. Viernes and R. J. Sassetti. Complement metabolism during membrane plasma separation. *Artif. Organs.*, **7**, 443–449 (1983).

3. J. G. Kadar and H. Borberg. Biocompatibility of extracorporeal immunoadsorption systems. *Transfus. Sci.*, **11**, 223–239 (1990).

Therapeutic Plasmapheresis (XII), pp. 451-455
T. Agishi *et al.* (Eds)
© VSP 1993

Effects on Coronary Atherosclerosis and Coronary Artery Bypass Grafting of Familial Hypercholesterolemia by Low Density Lipoprotein Apheresis Therapy

N. KOGA, T. SATO, K. WATANABE, S. SHIRAISHI and H. KUSABA

Koga Hospital, Kurume City 830, Japan

Key words: LDL apheresis; coronary atherosclerosis; regression; coronary artery bypass graft.

INTRODUCTION

Low density lipoprotein (LDL) apheresis is now widely used for severe familial hypercholesterolemia (FH) to remove increased LDL-cholesterol and to prevent the emergence and/or progression of coronary heart disease (CHD), which is the major cause of death in FH. In this report we have objectively evaluated the coronary angiogram of 13 patients and investigated the clinical effect of LDL apheresis in combination with lipid lowering drugs on native coronary artery stenosis and the patency of bypass grafts. Also we present the detailed pathological findings of one patient with FH who received long-term LDL apheresis before cardiac death.

MATERIALS AND METHODS

Angiographic regression study

   Patients. Thirteen FH patients consisting of two homozygous FH and 11 heterozygous FH, including six patients who received coronary artery bypass grafting (CABG), were studied. There were eight men and five women. The mean age was 42 years. Most patients had been treated with cholesterol-lowering drugs such as probucol, pravastatin, and cholestyramine in combination with LDL apheresis therapy.

   LDL apheresis. For the LDL apheresis treatment, double filtration plasmapheresis (DFPP) and a Liposorber system (KANEKA Corporation, Japan) were employed. The apheresis was regularly applied either once every 2 weeks, or 4 weeks for 50 months on average.

   Coronary angiography. We performed two angiographic evaluations with a mean interval between them of 42 months. The evaluation of coronary stenosis was determined using a Mypron I (Kontron Instruments) computer system using an edge-detecting method. The standard deviation (SD) of the repeat-measurement variance 3.7% and 3SD of 11.2%.

The pathological regression study of an autopsy case

Case history. A 42 year old male with heterozygous FH had received long-term LDL apheresis treatment before death occurred, presumably from an arrhythmia. His parents were cousins, and both his mother and younger brother suffered from FH. At age 30, he had suffered a myocardial infarction. At age 36 (1982), he was diagnosed with hyperlipoproteinemia Type IIa along with unstable angina and a left ventricular aneurysm. He consequently underwent LDL apheresis treatment at our hospital. At 37 years of age (8 months after the start of LDL apheresis), the patient underwent CABG of five coronary arteries, combined with a left ventricular aneurysmectomy. After CABG was performed, his clinical condition improved but premature ventricular contraction increased in frequency and became multifocal. In 1989 at age 42, he died suddenly, presumably due to ventricular fibrillation.

LDL apheresis. The patient had been treated for 4 years with a double filtration system (DFPP) and subsequently a Liposorber system for 2 years and 7 months.

Histopathological examination. Masson's trichrome resorcin fuchin staining (Gordon's stain) was employed for the histopathological examination of all step sections.

RESULTS

Angiographic regression study

The mean plasma total cholesterol (TC) levels of the patients was 513 mg/dl before the initiation of the treatment. During the period of the treatment with LDL apheresis, this value was reduced to 258 mg/dl of pretreatment and 63 mg/dl of post-treatment. A total of 116 segments in 13 patients were evaluated by computer analysis. Definite regression with a difference of at least 3SD (11.2%) by computer analysis was shown in nine (7.8%) segments. There were 105 (90.5%) of 116 segments was unchanged, and only two segments (1.7%) showed progression (Fig. 1). The mean value of percent stenosis was 28.1% initially and 27.2% finally. The mean change in percent stenosis of 116 segments was −0.90%, indicating regression. Regression occurred in five (38.5%)

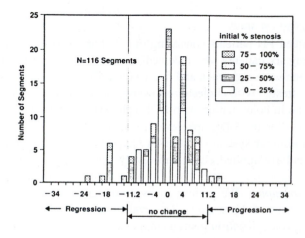

Figure 1. Changes of % stenosis in 13 FH cases by LDL apheresis.

of 13 patients, with no change in seven (53.8%) patients and one (7.6%) patient developed both regression and progression. The patency of the bypass grafts was beneficial, only one of 15 grafts was occluded. A 93% patency rate was obtained and two (13%) of 15 grafts developed new lesions.

Pathological regression study: case report

The clinical course of this patient is shown in Fig. 2. The TC level before the initiation of LDL apheresis was 638 mg/dl. During treatment, the time-averaged values ranged from 411 to 336 mg/dl for the first 4 years, and from 364 to 257 mg/dl for the sequential 2 years and 7 months.

Since specimens of the coronary arteries could be prepared by his sudden death, the serial step sections of all the coronary artery beds were examined histopathologically. In the native coronary arteries, we observed sclerotic lesions, without new and/or typical atheroma in the arterial wall, and only a few typical atherosclerotic lesions. There was a thickened intima and an eccentric thickened wall lesion rich in collagen fiber, suggesting a scarring of atheromatous plaque. Figure 3 shows angiograms of the proximal left circumflex artery (LCX) taken 5 years apart, showing the improvement of percent diameter stenosis from 34 to 20%. In the proximal site of the LCX where angiographic regression was documented, we observed a circumferentially thickened intima and a large eccentric thickened wall lesion with deficit in the media, as shown in Fig. 4. The eccentric thickened wall lesion was also rich in collagen fiber and there was a small necrotic center. A magnified view of Fig. 4 shows an accumulation of foam cells around the small necrotic center in the eccentric thickened wall lesion.

In the proximal site of the right coronary artery vein bypass graft which received PTCA, we observed an atheroma, accumulation of foam cells, intimal disruption and plaque proliferation. Intimal proliferation was observed in most of the vein bypass graft and in some sites, accumulation of foam cells was observed.

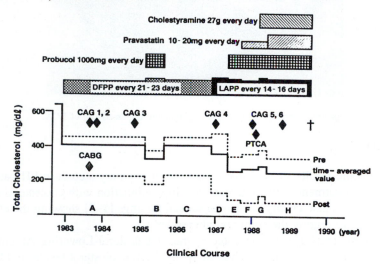

Figure 2. Clinical course and serum total cholesterol levels, time-averaged value of TC was shown by solid line, mean value of TC of the pretreatment by upper dotted line, and that of posttreatment by lower dotted line.

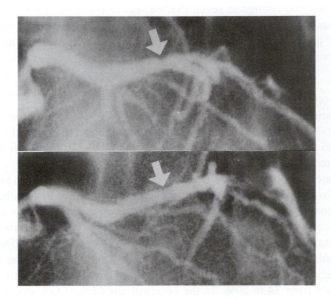

Figure 3. The LCX, which shows the angiographic regression obtained by LDL apheresis.

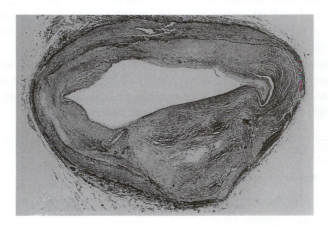

Figure 4. Autopsy specimen corresponding to the angiographic regressed site of LCX.

DISCUSSION

The angiographic results showed that regression of coronary steosis in FH patients can be induced by treatment with LDL apheresis in combination with cholesterol-lowering drugs. The results also clearly confirmed several findings [1–3] showing the efficacy of LDL apheresis to regress the coronary atherosclerosis.

Blankenhorn *et al.* [4] demonstrated in their Cholesterol-Lowering Atherosclerosis Study (CLAS) a reduction in total cholesterol and LDL cholesterol levels could not only prevent progress but even improve, native coronary atherosclerosis and restrain closing of bypass grafts. Our results obtained by LDL apheresis combined with lipid lowering drugs also restrain closing of bypass grafts in severe FH.

The qualitative changes in arterial walls in cases of hypercholesterolemia after such aggressive cholesterol-lowering therapy have remained obscured until now. In order to investigate the histopathological improvement that might occur in the arterial walls as the result of these therapies, we pathologically examined the coronary arteries of one FH patient who had received long-term LDL apheresis therapy combined with cholesterol-lowering drugs before sudden death. The findings revealed the process of scarring of atheromatous plaque, suggesting pathological regression, correlating well with the angiographic regression. We also observed the condensing of the thin and loose fibrous cap and the concomitant disappearance of atheromatous plaque. This further suggested that the formation of an eccentric thickened wall lesion rich in collagen fiber prevents atheromatous plaque from tearing off, which could cause an acute coronary event. It is noteworthy that clinical improvement may be demonstrated not only by angiographic reduction of stenosis but also by histopathological improvement in the stenotic lesions. Hence, even if widening of the stenotic lumen caliber is not present, one can expect a pathological improvement in the atherosclerotic lesion. It is concluded by this angiographic and pathological study that aggressive cholesterol-lowering therapy with LDL apheresis can induce 'true' regression of coronary atherosclerosis and also produce benefit to bypass grafts in FH patients.

REFERENCES

1. V. Hombach, H. Borberg, A. Gadzkowski *et al.* Regression of coronary arterosclerosis in familial hypercholesterolemia IIa by specific LDL plasma immunoadsorption. *Dtsch. Med. Wschr.*, 111, 1709–1715 (1986).

2. G. P. Thompson, M. Barbir, K. Okabayashi *et al.* Plasmapheresis in familial hypercholesterolemia. *Arterosclerosis*, 9, (Suppl. I), I-152–157 (1989).

3. N. Koga and K. Kohchi. LDL-apheresis and improvement in the coronary arterial stenosis of hypercholesterolemia: evaluation by computerized quantitative coronary angiography. *J. Therapy*, 70, 2282–2288 (1988) (in Japanese).

4. D. H. Blankenhorn, S. A. Nessim, R. L. Johnson *et al.* Beneficial effects of combined colestipol–niacin therapy on coronary atherosclerosis and coronary venous bypass grafts. *J. Am. Med. Ass.*, 257, 3233–3240 (1987).

Therapeutic Plasmapheresis (XII), pp. 457-461
T. Agishi *et al.* (Eds)
© VSP 1993

Reduction of Session Duration for Low Density Lipoprotein Apheresis using a New Sulflux (FS-08) Plasma Separator

T. NAGANO, H. IWAMOTO, K. SHIGEMITSU, T. SATO and N. KOGA

Koga Hospital, Kurume City 830, Japan

Key words: familial hypercholesterolemia; LDL apheresis.

INTRODUCTION

Familial hypercholesterolemia (FH) is frequently complicated with coronary heart diseases associated with coronary atherosclerosis, and so it has been highly anticipated to establish the procedure for prevention and treatment of this disorder. In recent years, potent lipid-lowering drugs that reduce low density lipoprotein (LDL), causative substances, and selective LDL apheresis have been developed, thus allowing the prevention and regression of coronary atherosclerosis. It is proclaimed that the lower the cholesterol level, the better for coronary heart disease (CHD). We have performed LDL apheresis by processing a large amount of plasma for FH patients with CHD and reported that LDL apheresis is effective in improving coronary atherosclerotic lesions by aggressively lowering serum LDL cholesterol levels [1, 2].

However, it takes a long time to process a large amount of plasma and so it is anticipated to shorten the time required for this procedure. Recently, we performed LDL apheresis using a plasma separator, Sulflux FS-05 (0.5 m^2) and its larger type, FS-08 (0.8m^2), and made a clinical assessment on the time required for processing 6 l of plasma, reliability of plasmapheresis, and the effectiveness and safety of this treatment.

PATIENTS AND METHODS

Five patients with severe FH (one homozygous patient and four heterozygous patients) as determined by LDL receptor assays were evaluated. Three patients were type IIa and two were type IIb according to WHO classification on hyperlipidemia. Three of them underwent coronary artery bypass grafting (CABG) surgery.

LDL apheresis was performed by a Liposorber LA-15 system comprising a plasma separator Sulflux FS-05 or FS-08 (Nikkiso Co., Japan), a selective LDL adsorption column Liposorber LA-15 (Kaneka Co., Japan) and an apheresis unit MA-01 (Yokogawa Electric Co., Japan).

Heparin at 2000–3000 units was administered initially and 500–1000 units/h were continuously injected.

An inner shunt in one case and femoral veins in four cases were used for withdrawing blood, and anterior brachial veins were used for returning blood in all cases. Blood flow rate (QB) was set to 120–150 ml/min and plasma flow rate (QF) was kept at 40–50 ml/min while transmembrane pressure (TMP) was controlled to below 30 mmHg. Six liters of plasma were processed for every treatment session.

The sieving coefficient (SC) was calculated for each liter of treated plasma by the following equation regarding blood total cholesterol (TC), triglyceride (TG), HDL cholesterol (HDL-C), total protein (TP), albumin (Alb), and immunoglobulin M (IgM).

$$SC = C_f/C_i$$

where C_f: concentration of solutes in separated plasma and C_i: concentration of solutes in blood at inlet of plasma separator.

Reduction rate during a procedure was determined for TC, TG, HDL-C, TP, Alb, and estimated for LDL-C using Friedewald formula.

Vital signs such as pulse rate, blood pressure and body temperature were checked during the treatment, and operating parameters were monitored and recorded every 1 l of plasma processed.

RESULTS

Figure 1 shows QB, QF and TMP for every liter of plasma processed during LDL apheresis. In the treatment using FS-05, TMP increased and QF decreased in seven out of 15 sessions (46.7%) when more than 4 l of plasma were processed. QF decreased down to 37.3 ± 0.6 ml/min when 6 l of plasma were processed. On the other hand, when

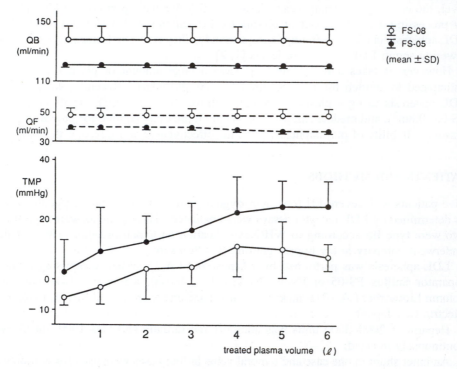

Figure 1. Changes in QB, QF and TMP using the FS-08 compared with those using the FS-05.

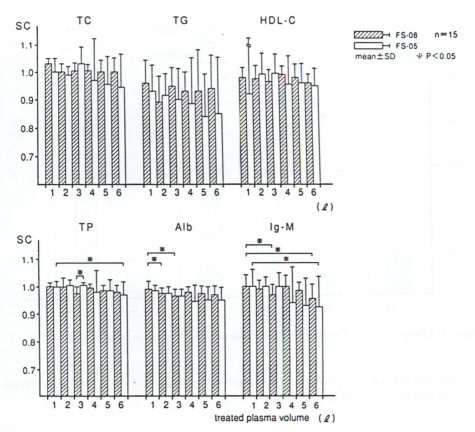

Figure 2. Changes in sieving coefficients for each 1 l of treated plasma volume using the FS-08 compared with those using the FS-05.

FS-08 was used, TMP remained low, with an average pressure of 10.9 ± 10.0 mmHg and QF stayed at a high level of approximately 47 ml/min. Consequently, it took an average of 173 ± 11.3 min for FS-05 and an average of 145.3 ± 13.0 min for FS-08 to process 6 l of plasma. This reduction of time, by approximately 28 min, was found to be statistically significant ($P < 0.001$).

SC for each plasma component is shown in Fig 2. SCs for TP, Alb, TC, HDL-C and IgM remained high, more than 0.95 during the entire procedure. However, SCs for TC, HDL-C and IgM had a tendency to decrease by approximately 0.05 as an increasing amount of plasma processed when FS-05 was used. SC for TG remained higher than 0.93 when FS-08 was used. However, it decreased below 0.90 when more than 4 l of plasma were processed by FS-05.

Regarding reduction rate of each plasma component such as TP, Alb and HDL-C, during each LDL apheresis, no significant differences were observed between FS-05 and FS-08. However, the reduction rate of TC was found to be $71.4 \pm 5.8\%$ with FS-05 and $75.0 \pm 3.3\%$ with FS-08 ($P < 0.05$), and that of LDL-C was $81.7 \pm 3.5\%$ with FS-05 and $85.3 \pm 2.8\%$ with FS-08 ($P < 0.005$). Thus FS-08 showed a significantly higher reduction rate for these parameters compared with FS-05, as shown in Fig. 3.

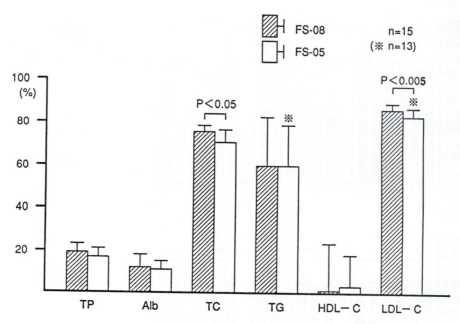

Figure 3. Changes of removal rates of plasma components by LDL apheresis using FS-08 and FS-05.

Only one transient hypotension was observed, probably caused from a vasovagal reaction due to pain at the needle sites.

DISCUSSION

The main purpose of LDL apheresis is clearly to prevent the progression of atherosclerosis and to induce regression of atherosclerosis. So our current goals are to remove a large amount of serum cholesterol to a TC level below 100 mg/dl by treating an average of 6 l of plasma. When using FS-05, two cases with type IIb showed elevated TMP as a function of time, and the QF/QB ratio dropped down to 10% to 33% of the level compared with at the start of the treatment. Consequently, it became necessary to treat patients for a long period of time. When FS-08, i.e. with a larger membrane surface area (0.8m²) was used, TMP was kept below 20 mmHg in all cases including these two cases, and the average treatment time was 145 min, which is about 28 min shorter compared with FS-05 ($P < 0.001$). Moreover, the procedure was tolerated well in all patients including three cases who previously underwent CABG. Clinically, it is extremely useful to shorten the treatment time while keeping the safety of treatment.

We assumed that the reduction rate of TC and LDL-C in a treatment session may decrease because the QF increased from 39.0 (FS-05) to 47.6 ml/min (FS-08) on average, but the reduction rate with FS-08 was found to be significantly higher compared with FS-05. We estimated that this is due to the high level of SC of lipids were kept up to 6 l of treated plasma with FS-08. Our data indicate that LA-15 has the ability to remove a sufficient quantity of TC and LDL-C even if QF is as fast as 40–50 ml/min.

CONCLUSION

We made an assessment on the clinical utility of a new plasma separator, Sulflux FS-08, in LDL apheresis for five FH patients. The results suggested that FS-08 is safe and useful to speed up the LDL apheresis procedure using Liposorber LA-15 selective LDL adsorption columns.

REFERENCES

1. R. Tatami and N. Koga. Regression of coronary artery disease as a result of intensive lipid-lowering therapy in patients with primary hypercholesterolemia. *Igakuno Ayumi*, **157**, 886–889 (1991).
2. N. Koga. Regression of coronary atherosclerosis by LDL-apheresis in patients with heterozygous familial hypercholesterolemia. *Igakuno Ayumi*, **157**, 895–901 (1991).

Therapeutic Plasmapheresis (XII), pp. 463-470
T. Agishi *et al*. (Eds)
© VSP 1993

Plasma Lipoprotein (a) Profile in Patients with Familial Hypercholesterolaemia Treated by Dextran Sulfate Cellulose Low Density Lipoprotein Apheresis and Plasma Exchange

C. STEFANUTTI, A. VIVENZIO, S. DI GIACOMO, C. COLOMBO,
C. ALESSANDRI and G. RICCI

*Instituto di Terapia Medica Sistematica, Haemoapheresis Unit,
University of Rome 'La Sapienza', Rome, Italy*

Key words: familial hypercholesterolaemia; LP(a); LDL apheresis; plasma exchange.

INTRODUCTION

Lipoprotein (a) [Lp(a)] was first described in 1963 by Berg [1]. However, only two decades later Morrisett *et al*. firmly suggested that high plasma Lp(a) concentration was associated with an high incidence of coronary heart disease [2]. Lp(a) is a glycoprotein containing Apo B100 and Apo(a). Lp(a) shows some properties which are common to those of other Apo B100-containing lipoproteins, namely low density lipoproteins (LDL). In particular, Lp(a) seems to be at least as atherogenic as LDL, but not necessarily correlated in terms of coronary risk prediction. There are evidences suggesting that plasma Lp(a) is an independent predictor of coronary heart disease risk, even in the presence of relatively low plasma LDL-cholesterol level [3]. Furthermore, it was

Table 1.

Hypolipidemic agent	Effect on plasma Lp(a) concentration	References
HMG-CoA reductase inhibitors	unchanged or ↑	Kostner, G. M., *et al*., *Circulation* (1989).
		Berg, K., *et al*., *Lancet* (1989).
		Thiery, J., *et al*., *Klin. Wochenschr.* (1988).
Plasmapheresis		
plasma exchange (conventional)		Schench, I., *et al*., *Klin. Wochenschr.* (1988).
HELP (LDL apheresis) (selective)		Amstrong, V. W., *et al*., *Eur. J. Clin. Inv.* (1989).
DSC (LDL apheresis) (selective)		Jones, P. H., *et al*., *Contr. Inf. Ther.* (1988).
Immuno (LDL apheresis) (selective)		Borberg, H., *et al*., *J. Clin. Apheresis* (1988).

Table 2.

Minimal plasma Lp(a) concentration which can be assessed in the laboratory by using different methods

Method	Lp(a) (mg/dl)
EID	5
RID	> 5
Nephelometry (IA)	5
ELISA	> 1
RIA	1
Most probable level of atherogenicity	> 30

also demonstrated that Lp(a) shares a close structural homology with plasminogen, and is similarly involved in the fibrinolytic system. Moreover, either plasma Lp(a) and plasminogen levels are genetically controlled by gene loci located on chromosome 6. This evidence was regarded as supporting the hypothesis that Lp(a) may play a role as a bridge between lipid metabolism and the haemocoagulatory system [3]. In 1986, Dahlen first reported evidence concerning the association between plasma Lp(a) level and the extent of coronary artery disease assessed angiographically [4]. Two years later, Hoff confirmed that plasma Lp(a) was related to restenosis in patients submitted to coronary

Table 3.

FH patients treated with plasmapheresis: LDL apheresis (LDL-A) and plasma exchange (PE)

	Patients	M/F	Age (years)	Lipoprotein phenotype	CHD	LDL-A (no.)	PE (no.)	Treatment (months)
Hoz	MD	M	6	IIa	−	28	29	28
	SM	M	34	IIa	+	107	63	57
Htz	□DNA	M	46	IIa	+	38	35	36
	□FG	M	42	IIa	+	28		14
	□PF	M	52	IIa	+	16		8
	□FA	F	48	IIa	−	32		16
	□LE	F	68	IIa	+	16		8
	□PN	M	45	IIa	+	0	32	16
	▲MJ	F	49	IIa	−	8		4
	▲AD	M	31	IIa	−	7		3.5
	▲CA	F	29	IIa	−	8		4
	▲SV	M	32	IIa	−	1		−
	▲CB	M	55	IIa	+	7	1	4
	▲CF	F	51	IIa	−	8		4

CHD, coronary heart disease;
Hoz, homozygous;
HTZ, Heterozygous;
□, non-responder;
▲, poor responder.

Table 4.

LDL apheresis. Lp(a), low levels: comparison between methods:[a] RID versus ELISA

	RID		ELISA (Immuno)	
	$\bar{x}$	SD	$\bar{x}$	SD
Pre	14.75	1.5	28.75	14.76[ns]
Post	9.0	1.41	11.75	7.93

[a] mg/dl; [ns] not significant.

Table 5.

LDL apheresis. Lp(a), high levels: comparison between methods:[a] RID versus ELISA

	RID		ELISA (Immuno)	
	$\bar{x}$	SD	$\bar{x}$	SD
Pre	36.75	13.37	35.75	6.07[ns]
Post	9.75	3.2	10.02	3.55

[a] mg/dl; [ns] not significant.

artery bypass surgery [5]. A number of drugs have been used in the attempt to reduce plasma Lp(a) levels. At present it is clear that only nicotinic acid, neomycin, stanozolol and some clofibric acid derivatives can influence plasma Lp(a) concentrations (Table 1) [6–8]. Thus, the possible use of several apheretical techniques for lowering Lp(a) in plasma was suggested (Table 1) [9–12]. We focused on this last possibility, and we carried out a study devoted to Lp(a) evaluation methodology and to the effect of dextran sulfate cellulose column LDL apheresis and conventional plasma exchange on plasma Lp(a) in patients with familial hypercholesterolaemia (FH) (Table 2).

MATERIAL AND METHODS

Eighteen patients with FH (two homozygous and 16 heterozygous) were submitted to therapeutic plasmapheresis (LDL apheresis and plasma exchange) since 1987 (Table 3). The patients were treated using two continuous flow cell separators:

(i) An automatic self-regenerating system (MA-01) using an hollow fiber plasma separator (Suflux FS-05) and two dextran sulfate cellulose columns (LA-15) (Kanegafuchi, Osaka, Japan) for selective apheresis (LDL apheresis).

(ii) A conventional centrifugal plasma exchanger unit (Dideco 'Vivacell' BT 798/A, Mirandola, Italy) with 20% albumin in saline (NaCl 0.9%) as replacement fluid solution for conventional plasmapheresis.

We determined plasma Lp(a) with two different laboratory methods (RID and ELISA), during three consecutive sessions, before/after plasmapheresis, and after 24 h and 7 days (Table 2).

Table 6.

Lp(a): LDL apheresis:[a] concentration variability in FH

	LDL apheresis			Plasma exchange		
	$\bar{x}$	SD	Δ%	$\bar{x}$	SD	Δ%
High levels						
pre	59.18	9.28		41.88	12.75	
post	24.9**	8.32	58	17.11**	7.60	59
Low levels						
pre	10.92	2.57		10.44	3.58	
post	5.57*	1.78	49	5.63*	1.83	46

[a] mg/dl; *$P < 0.01$; **$P < 0.001$.

Table 7.

Lp(a) time trend: LDL apheresis:[a] Htz and Hoz FH patients

	$\bar{x}$	(SD)	Δ%
Pre	48.5	23.38	
Post	23.25*	11.14	−52
24 h	30.0[ns]	14.16	−38 (+29)

[a] mg/dl; *$P < 0.001$; [ns] not significant.

Table 8.

Lp(a) time trend: plasma exchange:[a] Htz and Hoz FH patients

	$\bar{x}$	(SD)	Δ%
Pre	41.33	5.10	
Post	17.00**	3.60	−58
7 days	32.33*	4.16	−21 (+88)

[a] mg/dl; *$P < 0.05$; **$P < 0.001$.

RESULTS AND DISCUSSION

Plasma Lp(a) levels determined by two different laboratory methods showed a pronounced variability in patients affected by heterozygous FH, with the same clinical involvement of coronary arteries by atherosclerotic disease (Tables 4–5). Theoretically, the possible existence of Lp(a) isoforms, not assessed by the methods which have been used, might explain such a variability, at least in selected individuals belonging to this group. Nevertheless, two patients with homozygous FH, showed both high plasma levels of LDL and Lp(a), as reported elsewhere. Further comments on these figures, obtained

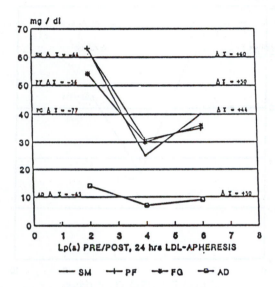

Figure 1. Lp(a) time trend (LDL apheresis).

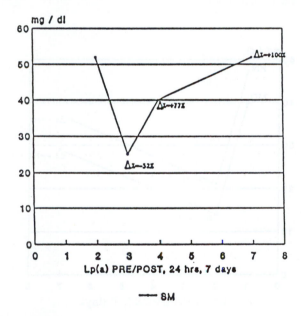

Figure 2. Lp(a) time trend (LDL apheresis).

in a cross-sectional frame, cannot be appropriate, since the evaluation has been done in a relatively small group. Both techniques, i.e. LDL apheresis and plasma exchange, with different mechanisms, can reduce plasma Lp(a), with high efficacy (Table 6). The reduction of Lp(a) obtained with apheretical techniques is obviously time-seized (Tables 7 and 8; Figs 1–4). This evidence should not necessarily be regarded as being a

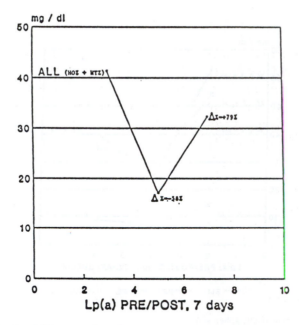

Figure 3. Lp(a) time trend (plasma exchange).

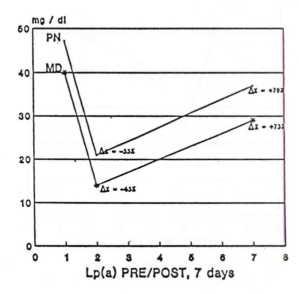

Figure 4. Lp(a) time trend (plasma exchange).

contraindication. The concept underlying the significance of using LDL apheresis in the treatment of monogenic inherited hyperlipoproteinemias is clearly that of a long-term and frequently performed lipoprotein lowering therapy.

CONCLUSION

Whether a contemporary decrease of all plasma apoprotein B100-containing particles, including those containing Apo (a), may be clinically favorable in terms of prevention of coronary heart disease, is still a matter of debate and should be further investigated. It is clear that, with few particular exceptions (nicotinic acid, neomycin, stanozolol, clofibric acid derivatives), only therapeutical plasmapheresis can easily and safely lower plasma Lp(a) concentration (Lp(a) apheresis).

Acknowledgments

This work was partially supported by a grant (no. 92.0000.4.41) of the Italian National Research Council, CNR–PF 'FATMA'.

REFERENCES

1. K. Berg. A new serum type system in man — the LP-system. *Acta Pathol. Microbiol. Scand.*, **59**, 369–375 (1963).

2. J. D. Morrisett *et al.* Lipoprotein (a): structure, metabolism and epidemiology. In: *Plasma Lipoprotein*, A. M. Gotto Jr (Ed.), pp. 129–151, Elsevier, Amsterdam (1987).

3. A. D. Bewu and P. N. Durrington. Lipoprotein (a): structure, properties and possible involvement in thrombogenesis and atherogenesis. *Atherosclerosis*, **85**, 1–14 (1990).

4. G. H. Dahlen *et al.* Association of levels of lipoprotein Lp(a), plasma lipids, and other lipoproteins with coronary artery disease documented by angiography. *Circulation*, **74**, 758–764 (1986).

5. H. F. Hoff *et al.* Serum Lp(a) level as a predictor of vein graft stenosis after coronary artery bypass surgery in patients. *Circulation*, **77**, 1238–1242 (1988).

6. M. Seed *et al.* Relation of serum lipoprotein (a) concentration and apolipoprotein (a) phenotype to coronary heart disease in patients with familial hypercholesterolaemia. *N. Engl. J. Med.*, **322**, 1494–1499 (1990).

7. G. M. Kostner *et al.* Lipoprotein Lp(a) and the risk for myocardial infarction. *Atherosclerosis*, **33**, 51–61 (1981).

8. J. Thiery *et al.* Serum lipoprotein Lp(a) concentrations are not influenced by an HMGCoA reductase inhibitor. *Klin. Wochenschr.*, **66**, 462–463 (1988).

9. Shenchi *et al.* Reduction of Lp(a) by different methods of plasma-exchange. *Klin. Wochenschr.*, **66**, 1197–1204 (1988).

10. V. M. Amstrong *et al.* The association between serum Lp(a) concentration and angiographically assessed coronary atherosclerosis. Dependence on serum LDL levels. *Atherosclerosis*, **62**, 249–257 (1986).

11. P. H. Jones. The use of combined LDL affinity apheresis utilizing dextran sulfate cellulose columns and hypolipidemic medication in patients with severe hypercholesterolaemia to assess regression of atherosclerosis. *Contr. Infus. Ther.*, **23**, 142–145 (1988).

12. H. Borberg *et al.* Treatment of familial hypercholesterolaemia by means of specific immunoadsorption. *J. Clin. Apheresis*, **4**, 59–65 (1988).

13. C. Stefanutti *et al.* Variables involved in the treatment of severe hyperlipoproteinemias by combined drug and LDL-apheresis treatment. *Atherosclerosis and Cardiovascular Disease*, **64**, 498–505 (1988).

14. C. Stefanutti *et al.* Dextran sulfate cellulose LDL-affinity apheresis in the treatment of severe familial hypercholesterolaemia and non-familial hyperlipoproteinemia. In: *Treatment of Severe Hypercholesterolaemia in the Prevention of Coronary Heart Disease – 2*, A. M. Gotto, M. Mancini, W. O. Richter and P. Schwandt (Eds), pp. 253–267 (1990).

15. C. Stefanutti *et al.* Extracorporeal atherogenic lipoprotein removal in patients with homozygous familial hypercholesterolaemia. In: *Treatment of Severe Hypercholesterolaemia in the Prevention of Coronary Heart Disease — 3*, O. Richter (Ed.), pp. 253–267 (1991).

Therapeutic Plasmapheresis (XII), pp. 471-479
T. Agishi *et al.* (Eds)
© VSP 1993

Long-term Treatment of Homozygous Familial Hypercholesterolaemia with Selective and Conventional Plasmapheresis

C. STEFANUTTI, B. MAZZARELLA, A. VIVENZIO, C. COLOMBO,
A. BUCCI and G. RICCI

*Istituto di Terapia Medica Sistematica, Haemoapheresis Unit,
University of Rome 'La Sapienza', Rome, Italy*

Key words: homozygous familial hypercholesterolaemia; Apo B100-containing lipoproteins; LDL apheresis;
plasma exchange.

INTRODUCTION

Familial hypercholesterolaemia (FH) is a genetically transmitted disease, characterized by high plasma cholesterol and low density lipoprotein (LDL) levels. The homozygous (Hoz) form is associated to the failure of LDL uptake by the Apo B/E receptor (LDL-receptor activity: minimal or absent), while heterozygous (Htz) FH shows about 50% of the physiological LDL receptor activity. The clinical feature of homozygous FH is composed of xanthomas, severe involvement of coronary arteries by premature atherosclerosis, myocardial infarction within the second decade of life. The former clinical therapeutic approach to homozygous FH was represented by drugs and/or surgical treatment (ileal bypass, veno-venous shunts), but showed to be almost unsuccessful. Since the last two decades, several clinical studies showed that the removal of plasma Apo B-containing lipoproteins by apheretical techniques, could effectively control the severe hypercholesterolaemia of these patients, leading to an improvement of coronary atherosclerosis.

STUDY OUTLINE

Two patients with homozygous FH were continuously treated by means of dextran sulfate cellulose affinity column LDL apheresis (DSC-LDL/A) and plasma exchange (PE). The first patient, S. M., has been submitted to therapeutical plasmapheresis since 1988, while the second patient, M. D., has been treated since 1990 (Table 1).

Table 1.

FH patients treated with plasmapheresis: LDL apheresis (LDL-A) and plasma exchange (PE)

	Patients	M/F	Age (years)	Lipoprotein phenotype	CHD	LDL-A (no.)	PE (no.)	Treatment (months)
Hoz	MD	M	6	IIa	−	28	29	28
	SM	M	34	IIa	+	107	63	47
Htz	□DNA	M	46	IIa	+	38	35	36
	□FG	M	42	IIa	+	28		14
	□PF	M	52	IIa	+	16		8
	□FA	F	48	IIa	−	32		16
	□LE	F	68	IIa	+	16		8
	□PN	M	45	IIa	+	0	32	16
	▲MJ	F	49	IIa	−	8		4
	▲AD	M	31	IIa	−	7		3.5
	▲CA	F	29	IIa	−	8		4
	▲SV	M	32	IIa	−	1		−
	▲CB	M	55	IIa	+	7	1	4
	▲CF	F	51	IIa	−	8		4

CHD, coronary heart disease;
Hoz, homozygous;
Htz, heterozygous;
□, non-responder;
▲, poor responder.

PATIENT DATA (S. M.)

S. M. is 35 years old. He has xanthomas and arcus corneae. Both parents have heterozygous FH with a plasma cholesterol concentration of 348–400 mg/dl. His sister, 43 years old, showed normal plasma cholesterol concentration (Fig. 1). The patient's skin fibroblasts were LDL-receptor defective. The genetic analysis of the restriction fragment length polymorphism's (RFLPs) confirmed the homozygosity of the patient (10). His initial plasma cholesterol level of 614 mg/dl, was little affected by diet and several drug combinations (cholestyramine 32 g/d, probucol 2 g/d, simvastatin 50 mg/d, pravastatin 50 mg/d, bezafibrate 600 mg/d). The extracorporeal treatment with DSC-LDL/A was begun at the age of 31 and is still on going now. Clinical evidence of coronary insufficiency, namely exercise angina, was observed on admission to our centre. A severe atherosclerosis involving all major arterial vessels was assessed by coronary angiography. Coronary angiography showed a proximal occlusion of the left anterior descending and a proximal significant stenosis of the circumflex. The right coronary artery, was completely occluded at the origin.

PATIENT DATA (M. D.)

M. D. is 7 years old. He has xanthomas and arcus corneae. His initial plasma choles-terol concentration of 800 mg/dl. Both parents are heterozygous FH with a plasma cholesterol concentration of 340–380 mg/dl. His brother, 10 years old, showed a plasma

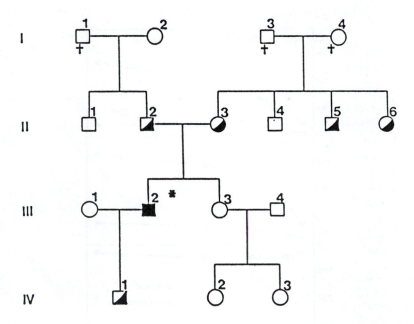

Figure 1. S. M., family pedigree.

cholesterol of 170 mg/dl (Fig. 2). The study of cultured skin fibroblasts showed a nearly absent LDL receptor activity (specific binding of ^{125}I-LDL/mg of cell protein/5 h: 20%; internalization: 22%; degradation: 14%) (Fig. 3).

The genetic study based on the analysis of RFLPs confirmed the patient's homozygosity by demonstrating haplotypes suggesting a point mutation of the gene encoding for the synthesis of LDL receptor (Fig. 4). Treatment with diet and several drug combinations failed to obtain an improvement of plasma atherogenic profile (cholestyramine 24 g/d, simvastatin 40 mg/d, bezafibrate 600 mg/d, gemfibrozil 1200 mg/d). The ex-

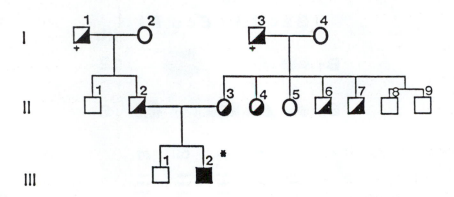

Figure 2. M. D., family pedigree.

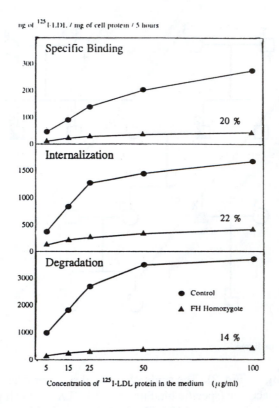

Figure 3. LDL receptor activity in cultured skin fibroblasts.

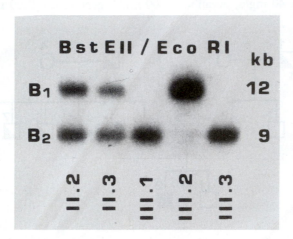

Figure 4. M. D., genetic analysis (see text for explanation).

tracorporeal treatment with DSC-LDL/A was begun on March, 1990, and is still on going now. The patient has been submitted to coronary angiography which failed to demonstrate an atherosclerotic involvement of the coronary arterial tree.

METHODS

The patients were treated using two continuous flow cell separators:
  (i) An automated self-regenerating system (MA-01) using a hollow fiber plasma separator (Sulflux FS-05) and two dextran sulfate cellulose columns (LA-15) (Kanegafuchi, Osaka, Japan) for selective apheresis (LDL apheresis);
  (ii) A conventional centrifugal plasma exchanger unit (Dideco 'Vivacell' BT 798/A, Mirandola, Italy) for plasmapheresis, using 20% albumin in saline (NaCl 0.9%) solution as replacement fluid.

The first patient (S. M.) was treated twice every month for 2 years, then every week (times treated: 180). During a single therapeutic session, which generally was 2.5–3.5 h, 3.5 l of plasma were processed. The second patient (M. D.) was treated twice every month (times treated: 54). A single therapeutic session was approximately 3 h, and the plasma volume which has been processed was of 2.5 l. Plasma total cholesterol (TOTc) and triglyceride (TG) levels were determined by enzymatic techniques (CHOD-PAP High Performance, TG-PAP Poli). HDL cholesterol (HDLc) was evaluated after precipitation of Apo B-containing lipoproteins with phosphotungstate $MgCl_2$. LDL cholesterol (LDLc) was determined after separation with a Beckman L5-65 preparative ultracentrifuge. Plasma apolipoprotein AI and B (Apo AI, Apo B) levels were determined by radial immunodiffusion (Lipo-Partigen Apo AI, Nor-Partigen Apo B, Behring).

RESULTS

A statistically significant acute reduction of plasma TOTc, LDLc, Apo B and TG levels was obtained in both patients by DSC-LDL/A and PE (P 0.001) (Table 2; DSC-LDL/A: Fig. 5). The treatment with DSC-LDL/A resulted in a slight acute reduction of plasma HDLc and Apo AI levels in both patients. PE was able to obtain a more pronounced decrease of plasma HDLc and Apo AI levels, as expected. Apo B showed a statistically significant reduction with both methods (Table 3). Patient S. M. showed a relevant decrease of preapheresis plasma cholesterol concentration, when the treatment was performed weekly (TOTc: −40%, LDLc: −47%). Plasma Apo B level showed a decrease of roughly 30%. Plasma HDLc and Apo AI levels rose slightly (Tables 2 and 3). The results given in Tables 2 and 3 are mean values estimated with data collected before and after the treatment with DSC-LDL/A and PE.

CONCLUSION

DSC-LDL/A and PE confirmed to be effective and well-tolerated for the treatment of homozygous FH. We have continuosly used these systems in the patients for over 48 and 27 months, respectively, at the time of this report. Plasma lipoprotein and apolipoprotein profile was improved and most atherogenic particles (Apo B100-containing lipoproteins) were reduced with apheretical techniques. HDLc and Apo AI were substantially unchanged in the first patient and showed only a slight decrease in the second, using

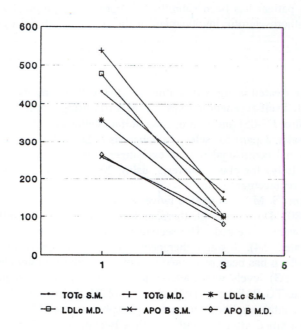

Figure 5. TOTc, LDLc and Apo B variations (DSC-LDL/A).

Table 2.

Mean plasma TOTc, HDLc and TG levels on DSC-LDL/A and PE treatment[a]

Patients	DSC-LDL/A						PE					
	$\bar{x}$			Δ%			$\bar{x}$			Δ%		
	TOTc	HDLc	TG	TOTc	HDLc	TG	TOTc	HDLc	TG	TOTc	HDLc	TG
S. M.[b]												
pre	434	53	117				443	42	86			
				62	7	45				61	42	33
post	165	49	64				170	24	58			
S. M.[c]												
pre	276	55	98				313	43	125			
				55	7	62				58	46	34
post	122	51	37				132	23	82			
M. D.												
pre	541	42	101				563	40	100			
				73	14	66				77	43	62
post	143	36	34				131	23	38			

[a] mg/dl; Δ%: $\frac{(pre + post)}{pre} \times 100$; $\bar{x}$: (pre + post)/2.
[b] 15 days interval.
[c] 7 days interval.

Table 3.

Mean plasma LDLc, Apo B and Apo AI levels on DSC-LDL/A and PE treatment

Patients	$\bar{x}$			Δ%		
	LDLc	Apo B	Apo AI	LDLc	Apo B	Apo AI
DSC-LDL/A						
S. M.[b]						
pre[a]	358	259	144	72	62	12
post	99	99	127			
S. M.[c]						
pre[a]	201	196	153	68	51	8
post	63	96	140			
M. D.						
pre	479	264	135	78	69	13
post	103	80	118			
PE						
S. M.[b]						
pre[a]	385	257	132	65	60	20
post	134	103	106			
S. M.[c]						
pre[a]	244	167	145	63	58	42
post	90	70	84			
M. D.						
pre	503	268	131	80	69	31
post	100	84	90			

[a] mg/dl; Δ%: $\frac{(pre-post)}{pre} \times 100$.

[b] 15 days interval.

[c] 7 days interval.

DSC-LDL/A (Fig. 6). On the contrary, the above mentioned lipoprotein and Apo AI showed a dramatic decrease during the treatment with PE (Tables 2 and 3). Therapeutical plasmapheresis, selective and conventional, showed to be the first choice treatment in these patients, severely affected by homozygous monogenic hypercholesterolaemia, with high coronary risk. Selective plasmapheresis showed a higher efficacy in reducing plasma Apo B100-containing particles. Plasma Apo AI-containing lipoproteins were slightly acutely reduced, but showed a clear increase on long-term treatment (data unpublished). A deeper acute reduction of Apo AI-containing lipoproteins was achieved by PE, as expected. Nevertheless, on long-term, the recovery of HDLc and Apo AI was almost sufficient even with PE. Undoubtedly DSC-LDL/A showed more advantages than PE. This can be assumed to be of significance for indefinitely treating such patients, in order of halting progression and/or achieving regression of arteriosclerotic lesions in the coronary arteries. We were unable to observe major side-effects with both techniques, continuously used with a relatively high frequency, on a yearly basis. The treatment did not influence the physical growth and the development of the younger patient, at least after 2.5 years. The major disadvantage of DSC-LDL/A clearly appeared to be the high cost, which is a very limiting factor in the diffusion of this useful and safe therapeutical tool.

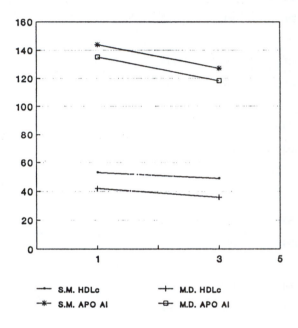

Figure 6. HDLc and Apo AI variations (DSC-LDL/A).

Acknowledgments
This work was partially supported by a grant (no. 92.0000.4.41) of the Italian National Research Council, CNR–PF 'FATMA'.

REFERENCES

1. G. R. Thompson *et al.* Assessment of long-term plasma-exchange for familial hypercholesterolaemia. *Br. Heart. J.*, **43**, 680–684 (1980).

2. H. Mabuchi *et al.* A new low density lipoprotein apheresis system using two dextran sulfate cellulose columns in an automated column regenerating unit (LDL continuous apheresis). *Atherosclerosis*, **68**, 19–28 (1987).

3. G. M. Berger *et al.* Three different schedules of low density lipoprotein apheresis compared with plasmapheresis in the patients with homozygous familial hypercholesterolaemia. *Am. J. Med.*, **88**, 94–102 (1990).

4. B. R. Gordon *et al.* Humoral immune response following extracorporeal immunoadsorption therapy of patients with hypercholesterolaemia. *Transfusion*, **30**, 327–332 (1990).

5. G. Schonfeld. The genetic dyslipoproteinemia — nosology update 1990. *Atherosclerosis*, **81**, 81–90 (1990).

6. P. H. Jones. The use of combined LDL affinity apheresis utilizing dextran sulfate cellulose columns and hypolipidemic medication in patients with severe hypercholesterolaemia to assess regression of atherosclerosis. *Contr. Infus. Ther.*, **23**, 142–145 (1988).

7. H. Borberg *et al.* Treatment of familial hypercholesterolaemia by means of specific immunoadsorption. *J. Clin. Apheresis*, **4**, 59–65 (1988).

8. C. Stefanutti *et al.* Variables involved in the treatment of severe hyperlipoproteinemias by combined drug and LDL-apheresis treatment. *Atherosclerosis and Cardiovascular Disease*, **64**, 498–505 (1988).

9. C. Stefanutti *et al.* Selective continuous removal of low density lipoproteins by dextransulfate cellulose column adsorption apheresis in the therapy of familial hypercholesterolaemia. *Contrib. Infus. Ther.*, **23**, 174–183 (1988).

10. C. Stefanutti *et al.* Dextran sulfate cellulose LDL-affinity apheresis in the treatment of severe familial hypercholesterolaemia and non-familial hyperlipoproteinemia. In: *Treatment of Severe Hypercholesterolaemia in the Prevention of Coronary Heart Disease — 2*, A. M. Gotto, M. Mancini, W. O. Richter and P. Schwandt (Eds), pp. 253–267 (1990).

11. C. Stefanutti *et al.* Extracorporeal atherogenic lipoprotein removal in patients with homozygous familial hypercholesterolaemia. In: *Treatment of Severe Hypercholesterolaemia in the Prevention of Coronary Heart Disease — 3*, O. Richter (Ed.), pp. 253–267 (1991).

12. D. Gairin *et al.* Lipoprotein particles in homozygous familial hypercholesterolemic patients treated with portocaval shunt and LDL-apheresis. *Clin. Chim. Acta*, **193**, 165–180 (1990).

Therapeutic Plasmapheresis (XII), pp. 481-484
T. Agishi *et al.* (Eds)
© VSP 1993

The Experience of Low Density Lipoprotein Apheresis in a Case of Steroid-Resistant Nephrotic Syndrome due to Focul Glomerular Sclerosis

S. MATSUNOBU, E. OZONO, A. NAKAZIMA, M. SUGA, K. UTSUMI,
T. NAKAMARA, M. SHIMIZU, H. KITAMURA, M. TAKEUCHI, M. KAWABE,
N. HAYAMA, Y. IINO, K. HARA and A. TERASHI

*Second Department of Internal Medicine, Nippon Medical School,
Tokyo, Japan*

Key words: focul glomerular sclerosis; nephrotic syndrome; hyperlipidemia; LDL apheresis.

INTRODUCTION

Pathogenesis of focul segmental glomerular sclerosis (FGS) is not definite. But secondary hyperlipidemia may be a risk factor in the progression of renal failure in FGS. We performed low density lipoprotein apheresis (LDL-A) in a patient with steroid-resistant nephrotic syndrome due to FGS. We report the clinical course of the case.

CASE

The patient was a 52 year old female, who was first admitted in 1989 with severe edema. First renal biopsy showed minor glomerular abnormality. So, we started steroid therapy. As a result, urinary protein excretion was reduced and incomplete remission was obtained. However, 1 month later, relapse of nephrotic syndrome occurred, so we performed a second renal biopsy and pathologic diagnosis was FGS. We performed pulse therapy by methylprednisolone again. As the therapy was not effective, we performed LDL-A. The laboratory data are given in Table 1.

METHODS

LDL-A was performed by using the specific sorbent of apoprotein B-containing lipoprotein, Liposorber LA-40, which was developed by Kanegafuchi Chemical Industrial Corp., Japan. The volume of plasma exchanged during each session was set at about 5 l. Direct puncture to veins was performed for blood access.

Table 1.
Laboratory data

	'89.4.1	'89.12.12	'91.11.6
WBC	7450	13220	9620
RBC	418×10^4	370×10^4	458×10^4
Hb (mg/dl)	13.3	11.1	12.5
Hct (%)	38.3	33.9	29.3
Plt	34.7×10^4	38.8×10^4	29.9×10^4
BUN (mg/dl)	70	15	28
Cr (mg/dl)	2.0	1.2	1.3
UA (mg/dl)	9.9	6.2	5.1
TP (g/dl)	4.3	5.5	4.5
Alb (g/dl)	1.5	3.0	1.9
Na (mEq/l)	137	136	133
K (mEq/l)	4.2	3.3	4.3
Cl (mEq/l)	106	98	95
Ca (mg/dl)	6.9	8.2	7.1
P (mg/dl)	–	3.1	4.1
T-ch (mg/dl)	573	297	586
TG (mg/dl)	453	203	497
β-Lip (mg/dl)	3006	1237	3342
LDL (mg/dl)	770	810	1336
VLDL (mg/dl)	1306	337	1086
HDL (mg/dl)	30	49	81
Lp(a) (mg/dl)	–	–	225
Ccr (ml/min)	30.0	50.6	26.9

RESULTS

After we performed a total of six procedures of LDL-A, incomplete remission was continued for about 1 year (Fig. 1).

In 1990, the patient was re-admitted with a relapse of nephrotic syndrome. We performed LDL-A every week with a combined drug treatment. However, severe edema was not under control. We performed LDL-A for 6 days and every week after that. As a result, the urinary volume increased and edema was reduced. Now, we perform LDL-A every 2 weeks, and reduction of edema is obtained (Fig. 2). Changes in serum lipids and lipoprotein by LDL-A are given in Fig. 3.

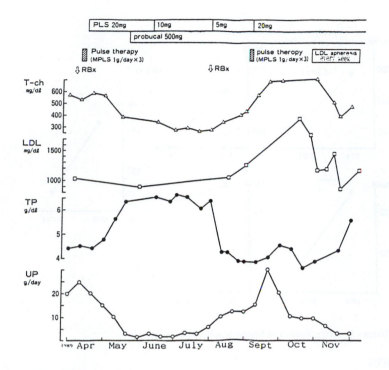

Figure 1. Clinical course on first admission.

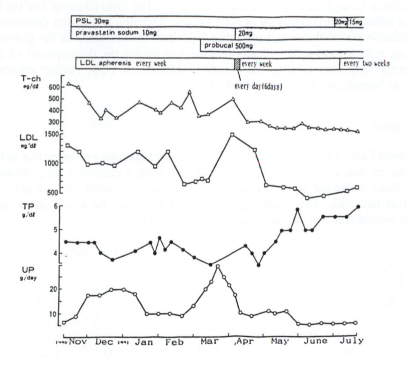

Figure 2. Clinical course on second admission.

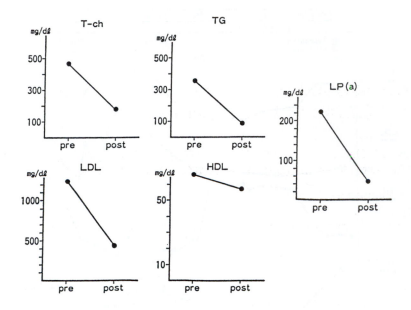

Figure 3. Changes in serum lipids and lipoprotein by LDL-A.

DISCUSSION

Hyperlipidemia in nephrotic syndrome is well known, but little attention has yet been paid to the influence on progression of renal failure. Recently, it has been demonstrated that reduction in serum cholesterol may alter deposition of cholesterol in the glomerular mesangium, reduce mesangial cell proliferation and inhibit the development of FGS. Many reports have demonstrated the benefit of LDL-A on FGS. Further studies are necessary to investigate the effect of LDL-A.

CONCLUSION

We performed LDL-A in a patient with steroid-resistant nephrotic syndrome due to FGS. Drug treatment was not successful, but by LDL-A with a combined drug treatment, urinary volume increased and a reduction of edema was obtained. No complications with LDL-A occurred. The result suggests that LDL-A may be a safe and effective therapy in steroid-resistant nephrotic syndrome due to FGS.

Therapeutic Plasmapheresis (XII), pp. 485-487
T. Agishi *et al.* (Eds)
© VSP 1993

Estimation of Distribution Volume of Low Density Lipoprotein (LDL) by LDL Apheresis

S. KOJIMA, M. HARADA-SHIBA, Y. TOYOTA, K. MURAKAMI, G. KIMURA, M. TSUSHIMA, M. KURAMOCHI, A. YAMAMOTO and T. OMAE

National Cardiovascular Center, Suita, Japan

Key words: low density lipoprotein; plasma volume; plasmapheresis; familial hypercholesterolemia.

INTRODUCTION

Hypercholesterolemia is one of the major risk factors for atherosclerotic cardiovascular disease. Although its pharmacological treatment became convenient due to the development of new antilipidemic drugs, plasmapheresis is indispensable for the treatment of severe hypercholesterolemia such as homozygous familial hypercholesterolemia (FH). Further, the lowering of serum cholesterol below the normal value is expected to lead to the regression of athelosclerosis which is mainly ascribed to hypercholesterolemia. In order to selectively remove low density lipoprotein (LDL), a column packed with dextran sulphate (DS) cellulose was devised. Since LDL apheresis with this column enabled us to decrease serum LDL levels without limitation, it is interesting to know whether the intensive removal of LDL with apheresis using this column causes excessive exclusion of cholesterol as compared with the decrease of plasma cholesterol reserve. In order to investigate whether excessive cholesterol is removed by LDL apheresis, the distribution volume of (VLDL + LDL)-cholesterol was measured based on the single pool model and was compared with the sum of plasma volume and the volume of extracorporeal circuit.

PATIENTS AND METHODS

Patients consisted of one homozygous and three heterozygous cases of FH and one case of unknown cause. Two of the patients were men and the other three were women, all between 16 and 57 years of age. Mean serum cholesterol level of these patients before apheresis was 272 ± 95 mg/dl (mean $\pm$ SD). All these patients were under regular LDL apheresis every other week. For LDL apheresis, we used a computer-controlled machine equipped with one plasma filter and two DS columns (MA01, Kanegafuchi Chemical Industry, Osaka, Japan). The total treated volume of plasma was 3000–6000 ml and it took 3–4 h for one apheresis session. Hemoglobin, hematocrit and serum concentrations of total cholesterol and HDL-cholesterol were measured at 0, 1000, 2000 and 3000 ml plasma treatment during LDL apheresis. The concentrations of (VLDL + LDL)-cholesterol were obtained by subtracting those of HDL-cholesterol from those of total cholesterol. Blood volume before apheresis was calculated according to the formula of Ogawa *et al.* [1] in Japanese volunteers:

$$BV = 168 \times H^3 + 50 \times W + 444 \text{ (for men)}$$
$$BV = 250 \times H^3 + 63 \times W - 662 \text{ (for women)}$$

where BV is blood volume (ml), H is body height (m), and W is body weight (kg) before apheresis. We found a good agreement between plasma volume estimated by this method and that directly measured by a dilution technique using indocyanine green dye [2]. Blood volume on the start of plasma filtration was estimated as follows:

$$\text{BVa} = \text{BVb} \times \text{Hgb/Hga}$$

where **a** is the value on the start of plasma filtration through the plasma filter, **b** is the value immediately prior to apheresis and Hg is the hemoglobin concentration. The entire plasma volume (PV) including the extracorporeal circulation was determined from blood volume and hematocrit (Ht) using the formula:

$$\text{PV} = \text{BV} \times (1 - \text{Ht}/100) + 250 \text{ (ml)}$$

where 250 ml corresponds to the volume of plasma from its separation to re-joining with blood. On the other hand, the distribution volume of LDL + VLDL was measured using the single pool model. The concentrations of (VLDL + LDL)-cholesterol, C, were expressed as a function of time, t: $C = C_0 \times \exp(-Kw \times t/V)$, where C_0 is concentration at the start of plasma treatment, V is the distribution volume of VLDL + LDL and Kw is clearance of (VLDL + LDL)-cholesterol which is almost equal to the plasma flow through the DS column. Logarithmic transformation of the above equation leads to $\ln C = \ln C_0 - Kw \times t/V$. The slope, a, which is equal to Kw/V, was determined by the least square method. V was accordingly calculated as a/Kw. Statistical comparison of paired data was undertaken by Student's t-test. The correlation between the two variables was evaluated using Pearson's coefficient of correlation. Values are shown as mean $\pm$ SEM.

RESULTS

The mean (VLDL + LDL)-cholesterol at 0, 1000, 2000 and 3000 ml plasma treatment was, respectively, 240.5 ± 43.8, 174.8 ± 30.8, 126.4 ± 27.5 and 92.3 ± 22.0 mg/dl. The entire plasma volume, the sum of intravascular plasma volume and extracorporeal plasma volume, was 2633 ± 199 ml, whereas the distribution volume of VLDL + LDL was 3065 ± 280 ml. Although the latter was significantly ($P < 0.01$) greater the former value, there was a close correlation ($r = 0.998$) between these two values (Fig. 1).

DISCUSSION

LDL apheresis using DS cellulose column is available for treatment of severe hypercholesterolemia resistant to the administration of drugs that lower serum cholesterol levels. The present study was aimed to estimate the distribution volume of

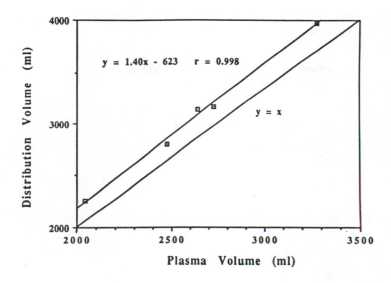

Figure 1. Correlation between plasma volume and distribution volume of VLDL + LDL.

(VLDL + LDL)-cholesterol using the single-pool model, based on the assumption that the amount of cholesterol generation was negligible compared with that of cholesterol removal by LDL apheresis. The subjects consisted of five patients with severe hyper-cholesterolemia; one homozygous and three heterozygous cases of FH, and one case of unknown cause. The distribution volume of (VLDL + LDL)-cholesterol was significantly ($P < 0.01$) greater than the sum of plasma volume and extracorporeal circulation volume, though there was a close correlation ($r = 0.998$) between these two values. These results indicate that the amount of cholesterol generation [3] might not be negligible during LDL apheresis or the single pool model might not be justified for the precise analysis of cholesterol kinetics. The distribution volume of (VLDL + LDL)-cholesterol should be assumed to be about 15% greater than the sum of plasma volume and extracorporeal circulation volume on deciding the apheresis volume of plasma in order to attain the goal in serum cholesterol level.

REFERENCES

1. R. Ogawa, T. Fujita and T. Fukuda. Normal value circulating blood volume in Japanese. Appendix. In: *Blood Volume and Extracellular Fluid Volume*, pp. 252–261. S. N. Albert (Ed.), T. Fujita (trans.). Shinko Koheki Co., Tokyo (1974).
2. B. C. Bradley and J. W. Barr. Determination of blood volume using indocyanine green dye. *Life Sci.,* 7, 1001–1007 (1968).
3. J. Joven, C. Villabona, E. Vilella *et al.* Abnormalities of lipoprotein metabolism in patients with the nephrotic syndrome. *N. Engl. J. Med.,* 323, 579–584 (1990).

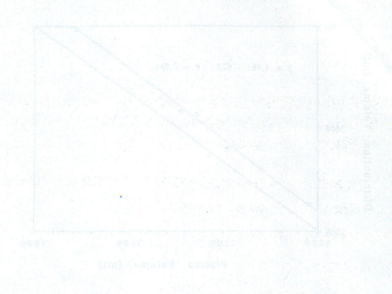

11
Emergency Apheresis

Therapeutic Plasmapheresis (XII), pp. 491-494
T. Agishi *et al.* (Eds)
© VSP 1993

Plasmapheresis in the Emergency Department

Y. ŌISHI, S. MATOBA, T. IIDA and C. TANIMURA

Kyoto Second Red Cross Hospital, Emergency and Critical Care Center, Kyoto, Japan

Key words: hemopurification; multiple organ failure; hepatic failure; continuous hemofiltration; plasma exchange.

INTRODUCTION

We performed hemopurification therapy in patients with various acute diseases at the emergency and critical care center of Kyoto Second Red Cross Hospital. These emergency cases were examined retrospectively to determine the effectiveness of hemopurification. We report here some findings obtained from this study.

CASES

Table 1.
Cases

Case	GOT (U)	GPT (U)	T-Bil (mg/dl)	AKBR	PT (%)	HPT (%)	Treatment	Other
MOF 1	407	1379	9.9	0.47	11.5	17.5	PE	BUN 107 mg/dl
MOF 2	904	1185	2.8	0.53	41.1	34.2	CHF HD	BUN 69.1 mg/dl
MOF 3	132	115	2.2	1.50	29	47	CHF HD	BUN 153 mg/dl
MOF 4	1406	2431	8.3	1.05	17	28	CHF HD	CPK 20724 IU/l
MOF 5	10950	1376	2.8	—	36	42	CHF HD	BUN 105.1 mg/dl

Case MOF-1 (62 year old male)
He developed multiple organ failure (MOF) following endotoxic shock. The condition occurred following sepsis caused by an uretheral stone and was initially treated with a respirator. Values of enzymes, such as GOT and GPT, were diminished by appropriate treatment, but values of prothrombin time (PT) and hepaplastin test (HPT) were diminished (11.5 and 17.5%, respectively), indicating that the stage of disorder of the coagulation system was advanced. In addition, the value of arterial ketone body ratio (AKBR) diminished to 0.47, suggesting that the patient developed a state of severe hepatic failure. Following these examinations, we decided that continuous hemofiltration (CHF) was not a suitable approach in this case, and thus plasma exchange (PE) therapy was initiated. We observed an immediate improvement in the patient's condition following the fourth application of PE.

Case MOF-2 (25 year old female)
She suffered from MOF, which was particularly marked by renal failure following acute parotiditis. Severe hepatic failure was confirmed by quantitative analysis of GOT (904 U), GPT (1185 U) and AKBR (0.53). We decided to proceed with treatment by CHF, since disorder of the coagulation system was not extreme as judged by values of PT and HPT (41.1 and 34.2%, respectively). Thus, instead of using PE, treating the patient by CHF and hemodialysis (HD) proved so effective that it saved her life despite the presence of severe renal and hepatic failure.

Case MOF-3 (52 year old male)
He developed MOF following a necrotizing fasciitis. Following admission into the hospital, he was in a state of septic shock and developed MOF, involving severe failure of the kidneys with DIC. The patient was treated by CHF and HD and attained a satisfactory prognosis.

Case MOF-4 (39 year old male)
He suffered from MOF following a malignant syndrome. He was presented with a state of renal and hepatic failure with DIC, which developed from a previous hypermyoglobinemia. Both CHF and HD were also performed in this case.

Case MOF-5 (30 year old male)
He suffered from MOF caused by traffic trauma. He was in a state of flail chest and hemorrhagic shock, and subsequently fell into MOF with DIC. Under respiratory control with a respirator, he developed lung-herniation, which complicated subsequent treatment. In addition, even after the CHF was complete, acute renal failure was so refractory that HD therapy continued for over a 1 month period. MOF was characterized by the following values of GPT (10950 U), GOT (1376 U), CPK (1975 U), LDH (28150 U), BUN (105 mg/dl) and total bilirubin (2.8 mg/dl). This condition was also controlled effectively by both CHF and HD instead of PE.

DISCUSSION

Hemopurification therapy is regarded as an effective treatment in emergency cases. In particular, PE, CHF and HD applied to cases of MOF with a high mortality are considered to be essential in saving lives, since these therapies prevent the complex deterioration of the disease process and allow sufficient time for each organ to recover its normal function. However, it remains uncertain whether cases of MOF should be primarily treated with either PE or CHF. With respect to application of PE, relative values of total bilirubin, AKBR, HPT and PT have been listed in many references [1, 2]. In addition, levels of these values reported in this study are summarized in Table 1. We feel that PE should be primarily administered in cases of fulminant hepatitis to remove unidentified toxic substances and to supply coagulation factors. On the other hand, for cases of MOF, particularly severe hepatic failure, it is thought that the application of PE should be restricted to cases where values of AKBR and PT fall below 0.70 and 15%, respectively. Application of PE to case MOF-1 was considered appropriate, as judged by the general values listed in other references and from our studies. Based on these criteria, PE was thought to be also applicable to cases MOF-2 and MOF-4.

However, both CHF and HD were found to be effective. Indeed, CHF was shown to be insufficient therapy in hemopurification for cases of hepatic failure because this treatment is known to remove soluble middle-sized molecular substances, but not protein-bound substances from blood. However, treatment of MOF, with CHF combined with intravenous hyperalimentation and administration of prostaglandin, plays a major role in gaining sufficient time to improve the condition of the emergency case [3]. This is because few of these situations fall into a state of severe hepatic failure, such as postoperative hepatic failure observed in cases of cirrhosis.

Therefore, in the emergency field, we consider the first choice of hemopurification therapy to be PE for cases of fulminant hepatitis, and CHF for cases of MOF.

CONCLUSION

Figure 1 illustrates how we decided upon hemopurification therapy in emergency cases. As a first choice of treatment, DHP was performed in cases of intoxication, and double filtration plasma pheresis (DFPP), free from infection, was used on patients with Guillain–Barré syndrome. Cases of fulminant hepatitis were primarily treated by PE to supply coagulation factors. Patients with MOF, whose major complications were renal failure, were treated with both CHF and HD. In contrast, patients with severe hepatic failure were treated with PE. Moreover, PE was applied to cases of fulminant hepatitis and hepatic failure, where values of AKBR and PT fell below 0.7 and 15%, respectively.

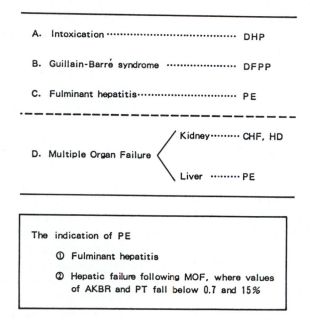

Figure 1. The indication of hemopurification.

REFERENCES

1. T. Tomiya, N. Inoue, I. Ogata *et al.* Plasma exchange in the treatment of fulminant hepatitis: evaluation of its effects on liver function. *The Saisin-Igaku*, **42**, 1619–1624 (1987).

2. Y. Ohtake, H. Hirasawa, T. Sugai *et al.* The indication of hemopurification for the patients with severe hepatic malfunction. *J. Intensive Care Med.*, **14**, 51–56 (1990).

3. R. H. Bartlett, J. R. Mault, R. E. Dechert *et al.* Continuous arteriovenous hemofiltration: improved survival in surgical acute renal failure. *Surgery*, **100**, 400–408 (1986).

Therapeutic Plasmapheresis (XII), pp. 495-498
T. Agishi *et al.* (Eds)
© VSP 1993

Endotoxin Removal by Plasma Perfusion over an Anion Exchange Resin in Obstructive Jaundice

J. TANAKA,[1] T. SATO,[2] P. S. MALCHESKY,[2] T. OHSHIMA,[2] K. SAWADA,[2] N. SATO[2] and K. KOYAMA[1]

[1]*Department of Surgery, Akita University School of Medicine, Akita, Japan*
[2]*Department of Biomedical Engineering and Applied Therapeutics,*
 The Cleveland Clinic Foundation, Cleveland, Ohio, USA

Key words: endotoxin removal; plasma perfusion; anion exchange resin; mononuclear cell transformation function; obstructive jaundice.

INTRODUCTION

Obstructive jaundice is frequently associated with systemic endotoxemia [1] and impaired cellular immune function [2]. Morbidity and mortality in patients with jaundice are especially high when systemic endotoxemia is present [3]. Plasma perfusion with a sorbent column has recently been applied to adsorb bilirubin and some other active substances so that replacement fluid such as albumin or fresh frozen plasma could be saved. This study evaluates the effect of plasma perfusion using an anion exchange resin on endotoxin removal and cellular functions in obstructive jaundice with endotoxemia.

MATERIALS AND METHODS

Obstructive jaundice was surgically created in male mongrel dogs by ligation and division of the common bile duct and cholecystectomy. Eight dogs were divided into two groups. The true treatment group ($n = 4$) was treated with on-line plasma perfusion over an anion exchange resin, BR-180 (Plasorba, Asahi Medical Co., Tokyo). Each dog received 10 treatments in 8 weeks. Three plasma volumes were treated. The plasma column temperature was maintained at 38 °C. The sham group ($n = 4$) underwent the same procedure without the sorbent column. Hematology and biochemistry were measured at pre- and posttreatment during the course of study. Plasma endotoxin levels were assayed by the synthetic chromogenic substance Boc-Leu-Gly-Arg-p-nitroanilide (Seikagaku Kogyo Ltd, Tokyo) with perchloric acid pretreatment. Mononuclear cells of the experimental animals with pooled normal plasma and those of normal dogs with plasmas from the true or sham group were evaluated for mitogen stimulated blastogenesis with phytohemagglutinin (PHA), concanavalin A (Con A) or pokeweed mitogen (PWM). These measurements were done at pre- and 7 (day of first perfusion), 21, 42, 63 postoperative days (POD).

RESULTS

All animals of the true group completed the protocol, while one dog of the sham group
died after three perfusions due to gastrointestinal bleeding and obstructive supprative
cholangitis found by autopsy.

Biochemical studies

The concentration of total bilirubin (T.Bil) increased in both groups on the 7th POD
before the first plasma perfusion. The reductions of T.Bil after each treatment were
significantly greater in the true group than in the shame group ($P < 0.01$). The concentrations of cholyglycine, that is a representative bile acid, were shown to increase
with the course for the sham group while those for the true group were shown not to
increase with a remarkable reduction after each treatment. Mean percentage reduction
of T.Bil was 43.7% and that of cholyglycine was 53.5%. However, the pretreatment
levels of T.Bil or cholyglycine for the true group were not significantly different from
the sham group.

Changes in plasma endotoxin levels

The mean plasma levels of endotoxin on 7 POD was 101.6 ± 32.7 pg/ml (normal:
<10 pg/ml). In the true group, mean percentage reduction of endotoxin was $77.9 \pm$
12.3% and pretreatment levels of endotoxin gradually decreased over the course to
57.7 ± 25.8 pg/ml on 63 POD. In contrast, the endotoxin levels in the sham group
steadily increased to 141.4 ± 14.6 pg/ml on 63 POD as shown in Fig. 1.

Mononuclear cell transformation functions (MNC-TFs)

MNC-TFs of the true group to the three mitogens were well maintained with a transient
suppression within the first week, while those in the sham group were shown to decrease

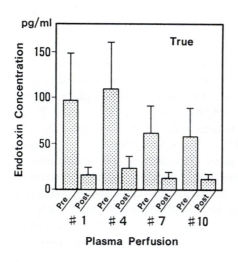 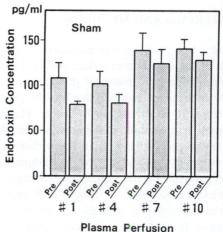

Figure 1. Changes in the concentration of plasma endotoxin (means $\pm$ SD).

after the 6th postoperative week. The plasmas from the sham group were shown to suppress the reactivities with mitogen stimulations of cells from the normal dogs over the course of study.

DISCUSSION

In the present study, it was confirmed that ligation of the common bile duct with cholecystectomy in dogs induced elevation of plasma endotoxin level as well as hyperbilirubinemia. Endotoxemia is believed to result from an increased absorption of intestinal endotoxin into the portal circulation due to the absence of bile salts in the gut [4, 5] with spill over into the systemic circulation due to impairment of the reticuloendothelial function by the Kupffer cells [6]. Endotoxin is well known to cause multiple organ failure (MOF), disseminated intravascular coagulation (DIC) and eventually fatal shock.

Endotoxins are derived from the outer cell membranes of Gram negative bacteria that consist of a polysaccharide component including the O-specific chain and core oligosaccharide and a lipid component termed lipid A. Since endotoxin is negatively charged because of the presence of lipid A, positively charged matrices can adsorb endotoxin through charge interaction. Positively charged filters have already been applied in depyrogenating biological fluids since most pyrogens have a low isoelectric point because of their phospholipid groups [7]. The use of the anion exchange column could therefore be effective in endotoxin removal.

Circulating lymphocyte function has also been shown to be impaired in patients with liver failure and cirrhosis [8, 9] and in obstructive jaundice [2]. This study evaluated the effect of plasma perfusion on cellular function and the suppressive effect of jaundiced plasma on normal mononuclear cells. Mean MNC-TF of the sham group over the course were significantly suppressed compared to the true group in spite of comparable high levels of bilirubin and bile acid at each pretreatment in both groups. Further jaundiced plasmas from the sham group were shown to suppress normal mononuclear cell function. Thus, it was found that nontreated jaundiced plasma has a immunosuppressive factor that can be removed by plasma perfusion treatment over the anion exchange resin.

CONCLUSION

Plasma perfusion over an anion exchange resin in obstructive jaundice effectively removed plasma endotoxin and improved impaired cellular functions. Clinical application of this resin for patients with endotoxemia could be beneficial.

REFERENCES

1. E. N. Wardle. Fibrinogen in liver disease. *Am. J. Surg.*, **109**, 741–746 (1974).

2. D. W. Vane, P. Redlich, T. Weber *et al.* Impaired immune function in obstructive jaundice. *J. Surg. Res.*, **45**, 287–293 (1988).

3. C. J. Ingoldby, G. A. D. McPherson and L. H. Blumgart. Endotoxemia in obstructive jaundice. *Am. J. Surg.*, **147**, 766–771 (1984).

4. M. E. Bailey. Endotoxin, bile salts and renal function in obstructive jaundice. *Br. J. Surg.*, **63**, 774–778 (1976).

5. J. A. Pain and M. E. Bailey. Measurement of operative endotoxin plasma levels in jaundiced and non-jaundiced patients. *Eur. Surg. Res.*, **19**, 207–216 (1987).

6. G. Drivas, O. James and N. Wardle. Study of reticuloendothelial phagocytic capacity in patients with cholestasis. *Br. Med. J.*, **1**, 1568–1569 (1976).

7. K. C. Hou, C. P. Gerba, S. M. Goyal *et al.* Capture of latex beads, bacteria, endotoxin, and viruses by charge-modified filters. *Appl. Environ. Microbiol.*, **40**, 892–896 (1980).

8. R. A. Fox, F. J. Dudley, M. Samuels *et al.* Lymphocyte transformation in response to phytohemagglutinin in primary biliary cirrhosis: The search for a plasma inhibitory factor. *Gut*, **14**, 89–93 (1973).

9. G. Holdstock, B. F. Chastenay and E. L. Krawitt. Studies on lymphocyte hyporesponsiveness in cirrhosis: The role of increased monocyte suppressor cell activity. *Gastroenterology*, **82**, 206–212 (1982).

Therapeutic Plasmapheresis (XII), pp. 499-503
T. Agishi *et al.* (Eds)
© VSP 1993

The Efficacy of Plasma Exchange in Intensive Care Medicine

T. SUGAI, H. HIRASAWA, Y. OHTAKE, S. ODA, H. SHIGA, K. NAKANISHI, K. MATSUDA, N. KITAMURA and H. UENO

Department of Emergency and Critical Care Medicine, Chiba University School of Medicine, Chiba, Japan

Key words: plasma exchange; intensive care medicine; hepatic failure; arterial ketone body ratio; osmolality gap.

INTRODUCTION

Blood purifications (BP) have been the essential therapeutic tools in intensive and critical care medicine. Various kinds of BP are applied independently or in combination depending upon the pathological conditions of the patients. Plasma exchange (PE) has advantages over other BP, because it is able not only to remove harmful substances with a wide range of molecular weights, but also to replace essential substances. We can also expect the enhancement of depressed self-defense mechanisms though the removal of depressant factors and replacement of opsonic proteins with PE. This study was undertaken to investigate the efficacy of PE and the criteria for initiation of PE for various pathological conditions treated in the ICU, putting emphasis on hepatic failure.

MATERIAL AND METHOD

The patients treated with BP in our ICU between August 1985 and April 1992 were entered to the study. The parameters expressing hepatic cellular function such as arterial ketone body ratio (AKBR) and serum osmolality gap (OG) were measured. Hepaplastin test (HPT) and total bilirubin (T.Bil) were also measured. The correlation between those parameters and outcome of the patients was studied.

RESULTS

During the past 7 years, 193 patients, about 11% of patients admitted in our ICU, were treated with eight different kinds of BP, such as continuous hemofiltration (CHF), continuous hemodiafiltration (CHDF), hemodialysis (HD), hemoadsorption (HA), plasma adsorption (PA), peritoneal dialysis (PD) and endotoxin adsorption (PMX), either applied independently or in combination. The number of cases treated with each BP are shown in Table 1. PE was applied 303 times on 75 cases. Multiple organ failure with hepatic failure and fulminant hepatitis were the two most common entities treated with PE, and they account for 76% of all cases. Other clinical entities treated with PE were thrombotic thrombocytopenic purpura (TTP), hemolytic uremic syndrome (HUS), Reye's syndrome, pancreatitis and severe sepsis. The survival rate of surgical and medical MOF with hepatic failure and fulminant hepatitis were 28, 44 and 48%, respectively (Table 2).

Table 1.
Blood purifications in ICU

Blood purifications		No. of cases
Continuous hemofiltration	(CHF)	65
Continuous hemodiafiltration	(CHDF)	86
Hemodialysis	(HD)	68
Plasma exchange	(PE)	75
Hemoadsorption	(HA)	18
Plasma adsorption	(PA)	14
Peritoneal dialysis	(PD)	2
Endotoxin adsorption	(PMX)	5
Total		193

Table 2.
Clinical entities treated with PE in ICU

Clinical entity	No. of cases	No. of PE	No. of survivors	Survival rate (%)
MOF with hepatic failure				
surgical	25	90	7	28
medical	9	22	4	44
Fulminant hepatitis	23	127	11	48
TTP, HUS	5	32	3	60
Reye's syndrome	3	3	3	100
Pancreatitis	3	6	2	66
Sepsis	2	4	1	50
Others	5	19	5	100
Total	75	303	36	48

The correlation between the AKBR measured before the initial PE and the outcome of hepatic failure patients was studied. The AKBR of survivors was significantly higher than those of non-survivors and there were no survivors among the patients whose AKBR was below 0.5.

The changes in acetoacetate (ACAC), β-hydroxybutyrate (BOHB) and AKBR with PE and also those values of fresh frozen plasma (FFP) were studied. Though the values of ACAC, BOHB and KBR of FFP was significantly lower than that of arterial blood, no significant changes of ACAC, BOHB and KBR with PE were observed, indicating that PE improved hepatic cellular function.

Studying the relationship between OG and Glasgow Coma Scale (GCS) of the hepatic failure patients, we found a significant correlation between them. The higher the OG, the lower the GCS. We found a significant correlation between the outcome of the hepatic failure patients and change in the OG with PE. Among the survivors, the preexisting large OG decreased into the normal range following the PE and remained within the normal range for 24 h. However, among the majority of the non-survivors the gap did not decrease into the normal range and among all the non-survivors the gap increased again above the normal values at 24 h after the PE.

The correlation between the change in HPT with PE and the outcome of the patients was investigated. The depressed hepaplastin value was improved with PE in both survivors and non-survivors immediately after the PE. However, at 24 h after PE the hepaplastin test remained improved among survivors; on the other hand, it deteriorated again among non-survivors.

DISCUSSION

It has been claimed that one of the reasons for the poor clinical result among the patients with hepatic failure treated with artificial liver support is the lack of an adequate method of assessment for hepatic function. We have proposed that organ failure such as hepatic failure is the summation of the cellular dysfunction in failing organs. From this point of view, it is reasonably assumed that hepatic cellular function should be monitored as the fundamental of hepatic function assessment. We have applied AKBR and OG for this purpose.

AKBR, the ratio of ACAC to BOHB of arterial blood, is an excellent parameter to evaluate the hepatic mitochondrial redox status [1]. The correlation between the AKBR before the initial PE and the outcome of hepatic failure patients clearly indicates that the AKBR is an excellent parameter to evaluate the hepatic cellular function and, therefore, to evaluate the hepatic function. The results also indicate that the AKBR can be used even as a prognostic index.

Since approximately 3200 ml of FFP was replaced, it seems to be reasonable to assume that those values in arterial blood decrease significantly after PE compared to those of pre-PE. However, no significant change in ACAC, BOHB and KBR with PE was observed. These results suggest that PE caused a drastic change in the redox status of the hepatocytes [2].

The OG is the difference between measured osmolality and predicted osmolality. It can express the amount of unmeasurable solute in patient's blood [3]. According to the correlation between OG and GCS, it is suggested that the blood purification which can lower the OG may be a beneficial treatment to recover the consciousness level of hepatic failure patients. The correlation between the outcome of the hepatic failure patients and change in the OG with PE indicates that the OG is a sensitive indicator to predict survivors from hepatic failure treated with PE.

Besides these two sensitive parameters for hepatic cellular function, HPT is an important parameter to evaluate hepatic protein synthesis. The correlation between the changes in HPT with PE and the outcome of the patients indicate that HPT is also very useful in the management of the acute hepatic failure.

Taking these results into consideration, we decided the criteria for the initiation of artificial liver support on acute hepatic failure as follows. First, AKBR is less than 0.7.

**ASSESSMENTS OF HEPATIC FUNCTIONS
AND INDICATIONS OF ARTIFICIAL LIVER SUPPORT IN CRITICAL CARE**

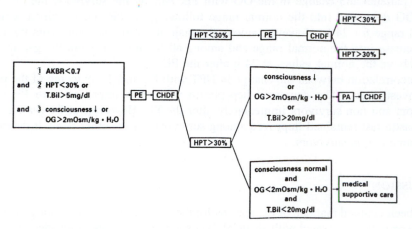

Figure 1. Assessments of hepatic functions and indications of artificial liver support in critical care.

Second, HPT is less than 30% or T.Bil is higher than 5 mg/dl. Third, the patient shows depressed consciousness level or OG is greater than 2 mOsm/kg/H$_2$O. Figure 1 shows the indication and the decision making chart for artificial liver support using the above parameters. When a patient shows all the criteria for the initiation of artificial liver support, PE is performed as the initial support. Then the patient is put on CHDF. The following day, HPT is re-evaluated. If his HPT is lower than 30%, the second PE is performed. On the other hand, if he shows one of the following sign or symptoms, namely depressed consciousness level, OG greater than 2 mOsm/kg/H$_2$O or bilirubin level greater than 20 mg/dl, PA is indicated as the second artificial liver support. If his HPT is over 30% following the initial PE and CHDF, and if his consciousness level is normal, OG is less than 2 and his bilirubin level is less than 20 concurrently, he seems to be in recovery stage from hepatic failure, and medical supportive care without any further artificial liver support is indicated.

PE consumes extensive FFP and has some adverse effects. Countermeasures for post-PE complications such as hypernatremia, metabolic alkalosis, bleeding tendency and hepatitis C have been developed. Hypernatremia and metabolic alkalosis were solved with simultaneous hemodialysis with low Na or low HCO$_3$-dialysate. Nafamostat mesilate as anticoagulant has decreased the rate of bleeding complications significantly. Now blood products can be routinely checked for the anti HCV antibody. Consequently, PE can be applied safely even to critically ill patients.

CONCLUSIONS

BP has been an essential therapeutic tool in intensive and critical care medicine. Since PE is able not only to remove large molecular substances but also to supplement useful substances, it has advantages over other BP. The efficacy of PE for hepatic failure and certain pathological conditions is widely accepted, and complications of PE are almost overcome. PE can be applied safely on even critically ill patients. However, from the view point of effective usage of FFP or cost–benefit ratio, we should review the indication of PE more cautiously.

REFERENCES

1. K. Ozawa, H. Aoyama, Y. Yasuda *et al.* Metabolic abnomalities associated with postoperative organ failure — a redox theory. *Arch. Surg.*, **118**, 1245–1251 (1983).
2. H. Inaba, H. Hirasawa and T. Mizuguchi. Serum osmolality gap in post operative patients in intensive care. *Lancet*, **2**, 1331–1335 (1987).
3. Y. Ohtake, H. Hirasawa, T. Sugai *et al.* The effects of plasma exchange on hepatic cellular metabolism. *Artif. Organs*, **14** (Suppl 2), 182–184 (1990).
4. H. Hirasawa, M. Odaka, T. Sugai *et al.* Prognostic value of serum osmolality gap in patients with multiple organ failure treated with hemopurification. *Artif. Organs*, **12**, 382–387 (1988).

Therapeutic Plasmapheresis (XII), pp. 505-508
T. Agishi *et al.* (Eds)
© VSP 1993

Regional Anticoagulant on Endotoxin Adsorption Therapy in Septic Multiple Organ Failure Patients

Y. TSUTAMOTO, K. HANASAWA, H. AOKI, T. TANI, Y. ENDO,
K. MATSUDA, T. YOSHIOKA, K. NUMA, H. ARAKI,
T. YOKOTA and M. KODAMA

*First Department of Surgery, Shiga University of Medical Science,
Seta, Otsu, Shiga 520-20, Japan*

Key words: nafamostat mesilate (FUT-175); herarin; DHP; PMX-F; regional anticoagulant.

INTRODUCTION

The surface structures of blood-perfused artificial organs activate various proenzymes in coagulation and complement systems. An ideal anticoagulant for artificial organs should inhibit the activation of all enzymes in the blood–material interactions, and only activate in the circuit. Until recently, heparin has been the most popular anticoagulant; however, it is not ideal. Despite intensive supportive care, there is mortality among septic patients. Removing endotoxin directly from the blood, we developed a material consisting of Polymyxin B which is immobilized on polystyren fibers (PMX-F) [1].

In this paper, we report on the application of nafamostat mesilate [2] during direct hemoperfusion with Polymyxin B immobilized fiber as an anticoagulant.

PATIENTS AND METHODS

Patient profiles

PMX-F treatment was initiated for the patients who did not respond to conventional therapy as shown Table 1. We used PMX-F for 17 septic patients of multiple organ failure (MOF). Using heparin or nafamostat mesilate as an anticoagulant, PMX treatment were performed 37 times overall in these 17 patients. The mean age was 63 years. The number of failed organs was between two and five. Four patients were diagnosed to have DIC (nos 6, 7, 12 and 14). Ten out of the 17 patients had thrombocytopenia (a count of less than 100 000). Six out of these 10 were treated using nafamostat mesilate as an anticoagulant. Heparin was used on the remainder. The adsorbence column used clinically contained 53 g of PMX-F fiber bound covalently to 370 mg of Polymyxin B and could hold 170 ml of blood. The column was sterilized in a pressurized steam autoclave at 120 °C and passed various pressure and leakage tests. Direct hemoperfusion with PMX-F was carried out for 2 h at a blood flow rate of 80–100 ml/min. Anticoagulant heparin was infused continuously at 2000 U/h following a bolus infusion of 3000 U at initiation. Nafamostat mesilate was infused continuously at 30 mg/h following a bolus infusion of 20 mg at initiation.

Table 1.
Septic MOF cases

No.	Disease	Pathogenic bacteria	No. of failed organs	Anticoagulant
1	Pneumonia	*S. aureus* xantho	2	heparin[c]
2	Rupture of trans. colon	*E. coli* bacteroides	3	heparin[c]
3	Meningitis	Enterococcus	2	heparin
4	Torsion of sigm. colon	ND[b]	5	heparin
5	Subphrenic abscess	Bacteroides	2	heparin
6	SMAO[a]	*P. aeruginosa*	4	FUT-175[c]
7	Rupture of sigm. colon[a]	Enterobacter	2	FUT-175[c]
8	Duodenal rupture	Lactobacillus	3	FUT-175[c]
9	Ileus pneumonia	*P. enterococcus*	2	FUT-175[c]
10	Injury of liver and pancreas	*P. e. coli*	4	FUT-175[c]
11	Rupture of sigm. colon	*E. coli*	2	FUT-175[c]
12	Sepsis after total pancreatectomy[a]	Enterobacter	3	FUT-175[c]
13	Rupture of sigm. colon	*Staph. A*	3	FUT-175
14	Pneumonia[a]	ND[b]	5	FUT-175
15	Perforation of stomach	*S. aureus*	3	FUT-175
16	Duodenal rupture	*E. coli*	5	FUT-175
17	Obstructive enterocolitis	Enterobacter	5	FUT-175

[a] DIC; [b] not detected; [c] survivor.

Endotoxin measurement
Heparinized blood samples were collected before and at 30 min during treatment. Endotoxin concentration was determined by the endospecy test (Seikagaku-kogyo, Osaka, Japan) with new-PCA pretreatment [3].

RESULTS

Changes of platelet counts
We compared the changes of platelet counts during hemoperfusion. Figure 1 shows the changes of percent value. At 120 min, the nafamostat group had increased the percent value of platelets significantly compared with the heparin group. Thus we could do PMX hemoperfusion safely in patients who had a bleeding tendency or thrombocytopenia.

Endotoxin levels
The endotoxin concentrations at the inlet and outlet of the column were determined by endospecy with new-PCA pretreatment, at 30 min after initiation of treatment and at the conclusion of treatment. The mean value decreased from 80 pg before treatment to 21 pg after treatment. The mean concentration at the column inlet was 30 pg and that at the outlet was 25 pg. There were significant differences between the pre- and post-treatment values.

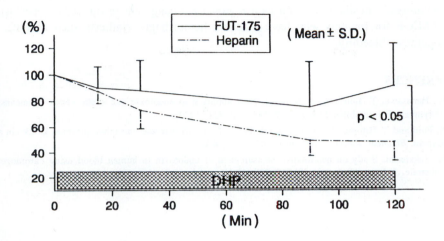

Figure 1. Changes of platelet counts.

Effects of PMX-F treatment
No serious complication such as unexpected hemorrhage, which has often been observed during or after DHP, occurred in our treatment series. Nine out of the 17 patients (53%) clinically improved and survived.

CLINICAL REPORTS

Clinical application of PMX-F treatment with nafamostat mesilate in 64 year old man. He had sigmoid colon cancer and had developed panperitonitis due to perforation of the sigmoid colon. As a result, an emergency operation had been done. He had severe coagulopathy. The day after operation, PT had been prolonged to 18.5 s and APTT to 120 s. FDP had increased to 72.5 mg/ml and fibrinogen had dropped to 120 mg/dl. This was evidence of disseminated intravascular coagulation. The treatment with PMX was performed on that day and we did not experience any exacerbation of hemorrhagic diathesis. Another clinical application of PMX with nafamostat mesilate. He had a good clinical course for about 10 days total pancreatectomy for pancreatic advanced cancer infiltrated to portal vein. However, from the 16th day his platelet counts suddenly dropped to 20000 and there began to be evidence of DIC. He received a transfusion of platelets and AT-3 as well but platelet counts did not recover. At this time PMX treatment was performed and then began to increase slightly. However, from the 23th day, these again began to drop gradually. So platelets were transfused once more, but when they did not recover, PMX was performed on the 25th day. From the 30th day the platelet counts gradually recovered, and the patient improved and was subsequently discharged.

CONCLUSIONS

We showed that PMX treatment for septic patients with (MOF) could significantly decrease the mean serum endotoxin level after 2 h. Nine out of 17 patients with

MOF had clinical improvement and survived. This clinical study also revealed that thus nafamostat mesilate is useful as a regional anticoagulant in direct hemoperfusion with PMX-F for patients who have a severe hemorrhagic diathesis such as DIC, or post-operative bleeding.

REFERENCES

1. K. Hanasawa, T. Tani and M. Kodama. New approach to endotoxic and septic shock by means of Polymyxin B immobilized fiber. *SGO,* **168**, 323–331 (1989).
2. S. Fujii and Y. Hitomi. New synthetic inhibitors of C1r, C1 esterase, thrombin, plasmin, kallikrein and trypsin. *Biochem. Biophys. Acta,* **661**, 342–345 (1981).
3. K. Takahashi. Study on quantitative measurement of endotoxin in human blood using chromogenic substrate. *J. Iwate Med. Ass.,* **40**, 213–220 (1988).

Therapeutic Plasmapheresis (XII), pp. 509-512
T. Agishi *et al.* (Eds)
© VSP 1993

Plasmaperfusion Through Activated Charcoal Increases Oxygen Extraction in Septic Shock

L. N. SZTERLING, C. FERNANDES, N. AKAMINE, N. HAMERSCHLAK, M. C. NETO, O. SANTOS and E. KNOBEL

Albert Einstein Hospital, São Paulo, SP, Brazil

Key words: plasmapheresis; septicemia; charcoal; plasmaperfusion; shock.

INTRODUCTION

The septic patient is normally treated after the etiologic diagnosis is made and the gateway of the infection is identified. The right handling of modern antimicrobials undoubtable contributes to a lower mortality in septicemia.

Nevertheless, there is a significant group of patients who evolve — despite intensive care — to a progressive deterioration of organs or systems, the so-called Multiple Organs Failure Syndrome. This is a case of sky-high mortality, when the handling of the patient becomes critical in terms of survival. The hemodynamic monitorization with the Swan-Ganz catheter, as well as the readings of the gasimetric parameters, give us important information concerning the systemic alterations occurring in these patients.

It is well-known that one of the most important mechanisms that keep the septic patient under shock is related to the presence of endotoxins with the consequent liberation of mediators from patient's cells, induced by endotoxin.

Gotloib, from Israel [1], documented the improvement in respiratory insufficiency of 24 patients who suffered from the Adult Respiratory Distress Syndrome who had been subjected to hemofiltration, associating their improvement to the clearance of vasoactive peptides. Bende, from Hungary [2], documented the elimination of endotoxins in the blood with the usage of hemoperfusion in activated charcoal with an experimental model. And Werdan, from the University of Munich [3], dealt with septic patients mentioning the benefit of plasmapheresis in those patients whose antibiotic therapy had been ineffectual, through a study that included 27 patients.

OBJECTIVES

Our main objective was to test the utilization of plasmaperfusion by using the charcoal filter, so as to verify the observable changes in the hemodynamic patterns, as well as the oxygen consumption, in critical patients.

APPARATUSES AND METHODS

Ten septicemic patients admitted at the Intensive Care Unit of Albert Einstein Hospital, in Sao Paulo, were studied (six males and four females, their ages ranging from 22 to 62). They all showed clear signs of clinical deterioration the shock settled and needing vasoactive drugs to keep their hemodynamic stability.

The patients were monitorized with the Swan-Ganz catheter; the indexes were estimated according to the body surface; the cardiac debt was obtained by thermodilution; gasimetric studies were corrected according to the temperature; and standard formulas were used to calculate both the hemodynamic variables and the transport of oxygen.

When patients showed evidence of low oxygen consumption — associated to a chart of persistingly rising of the lactate — it was decided that the ideal procedure would be to make them undergo a plasma perfusion through an activated charcoal filter.

A double-lumen Shilley-like catheter was inserted in the subclavian vein. The plasmapheresis was carried out with apparatuses of discontinuous flow (Hemonetics or Diddeco). As the plasma flows out of the bowl, it is deviated by means of a peristaltic pump — setting up a second system — to the activated charcoal filter (Gambro.) previously washed with two solutions: one liter of dextrose 10% and 1 l of normal saline.

The filtered plasma is then conducted to a reinfusion bag, where it meets the red blood cells coming from the processor, and together they return to the patients. The cycle is repeated until about two plasma volumes are attained.

The ACD-A formula was used as anticoagulant on a 10% basis and careful verifications of the blood pressure were made. Whenever the patient had been submitted to hemofiltration due to renal failure, a plasmaperfusion was carried out by utilizing the arterial and venous connections of the hemofiltration filter itself, in such a way that we had three parallel systems going on at the same time. The *hemofiltration* allowing a flow to the *plasmapheresis*; and the plasmapheresis furnishing material to the *plasmaperfusion*. The procedure was repeated every other day, whenever there was evidence of an improvement — until stabilization was reached — or until the patient came to an extreme degree of clinical worsening. Readings were obtained before and about 90 min after the procedures.

RESULTS

There was no problem with the blood flow in all patients studied, the mean time spent being, 2.5 h. There was no need for volume replacement.

Table 1 shows the main hemodynamic variables obtained. One can notice that there were no significant changes in the cardiac index, in the filling pressures and/or in relation to oxygen transportation, nevertheless we call attention to the index of oxygen extraction, which was significantly better after the procedures.

Table 1.
Swan-Ganz catheter — results

	Baseline	Follow-up
Cardiac index (l/min/m)	4.5 ± 1.0	4.4 ± 1.0
Wedge pressure (mmHg)	15.3 ± 3.6	16.3 ± 3.4
Left ventricular systolic work index (kg/min/m^2)	44.2 ± 13.1	44.1 ± 14.4
Oxygen delivery (ml/min)	676 ± 148	632 ± 167
Oxygen consumption (ml/min)	123 ± 38	149 ± 40
Oxygen extraction (%)	18 ± 6	25 ± 8*

*$P < 0.05$.

No hemolysis was observed, once the erythrocytes are deviated from the filter through plasmapheresis, and the degree of trombocytopaenia observed did not concern us clinically.

DISCUSSION

We know that some active substances have the capacity for being absorbed in different surfaces [4], and we know that charcoal is able to remove substances with a molecular weight under 5000 daltons [5]. Among known substances we can mention histamine, serotomine, PGE, tromboxane, bradykinin, etc. (Table 2). We cannot yet tell exactly which of the substances involved in the septic shock are being removed in this system.

Table 2.
Weight of mediators

Substance	Daltons
Histamine	127
Serotonine	210
PGE	600
Tromboxane	600
Leukotrienes	600
B-Endorphin	4056
MDF	1000
Bradykinin	1060

We suppose the increase of the oxygen extraction index is due to a redistribution of the blood flow and/or to an increase of the metabolic activity in the cells, induced by the undertaken procedures. This can surely be modifying the natural course of the infected and seriously ill patient. We hope that we will be able to answer some questions which remain unanswered, in the future: What substances are we dealing with? What is the ideal amount of plasma to be processed? What is the frequency of the procedure? When to start the procedure? Are not we possibly indicating the procedure too late?

Acknowledgments
The authors thank all colleagues who work at Albert Einstein Hospital's Blood Bank and Intensive Care Unit for their help.

REFERENCES

1. L. Gotloib, E. Barzilay, A. Shostak *et al.* Hemofiltration in septic ARDS. The artificial kidney as an artificial endocrine lung. *Resuscitation*, **13**, 123–132 (1986).

2. S. Bende and L. Bertók. Elimination of endotoxin from the blood by extracorporeal activated charcoal hemoperfusion in experimental canine endotoxin shock. *Circ. Shock*, **19**, 239–244 (1986).

3. K. Werdan, G. Pilz and S. Kääb. Hemodynamic effects during treatment of sepsis and septic shock with immunoglobulins and plasmapheresis. *Second Vienna Shock Forum*, pp. 1025–1030 (1989).

4. G. K. Bysani, J. L. Shenep, W. K. Hildner *et al.* Detoxification of plasma containing lipopolysaccharide by adsorption. *Crit. Care Med.*, **18**, 67 (1990).

5. B. Ditter, R. Urbaschek and B. Urbaschek. Ability of various adsorbents to bind endotoxins *in vitro* and to prevent orally induced endotoxemia in mice. *Gastroenterology*, **84**, 1547–1552 (1983).

Therapeutic Plasmapheresis (XII), pp. 513-518
T. Agishi *et al.* (Eds)
© VSP 1993

Emergency Plasmapheresis

M. TAKAHASHI, N. KAMII, K. ONODERA, H. WITMANOWSKI, J. MEGURO,
K. KUKITA, M. YONEKAWA and A. KAWAMURA

*Department of Surgery, Sapporo Hokuyu Hospital, Artificial Organ
and Transplantation Hospital, Sapporo, Japan*

Key words: plasma exchange; cryofiltration; double filtration plasmapheresis.

INTRODUCTION

Emergency plasmapheresis is required for the treatment of fulminant hepatic failure, multiple myeloma (MM) and rhabdomyolysis to prevent further progression and complication. This report presents the efficacy of plasmapheresis in these diseases.

MATERIALS AND METHODS

Nineteen patients with fulminant hepatic failure (FHF) were treated with plasmapheresis; 18 patients with plasma exchange (PE), 14 with cryofiltration (Cryo) and one with bilirubin adsorption (BA).

Sixteen patients with MM were treated with plasmapheresis; three patients with PE, 14 with Cryo and two with double filtration plasmapheresis (DFPP). Thirteen patients had renal failure and nine patients required hemodialysis. Two patients with rhabdomyolysis were treated with Cryo, one of whom had a complicated renal failure.

In the PE procedures, large amounts of fresh frozen plasma (FFP) (4–6 l) were required for each treatment. The Cryo system was constructed from a plasma separator, cryofilter and cooling chamber. The DFPP system was constructed from a plasma separator and plasma filter. In the Cryo and DFPP procedures, the plasma volume processed per each treatment was 4 l.

RESULTS

Fulminant hepatic failure
We had 11 females and eight males. The average age was 40.2 years old and survival rate was 36.8%. Comparing surviving and non-surviving cases, the etiology, the sex and the age were not significantly different between the two groups. At the point of frequency of plasma exchange, there were no significant differences between the two groups. Most patients of the non-surviving group were treated with hemodialysis to correct the electrolytes and to reduce brain edema (Table 1).

Table 1.
Treatment of fulminant hepatic failure

	PE	PE Cryo	PE Cryo BA	Cryo	with HD	Improvement of consciousness
Survival	0	5	1	1	2	7
$(n = 7)$		$\begin{pmatrix} 5.4 \pm 4.5 \\ 5.6 \pm 2.6 \end{pmatrix}$	$\begin{pmatrix} 3 \\ 6 \\ 2 \end{pmatrix}$	(2)	(28.5%)	(100%)
Dead	5	7	0	0	8	9
$(n = 12)$	(7.6±6.3)	$\begin{pmatrix} 5.6 \pm 3.8 \\ 2.1 \pm 1.0 \end{pmatrix}$			(66.7%)	(75%)

About the complication: four cardiac failure, one severe urticaria and one anaphylactic shock were observed. But no complications of Cryo were observed. The values of liver CT volume of survivors and non-survivors on admission day were 1200±240 and 710 ± 315 ml, respectively. On the 7th day of over 10 day survivors, the differences of the liver volume between the two groups were significant (Fig. 1). Liver CT volume of most survival cases increased gradually by every week, but those of non-surviving cases did not increase (Fig. 2).

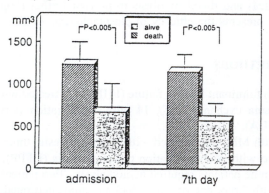

Figure 1. Changes of liver CT volume.

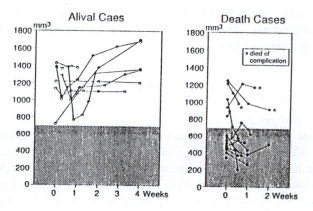

Figure 2. Changes of liver CT volume.

Multiple myeloma

Eight females and males were treated with emergency plasmapheresis. The average age was 60 years old. Treatment type were one case of PE alone, two of PE and Cryo, 11 of Cryo and DFPP, and one of DFPP alone. The prognosis of 13 patients with renal failure was poor. Only two patients who did not require hemodialysis survived. Eleven patients died of myeloma or complications other than renal failure within 6 months. Three patients without renal failure survive now (Fig. 3). The average removal of total protein, IgG and IgA were 16.8, 19 and 24%, respectively (Fig. 4). The blood viscosity in one case was reduced to 75% after five Cryo procedures. Of 10 patients who were undergoing hemodialysis, only one patient could be released from hemodialysis. Her serum BUN was 96 mg/dl, serum creatinine was 11.8 mg/dl, and daily diuresis was less than 100 ml on admission. By frequent Cryo and hemodialysis, urinary volume increased and serum creatinine was gradually lowered. Following 13 Cryo treatments, she was given five DFPP treatments. She recovered well enough to stop dialysis treatment after 40 days (Fig. 5).

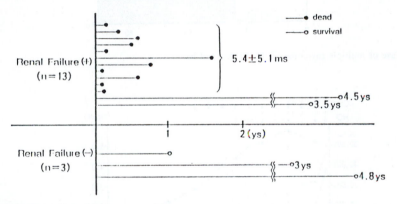

Figure 3. Renal failure and prognosis of multiple myeloma patients.

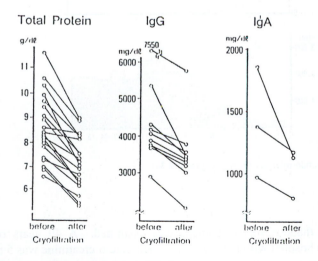

Figure 4. Protein removal from plasma by cryofiltration.

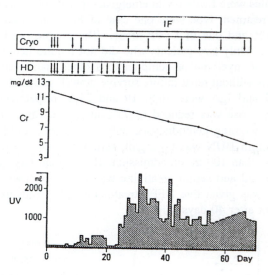

Figure 5. Case of multiple myeloma (T. N. 43 year old F).

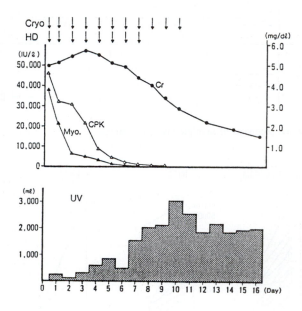

Figure 6. Case of rhabdomyolysis (T. K., 49 year old M).

Rhabdomyolysis

One of the two rhabdomyolysis patients was examined. A 49 years old man was transferred to our hospital with left leg trauma. His serum creatinine was 5 mg/dl, serum myoglobin and creatinine phosphokinase were very high and daily diuresis was almost zero on admission. By frequent Cryo and hemodialysis, urinary volume increased and serum myoglobin and CPK were markedly decreased. The serum creatinine decreased to within normal limits after 16 days (Fig. 6).

DISCUSSION

PE has been the first choice for FHF in recent years and this treatment effectively improved consciousness in our cases. The aim of Cryo is to reduce the antibodies and the immunomodulation, and we think it is worth-while for FHF patients after consciousness improves [1]. As an indicator of the prognosis of the patient with FHF, the liver volume calculated by CT was very useful [2]. If the liver CT volume is more than 700 ml at any point, we can predict good prognosis of the patients. We lost four patients complicated by cardiac failure. First we used large amounts of FFP (6 l), and this was the main reason for cardiac failure. After this experience, we have used 4 l FFP, and we have not experienced such complications.

PE has been considered the most rational way to remove large amounts of light chains that are thought to play a major causative role in renal damage due to multiple myeloma [3]. However, there are some risks of viral infections and complication with PE [4]. Furthermore, PE is costly and requires large volumes of FFP. To avoid such risks, we have applied Cryo and DFPP. These procedures can remove macromolecules such as fibrinogen and immunoglobulin from plasma, and retain the relatively small molecular components in plasma without FFP [5]. Although the efficiency of light chain reduction by Cryo compared with PE has not been clarified yet, we have detected light chains in cryogel [6]. In addition, there is a possibility that the decrease of blood viscosity, which is a consequence of the reduction in macromolecules is a result of Cryo and DFPP, supports renal circulation.

More than 50% of patients with multiple myeloma have renal failure at the time of diagnosis and uremia is the second most common cause of death [7]. At the time of diagnosis, the possibility of recovery from renal failure cannot be evaluated, so early treatment with a combination of hemodialysis and Cryo is recommended in cases of renal failure due to multiple myeloma [8].

The same treatment is recommended in cases of renal failure due to rhabdomyolysis. About the plasmapheresis for rhabdomyolysis, some reports recommend PE [9] and some reports do not [10]. To the best of our knowledge Cryo has not been previously attempted in the treatment of rhabdomyolysis associated myoglobin-induced damage of the kidney. As evidenced by the case history presented Cryo may be considered an adjunct to conventional therapy whenever risk of renal damage is imminent.

REFERENCES

1. M. Yonekawa, H. Witmanowski, K. Kukita, J. Meguro, A. Kawamura, K. Takeda, M. Takahashi and H. Furui. Indication and efficacy of plasmapheresis in acute hepatic failure. *Proc. Jpn. Soc. Ther. Eng.*, 3, 158–161 (1991).
2. K. Kukita, J. Meguro, M. Yonekawa, A. Kawamura, N. Abe, K. Seto, N. Kobayashi, T. Irie, T. Higa, M. Kasai, T. Ariyama and K. Makita. The relationship between prognosis and periodic liver CT volume change in patients with fulminant hepatitis. *Geka*, 51, 290–293 (1989).
3. P. Zucchelli, S. Pasquali, L. Gagnoli and G. Ferrari. Controlled plasma exchange trial in acute renal failure due to multiple myeloma. *Kidney Int.*, 33, 1175–1180 (1988).

4. M. Yonekawa, J. Meguro, K. Kukita, A. Kawamura, N. Abe, K. Seto, N. Kobayashi, T. Irie, K. Kawamura, T. Higa, M. Kasai, T. Ariyama, H. Furui and K. Makita. Positive and negative effect of plasma exchange. *Artif. Organs*, **14**, 185–187 (1990).

5. M. Yonekawa, A. Kawamura, K. Kukita, J. Meguro, K. Kawamura, N. Kobayashi, K. Imai, S. Takahashi and T. Komai. Cryofiltration for treatment of immune complex diseases. In: *Therapeutic Plasmapheresis (VIII)*, pp. 167–170, ISAO Press, Cleveland (1988).

6. K. Kukita, J. Meguro, M. Yonekawa, A. Kawamura, H. Furui, K. Makita, N. Abe, K. Seto, T. Irie, T. Naohara, K. Kawamura, T. Higa, M. Kasai and S. Takahashi. Therapeutic trials of cryofiltration in patients with myeloma kidney. In: *Therapeutic Plasmapheresis (IX)*, pp. 56–60, ISAO Press, Cleveland (1989).

7. R. A. De Fronzo, C. R. Cooke, J. R. Wright and R. L. Humphrey. Renal function in patients with multiple myeloma. *Medicine*, **57**, 151–166 (1978).

8. M. Yonekawa, H. Witmanowski, K. Kukita, J. Meguro, A. Kawamura, K. Kawamura, T. Higa, M. Kasai, K. Takeda, M. Takahashi and H. Furui. Efficacy of plasmapheresis in patients with multiple myeloma. In: *Therapeutic Plasmapheresis (X)*, pp. 573–576, ISAO Press, Cleveland (1990).

9. W. P. Paaske, P. Gagl, J. E. Lorentzen and K. Olgaard. Plasma exchange after revascularization compartment syndrome with acute toxic nephropathy caused by rhabdomyolysis. *J. Vasc. Surg.*, **7**, 757–758 (1988).

10. J. J. Cornelissen, W. Haaustra, H. J. T. M. Haarman and R. H. W. M. Derksen. Plasma exchange in rhabdomyolysis. *Intensive Care Med.*, **15**, 528–529 (1989).

Therapeutic Plasmapheresis (XII), pp. 519-522
T. Agishi *et al.* (Eds)
© VSP 1993

Treatment of Septic Shock by Extracorporeal Elimination of Endotoxin using Fiber-immobilized Polymyxin B

H. AOKI, T. TANI, K. HANASAWA, Y. ENDO, K. MATSUDA, T. YOSHIOKA, K. NUMA, H. ARAKI, Y. TSUTAMOTO and M. KODAMA

First Department of Surgery, Shiga University of Medical Science, Otsu, Shiga, Japan

Key words: septic shock; endotoxin; multiple organ failure; polymyxin B; hemoperfusion.

INTRODUCTION

Septic shock, a life threatening complication of serious Gram-negative bacterial infection, is a major cause of irreversible hypotension, multiple organ failure (MOF) and death [1]. Despite the use of potent antibiotics and intensive supportive care, the mortality rate in patients with septicemia or septic shock remains high. Septic shock is considered to be caused by entry of endotoxin into the body in Gram-negative infection. Polymyxin B is long known to neutralize the various biological activities of endotoxin [2]. However, polymyxin B that enters into the body has renal toxicity and neurotoxicity. We chemically immobilized polymyxin B on insoluble fibrous carriers in 1983 and have developed a method to adsorb and remove endotoxin in the blood without releasing polymyxin B [3, 4]. In this study, DHP using polymyxin B immobilized fiber column was used for one to several sessions in a patient with severe septicemia or septic MOF, and its effects were evaluated by a multi-center clinical study.

SUBJECTS AND METHODS

A clinical study was carried out at six institutions during the 2-year period from February, 1989. PMX for 2 h was performed 1–7 times in patients with severe septicemia or septic MOF in whom other treatment methods were not effective. We evaluated the changes in various circulatory parameters, symptoms of septic shock and blood endotoxin concentration after this treatment, and the survival rate.

RESULTS

DHP was performed for 61 sessions in 42 patients, of whom 38 had septic MOF. Twenty five patients had Gram-negative bacterial infection, and eight had Gram-positive bacterial infection. Twenty-two of the 42 patients survived. DHP was performed once in 30 patients and 2–7 times in another 12 patients. At the time of the initiation of this treatment, 33 patients were receiving an anti-hypotensive drug and 36 were under artificial ventilation via endotracheal intubation. Treatment effects were evaluated after

50 DHP in patients showing a blood endotoxin concentration of 9.8 mg/ml. The endotoxin concentration (mean ± SE; pg/ml) was 85.0 ± 27.2 immediately before treatment
but significantly decreased to 57.5 ± 28.4 after treatment ($n = 50$) and to 28.2 ± 4/4 on
the next day ($n = 23$) ($P < 0.01$). The endotoxin concentration at the inlet and outlet
of the PMX also significantly decreased 30 min after the initiation of DHP (Fig. 1).
The dosage of the antihypotensive drug could be reduced after treatment in six of the
33 patients, and drug was discontinued in eight. Artificial ventilation was discontinued
in three patients. As antipyretic effects, in patients with a body temperature of 38 °C or
more before treatment ($n = 21$), the mean value was 38.9 ± 0.2 °C before treatment but
significantly decreased to 38.4 ± 0.2 °C immediately after treatment and to 38.0 ± 0.2 °C

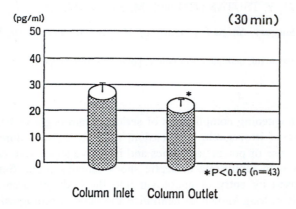

Figure 1. Endotoxin concentration.

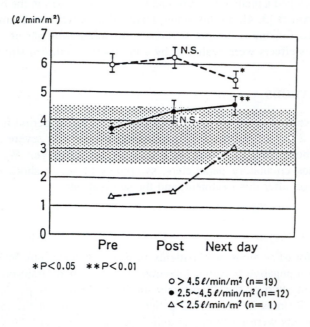

Figure 2. Changes of CI.

on the next day ($P < 0.01$ each). In patients in whom the systolic arterial pressure (mmHg) was maintained at 90 or more with an anti-hypotensive drug ($n = 28$), the mean value was 125 ± 4.7 before treatment but significantly increased to 128 ± 4.7 on the next day ($P < 0.01$). In patients with values less than 90, the mean pressure also significantly increased both immediately after treatment and on the next day. In patients with a pre-treatment cardiac index (CI: $l/min/m^2$) of 2.5 or less, the mean value was 1.3 immediately before treatment but significantly increased to 3.1 on the next day ($P < 0.01$). In patients in a hyperdynamic state showing a pre-treatment value of 4.5 or more ($n = 19$), the mean value was 6.0 ± 2.2 immediately after treatment but decreased to 5.5 ± 0.3 on the next day ($P < 0.05$) (Fig. 2). In patients in a hyperdynamic state showing a pre-treatment systemic vascular resistance (SVR: dyne s cm^{-5}) of less than 1000 ($n = 18$), the mean value was 647 ± 36.5 immediately before treatment, 729 ± 51.4 immediately after treatment, but 839 ± 71.4 on the next day ($P < 0.01$); the systemic vascular resistance significantly increased, showing a tendency to normalization. As side effects of PMX, the platelet count decreased but began to increase before the termination of DHP and recovered to the pre-DHP level on the next day. In patients with a platelet count of less than 50 000, the value did not decrease and rather increased. There was no increase in bleeding tendency or danger of hemorrhage during treatment.

DISCUSSION

In recent years, the mechanism of septic shock has been clarified, and the involvement of many mediators and cytokines has been suggested. Treatment methods to inhibit each mediator or cytokine have been developed and reported. Anti-LPS antibody treatment has been developed by the Centcore and Xoma Co. Ziegler *et al.* [5] reported the effects of a single administration of monoclonal antibody in a large-scale clinical study. However, in their reports, improvement in symptoms of endotoxemia by removal of endotoxin and improvement in the endotoxin concentration were not evaluated, and the mechanism of the effects of anti-LPS antibody was not clarified. In our study, patients had intractable disease that did not respond to various other methods. Thirty-eight of 42 patients had MOF, 33 were receiving anti-hypotensive drug and 36 were under artificial ventilation via endotracheal intubation. The subjects in our study had very severe conditions. The survival rate by PMX therapy was more than 50% (22/42). PMX treatment markedly alleviated symptoms of sepsis syndrome. A study on endotoxin infusion in humans has shown marked changes in circulatory parameters such as blood pressure, CI and SVR, and parameters of metabolism such as lactic acidosis [6]. In our study, similar abnormalities were observed. After PMX treatment, the use of an anti-hypotensive drug was discontinued, or its dosage was reduced in many patients. Abnormal endotoxin concentration before treatment significantly decreased after treatment. The endotoxin further decreased on the next day, the elimination rate being 66%. This clinical study on PMX treatment is the first to confirm responses to the removal of endotoxin from the blood and at least demonstrates that reduction or elimination of endotoxin in the blood is useful for treating severe septicemia. A side effect of PMX treatment is a decrease in the platelet count. However, the platelet count slightly increased in patients showing a value of 50 000 or less. This suggests that PMX treatment is effective in patients in critical conditions with DIC as a complication. No patient showed aggravation of bleeding tendency or bleeding after DHP. Further studies are needed on the duration and frequency of DHP.

CONCLUSION

Removal of endotoxin in the blood using PMX was effective for severe septicemia or septic MOF, and the effects were observed within 24 h. Various symptoms due to endotoxin were alleviated after this treatment.

REFERENCES

1. B. E. Kreger, D. E. Craven and W. R. Mccabe. Gram-negative bacteremia. Reevaluation of clinical features and treatment in 612 patients. *Am. J. Med.*, **68**, 344–355 (1980).
2. J. D. Palmer and D. Rifkind. Neutralization of the hemodynamic effects of endotoxin by polymyxin B. *Surg. Gynecol. Obstet.*, **138**, 755–759 (1974).
3. H. Aoki, T. Yoshioka and T. Tani. Fundamental study on detoxifying capacity by endotoxin adsorbing materials. *Jpn. J. Artif. Organs.*, **17**, 583–586 (1988).
4. K. Hanasawa, T. Tani and M. Kodama. New approach to endotoxic and septic shock by means of polymyxin B immobilized fiber. *Surg. Gynecol. Obstet.*, **168**, 323–331 (1989).
5. E. Ziegler, C. J. Fisher, C. L. Sprung *et al*. Treatment of Gram-negative bacteremia and septic shock with HA-1A human monoclonal antibody against endotoxin. *N. Engl. J. Med.*, **324**, 429–436 (1991).
6. A. F. Suffredini, R. E. Fromm, M. M. Parker *et al*. The cardiovascular response of normal human to the administration of endotoxin. *N. Engl. J. Med.*, **321**, 280–287 (1989).

12
Immunoadsorption

Therapeutic Plasmapheresis (XII), pp. 525-529
T. Agishi *et al*. (Eds)
© VSP 1993

Clinical and Technical Problems in the Treatment of Myasthenia Gravis by Immunoadsorption

M. NISHIMURA and N. FUJII

Asou Iizuka Hospital, Iizuka, Japan

Key words: immunoadsorption; Myasthenia gravis.

INTRODUCTION

Myasthenia gravis (MG) is a well-known autoimmune disease, characterized by muscle weakness due to impaired neuromuscular transmission. Autoantibodies against acetyl-choline receptor (AchR) are detected in about 90% of MG patients [1]. Recently, it is said that immunotherapy using immunoadsorbent columns bring about clinical success in the treatment of MG, especially in serious situations. However, several problems exist with this alternative therapy. We have treated five MG patients in the past 2 years.
    We report on the clinical and technical problems in this interesting therapy.

PATIENTS AND METHODS

We treated five MG patients between May 1990 and June 1991. Of these patients (two males, three females), thymectomies were done in three patients (cases 1–3) preceding immunoadsorption therapy, the remainder (cases 4 and 5) received this treatment as a pre-operative therapeutic method. The age distribution was 22–59 years, with a mean of 37.4 years. According to Osserman's classification, they were in group 2A or 4 (Table 1). Treatment was carried out using plasmaflo AP-05H plasmaseparators and TR-350 immunoadsorbent columns produced by Asahi Medical Co. TR-350 consist of micro spheres of synthetic resin embedded in a polyvinyl alcohol gel with tryptophan as a ligand.

Table 1.
Patient profiles

Case	Sex	Age	Years of disease	Thymectomy	Anti AchR Ab	Classification Osserman	Previous therapy
1	M	46	7	+	+	4	prednisolone
2	F	25	1	+	+	2A	ambenonium
3	F	22	2	+	−	2A	prednisolone
4	F	35	9	−	+	2A	pyridostigmine
5	M	59	2	−	+	2A	ambenonium

Blood flow was maintained at 120–150 ml/min and plasma flow through the immunocolumn was 30–40 ml/min.

The interval between each session was 1–2 weeks. Total perfused plasma volume was 1800–2800 ml per session. Before each plasma perfusion, the next day and one month later, the following laboratory tests were obtained: anti-AchR binding antibody, anti-AchR blocking antibody, fibrinogen and lymphocyte subsets. The normal range of anti-AchR binding antibody is under 0.16 pmol/ml and that of anti-AchR blocking antibody (binding rate) is over 90%. Statistical analyses were not done because of the small number of patients.

RESULTS

After each session, all of the patients showed an early clinical improvement in bulbar symptoms and limb power.

Table 2.
Clinical outcomes

Case	No. of sessions	Total perfused plasma volume (ml)	Relapse within 3 months	Treatments when relapsed	Outcomes after 6 months
1	2	5000	–		remission
2	2	5000	–		remission
3	3	7700	+10 days after	increase of drugs	remission
4	3	6200	+17 days after	increase of drugs	remission
5	1	2000	+ 5 days after	increase of drugs	remission

Although three of them relapsed within a month, to be exact 5–17 days, they recovered and attained to remission for the sake of an increase of steroids or other drugs (Table 2). Anti-AchR binding antibody decreased on the next day with the mean reduction rate of 49%. On the other hand, serum concentration of anti-AchR blocking antibody (binding rate) altered, unexpectedly, from 89.9 to 67.8% for the session. The reduction rate was 24.6% and slightly recovered 1 month later. The concentration of fibrinogen decreased to about half that at the beginning of session, from 271.2 to 151.2 mg/dl. As to lymphocyte subsets, four patients were evaluated.

OKT3 and OKT4A changed in various manners 1 month later, OKT8 was slightly raised in all and OKT4A/OKT8 decreased in all except one (Figs 1–4).

DISCUSSION

All our patients showed both clinical improvements and a decrease in anti-AchR binding antibody concentration, which eventually reached previous levels.

In spite of the recovery of that antibody, they could get along. It seemed that the causative antibodies of MG are heterogenous [2].

Drugs may act effectively after immunoadsorption therapy. However, the ability of autoantibodies adsorption is limited. Contrary to our expectation, anti-AchR blocking

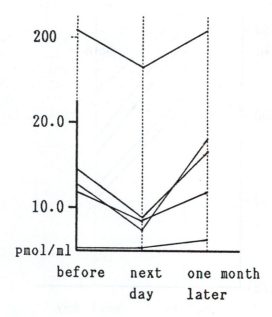

Figure 1. Anti-AchR binding antibody.

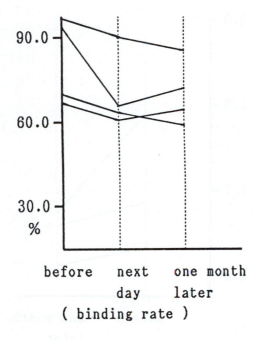

Figure 2. Anti-AchR blocking antibody.

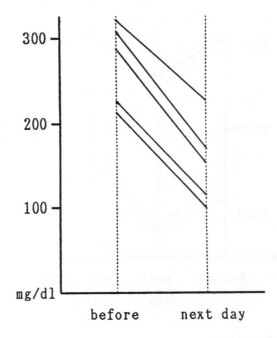

Figure 3. Fibrinogen.

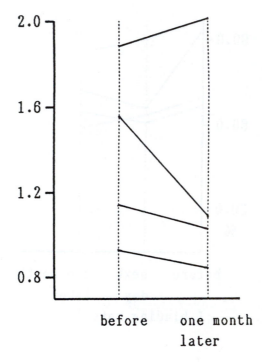

Figure 4. OKT4A/OKT8.

antibody (binding rate) also decreased. Adsorption of fibrinogen was prominent. We were troubled by the increase of pressure at the inlet of a column by fibrin formation. Immunoadsorption does not have important effects on T lymphocytes.

REFERENCES

1. P. C. Dau *et al.* Plasmapheresis and immunosuppresive drug therapy in myasthenia gravis. *N. Eng. J. Med.*, **297**, 1134–1140 (1977).

2. A. D. Roses *et al.* No direct correlation between serum antiacetylcholine receptor antibody levels and clinical state of individual patients with myasthenia gravis. *Neurology*, **31**, 220–224 (1981).

Therapeutic Plasmapheresis (XII), pp. 531-534
T. Agishi *et al.* (Eds)
© VSP 1993

Immmunoadsorption Plasmapheresis and Plasma Exchange in Guillain–Barré Syndrome

T. SHINODA, C.-S. KOH,[1] H. ARAKURA, E. YAMAGAMI,
M. KATAKURA and N. YANAGISAWA[1]

*Department of Artificial Organ Treatment and [1]Department of Medicine (Neurology),
Shinshu University School of Medicine, Matsumoto, Japan*

Key words: Guillain–Barré syndrome; immunoadsorption plasmapheresis; plasma exchange; immediate effect; long-term effect.

INTRODUCTION

Plasma exchange (PE) [1–3] and high-dose steroid therapy [4] has been considered as the first choice of treatment for Guillain–Barré Syndrome (GBS). On the other hand, the therapeutic value of immunoadsorption plasmapheresis (IAPP) for GBS was recently reported [5–7]. The present study was designed to critically compare the effectiveness of IAPP and PE as the treatment of GBS in a prospective manner.

PATIENTS AND METHODS

Six patients with GBS (four men and two women, age 34–76 years) were treated with IAPP and another five patients with GBS (four men and one woman, age 12–47 years) were treated with PE (Table 1); the results of PE therapy of the five patients were previously reported [3]. All patients agreed to participate in the study with informed consent. The age was significantly different between the two patient groups (P < 0.05 by Mann–Whitney test). The criteria to start IAPP in patients with GBS were exactly the same as in the case of PE [3]; (i) within 14 days from the onset, (ii) in Grades 4 or 5 according to the grading scale of the Guillain–Barré Syndrome Study Group [1], and (iii) not receiving corticosteroids.

The protocol for IAPP was essentially the same as that for PE [3] except for using an adsorption column (PH-350; Asahi Medical, Tokyo, Japan) instead of 4.4% diluted albumin solution (Plasma Protein Fraction, Baxter Healthcare, Glendale, CA) as replacement fluid. The IAPP and PE were made two sessions or more per week (every day for severe cases). The plasma volume processed in IAPP was 35 ml/kg body weight/session or more. The same plasma separators (AP-05, OP-05; Asahi Medical, Tokyo, Japan or FS-05; Kanegafuchi Chemical, Osaka, Japan) and control machines (KEM-21; Nikkiso, Tokyo, Japan or KL-30; Kawasumi Laboratories, Tokyo, Japan) were used in both treatments.

The efficacy of IAPP and PE was judged by clinical signs and symptoms. Immediate effects were qualitatively classified into four classes: (−): progression in spite of treatments, (±): a little improvement in a plateau phase, (+): cessation of the progress and (++): evident improvement in both progress and plateau phases. Long-term effects were evaluated by the following three points; the Grades at 4 weeks and 6 months after the first treatment, and the time needed to reach Grade 2. Statistical analyses were made by chi-square tests or Mann–Whitney tests for appropriate cases.

RESULTS

Immediate effects of IAPP and PE therapies were comparable (Table 1). Immediate improvement was seen in respiratory paralysis, bulbar palsy and muscle weakness of the face and extremities. Improvement was not evident in one patient in each group: both patients were in a plateau phase (14 and 6 days from the onset, respectively).

Table 1.
Immediate effect

Case no.	Age (years)	Sex	Grade	Onset (days)	Phase	Immediate effect	Sessions by the effect
IAPP Group							
1	34	F	4	−12	progress	++	1
2	76	M	4	−10	progress	++	1
3	54	F	4	−14	plateau	±	2
4	39	M	4–5	−3	progress	++	2
5	75	M	4	−14	progress	++	2
6	68	M	4–5	−8	progress	++	1
PE Group							
7	47	M	4	−6	plateau	±	2
8	20	M	4–5	−6	progress	+	3
9	12	M	4	−10	progress	++	1
10	17	F	4	−5	progress	++	2
11	12	M	5	−3	progress	++	1

M male; F female.

Long-term effects of the two treatments were also comparable with respect to the Grades at 4 weeks and 6 months (Fig. 1). On the other hand, the time to reach Grade 2 seemed to be shorter in the IAPP Group (14, 14 and 21 days vs 28, 42, 150, 150 and 450 days in the PE Group), although only three patients were available in the IAPP group for the comparison. Concerning the remaining three patients, one patient (case 3) did not reach Grade 2 within the follow-up period of 6 months, and another two patients (cases 5 and 6) were not followed up for more than 4 weeks in the IAPP Group.

Two patients (one in each group, cases 3 and 7) in a plateau phase at the initiation of the treatments did not reach Grade 3 by 4 weeks and Grade 2 by 6 months. An additional patient in the IAPP Group (case 5) was in progress at the initiation of IAPP and showed an immediate effect but did not reach Grade 3 by 4 weeks. Others reached Grade 3 or less by 4 weeks and Grade 2 or less by 6 months.

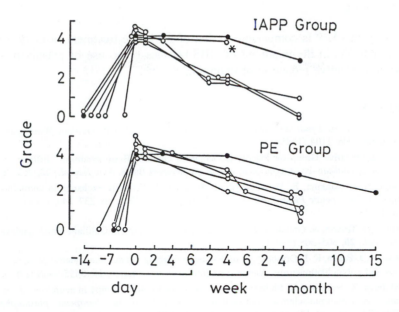

Figure 1. Clinical course. IAPP or PE were started on day 0. Open and closed circles shows patients in progressive and plateau phases, respectively.

Transient hypotension, which was easily recovered by saline infusion, was the only adverse effect observed in both treatments. Reduction rates of immunoglobulins by IAPP and PE were examined in one patient (case 5) who received both treatments. The rates were 27 and 64% for IgG, 15 and 64% for IgA and 39 and 70% for IgM, respectively.

DISCUSSION

The present study indicates that the efficacy of IAPP in the treatment of GBS is comparable to that of PE with respect to both immediate and long-term effects. Although the study was not a randomized trial, the two treatment groups were comparable with respect to clinical status, except for age.

The clinical courses of cases 3 and 7 suggest the hypothesis that both IAPP and PE are ineffective in patients with GBS in a plateau phase even though the onset of neurological symptoms is very recent. In other words, IAPP and PE protect the development of neural injury in GBS by removal of humoral pathogenic factor(s) or modulation of cellular immunity, but do not accelerate the recovery of the established neural injury. This hypothesis may be also suggested from the fact that high-dose steroid therapy [4] but not conventional steroid therapy [8] is effective in the treatment of GBS. The former may more effectively remove humoral factor(s) or modulate cellular immunity in the early stage of GBS. Thus, it may be critical in the treatment of GBS to prevent the progression of neural injury during the early stage of the disease before the injury becomes too severe and unresponsive to the therapeutic maneuvers.

The result of long-term follow-up suggests that the grade at 4 weeks predicts patients' prognosis. The prognosis may be poor unless patients do not reach Grade 3 or less by 4 weeks with IAPP or PE treatment.

CONCLUSIONS

The efficacy of IAPP is comparable to that of PE in the treatment of GBS. IAPP may be superior to PE in the treatment of GBS because of no use of plasma preparations and less non-selective reduction of immunoglobulins.

REFERENCES

1. The Guillain–Barré Syndrome Study Group. Plasmapheresis and acute Guillain–Barré syndrome. *Neurology*, **35**, 1096–1104 (1985).

2. French Cooperative Group on Plasma Exchange in Guillain–Barré syndrome. Efficiency of plasma exchange in Guillain–Barré syndrome: role of replacement fluids. *Ann. Neurol.*, **22**, 753–761 (1987).

3. T. Shinoda, H. Arakura, E. Yamagami *et al.* Reappraisal of plasma exchange in Guillain–Barré syndrome. In: *Therapeutic Plasmapheresis (IX)*, N. Koga *et al.* (Eds), pp. 237–240, ICAOT Press, Cleveland (1991).

4. A. Haaß, N. Trabert, N. Greßnich *et al.* High-dose steroid therapy in Gulillain–Barré syndrome. *J. Neuroimmunol.*, **20**, 305–308 (1988).

5. J. Nikolay, J. Braun, K. F. Druschky, *et al.* Klinische erfarung mit der immunoadsorption bei myasthenia gravis und polyradikuloneuritis. *Nieren- und Hochdruckkrankheiten*, **16**, S455-S460 (1987).

6. N. Shibuya, K. Nagasato, K. Shibayama *et al.* Immunoadsoption therapy in neurologic diseases: myasthenia gravis, multiple sclerosis, and Guillain–Barré syndrome. In: *Therapeutic plasmapheresis (VI)*, T. Oda (Ed.), pp. 122–128, ISAO Press, Cleveland (1987).

7. K. Ujiie, H. Kamet..ni, M. Suenaga *et al.* Efficiency of immunoadsorption plasmapheresis in Guillain–Barré syndrome. In: *Therapeutic Plasmapheresis (IX)*, N. Koga *et al.* (Eds), pp. 227–231, ICAOT Press, Cleveland (1991).

8. R. A. C. Hughes, J. M. Newsom–Davis, G. D. Perkin *et al.* Controlled trial of prednisolone in acute polyneuropathy. *Lancet*, **2**, 750–753 (1978).

Therapeutic Plasmapheresis (XII), pp. 535-539
T. Agishi *et al.* (Eds)

Red Cell Mediated Adsorption of Immune Complexes

K. TSUKUI, K. SHINOZAKI and K. NISHIOKA

Central Blood Center, The Japanese Red Cross, Japan

INTRODUCTION

Complement receptor type 1 (CR-1) is a receptor for C3b or C4b. It is a single polypeptide with four LHRs (A, B, C, D) and each LHRs has seven SCRs consisting of 60–70 amino acids [1]. As the red cell is the major constituent of blood cells, over 95% of CR-1 molecules are present on red cells [2].

Red cells have a primary roll to clear immune complexes by carrying them to hepatic macrophages by means of CR-1 [3, 4]. Although red cells from healthy individuals have 500–1000 CR-1 molecules on average [5, 6], red cells from patients with SLE or other autoimmune diseases, with rheumatic diseases or with severe infectious diseases show decreased activities of CR-1 [7–10]. Thus, transfusion of red cells with high CR-1 activities into these patients should be an effective therapy [10]. For this reason, to serve red cells for these patients, we analyzed the amount of surface CR-1 molecules of red cells from healthy blood donors.

MATERIALS AND METHODS

Red cells

Red cells from blood grouping tests were routinely used. The cells were washed with Dulbecco's phosphate buffered saline without Ca^{2+} and Mg^{2+} plus NaN_3 (0.01%). After washing 3 times, cell hematocrit was adjusted to 2% by the same buffer. For time kinetic analysis, blood was stored at 4 °C in CPD. After appropriate days of storage, small amounts were collected by syringes.

Antibodies

Mouse anti-CR-1 monoclonal antibody (moAb; clone C3RTo5) and goat $F(ab')_2$ fraction of anti-mouse IgG FITC antibodies (GAMIgG–FITC) were purchased.

Flow-cytometric (FCM) analysis

Twenty microliters of washed red cell preparations was inoculated with 30 μl of anti-CR-1 moAb (final concentration, 10 μg/ml) together with cytocharasin B (10 μg/ml) and gelatine (0.1%). After 30 min at 20 °C, red cells were washed 3 times and further inoculated with GAMIgG–FITC. After 60 min at 4 °C in the dark, cells were washed again and submitted for FCM analysis. As a negative control for first antibody, monoclonal mouse IgG was used.

Density separation of red cell fractions
Red cells were prepared mostly according to Lutz *et al.* [11]. In brief, blood mixed with
CPD was inoculated with a half volume of PBS(−)–NaN$_3$ plus 0.05 mM EDTA, and
passed through a Sephadex G-25 column at room temperature. Red cells were collected
and washed twice, then the hematocrit adjusted to 30%. Percoll was adjusted to an
initial density of 1.106 and salt concentration physiologically by adding concentrated
PBS(−), and adjusted the pH to 7.4. Red cell suspensions (500 μl) were gently applied
to 8.5 ml of Percoll in centrifugation tubes, and centrifuged in a Hitachi CR20B2
high speed centrifuge with a RPR18-3 angle rotor at 27000 *g* (bottom) for 30 min at
10 °C. Density marker beads were applied on Percoll of another tube and centrifuged
simultaneously.

RESULTS

Influence of F/P molar ratio of the second antibody (GAMIgG–FITC)
Results of FCM analysis were extremely affected by F/P molar ratio of the second
antibodies. Comparison between analyses of the same test preparation showed that the
second antibody with high F/P molar ratio was apt to show a higher value of CR-1

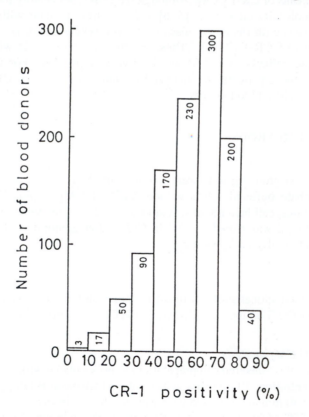

Figure 1. Distribution of Japanese healthy blood donors on CR-1 positivities. Red cells from 1100 Japanese
healthy blood donors were analyzed on CR-1 positivities by FCM. Numbers populated within 10% intervals
were indicated.

positivity, and resulted in showing very little differences between preparations. So, when the second antibodies, having a F/P molar ratio of 3.52 or 0.53, were used, values of 90.6% or 64.2% were obtained as the respective CR-1 positivities against the same red cell preparation. Thus, in order to compare the amount of surface CR-1 between preparations, second antibodies (F/P molar ratio, 2.5) were used hereafter.

CR-1 positivities of 1100 Japanese healthy blood donors

Analysis of CR-1 positivities against 1100 Japanese healthy blood donors is shown in Fig. 1. As indicated, around 70% of donors were distributed into up to 50% CR-1 positive groups. Within this group, about one fifth of donors showed the highest CR-1 positivities (>70%).

Change of surface CR-1 positivities during storage

Surface CR-1 positivities were analyzed if a change of the positivities occurred during storage at 4 °C. In Fig. 2, analysis of surface CR-1 periodically examined up to 37 days is shown for four red cell preparations. As indicated, irrespective of the level of CR-1 positivities, each preparation showed very little change during the period of storage.

Populational difference of CR-1 positivities

Even in a single preparation, the fluorescence intensity was widely distributed. Highly positive preparations contained a large amount of high intensity fractions and lower positive preparations showed a reverse correlation. Whether these distributions among preparations were caused by the existence of concomitant aged cell populations or not,

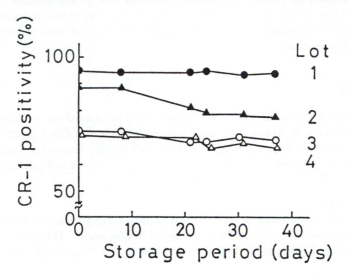

Figure 2. Effect on storage on CR-1 positivities. Red cells from four blood donors of different CR-1 positivities were stored at 4 °C under usual storage condition of blood for transfusion. On days 0, 8, 21, 24, 31 and 37, 2 ml samples were collected by syringe and analyzed for CR-1 positivities. Each symbols indicates individual preparations.

red cell fractions were separated by Percoll gradient and the CR-1 reactivity measured in each fraction. Although 10–20% differences between major fractions (light) and minor fractions (dense) were observed for CR-1 positivities, decay of the positivities was hardly observed on all six density separated fractions.

DISCUSSION

The effectiveness of red cell transfusion has already been observed in patients with SLE, rheumatoid arthritis and thrombotic thrombocytopenic purpura [10]. To perform the red cell transfusion protocol more effectively, analysis of surface CR-1 positivities was necessary to submit highly CR-1 positive red cells. If up to 70% of red cell preparations are highly positive and around 20% are extremely high on the CR-1 existencies as mentioned in this paper, half or more preparations of red cells from healthy Japanese volunteers should be able to be used for the purpose of this therapy, and around 20% for special cases. These red cells need not always be fresh, because 37 days storage affected least changes on CR-1 positivities at the usual 4°C condition. Red cells live for around 120 days *in vivo*, so even a single preparation of red cells should contain young to scenecent populations [11]. Definitely, many bands were separated on spontaneous Percoll gradient, but (i) 10–20% differences were observed between light and dense fractions on CR-1 positivities, (ii) decay of CR-1 hardly occurred in the all six fractions and (iii) only very little change of red cell amounts between separated bands were observed until 3 weeks storage, so large population of red cell preparations from Japanese healthy volunteers should be able to be used for the purpose of therapies to eliminate circulating immune complex.

For patients with AIDS, immune adherence activity of red cells by means of CR-1 was extremely decreased [12] and complement-opsonized HIV in the absence of antibody enhances infection of the virus into T cells [13], it is possible that transfusion of red cells of high CR-1 positivities adsorb the opsonized virus and immune complex, and improve the disease state.

CONCLUSION

From the results, it was concluded that: (i) about 70% of individuals were in the highly CR-1 positive group in which 20% were extremely high, (ii) CR-1 positivity on red cells was stable up to 3 weeks storage at 4°C, (iii) density separation indicated little affect of aged cell population on CR-1 positivities of the whole cell population.

Acknowledgments
We thanks to Dr Yahagi and Miss Miyazaki, Ortho Diagnostics, for their kind help with the FCM technique, and Mr Aoyama and Mr Kawamoto, Director and Chief of Diagnosis Section, Kawasaki Red Cross Blood Center, for their useful discussions.

REFERENCES

1. L. B. Klickstein, W. W. Wong, J. A. Smith *et al.* Human C3b/C4b receptor (CR-1). Demonstration of the long homologous repeating domains that are composed of the short consensus characteristic of C3/C4 binding proteins. *J. Exp. Med.*, **165**, 1095–1112 (1987).

2. I. Siegel, T. L. Liu and N. Gleicher. The red cell immune system. *Lancet*, i, 556–559 (1981).

3. J. B. Cornacoff, L. A. Hebert, W. L. Smead *et al.* Primate erythrocyte–immune complex-clearing mechanism. *J. Clin. Invest.*, 71, 236–247 (1983).

4. K. A. Davies, V. Hird, S. Stewart *et al.* A study of *in vivo* immune complex formation and clearance in man. *J. Immunol.*, 144, 4613–4620 (1990).

5. D. T. Fearon. Identification of the membrane glycoprotein that is the C3b receptor of the human erythrocyte, polymorphonuclear leukocyte, B lymphocyte, and monocyte. *J. Exp. Med.*, 152, 20–30 (1980).

6. J. C. Edberg, E. Wright and R. P. Taylor. Quantitative analysis of the binding of soluble complement fixing antibody/dsDNA immune complexes to CR-1 on human red blood cells. *J. Immunol.*, 139, 3739–3747 (1987).

7. G. D. Ross, W. J. Yount, M. J. Walport *et al.* Disease associated loss of erythrocyte complement receptors (CR-1, C3b receptors) in patients with systemic lupus erythematosus and other diseases involving autoantibodies and/or complement activation. *J. Immunol.*, 135, 2005–2014 (1985).

8. M. J. Walport and P. J. Lachmann. Erythrocyte complement receptor type 1, immune complexes, and the rheumatic diseases. *Arthritis Rheum.*, 31, 153–158 (1988).

9. F. A. Tausk, J. A. McCutchan, R. D. Schreiber *et al.* Deficiency of erythrocyte C3b receptor (CR-1) in AIDS and AIDS related syndromes. *Biosci. Rep.*, 6, 81–86 (1986).

10. Y. Inada, M. Kamiyama, T. Kanemitsu *et al. In vivo* binding of circulating immune complexes by C3b receptors (CR-1) of transfused erythrocytes. *Ann. Rheum. Dis.*, 48, 287–294 (1989).

11. H. U. Lutz, P. Stammler, S. Fasler *et al.* Density separation of human red blood cells on self forming Percoll® gradients: correlation with cell age. *Biochem. Biophys. Acta*, 1116, 1–10 (1992).

12. N. Madi, G. Steiger, J. Estericher *et al.* Abnormal immune adherence and elimination of hepatitis B surface antigen/antibody complexes in patients with AIDS. *J. Immunol.*, 148, 723–728 (1992).

13. V. Boyer, C. Desgranges, M. A. Traubaud *et al.* Complement mediates human immunodeficiency virus type 1 infection of a human T cell line in a CD4⁻ and antibody-independent fashion. *J. Exp. Med.*, 173, 1151–1158 (1991).

Therapeutic Plasmapheresis (XII), pp. 541-545
T. Agishi *et al*. (Eds)
© VSP 1993

Adsorption of Anti-RNP and Anti-ss-DNA Antibodies

S. KURE, K. YAMANE, R. MURAYAMA, H. ASARI and S. TAKASHIMA[1]

Second Department of Anesthesiology, Toho Ohashi Hospital,
School of Medicine Tokyo, Japan
[1]*Co-operative Research Center, Okayama, Japan*

Key words: Anti-RNP antibody; Anti-ss-DNA antibody; plasmapheresis; adsorption; batch method.

INTRODUCTION

Antibodies to ribonucleoprotein (RNP) and DNA are characteristically present in au-toimmune disease patient serum. These autoantibodies serve as important diagnostic and prognostic markers in the disease. Recent observations indicate that human and murine monoclonal anti-double-stranded DNA (dsDNA) antibodies are also able to react with several cross-reactive moieties, such as cardiolipin and other phosphodiester-linked groups [1].

Furthermore, there have been reports that anti-dsDNA antibodies are able to bind to molecules bearing repeating negatively charged groups such as hyaluronic acid, chon-droitin sulphate, heparan sulphate and dextran sulphate [2, 3]. However, Aotsuka re-ported that no adsorbent was able to adsorb anti-RNP antibodies and single-stranded DNA (ss-DNA) antibodies could be adsorbed only by dextran sulphate, polyacrylic acid and sulphic acid to some extent [4]. Although double membrane filtration plasmaphere-sis is still the most effective treatment for autoimmune disease patient with mainly SLE, it will be important to identify adsorbents which could adsorb anti-RNP antibodies for mixed connective tissue disease. In this study, several adsorbents with were very differ-ent pore sizes, surface areas and ionic charge distributions on the surface were examined by batch methods to ascertain whether they could adsorb both anti-RNP and anti-ss-DNA antibodies from patient serum.

MATERIALS AND METHODS

Sera
Serum samples were obtained from autoimmune disease patients countaining high titers of anti-RNP and anti-ss-DNA antibodies.

Adsorbents
All of the adsorbents are in use in the chemical industry field. These adsorbents are classified into four categories such as molecular sieve, solid acid, fraipontite and anionic, cationic exchanging resin (AER, CER). Zinc almina silicate consists of a scattered two-layer crystal fraipontite surrounding non-crystal silica particles. Fraipontite has acidic adsorbent activity on one side and basic activity on the other side.

Anti-RNP and anti-ss-DNA antibody assay
The assay was performed by commercially available ELISA kits for the anti-RNP antibody (MBL, Japan) and the anti-ss-DNA antibody (Fujirebio, Japan). The adsorption experiment was carried out by the batch method. Each adsorbent (0.1, 0.3 g) was added to 0.75 ml saline in a test tube and devaporized by autoclaving. Sample serum (0.75 ml) was mixed with the adsorbent on a waverotar for 60 min at room temperature. After centrifugation (3000 r.p.m., 3 min), the supernate was filtrated by a microfilter (pore size; 0.45 μm). Calorimetric measurements were taken with an automatic ELISA reader (Toso, Japan) using a 450 nm filter for both antibodies.

Acidity and basicity on the surface of each adsorbent
Measurement of ionic charge distribution was calculated by the titration method; 0.1 g of each adsorbent was added to 5 ml of 0.01 N NaOH (HCl) solution in a test tube. The adsorbent was degased under reduced pressure for 1 h at room temperature. Then, 1 ml of the solution was titrated with 0.01 N HCl (NaOH) solution by a microsyringe using phenolphtalein as an indicator. The number of $H^+(OH^-)$ on its surface was indicated as Avogadro's number.

Blood compatibility of zinc almina silicate
Non-coated zinc almina silicate silicate powder (AP, HP) and granules (AG, HG) coated with polyhydroxyethylmetacrylate (PHEMA) were examined. After devaporization, 0.3 g of each adsorbent was added to 9 ml of normal adult serum with 0.4 ml sodium citrate and incubated for 60 min at body temperature. PHEMA-coated active carbon was taken as positive control. Blood coagulating factors [2–13] and serum compliments were measured for each samples.

Table 1.
Adsorption ratio of anti-RNP antibody, anti-ss-DNA antibody and albumin

Adsorbents	Vol	Anti-RNP	Anti-ss-DNA	Albumin
	g	Ab (%)	Ab (%)	(%)
alumina (acidic)	0.3	6.4	15.5	< 1
alumina (basic)	0.3	10.9	15.6	9.0
alumina (neutral)	0.3	13.4	15.5	18.2
Zeolite (10 nm)	0.3	7.9	18.9	22.7
Hydroxyapatite	0.3	33.0	6.9	41.0
Silica alumina	0.3	16.7	15.5	18.2
AER (51–51)③	0.1	7.1	15.6	13.6
CER (IR-120B)①	0.3	23.4	< 1	< 1
CER (IRC-84)②	0.3	18.2	< 1	< 1
Mizukanite AP⑤	0.1	92.0	84.5	36.3
Mizukanite HP④	0.1	86.0	56.9	18.2
Control		202.6	58.0	22.0
		(U/ml)	(U/ml)	(g/dl)

RESULTS

Powdered zinc alumina silicate (AP, HP) adsorbed both antibodies most effectively; adsorption ratios were 92.0, 86.0% for anti-RNP and 84.5, 56.9% for anti-ss-DNA, respectively (Table 1). These adsorbents also bound albumin but the removal ratio was less than 30% (mean; 27.2%). Hydroxyapatite, which is a very popular dental material, was able to adsorb anti-RNP antibody to some extent. Zinc alumina silicate showed that it was bi-chargic material on whose surface acidic points and basic points are located in equally amounts. Silica alumina also revealed the same property but its adsorption ratio was much lower than zinc alumina silicate (Figs 1 and 2). Blood compatibility

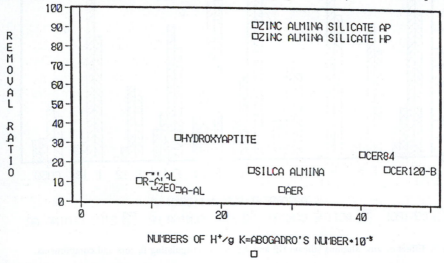

Figure 1. Relationship between removal ratio (%) of anti-RNP antibody and acidity (K) on the surface of each adsorbent.

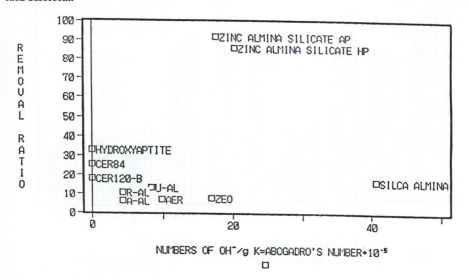

Figure 2. Relationship between removal ratio (%) of anti-RNP antibody and basicity (K) on the surface of each adsorbent.

of powdered zinc alumina silicate (AP, HP) was not satisfactory (Fig. 3). Coagulating factors including serum compliments were reduced in level after incubation with the adsorbents. The volume ratio of adsorbent to serum was 1:30 (w/v). However, PHEMA-coated granular zinc alumina silicate (AG, HG) improved all of the discompatibility of AP and HP. This tendency was clearer in PHEMA-coated HG than AG (Fig. 4).

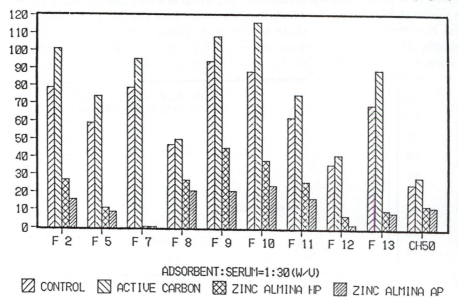

Figure 3. Effect of zinc alumina silicate HP and AP on the coagulating factors and compliments.

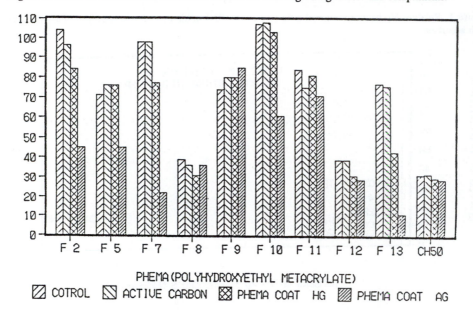

Figure 4. Effect of PHEMA-coated zinc alumina silicate HG and AG on coagulating factor and compliment adsorbent: serum = 1:30(w/u).

DISCUSSION

Mechanism of adsorption depends proportionally on pore size, surface area and ionic charge distribution of adsorbent. Our results show that zinc alumina silicate (AP, HP) adsorbed both anti-RNP and anti-ss-DNA antibodies. Although the precise mechanism is still unknown, its unique property of equal bi-chargic units which is different from negatively charged units may play a major role in the adsorption. This was confirmed by the fact that several pore sizes of Zeolite (molecular seive) could no longer make any difference to the binding capacity. PHEMA is a very useful coating substance which is now in use with active carbon for selective removal for drug abuse patient. In the same way, PHEMA coating improved the biocompatibility of zinc alumina silicate, but problems of reduction of binding capacity by coating still remain. The best treatment for autoimmune disease patients intractable to steroid theraphy is now double membrane filtration plasmapheresis. However, selective removal of anti-nuclear antibodies by immunoadsorption is thought to be an ideal therapy [5]. Zinc alumina silicate coated with PHEMA will be examined further as an ideal adsorbent for immunoadsorption in the future.

CONCLUSION

Zinc alumina silicate is a most effective adsorbent for anti-RNP and anti-ss-DNA antibodies and its biocompatibility is improved by PHEMA coating. Although its adsorption mechanism remains unknown, its bi-chargic units may play an important role in the adsorption.

REFERENCES

1. E. M. Laffer, J. Rauch, J. C. Andrzejewski *et al.* Polyspecific monoclonal lupus autoantibodies reactive with polynucleotides reactive with both polynucleotides and phospholipids. *J. Exp. Med.*, 153, 897–909 (1981).
2. P. Faaber, P. J. A. Capel, T. P. M. Rijke *et al.* Cross-reactivity of anti-DNA antibodies with proteogly-cans. *Clin. Exp. Immunol.*, 55, 502–508 (1984).
3. P. Faaber, T. P. M. Rijke, B. A. V. Levinus *et al.* Cross-reactivity of human and murine anti-DNA antibodies with heparan sulfate. *J. Clin. Invest.*, 77, 1824–1830 (1986).
4. S. Aotsuka, T. Funahashi, N. Tani *et al.* Adsorption of anti-ds DNA antibodies by immobolized polyan-ionic compounds. *Clin. Exp. Immunol.*, 79, 215–220 (1990).
5. M. Kinoshita, S. Aotsuka, T. Funahashi *et al.* Selective removal of anti-double-stranded DNA antibodies by immunoadsorption with dextran sulphate in a patient with lupus erythematosus. *Ann. Rheumatic Dis.*, 48, 856–860 (1989).

Therapeutic Plasmapheresis (XII), pp. 547-549
T. Agishi *et al.* (Eds)
© VSP 1993

Effect of a Selective Apheresis Column (SL-01) on Systemic Lupus Erythematosus

S. NAGANUMA, T. AGISHI, K. OTA and T. SANAKA

Kidney Center, Tokyo Women's Medical College, Tokyo, Japan

Key words: systemic lupus erythematosus; adsorption; anti-DNA antibody; anti-cardiolipin antibody.

INTRODUCTION

Although the etiology of systemic lupus erythematosus (SLE) is unknown, antibodies including anti-DNA antibody, are thought to play an important part in pathognomonic mechanisms. Active SLE is treated by steroid and immunosuppressants; however, these have many side-effects. Plasmapheresis has been used for the treatment of SLE resistant to drug therapy. However, its effects are controversial because of not selectively removing pathogenic factors and rebound phenomenon.

In the current study, the effectiveness and safety of a selective adsorption column (SL-01) attached to filtration plasmapheresis on SLE were evaluated.

MATERIAL

Two SLE patients with high titers of anti-DNA and/or anticardiolipin antibodies (aCL), who satisfied ARA criteria (1982) for SLE resistant to steroid therapy, were selected for this study. Prednisolone was used and its dose was unchanged during the plasmapheresis treatment.

METHOD

Adsorption apheresis had been done utilizing a SL-01 column [dextran sulphate cellulose beads (DS), Kaneka, Japan] installed in a reciprocative double column system (MA-01). About 4000 ml of plasma processed by a membrane plasma separator (polysulphone, 0.5 m^2) was led into the adsorption system. The schedule of the adsorption apheresis was as follows; five apheresis treatments once weekly (case 1), eight apheresis treatments once weekly (case 2), during 8 weeks.

Titers of anti-DNA, aCL (by RIA) and other laboratory markers were measured pre and post each LDL apheresis treatment.

RESULT

Changes in titers of anti-DNA after adsorption plasmapheresis
As shown in Fig. 1, titers of anti-DNA significantly decreased after adsorption plasma-pheresis. Reduction rates of anti-DNA antibody were 47% (case 1) and 38% (case 2) on the basis of the titers before and after apheresis, while the adsorption rates between the antibody adsorbed on the columns and all that introduced to the columns were 56% (case 1) and 57% (case 2).

Changes in aCL titers after adsorption plasmapheresis
Titers of aCL significantly removed by 32% (case 2) before and after the apheresis. aCL in case 1 had a low titer.

Clinical manifestations and the rebound phenomenon after adsorption plasmapheresis
As shown in Table 1, discoid rash, Raynaud's phenomenon and arthralgia improved after the plasmapheresis treatment. Proteinuria and urine casts improved, but low com-plementemia did not improve in case 1.

Changes in biochemical data after apheresis
Although each immunoglobulin level slightly decreased after apheresis, the changes were within the normal range. Other clinical data, apart from cholesterol, after the therapy were maintained almost equal to those before the treatment.

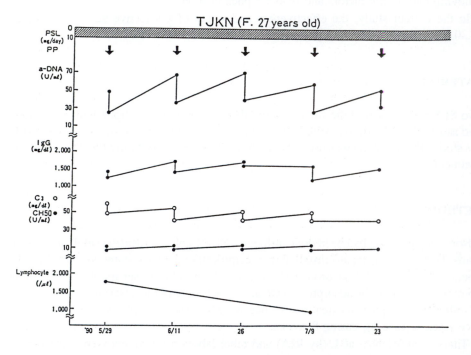

Figure 1. Clinical course in SLE patient treated by plasmapheresis.

Table 1.
Effect on clinical manifestation after adsorption

Patients	KN		KA	
Age	27		30	
Sex/body weight	F/48		F/44	
Disease duration	8		9	
Steroid (mg/day)	10	10	25	25
Immunosuppressants			+	+
Treatment no.	5		8	
	before PP	after PP	before PP	after PP
Face erythema	−	−	+	−
Disk rash	−	−	+	−
Photosensitivity	+	+	−	−
Arthralgia	+	+	−	−
Proteinuria	+	+	+	+
Casts	+	+	+	−
Lymphopenia	+	+	−	−
LE cell	+		−	
Anti-DNA antibody (U/ml)	48	50	109	200
Anti-nuclear antibody (X)	320	640	80	+

DISCUSSION

DS columns have been used widely as specific adsorbents for low density lipoprotein in familial hypercholesterolemia. It was found that anti-DNA had a high affinity for DS which had repetitive negatively charged units, and the titers of anti-DNA in SLE decreased after plasmapheresis using DS columns.

Recent attention has focused on the presence of cardiolipin and its possible role in recurrent thrombosis, thrombocytopenia in SLE. Smeenk *et al.* found that anti-DNA was less antigen specific and tended to cross-react with cardiolipin. Thus, an adsorbent DS column adsorbs not only anti-DNA but also aCL. In this study anti-DNA and aCL significantly decreased. However, there was a rebound phenomenon in the titers of autoantibodies over longer than a 1 week interval.

Clinical manifestations, which include rash, erythema and Raynaud's phenomenon, were improved. Indications for plasmapheresis, including the duration and number of treatments, volume of plasma processed, combination therapy including steroids and immunosuppressants, and the stage of active and/or severe SLE, require further study.

In conclusion, adsorbent plasmapheresis can remove anti-DNA and aCL antibody selectively and safely.

REFERENCE

1. H. Hashimoto, H. Tsuda, Y. Kanai, S. Kobayashi *et al.* Selective removal of anti-DNA and anticardiolipin antibodies by adsorbent plasmapheresis using dextran sulphate columns in patients with systemic lupus erythematosus. *J. Rheumatol.*, **18**, 545–551 (1991).

Therapeutic Plasmapheresis (XII), pp. 551-555
T. Agishi *et al.* (Eds)
© VSP 1993

Immunoadsorption (TR-350) in Guillain–Barré Syndrome

M. IWAHASHI, T. MAEDA, K. OHNISHI,
M. FUKUHARA and K. TANEMOTO

Department of Internal Medicine, Kobe Rosai Hospital, Kobe, Japan

Key words: immunoadsorption; TR-350; Guillain–Barré syndrome; plasmapheresis; circulating factor.

INTRODUCTION

Guillain–Barré syndrome (GBS) is a demyelinating disorder, which is thought to be related to abnormalities of both humoral and cellular immune mechanisms [1, 2]. The recent multicenter study showing plasmapheresis to be an effective treatment in these patients has increased speculation that antibodies or other circulating factors may play a role [3]. We employed immunoadsorption therapy (IAT) using TR-350 instead of plasmapheresis to treat GBS in an acute stage. The purpose of this study is to identify the clinical efficacy of IAT for removing these factors from the plasma, through the clinical course of one case with excellent results.

PATIENT

A 16 year old girl had a common cold on October 3, 1991, and took OTC medicine. The symptoms subsequently improved. On October 22, however, she developed heaviness in the knees and palsy in the distal parts of the feet. On October 23, she found it difficult to climb the stairs and on October 26 she started finding it difficult to walk. She then consulted LMD and was subsequently referred to our hospital. On October 27 she was admitted to our hospital for detailed examination and therapy. At the time of admission, mild bilateral facial palsy was noted, together with paralysis in the distal end of the lower extremities and bilateral muscle weakness. Deep reflex was absent, but no pathological reflex was noted. In the electromyogram, fibrillation potentials were detected and conduction velocities of the peripheral motor fibers were reduced in the lower extremities. Blood examination on admission showed ESR of 30 mm/h, ASLO of 53 and a 4-fold increase in anti-myelin antibody. No abnormalities were found in the blood gas analysis and urinalysis, and no significant increase in anti-virus antibody was noted. Lumbar cerebrospinal fluid was watery clear, and the internal pressure of the fluid was 130 mmH$_2$O. The fluid showed 109 mg/dl protein, 62 mg/dl sugar and 2 lymphocytes/3 (F), showing albuminocytologic dissociation. The immunoglobulin classes contained in the fluid were IgG, 96 mg/dl; IgA, 2.4 mg/dl; and IgM, 0.3 mg/dl. The myelin basic protein level was 1.1 ng/dl.

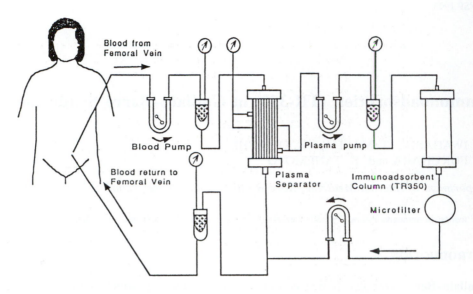

Figure 1. Catheter placement and extracorporeal circuit in immunoadsorbent plasma perfusion.

METHODS

IAT was performed with a Plasort 1000 (Fig. 1). Blood access was through a double-lumen catheter placed in the femoral vein. Cell components were separated by a plasma separator Plasmaflo OP-08 (Asahi Medical Co. Ltd), following a blood pump. Separated plasma was processed in an immunoadsorbent column and returned to the femoral vein together with the cell components. The immunoadsorbent column was TR-350 (Asahi Medical Co. Ltd), a hydrophobic adsorbent column in which tryptophan is fixed as a ligand in polyvinyl alcohol gel. Blood flow rate was 1000 ml/min and plasma flow rate was 30 ml/min. The amount of plasma processed in one treatment of IAT was 2500–3000 ml in 2 h. Nafamostat mesilate was used as an anticoagulant at a rate of 50 mg/h. In order to evaluate clinical improvement, changes in subjective symptoms were studies as well as objective signs including blood gas analysis, pulmonary function, electromyogram, lumbar cerebrospinal fluid, serum protein fraction, immunoglobulins, and serum C3 and C4. To evaluate the efficacy of this adsorption system, serum protein fraction, immunoglobulins, and serum C3 and C4 were also measured before and after IAT. (See Tables 1–3 and Figs 2–4).

Table 1.
Changes of blood gas analysis

	Day 5 (room air)	Day 15 (room air)	Day 16 (room air)	Day 16 (FiO$_2$: 30%)	Day 24 (room air)
PH	7.397	7.441	7.384	7.406	7.398
PO$_2$ (mmHg)	90.1	90.9	53.7	86.7	110.1
PCO$_2$ (mmHg)	38.5	36.8	41.8	38.5	39.4
O$_2$sat. (%)	96.7	97.2	86.9	96.5	98.1

Table 2.
Changes of lung function

	Day 18	Day 19	Day 24	Day 25
VC (cc)	1730	1840	2530	2480
%VC (%)	56.5	60.1	82.7	81.1
FEV 1.0 (cc)	840	720	2530	2000
FEV 1.0% (%)	48.5	39.1	74.3	80.7
TLC (cc)	3060	3060	3060	3060
V 25/Ht (l/s)	0.33	0.25	0.40	0.44

Table 3.
Electrophysiologic investigation

	Day 10	Day 30	Day 45
MCV (m/s)			
Upper extremities (N. ulnaris)	38.3	52.1	45.1
Lower extremities (N. peroneus)	42.4	24.7	45.3
SCV (m/s)			
Upper extremities (Nn. digitales dorsales)	31.4	52.1	
Lower extremities (N. suralis)	42.9	53.3	

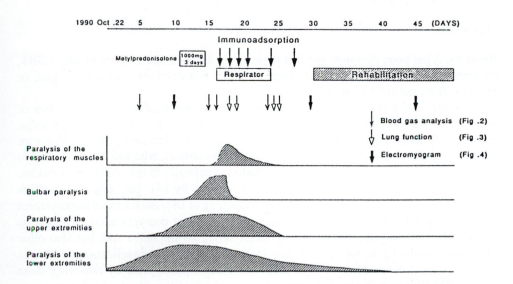

Figure 2. Clinical course. The day heaviness of the knees appeared is defined as day 1.

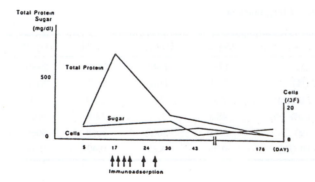

Figure 3. Transition of lumbar cerebrospinal fluid findings.

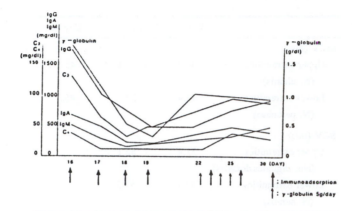

Figure 4. Changes in plasma fractions through the clinical course.

DISCUSSION

Recently, it has been demonstrated that plasmapheresis is an effective treatment in GBS, by removing demyelinating factors such as antimyelin antibody, immunocomplex or protease from patient's plasma [4–7].

However, plasmapheresis requires a large volume of substitution serum and a lack of substitution was pointed. It also has some complications such as infection and allergic reactions. In this study, we performed a trial IAT using TR-350 on a patient with severe GBS at an acute stage instead of plasmapheresis. The patient, who had not responded to pulse corticosteroid therapy and who had developed paralysis of the respiratory muscles, showed dramatic improvement in signs and symptoms by IAT. She was able to drink water with a straw unaided only 2 h after the beginning of IAT. Such a rapid improvement in muscles paralysis suggested an initiation mechanism of demyelination. It might be thought that not only the demyelinating factor acting on the nerve root but also other unknown circulating factors play a role in the initiation of demyelination. IAT was thought to be a much more useful treatment for acute phase GBS by removing these factors than plasmapheresis. Furthermore, the analysis of the adsorbed substance may elucidate the pathological substance or mechanism in the future.

CONCLUSION

We performed a trial IAT using TR-350 to a patient with GBS instead of plasmapheresis. We thought IAT was a much more useful treatment for GBS than plasmapheresis.

REFERENCES

1. P. R. Brette *et al.* Treatment of acute polyneuropathy by plasma exchange. *Lancet*, **2**, 1100 (1978).

2. M. Yoshioka *et al.* Treatment of the Guillain–Barré syndrome in childhood by plasmapheresis. In: *Therapeutic Plasmapheresis* (V), T. Oda (Ed.), pp. 451–454. Schattauer, Stuttgart (1986).

3. A. A. Ilyas *et al.* Serum antibodies to gangliosides in Guillain–Barré syndrome. *Ann. Neurol.*, **23**, 440–447 (1988).

4. The Guillain–Barré syndrome study group. Plasmapheresis and acute Guillain–Barré syndrome. *Neurology*, **35**, 1096–1104 (1985).

5. French Cooperative Group on Plasma Exchange in Guillain–Barré Syndrome. Efficiency of plasma exchange in Guillain–Barré syndrome: role of replacement fluids. *Ann. Neurol.*, **2**, 753–761 (1987).

6. G. M. McKhann *et al.* Plasmapheresis and Guillain–Barré syndrome: analysis of prognostic factors and the effect of plasmapheresis. *Ann. Neurol.*, **23**, 347–353 (1988).

7. B. H. Waksman and R. D. Adams. Allergic neuritis: an experimental disease of rabbits induced by the injection of peripheral nerve tissue an adjuvants. *J. Exp. Med.*, **102**, 213–236 (1955).

Therapeutic Plasmapheresis (XII), pp. 557-560
T. Agishi *et al*. (Eds)
© VSP 1993

Immunoadsorption Plasmapheresis and Plasma Exchange in Miller Fisher Syndrome

C.-S. KOH, T. SHINODA,[1] K. SHIMADA, A. INOUE and N. YANAGISAWA

Departments of Medicine (Neurology) and [1]Artificial Organ Treatment, Shinshu University School of Medicine, Matsumoto, Japan

Key words: Guillain–Barré syndrome; Miller Fisher syndrome; immunoadsorption plasmapheresis; plasma exchange.

INTRODUCTION

Miller Fisher syndrome (MFS) is characterized by the acute onset of ophthalmoplegia, ataxia and areflexia [1]. Spontaneous resolution is also a hallmark of MFS. However, complications, death or residual disability are pronounced at peak deficit, and plateau phase is protracted. Therefore, an effective treatment is needed. The exact pathogenesis of MFS has not been clarified, although MFS is considered to be the ophthalmoplegic form of Guillain–Barré syndrome (GBS). Immunologic studies have shown that it may be caused by cell-mediated immunity to peripheral antigens but not to central myelin antigens. Corticosteroids have shown no benefit. On the other hand, the therapeutic value of plasma exchange (PE) for MFS was reported [2, 3]. The efficacy of immunoadsorption plasmapheresis (IAPP) was compared to that of PE as a treatment for MFS in the present study.

PATIENTS AND METHODS

Two female patients with MFS were treated with IAPP and another two patients with MFS (one female and one male) were treated with PE (Table 1). All patients agreed to participate in the study with informed consent. The criteria to start IAPP in patients with MFS were exactly the same as in the case of PE; (i) within 14 days from the onset, (ii) in the phase of progress and (iii) not receiving corticosteroids. The protocol for IAPP was essentially the same as that for PE except for using an adsorption column (PH-350; Asahi Medical, Tokyo, Japan) instead of 4.4% diluted albumin solution (Plasma Protein Fraction, Baxter Healthcare, Glendale, CA) as replacement fluid. IAPP and PE were performed two sessions or more per week. Plasma volume processed in IAPP was 35 ml/kg body weight/session or more. The same plasma separators (AP-05, OP-05; Asahi Medical, Tokyo, Japan or FS-05; Kanegafuchi Chemical, Osaka, Japan) and control machines (KEM-21; Nikkiso, Tokyo, Japan or KL-30; Kawasumi Laboratories, Tokyo, Japan) were used in both treatments. The efficacy of IAPP and PE was judged by clinical signs and symptoms. An immediate effect was qualitatively classified into four classes; (−): progression in spite of treatments; (±): a little improvement in a plateau phase; (+): cessation of the progress; and (++): evident improvement in both progress and plateau phases. Long-term effects were evaluated by the following two points; (i) period of time to be able to walk 20 m from the first treatment and (ii) period of time to recover from ophthalmoplegia from the first treatment.

RESULTS

An immediate effect of IAPP and PE therapies was equally comparable (Table 2). Immediate improvement was seen in all cases treated with IAPP or PE, in ataxia, ophthalmoplegia and even in bulbar palsy in some cases. Long-term effects of IAPP seem to be better than those of PE. Two patients with MFS treated with IAPP were able to walk 20 m very shortly after the first IAPP treatment (Table 2). Both the period of time to be able to walk and the period of time to recover from ophthalmoplegia after the first treatment were much shorter in the IAPP treated group than in the PE treated group. Two cases treated with PE were injected intravenously with gamma globulin after PE to prevent secondary infection. Two cases treated with IAPP were not particularly treated after IAPP. No side-effects were observed during the treatment and in the course of follow up.

Table 1.
Patient profiles

Case	Age/sex	Neurological signs and symptoms[a]	Days from the onset	Cerebrospinal fluid	
				CC (/mm^3)	TP (mg/dl)
IAPP group					
1	52/F	A O AR B	10	1	30
2	46/F	A O AR	6	8	378
PE group					
3	53/F	A O AR B	11	1	146
4	59/M	A O AR	13	1	155

[a] A, ataxia; O, ophthalmoplegia; AR, areflexia; B, bulbar palsy.

Table 2.
Effects of IAPP and PE in the treatment of MFS

Case	Age/sex	Phase	Days from the onset	Immediate effect	Long-term effect (days)	
					(a)	(b)
IAPP group						
1	52/F	progress	10	++	4	3
2	46/F	progress	6	++	9	2
PE group						
3	53/F	progress	11	++	14	22
4	59/M	progress	13	++	14	14

DISCUSSION

MFS is generally agreed to be a variant of acute inflammatory polyneuropathy or GBS [1]. The pathological findings in GBS consist of multifocal infiltrates of inflammatory cells in the spinal roots and peripheral nerves associated with segmental demyelination and variable axonal destruction [2]. The anatomopathology of the lesion in MFS remains obscure [3], but it may be an acute intra-axial and extra-axial inflammation in the midbrain [4, 5]. The exact pathogenesis of GBS or MFS is not clarified. However, there is increasing evidence that immunological factors are involved in the pathogenesis of GBS and MFS [6]. In these four cases of MFS, both IAPP and PE resulted in a dramatic improvement with ultimate remission. The IAPP or PE was done in an acute exacerbating phase and the patients did not show a plateau phase of the disease, which is commonly observed in the natural course. We suggest that the rapid clinical effect by IAPP or PE is directly attributed to removal of a pathogenic humoral factor, especially immunoglobulins or immune complexes [7]. There are increasing reports that PE is beneficial in inflammatory polyneuropathy including MFS when it is carried out early in the course of the disease [8, 9]. No significant difference has been reported in GBS between the group that received albumin and the group that received fresh frozen plasma as replacement fluids [10]. Although this study was performed in only a small number of patients, IAPP resulted in better long-term effects than PE. Further studies are needed to confirm this point. Given its risk and the lack of its clear superiority over IAPP, we recommend that IAPP should be applied first to treat MFS rather than PE.

CONCLUSIONS

The efficacy of IAPP was compared with that of PE in the treatment of MFS. IAPP and PE were equally effective for the cessation of progression and improvement of clinical signs and symptoms in patients with MFS. IAPP may be superior to PE in the treatment of MFS because of no use of plasma preparations and less non-selective reduction of immunoglobulins.

REFERENCES

1. M. Fisher. An unusual variant of acute idiopathic polyneuritis (syndrome of ophthalmoplegia, ataxia and areflexia). *New. Engl. J. Med.*, **255**, 57–65 (1956).
2. B. G. W. Arnason. Acute inflammatory demyelinating polyradiculopathies. In: *Peripheral Neuropathy*, 2nd edn, P. J. Dyck *et al.* (Eds), pp. 2050–2100, W. B. Saunders, Philadelphia (1984).
3. M. S. Philips, S. Stewart and J. R. Anderson. Neuropathological findings in Miller Fischer syndrome. *J. Neurol. Neurosurg. Psychiatry*, **47**, 492–495 (1984).
4. I. Derakhshan, J. Lofti and B. Kaufman. Ophthalmoplegia, ataxia and hyporeflexia (Fisher's syndrome) with a midbrain lesion demonstrated by CT scanning. *Eur. Neurol.*, **18**, 361 (1979).
5. A. N. Al-Din, M. Anderson, B. R. Bickerstaff and I. Harvey. Brain stem encephalitis and the syndrome of Miller Fisher. A Clinical Study. *Brain*, **105**, 481–495 (1982).
6. P. O. Behan and N. Geschwind. The ophthalmoplegic form of the Guillain–Barré syndrome: an immunologic study. *Acta Ophthalmol.*, **51**, 529–535 (1973).
7. N. Kobayashi, K. Okudaira, Y. Miyamoto, Y. Yamada, T. Yamada, H. Doyoshita, A. Nozawa, H. Yoshizawa and K. Takahashi. Plasma cleaning using immunosorbent IM-P for patients with rheumatoid arthritis. *Ther. Plasmapheresis*, **4**, 153–157 (1984).

8. R. Littlewood and S. Bajada. Successful plasmapheresis is in the Miller Fisher syndrome. *Br. Med. J.*, **282**, 778 (1981).

9. T. Shinoda, H. Arakura, E. Yamagami, T. Shirota, M. Katakura, Y. Hara, K. Miyagi, S. Miyazawa, Y. Takei, C.-S. Koh and N. Yanagisawa. Reappraisal of plasma exchange in Guillair–Barré syndrome. In: *Therapeutic Plasmapheresis (IX)*, N. Koga, N. Inoue and S. Nakagawa (Eds), pp. 237–240, ICAOT Press, Cleveland (1991).

10. French Cooperative Group on Plasma Exchange in Guillain–Barré Syndrome. Efficiency of plasma exchange in Guillain–Barré syndrome: role of replacement fluids. *Ann. Neurol.*, **22**, 753–761 (1987).

Therapeutic Plasmapheresis (XII), pp. 561-564
T. Agishi *et al*. (Eds)
© VSP 1993

Clinical Application of a New Immunoadsorbent PC-2 Column

Y. SUZUKI, M. OHARA, K. YOKOYAMA, K. ARIZONO, Y. UBARA, S. HARA, Y. OGURA, O. OTSUBO and N. MIMURA

Kidney Center, Toranomon Hospital, Tokyo, Japan

Key words: immunoadsorbent; immunoglobulin G; immune complex; pemphigus; anti-acethylcholine receptor antibody.

INTRODUCTION

Recently, several immunoadsorbents have been developed and have come to be available for selective plasma purification therapy [1, 2]. We have developed a new ligand-free adsorbent PC-2 and already reported its performance *in vitro* and safety in canine *ex vivo* test [3, 4]. In this paper, eight clinical cases successfully treated using immunoadsorbent PC-2 are reported.

MATERIALS AND METHODS

Newly developed immunoadsorbent, PC-2, was prepared from Sepharose CL-4B, cross-linking with hexamethylene-diisocyanate. PC-2 is spherical in shape and the mean diameter is 55 μm. Though PC-2 have neither biological nor chemical ligand, it

Table 1.
Clinical Findings of Eight Clinical Cases Treated by Immunoadsorption using PC-2

Case no.	Disease	Sex	Age (years)	Clinical findings
1	RA	M	61	improvement of arthralgia and lumbago, recovery of the joint movements
2	MG	M	54	no significant change (anti-AchR Ab (−))
3	Pem	F	64	improvements of skin rash
4	GS	F	69	recovery of muscular strength, enabling to standing up
5	GS	M	59	enabling to move the upper extremity
6	SLE	F	60	improvement of general symptom and arthralgia
7	SLE	F	43	improvement of arthralgia and myalgia
8	RA	M	63	disappearance of arthralgia

RA, Rheumatoid Arthritis; MG, Myasthenia Gravis; Pem, Pemphigus;

GS, Guillain–Barré Syndrome; SLE, Systemic Lupus Erythematosus.

can widely adsorb the pathogenic substances which belong to the IgG fraction in blood. From 200 to 300 ml of the gel was packed in a cylindrical column and sterilized by autoclave before use.

Table 1 shows the eight clinical cases having undergone treatment by PC-2. They were Rheumatoid Arthritis, Myasthenia Gravis, Pemphigus, Guillain–Barré Syndrome and Systemic Lupus Erythematosus.

Plasma adsorption therapy was performed using blood circuit and polypropylene hollow fiber membrane was used as plasma separator. Heparin was used as an anti-coagulant. A volume of 2500 ml of plasma was processed at each treatment.

RESULTS AND DISCUSSIONS

A total of 33 plasma adsorption treatments using PC-2 were performed for five diseases of eight patients and no side-effects were observed.

As shown in Table 1, in seven cases, clinical findings improved as follows, namely disappearance of arthralgia and recovery of range of joint movements in the cases of Rheumatoid Arthritis, improvements of skin rash in the case of Pemphigus, recovery of muscular strength of the extremities in the cases of Guillain–Barré Syndrome, and disappearance of arthralgia and myalgia in the cases of Systemic Lupus Erythematosus.

In one case of Myasthenia Gravis, however, clinical findings were not changed. In this case, the patient had already been subjected to thymectomy, and anti-acetylcholine receptor antibody was negative.

Figure 1 shows the averaged reduction rates of IgG, albumin, total protein, IgA, IgM, IgE and immune complex, after 27 treatments. IgG and immune complex could be selectively reduced as compared with other plasma components.

The results indicate that plasma adsorption therapy using PC-2 is effective for the treatments of these immune diseases.

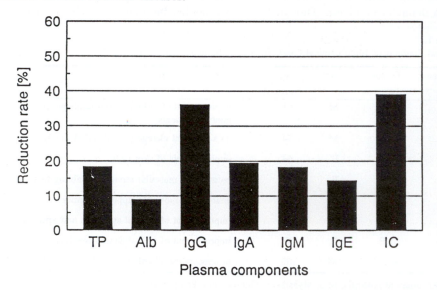

Figure 1. Reduction rate of plasma components by PC-2 immunoadsorption treatment (average of 27 treatments).

CASE REPORT: CASE 3, PEMPHIGUS

The patient was a 65 years old housewife, and her chief complaint was erythema in the whole body and bullae formation in the legs. The past and family history were not contributory. On June 22, 1990, she suffered from sudden eczematous eruption in the upper arm and it gradually extended to the whole body with bullae formation in the both legs. On July 16, she was hospitalized.

On admission, erythema were observed on the whole body including face. Bullae of 2 cm in diameter were observed on the both legs. Laboratory findings showed several abnormalities, namely high LDH of 623 HU, high CRP of 6.8 mg/dl, WBC of 9900/mm^3 (eosin: 15%), high RF titer of 309 U/ml, and high IgM level of 413 mg/dl. Epithelial basement membrane Ab was negative, but epithelial intracellular Ab was positive. Skin biopsy revealed pemphigus with pustule formation.

Figure 2 shows the clinical course after admission. After admission, prednisolone was started and eruption was improved somewhat. But, depending on the reduction of the dose of prednisolone, eruption began to reappear. Therefore, plasma exchange treatment was carried out three times in November 1990, and improvement of eruption was achieved. However, in January 1991, succeeding immunoadsorption treatment using PC-2, had to be performed three times and eruption was improved. In March 1991 too, plasma adsorption treatment using IM-TR350 was carried out three times, and eruption was improved. In addition, in order to improve eruption and decrease the dose of corticosteroid, plasma adsorption treatment using PC-2 were carried out two times, and good results were obtained.

The reduction rate (mean ±SD) of plasma components of the patient using PC-2 and IM-TR350 were studied. The reduction rates of IgG were about 50% in both adsorbent.

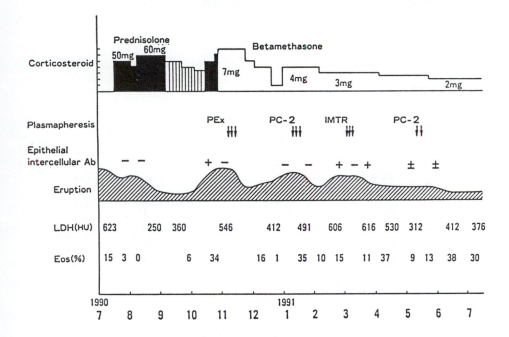

Figure 2. Clinical course of case 3 (Pemphigus, female, 65 years old).

Although the reduction rates of IgA and IgM in PC-2 were as low as those of TP and Albumin, the reduction rates of IgA and IgM in IM-TR were as high as the those of IgG.

The results that PC-2 could most specifically adsorb IgG compared to the other proteins, achieved concurrent improvements of skin rash, suggested that PC-2 could adsorb IgG class pathogenic Ab in Pemphigus. Immunoadsorbent PC-2 would be effective for the treatment of Pemphigus.

CONCLUSION

On the basis of the above findings, it was concluded that,

(i) PC-2 could specifically adsorb IgG compared with other proteins.

(ii) Immunoadsorption treatment by PC-2 would be effective for the treatments of these immune disease.

REFERENCES

1. T. Shibamoto, T. Akiba, M. Maeda *et al.* Study of immunoadsorption therapy in five severe cases of myasthenia gravis. In: *Therapeutic Plasmapheresis (IX)*, N. Koga, N. Inoue and S. Nakagawa (Eds), pp. 209–213, ICAOT Press, Cleveland (1991).

2. N. Takanashi, K. Uchida, S. Miki *et al.* Effect of immunoadsorbent therapy on four immunoneuropathic patients. *ibid*, 217 (1991).

3. Y. Suzuki, Y. Ogura, O. Otsubo *et al.* Studies on adsorptive capability for some pathogenic reactant by newly developed immunoadsorbent PC-2. *Jpn. J. Artif. Organs*, **20**, 308–313 (1991).

4. Y. Suzuki, T. Yanagisawa, H. Hasegawa *et al.* Adsorption of anti-acetylcholine receptor antibody by newly developed immunoadsorbent. *Artif. Organs*, **14** (Suppl. 2), 134–137 (1990).

Therapeutic Plasmapheresis (XII), pp. 565-568
T. Agishi *et al.* (Eds)
© VSP 1993

Establishment of On-line Closed Antibody Elimination Plasmapheresis System Applying Red Blood Cells as Adsorbents — Application to the Treatment of P Incompatible Pregnancy

Y. UEDA,[1,4] M. UEDA,[1,4] M. UKITA,[3] T. INOUE,[3] F. OWAKI,[4]
S. WATANABE,[4] Y. IKEDA,[4] Y. YAGIRI,[4] Y. KIRITA,[5] A. SUEOKA,[5]
Y. YOSHIDA,[1] K. ITO,[2] M. OKUMA[1] and H. UCHINO[1]

[1]*The First Division, Department of Medicine, Kyoto University, Japan*
[2]*Transfusion Service, Kyoto University, Japan*
[3]*Department of Gynecology and Obstetrics, Kurashiki Central Hospital, Japan*
[4]*Transfusion and Haemapheresis Center, Kurashiki Central Hospital, Japan*
[5]*Kuraray Co., Ltd, Japan*

Key words: habitual abortion; P incompatible pregnancy; anti-P antibody; red blood cells; immunoadsorption.

INTRODUCTION

We have already reported batch type anti-red cell antibody elimination plasmapheresis treatments using red blood cells as adsorbents for M [1], D [2, 3] and P [4] incompatible pregnancies. Recently, we have established a new on-line closed plasmapheresis system applying an antibody elimination method using red blood cells as adsorbents, and applied it to the treatment of P incompatible pregnancy. In this paper, details of our new system and the results of clinical application will be shown.

CLINICAL HISTORY OF THE PATIENT

The patient (M.T.) was a 33 years old Japanese woman. Her parents were second cousins to each other. She experienced three consecutive abortions at 9–12 weeks of gestation with no successful pregnancies. She consulted Osaka University Hospital of her habitual abortions and it was found that there were no etiologic factors associated with early abortions except that her blood type was P_1^k and she had anti-P antibodies in her serum. Because the possibility was strongly suggested that anti-P antibodies generated in the maternal blood disturbed the fetomaternal environment and caused repetitive abortions, the need for therapeutic plasmapheresis to remove anti-P antibodies in her next pregnancy was anticipated. In January 1991, she was diagnosed at 6 weeks of gestation and admitted to Kurashiki Central Hospital. On admission, her serum anti-P titer was 1:1024 by indirect antiglobulin test. On her second day of admission, 7 weeks and 1 day of gestation, therapeutic plasmapheresis to remove anti-P antibody in the maternal blood was commenced.

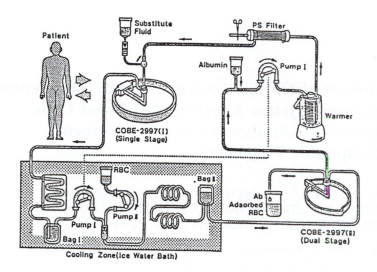

Figure 1. Flow diagram of on-line anti-P antibody elimination plasmapheresis system applying red blood cells as adsorbents.

MATERIALS AND METHODS

Several experiments were performed to investigate the optimal conditions of incubation. Based on the results of these experiments, we established the optimal condition as follows: red cells to plasma ratio, 1:5; temperature, 4 °C; time for incubation, 2–5 min. Figure 1 shows the flow diagram of our system. The patient's blood was separated into concentrated red cells and plasma by the first COBE 2997. Cooled plasma driven by the blood pump I, flowed into the drip chamber and was mixed with P positive leucocyte poor, washed and concentrated red cells obtained from Okayama Red Cross Blood Center which had also been cooled in the ice water bath and driven by the blood pump II. The mixture passed through the coiled tubes, the total priming volume of which was 76 ml at the flow rate of 36 ml per minute, and flew into the second COBE 2997 which was equipped with a dual stage channel. In the second centrifuge, the mixture of the patient's plasma and P positive red blood cells was separated again. The processed plasma was delivered to the membrane plasma separator (polysulfone membrane separator, Kuraray Co., Ltd, Osaka, Japan) through the blood pump I on which double tubing was performed. A substitute fluid line was placed between the second centrifuge and the blood pump I, and 5% albumin solution was used as a substitute fluid to adjust the plasma flow rate. All the cell components in the processed plasma were removed while passing through the membrane plasma separator and the cell free plasma was returned to the patient through the first centrifuge.

RESULTS

Figure 2 shows the changes of anti-P titer. Seven times of plasma exchange and three times of antibody elimination were performed. Anti-P reduction rate of our new system

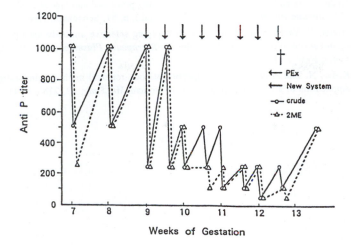

Figure 2. Changes of anti-P titer in association with therapeutic plasmapheresis. Intrauterine fetal death was recognized in 12 weeks and 5 days of gestation.

was comparable to that of plasma exchange. Plasma components other than anti-P antibodies were well retained during the new procedure. No elevation of plasma hemoglobin concentration nor C3d concentration could be detected. Although plasmapheresis was performed very smoothly, the fetal heart became suddenly inaudible and fetal death was recognized at 12 weeks and 5 days of gestation.

DISCUSSION

The reason why intrauterine fetal death occurred in spite of repetitive therapeutic plasmapheresis in this case is obscure. But in reported cases of P incompatible pregnancy, successfully treated with plasmapheresis, anti-P titer was kept lower than that of our case. As far as this patient is concerned, more intensive plasmapheresis will be necessary on her next pregnancy. The possibility of infection resulting from the blood used for immunoadsorption could not be excluded completely. But screening tests for hepatitis B, hepatitis C, acquired immunodeficiency syndrome, adult T cell leukemia and syphilis had already been performed for the donated blood before clinical applications. The infused blood was washed before incubation and all of the cell components of the incubated blood were completely eliminated by the membrane plasma separator. The possibility of infections caused by incubated blood was considered to be very small. Our new system is applicable to eliminate anti-red cell antibodies other than anti-P antibodies in circulation, by applying appropriate conditions of incubation to eliminate the pathologic antibodies. Until purified or synthetic adsorbents of anti-P antibodies become available easily, abundantly and inexpensively, red blood cells will be applied as the specific adsorbents of anti-P antibodies from now on.

REFERENCES

1. H. Yoshida, Y. Yoshida, K. Tatsumi and T. Asoh. A new therapeutic antibody removal method using antigen positive red cells. Application to M incompatible pregnant woman. *Vox Sang*, **43**, 35 (1982).

2. Y. Ueda, M. Ueda, N. Yamada *et al.* Plasma exchange using processed autologous fresh frozen plasma (PAFFP). In: *Therapeutic Plasmapheresis (III)*, T. Oda (Ed.), p. 81, Schattauer, New York (1983).

3. M. Ueda, Y. Ueda, Y. Yagiri *et al.* Plasmapheresis applying selective antibody adsorption using red blood cells, against severe rhesus alloimmunization. In: *Therapeutic Plasmapheresis (IV)*, T. Oda (Ed.), p. 183, Schattauer, New York (1985).

4. H. Yoshida, K. Ito, N. Emi *et al.* A new therapeutic antibody removal method using antigen-positive red cells II. Application to a P-incompatible pregnant woman. *Vox Sang*, **47**, 216 (1984).

Therapeutic Plasmapheresis (XII), pp. 569-571
T. Agishi *et al.* (Eds)
© VSP 1993

Significance of Immunoadsorption Therapy in Patients with Systemic Lupus Erythematosus: Analysis of Serum Autoantibody and Immune Complexes by a Isoelectric Focusing Column

A. SAGAWA, N. OGURA, T. ATSUMI, S. JODO, Y. AMASAKI, T. NAKABAYASHI, K. OHNISHI and A. FUJISAKU

The Second Department of Internal Medicine,
Hokkaido University School of Medicine, Sapporo 060, Japan

Key words: systemic lupus erythematosus; anti-DNA antibody; immune complex; isoelectric focusing; spectrotype.

INTRODUCTION

Systemic lupus erythematosus (SLE) is an autoimmune disease manifested by the production of autoantibodies [1]. Among these autoantibodies, anti-DNA antibodies play a major role since the resulting DNA/anti-DNA immune complexes cause glomerulonephritis and other autoimmune local lesions in SLE [2].

Immunoadsorption therapy using the PH350 Immusorba column was applied in the case of a patient with SLE who had been resistant to steroid therapy [3, 4]. Serum autoantibody repertoires, especially regarding anti-DNA antibody and the change in the levels of these autoantibodies and immune complex, were analyzed during the course of this therapy.

MATERIALS AND METHODS

PH350 Immusorba column (phenylalanine coated column, Asahi Medical, Tokyo). Preparative isoelectric focusing (IEF): Rotofor column (Bio-Rad, USA). ELISA for anti-DNA antibody measurement: ds-DNA or ss-DNA coated plate. ELISA for immune complex detection: monoclonal IgG rheumatoid factor (MRL mouse) coated microplate (Nissui, Japan).

RESULTS

IEF of anti-DNA
IgG anti-DNA antibodies were focused to two distinct pH regions; one was the acidic region at around pH 5.7 and the other to a far basic region at around pH 9. Whereas IgA and IgM class anti-DNA antibodies were focused to a relatively restricted acidic region.

IEF of immune complexes
Immune complexes were focused to the same basic region as a fraction of IgG anti-DNA antibodies did.

Clinical course of SLE
A patient with SLE has been treated with high-dose prednisolone, 60 mg per day for more than 12 weeks and with 50 mg of azathiopurine. In spite of long-term steroid therapy, her anti-DNA antibody level has been kept high and psychological disturbance appeared. Therefore immunoadsorption therapy was introduced. Patient plasma (2000 ml) was perfused in 120 min at one operation. No plasma specimen other than own plasma from the immunoadsorption column was infused into the patient. After the first immunoadsorption therapy, the level of anti-DNA antibodies was immediately decreased.

Change of anti-DNA titer by PH350 column
The result clearly shows that the anti-DNA antibody titer of blood specimens from the inlet of the column gradually decreased according to the volume of perfused plasma. On the contrary, the anti-DNA antibody titer from the outlet of the column increased according to the perfusion volume.

IEF of SLE serum of pre- and post-PH350 column
Before passing the column, the pH distribution of anti-DNA antibodies was widely spread and, especially, shown in two peaks. Whereas, after passing the immunoadsorbent column, the total level of anti-DNA antibodies decreased markedly, especially at high pH range. So-called cationic anti-DNA antibodies were removed from the circulation.

PH10 column elution pattern
In order to clarify the substance bound to this column, we made a small column (PH10 column) packed with same gel as the PH350 column. After washing the column with Tris buffer, elution was performed with stepwise increases of NaCl concentrations. First, elution was with 0.15 M NaCl, next with 0.5 M NaCl and finally with 2 M NaCl. At first step elution with 0.15 M NaCl, a relatively high peak was noted. Then, with 0.5 M NaCl, a smaller peak was noted. No more protein peak was noted with 2 M NaCl solution. In case of normal sera the obtained protein peak pattern was almost the same as in SLE.

IgG and anti-DNA titer of PH column eluate
Anti-DNA antibody activity was detected in both peaks from the SLE patient. A second peak with 0.5 M NaCl showed a higher anti-DNA activity ratio against IgG concentration compared with the first peak.

IEF of PH column eluted samples

Eluted samples were 50 or 100 times concentrated and applied to the IEF plate. The focusing pattern of the protein with 0.15 M NaCl elution showed a relatively wide spread distribution at alkaline pH. Whereas, the focusing pattern of the protein with 0.5 M NaCl elution was restricted to the high alkaline pH range. No oligoclonal band staining was noted. This second peak seems to mainly consist of so-called cationic anti-DNA antibodies. Anti-DNA antibodies of this nature bound to PH10 column strongly.

DISCUSSION

In this report, spectrotypes of anti-DNA antibodies of IgG, IgA and IgM classes, and immune complexes were studied by IEF. By electrofocusing, both IgA and IgM anti-DNA antibodies were focused to relatively restricted acidic regions. In contrast, IgG anti-DNA antibodies were focused to two distinct pH regions; one was the acidic region, similar to that where IgA and IgM antibodies migrated (pH 3.2–6.0), and the other was the far basic region between pH 7.8 and 10.0. Immune complexes were focused to the same basic region as a fraction of migrated IgG. Use of the PH column selectively eliminated anti-DNA antibodies and immune complexes from the circulation. Anti-DNA antibodies of IgG class, especially those focused to the alkaline pH region (cationic antibodies) bound to the phenylalanine (PH) column with high affinity. From these results, it was inferred that anti-DNA antibodies of IgG class, especially those having a high basic charge (cationic antibodies), showed a tendency to form immune complexes and that the cationic antibodies may participate in the pathogenesis of tissue injury, especially glomerulonephritis, in SLE. If this cationic anti-DNA has pathogenic character, as reported previously, this immunoadsorption column has an important role in removing especially pathogenic anti-DNA antibodies. Also, analysis of the distribution of anti-DNA antibodies according to pH by the IEF method is a very useful method for detailed studies.

REFERENCES

1. A. Sagawa and N. Abdou. Suppressor-cell antibody in systemic erythmatosus. *J. Clin. Invest.*, **63**, 536–539 (1979).

2. M. P. Madaio, J. Carlson, J. Cataldo *et al.* Murine monoclonal anti-DNA antibodies bind directly to glomerular antigens and form immune deposits. *J. Immunol.*, **138**, 2883–2889 (1987).

3. A. Sagawa, Y. Baba, Y. Amasaki *et al.* Significance of immunoadsorption therapy in patients with systemic lupus erythematosus: analysis of serum autoantibody repertoires by isoelectric focusing column. In: *Therapeutic plasmapheresis (VIII)*, ISAO Press, Cleveland (1989).

4. Y. Amasaki, A. Sagawa, Y. Baba *et al.* Effect of immunoadsorption therapy on lupus nephritis using immunoadsorbent PH 350 column. In: *Therapeutic plasmapheresis (VIII)*, ISAO Press, Cleveland (1989).

Therapeutic Plasmapheresis (XII), pp. 573-576
T. Agishi *et al.* (Eds)
© VSP 1993

Development of a Specific Immunoadsorbent Containing Immobilized Synthetic Peptide of Acetylcholine Receptor for Treatment of Myasthenia Gravis

S. NAKAJI, K. OKA, M. TANIHARA, K. TAKAKURA and M. TAKAMORI[1]

Kuraray Co., Ltd, Kurashiki, Japan,
[1]*Kanazawa University School of Medicine, Kanazawa, Japan*

Key words: myasthenia gravis; immunoadsorption; acetylcholine receptor; synthetic peptide; blocking antibody.

INTRODUCTION

Myasthenia gravis (MG) is an autoimmune disorder in which neuromuscular transmission is impaired by antibodies against the nicotinic acetylcholine receptor (AChR) in skeletal muscle. In order to remove anti-AChR antibodies, plasma exchange and double filtration plasmapheresis have been used. However, these methods have the disadvantages that loss of useful plasma components is inevitable and supply of replacement fluid such as fresh frozen plasma or albumin preparations is required. Therefore, recently the clinical significance of immunoadsorption has increasingly been recognized.

Anti-AChR antibodies are classified into two subclasses; binding antibody and blocking antibody. These antibodies cause the acceleration of AChR degradation, complement-mediated lysis of post-synaptic membrane and blockade of ACh-binding with AChR. The blocking antibody is known to prevent the ACh-binding with AChR, thereby inducing MG. Takamori *et al.* [1, 2] reported that the α183–200 segment of the *Torpedo californica* AChR is the ACh-binding site recognized by a blocking antibody.

Based on their study, we have developed a new immunoadsorbent column for MG treatment (Medisorba MG) by using the synthetic peptide (*Torpedo* α183–200) as an affinity ligand to specifically remove the blocking antibodies.

MATERIALS AND METHODS

Adsorbent

The synthetic peptide *Torpedo californica* α183–200 (Fig. 1) synthesized by a solid-phase procedure was used as a ligand. The peptide was covalently immobilized on porous cellulose beads (diameter 250 μm). The amount of the immobilized peptide was 35 mg/50 ml beads.

183
H-Lys-Lys-Gly-Trp-Lys-His-Trp-Val-Tyr-Tyr-Thr-Cys-Cys
200
-Pro-Asp-Thr-Pro-Tyr-Leu-Asp-Lys-Lys-Gly-OH

Figure 1. Amino acid sequence of the synthetic peptide corresponding to *Torpedo* α183–200.

In vitro study
Blocking antibody. The patient plasma (200 μl) was treated with 50 mg of peptide-bound adsorbent for 3 h at 37°C. A glycine-bound adsorbent was used as a control. The blocking antibody titer was measured by α-bungarotoxin binding inhibition assay.

Plasma protein. Healthy human plasma (5 ml) was treated with 250 mg of the peptide-bound adsorbent for 3 h at 37°C, and then the plasma protein levels were measured.

Immunoadsorbent device
Immunoadsorbent Medisorba MG consists of a small column, packed with 50 ml of peptide-bound adsorbent and sterilized by autoclaving. The safety of the device has been confirmed by various toxicity tests including acute and subacute toxicity, cytotoxicity, mutagenicity and immunogenicity tests.

Clinical evaluation
Seventy-seven treatments of plasma immunoadsorption were performed for 19 patients with MG. The immunoadsorption treatment was carried out 3 times/week [3].

RESULTS AND DISCUSSION

Figure 2 and Table 1 show the results of an *in vitro* study on adsorption of blocking antibody and on adsorption of plasma proteins, respectively. The clinical results of changes in blocking antibody obtained with the 36 immunoadsorption treatments are represented in Fig. 3. From both the *in vitro* study and clinical evaluation it was demonstrated that the peptide-bound adsorbent removed specifically blocking antibody without significantly reducing plasma proteins such as albumin and IgG. The removal rates obtained with clinical studies are as follows: blocking antibody 40.2%, binding antibody 12.4%, total proteins 5.7%, albumin 2.4%, IgG 10.2%. Figure 4 shows the changes in blocking antibody (anti-peptide antibody) and IgG level over a period of 35 days. Blocking antibody titer was reduced remarkably after the treatments contrary to the slight change in IgG level, and remained at a low level for the observation period. It is suggested that this immunoadsorption treatment provides promise for the long-term effect without occurrence of rebound. Clinical treatments improved effectively the myasthenic state. The improvement was found in 78% of the cases and no adverse effects were observed in any case of treatment.

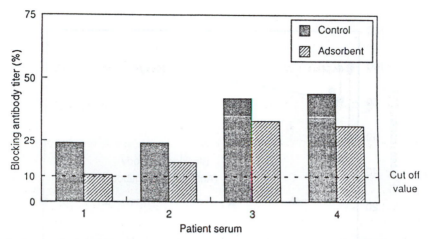

Figure 2. Changes in blocking antibody titer by adsorption treatment (*in vitro*). Adsorbent: synthetic peptide *Torpedo* α183–200 bound to porous cellulose beads. Control: glycine bound to porous cellulose beads.

Table 1.
Effect of adsorption treatment on plasma protein levels (*in vitro*)

	Adsorbent	Control
Alb (g/dl)	3.8	3.7
IgG (mg/dl)	1060	1120
IgA (mg/dl)	207	196
IgM (mg/dl)	113	105
C3 (mg/dl)	60	60
C4 (mg/dl)	19	22
TP (g/dl)	5.6	5.6
A/G	2.08	2.01

Adsorbent: synthetic peptide *Torpedo* α183–200 bound to porous cellulose beads. Control: without adsorbent.

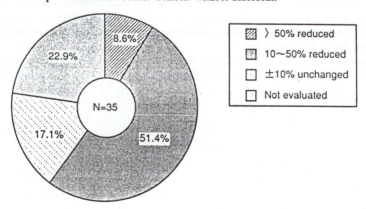

Figure 3. Changes in blocking antibody titer after plasma immunoadsorption on treatments in clinical study (Kanazawa University).

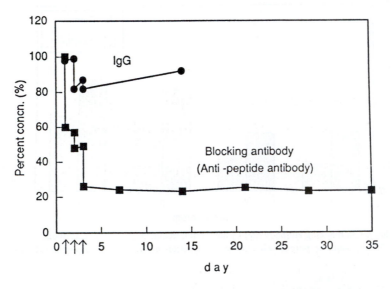

Figure 4. Changes in IgG and blocking antibody (anti-peptide antibody) levels. Arrows indicate the plasma immunoadsorption treatments.

CONCLUSION

We have developed the new immunoadsorbent containing immobilized synthetic peptide of AChR (*Torpedo* α183–200) for MG treatment. Medisorba MG showed the specific removal of blocking antibody, one of the antibodies involved in the pathogenesis of MG, without reducing significantly plasma protein levels. The clinical usefulness of the immunoadsorbent has been demonstrated for the MG treatment.

REFERENCES

1. M. Takamori, S. Okumura, M. Nagata *et al.* Myasthenogenic significance of synthetic α-subunit peptide 183–200 of *Torpedo californica* and human acetylcholine receptor. *J. Neurol. Sci.,***85**, 121–129 (1988).
2. M. Takamori, S. Okumura, Y. Ide *et al.* A synthetic peptide, *Torpedo californica* α183–200 of the acethylcholine receptor as a tool for immunoadsorption via plasma perfusion in myasthenia gravis. *Artif. Organs Today*, **1**, 53–60 (1991).
3. Y. Ide, S. Okumura and M. Takamori. Treatment of myasthenia gravis with a specific immunoadsorbent bound to acetylcholine receptor peptide α183–200. *Ther. Plasmapheresis*, **9**, 147–152 (1991).

Therapeutic Plasmapheresis (XII), pp. 577-580
T. Agishi *et al.* (Eds)
© VSP 1993

Extracorporeal Granulocyte Depletion System for the Treatment of Tumor Bearing Hosts

T. KOMAI, T. NAKAMURA, K. MIYAMOTO, M. YONEKAWA,[1] K. KUKITA,[1]
A. KAWAMURA,[1] T. TABUCHI,[2] T. SOMA,[2] K. URANO,[3]
T. MIZUTA[3] and S. ADACHI[3]

Faculty of Engineering, Mie University,
[1]*Sapporo Hokuyuu Hospital, Artificial Organ and Transplantation Institute,*
[2]*Kasumigaura Hospital, Tokyo Medical College*
[3]*Japan Immunoresearch Laboratories, Japan*

Key words: granulocyte depletion; tumor reduction; extracorporeal; experimental therapy.

INTRODUCTION

Experiments on murine tumor models and a survey of Granulocytes (Gr) and lympho-cytes (Ly) count in cancer patients disclosed a strong correlation between Gr count and tumor growth. While Ly count was not related to tumor growth, the correlation between tumor growth and the hematological parameters increased by using the Gr to Ly ratio (G/L). In an attempt to clarify these relationships, we designed and constructed a device depleting Gr in cancer patients by an extracorporeal blood circulation system and applied this system on rabbits, either normal or transplanted with VX2 Shope papilloma-derived tumor cell line.

EXPERIMENT

Investigation of the resin which absorbed Gr selectively from whole blood
Six different materials, including Nyrone, Tefrone, Polystyrene, Glass and Cellulose acetate, were examined for use as Gr adsorbent *in vitro, exo vivo* and *in vivo*. Cellulose acetate (CA) beads were found to adsorb Gr most selectively and not Ly.

Extracorporeal Gr depletion system (EGDS)
Venous blood obtained from the right earlobe vein of a rabbit using an indwelling needle was perfused with a peristatic pump through the plastic column in which CA beads were loaded and returned to the left earlobe artery.

Establishment of the cell line

VX2 Shope papilloma cells were kindly supplied by Dr H. Nakazawa, Kidney Center, Tokyo Women's Medical college. The tumor had been serially passaged *in vivo* in Japanese white female rabbits (Kitayama, Minowa, Japan) weighing from 2.5 to 3.0 kg. The transplanted tumor in rabbit was excised, washed, collagenase-treated and passed through a mesh. The preparation was transferred and primary cultured *in vitro*. Changing the medium every 2 days, the adherent monolayer in the culture was detached by treating with trypsin, washed twice with RPMI 1640, then suspended in the medium at 2×10^5 cells/ml. After it was harvested and checked for transplantability, 1×10^7 cells, suspended in 0.5 ml of 0.85% NaCl solution, were transplanted into a rabbit. Like the parent tumor, cells were highly metastatic to lung. The VX2 cell line, thus established, was maintained in liquid nitrogen until use.

Preparation of VX2 cells for transplantation

The frozen cells were rapidly heated to 37 °C, washed 3 times in RPMI 1640. Then suspended in the medium at 2×10^5 cells/ml. The cells were cultured in 6-well flat bottom plates at 2 ml/well and serially passaged. The final culture contained 0.8–1.2 cells/plate.

Animals

Twenty-eight female rabbits weighing 2.6 to 2.9 kg were used. Nine rabbits received no tumor transplantation. The animals were then transplanted with 1×10^7 cells of VX2 suspended in 0.5 ml of 0.85% NaCl by injection. The rabbits were placed in cages individually and were fed a standard diet. After 2 weeks, rabbits with a major axis of tumor exceeding 20 mm were considered to be established tumor bearing (TB) animals. Sixteen of the above 19 rabbits were divided into three experimental groups: (i) eight rabbits were subjected to EGDS treatment (EGDS rabbit), (ii) eight others received no treatment (Control rabbits) and (iii) three rabbits were used to test the hypothesis that granulocytosis exacerbates malignant tumor growth (TB rabbits). Nine additional rabbits received no VX2 transplantation and served as a negative control for evaluating the effect of the experimental system. Six of them served as blood donors for assessing changes in WBC, Gr, Ly and G/L ratios before and after passage through the system. The three others received EGDS sessions and were used to observe WBC and G/L values before during, and after EGDS.

Treatment of rabbits with EGDS

EGDS rabbits received the treatment for 13 weeks at a rate of twice a week for the first 3 weeks and once a week thereafter. The blood flow was set at 1.5 ± 0.2 ml/min for 1 h which corresponded to half of the total blood of the test rabbit that was circulated. Peripheral blood was sampled from the syringe connected to the EGDS before treatment, at the end of treatment, and at 1 and 24 h after the completion of treatment. The tumor size (TS) was evaluated by measuring bidirectional sizes of the tumor before each treatment using a vernier caliper.

RESULTS

The tumor size was strongly correlated with the number of WBC, Gr and G/L, which were statistically significant. The differences among the input and output of these numbers and ratio were also statistically significant, whereas that of Ly was not. The highest decrease on percentage from input to output was found at 75% in Gr, then 44.% in WBC. The least decrease was at 27% in Ly. In normal rabbit, WBC was considerably reduced (23.3%) immediately after the EGDS treatment, and increased to 63.0% after 1 h of the treatment, then recovered approximately to the original value. In the EGDS treated group, the number of WBC and Gr were maintained at low levels, while that of Ly showed no marked variation among the sessions, indicating that EGDS treatment did not adsorb Ly significantly. The tumor growth was markedly inhibited in the treated group whereas the increase in the control demonstrated a fast growth malignancy. Also, all the control rabbits developed a severe necrosis by which the tumor size of four out of eight control rabbits become non-measurable. Those four rabbits subsequently died of the tumor on days 33, 48, 69 and 70. The maximum survival in the control group was 121 days. Two EGDS rabbits showed complete remission with total regression of the tumors after 46 and 75 days. The tumors of the other EGDS rabbits either slowly decreased in size or remained stable.

DISCUSSION

Leukocytosis — mainly granulocytosis — has long been known to be associated with malignancy, and was thought to be caused by an infection. However, leukocytosis was often observed in cancer patients with no clinical sign of infection. The detail on this phenomena is still ambiguous, some investigators reported that peripheral Gr had a cytotoxic effect on cancer cells. A clinical survey of gastric cancer cases showed that the Gr count increased with the progression of the disease. Furthermore, experiments on murine models showed that the proliferation of granulocytes induced by i.p. injection of GM-SFS accelerated the growth of the tumor transplantation. On the other hand, murine mammary carcinoma cells transplanted into mice induced granulocytosis which seemed to be caused by stimulating of granulocytes by the tumor cell-secreted G-CSF. Our result clearly demonstrates a correlation between tumor growth and granulocytosis. Moreover, the highest correlation coefficient was found between the G/L ratio and tumor size. One possible explanation of this phenomenon is that both Gr and Ly are involved in the process of tumor growth and reduction, and that the G/L ratio reflects the condition of the patient. This view agrees with findings of Ietomi who conducted a survey of the G/L ratio in gastric cancer cases. They found that cancer patients with a high G/L ratio at the beginning of therapy died earlier than those with a lower G/L ratio. We have a histopathological result with VX2-transplanted rabbits that the Gr invaded into tumor as if it was forming a barrier preventing Ly reaching the affected site. This suggests a possibility that granulocytosis is the real cause of the tumor growth since Ly can not react with the tumor, and this suggestion is consistent with the inhibition of cytotoxic/killer lymphocytes and NK cells by Gr. Also, this suggests that Gr possesses a promoting effect on tumor growth. Shau *et al.* also reported that Gr inhibited *in vitro* LAK induction caused by IL-2. Petrie *et al.* reported that inhibition of cytotoxic T cells by Gr was dependent on the Gr count. Recently, Ishikawa *et al.* reported that proliferation of Gr promoted metastasis of B16 melanoma transplantation to the lungs. Similarly, injection of PMN (polymorphonuclear) cells enhanced metastasis in a dose-dependent fashion. Our results showed that depletion of Gr resulted in a reduction of tumor size. Our study suggests that there might be a physiological range for the G/L ratio, within which tumor size would be stable. Above this range, the tumor grows; below this range, the tumor regresses. Thus results from the experiments on rabbit tumor models demonstrated the ability of EGDS to maintain the Gr count at a low level. Most interestingly, tumor-bearing rabbits which were subjected to EGDS treatment showed sign of recovery, and two of the rabbits were completely cured. These findings show that tumor growth is inhibited by this novel cancer therapeutic device Extracorporeal Granulocyte Adsorption System.

Therapeutic Plasmapheresis (XII), pp. 581-583
T. Agishi *et al.* (Eds)
© VSP 1993

Plasma Immunoadsorption Therapy in Fisher's Syndrome

H. SHIMIZU,[1] K. ISHIKAWA,[1] K. HIRABAYASHI,[1] T. ATSUMI,[1] A. ASHIKI,[2]
S. TAKAHASHI[2] and K. IYODA[3]

Departments of [1]Neurology and [2]Urology, and [3]Section of Hemodialysis,
Seirei Hamamatsu General Hospital, Hamamatsu, Shizuoka, Japan

Key words: immunoadsorption; Fisher's syndrome.

INTRODUCTION

Fisher's syndrome is characterized by the three classical symptoms, ataxia, areflexia and external ophthalmoplegia. Immune mechanisms, especially those induced by humoral factors, may be important in the pathogenesis of Fisher's syndrome as well as in Guillain–Barré syndrome (GBS).

Recent trials with plasmapheresis in GBS have been reported to shorten the duration and severity of this syndrome [1, 2]. Therefore, we treated two patients with Fisher's syndrome using immunoadsorption instead of plasmapheresis, since it required no supplementation of albumin and there was no risk of infection being delivered by blood materials. We discuss the effect of immunoadsorption in the treatment of this syndrome.

METHODS

Two patients received three treatments of immunoadsorption on a daily basis. Both patients had a Vas-Cath inserted in their subclavian vein. The plasma immunoadsorption machine used was KM8800 (Kuraray Co. Ltd) with Plasmacure (plasma separator, Kuraray Co. Ltd) and PH-350 (plasma immunoadsorbent column, Asahi Medical Co. Ltd) (Fig. 1). PH-350 is a synthetic resin that consists of a polyvinyl alcohol gel which has bound phenylalanine as a ligand. The average daily immunoadsorbed plasma volume was 2.4 l and a total of 7.2 l was immunoadsorbed during 3 days. The exchange was not followed by either infusion of albumin or fresh frozen plasma for replacement.

Total protein, albumin, IgG, IgM, IgA contents were measured before and after immunoadsorption.

Case 1
A 64 year old male was admitted with a 4-day history of a progressive gait disturbance and diplopia. Fourteen days before admission he had an episode of an upper respiratory tract infection for 4 days.

Neurological examination revealed restricted eye movements in all directions, nasal voice, areflexia, mild dysesthesia of the palms, moderate diminution of vibration sensation of the lower limbs, dysmetria on finger–nose testing and heel–knee testing, and

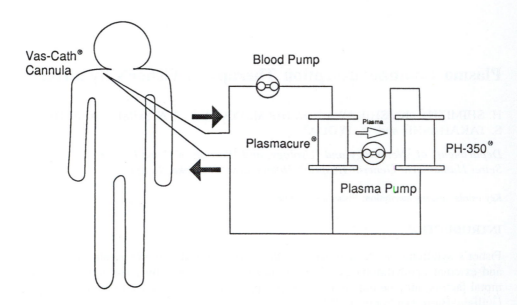

Figure 1. Circuit diagram.

moderate truncal ataxia. The CSF protein was 37 mg/dl with a normal cell count. Nerve conduction velocities and compound muscle action potentials were normal. The head MRI was normal.

Initial treatment with methylprednisolone pulse therapy followed by steroid therapy did not improve his clinical picture, but ophthalmoplegia and ataxia were deteriorated, so he received immunoadsorption therapy. After immunoadsorption, external ophthalmoplegia became mildly improved and there was no progression of clinical features. He slowly improved and fully recovered in 3 months.

Case 2

A 40 year old male was admitted with a 1-day history of an acute progressive diplopia. Thirteen days before admission he had an episode of upper respiratory tract infection for 3 days.

Neurological examination revealed restricted eye movement in all directions, especially lateral gaze, hyporeflexia and mild dysmetria on heel–knee testing. The CSF protein was 38 mg/dl with normal cell count. Nerve conduction velocities and compound muscle action potentials were normal. The head MRI was normal.

Initial treatment with methylprednisolone pulse therapy did not improve his clinical picture. Ophthalmoplegia was deteriorated. Bilateral facial palsy and dysesthesia of both hands occurred, so he received plasma immunoadsorption therapy. After immunoadsorption, external ophthalmoplegia became mildly improved and there was no progression of clinical features. He gradually improved and fully recovered in 3 months.

Table 1.

Protein and immunoglobulin before and after immunoadsorption

	Before	After	Rate (%)
Case 1			
IgG (mg/dl)	1565	675	43.1
IgA (mg/dl)	283	228	80.6
IgM (mg/dl)	78	51	65.4
T. P. (mg/dl)	5.5	5.3	96.4
Alb. (mg/dl)	3.1	3.2	103.2
Case 2			
IgG (mg/dl)	1048	784	74.8
IgA (mg/dl)	268	221	82.5
IgM (mg/dl)	149	112	75.2
T. P. (mg/dl)	5.9	5.0	84.7
Alb. (mg/dl)	3.9	3.4	87.2

RESULTS (TABLE 1)

After treatment, serum IgG content decreased 59% (mean) and serum IgM content decreased 70% (mean).

The adsorption rate of immunoglobulin in each case was different. We could not find any explanation for the difference. However, compared with albumin, the decrease of immunoglobulin was significant.

DISCUSSION

The clinical features of these cases showed Fisher's syndrome. Fisher's syndrome is thought to be an immunological disorder mainly involving the peripheral and cranial nerves. Recently, anti-GQ1b gangliooside antibody was detected in the serum and CSF of patients with Fisher's syndrome as a possible pathogenetic antibody (K. Mizoguchi, personal communication).

After immunoadsorption, clinical improvement and a decrease of IgG were observed in both cases. Removal of immunoglobulin, which contains the unknown pathogenic antibody, could diminish the dysimmune process of this syndrome.

We feel that immunoadsorption would be efficacious in treating Fisher's syndrome especially in the acute phase. In conclusion, immunoadsorption is beneficial in stopping the progression, improvement of clinical signs and is safe.

REFERENCES

1. The Guillain–Barré Syndrome Study Group. Plasmapheresis and acute Guillain–Barré syndrome. *Neurology*, **35**, 1096–1104 (1985).
2. French cooperative group on plasma exchange in Guillain–Barré syndrome. Efficiency of plasma exchange in Guillain–Barré syndrome: role of replacement fluids. *Ann. Neurol.*, **22**, 753–761 (1987).

13
Extracorporeal Immunomodulation

Therapeutic Plasmapheresis (XII), pp. 587-590
T. Agishi *et al.* (Eds)
© VSP 1993

A Novel Approach to the Original SAC Immunoadsorption as a Modality for Cancer Treatment

A. SOBKO, A. SEMERNIKOV, S. KHUTORNOY and V. NIKOLAEV

Section of Artificial Organs and Medical Biotechnologies,
Kavetsky Institute for Experimental Pathology, Oncology and Radiobiology,
Ukrainian Academy of Science, Kiev, Ukraine

Key words: protein A; SAC; immunoadsorption; immunomodulation.

INTRODUCTION

Since the middle 1970s oncologists' attention have been focused on protein A immunoadsorption [1]. Because of its high toxicity, dangerous to patients' life, a *Staphylococcus aureus* Cowan 1 (SAC) suspension used earlier was substituted with an immobilized form of pure protein A [2]. This enabled the frequency and gravity of side reactions to be sharply reduced but had a negative effect on therapeutic properties of the immunoadsorbent as far as malignant diseases are concerned [3]. Proceeding from these observations, one could assume that the development of an antitumor effect is determined not only by the removal of circulating immune complexes (CIC) and suppressive IgG but also by the immunomodulating effect of other components of a SAC cell wall (enterotoxins, glycoproteins) [3]. To reduce side effects associated with the extremely low biocompatibility of SAC and, if possible, to retain its therapeutic properties to a certain extent, we developed a binary carbon–bacterial immunoadsorbent (BIA) [4]. It is a fibrous activated carbon matrix (ACFM) with an extremely developed porosity (the specific surface area is about $2500 \mathrm{m}^2/\mathrm{g}$) and very high adsorption capacity for substances with a molecular weight up to 20–30 kDa where devitalized SAC cells are immobilized.

MATERIALS AND METHODS

The experiments were performed in dogs with spontaneous mammary adenocarcinoma. Single or double on-line plasmoadsorption (PA) of the total plasma volume was performed with an interval of 7–14 days. The antitumor effect was classified on a four-point scale accounting for regression and healing of ulcerated surfaces [6]. Characteristics of acid–base and electrolytic blood status, total protein and its fractions, osmometry of blood plasma, blood cell counting and hematocrit were determined by conventional methods. The concentration of IgG in blood plasma was determined by modified rocket immunoelectrophoresis [7]. The total level of small and middle molecules (SMM) in blood plasma ultrafiltrates was determined by HPLC. The CIC levels were analyzed nephelometrically at $\lambda = 450 \mathrm{nm}$. To determine the tumor specific reactivity of lymphocytes in dogs, a Leukocyte Adhesion Inhibition Test (tube-LAI) was used [9].

RESULTS

Plasmoadsorption was performed in 13 dogs with histobiologically confirmed malignant mammary tumors of third and fourth stages (Table 1). Any significant changes in acid–base and electrolytic balance in tumor-bearing animals were not revealed during plasmoperfusion on two types of adsorbent, except for a certain reduction in the Ca^{2+} level after IA on BIA (from 2.41 to 1.96 mM/l). The results of investigations of a PA effect on systemic and local levels of IgG, CIC and SMM are summarized in Table 2. The data on the LAI index in dogs with cancer before and after PA are given in Fig. 1.

Table 1.

Plasmaimmunoadsorption results in dogs bearing mammary adenocarcinoma

Sorbent type				BIA						ACFM			
Dog (no.)	1	2	3	4	5	6	7	8	9	10	11	12	13
Bulk of tumors (cm³)	234	159	1428	85	189	923	98	189	240	71	171	102	58
Regression	2+	1+	1+	2+	—	1+	3+	—	—	1+	1+	—	1+
Healing of ulcers	4+	—	—	4+	—	—	—	—	—	1+	—	—	—
Stabilization (months)	5.5	7.0	0.8	2.5	—	1.2	≫9	—	—	4.0	5.1	—	≫6

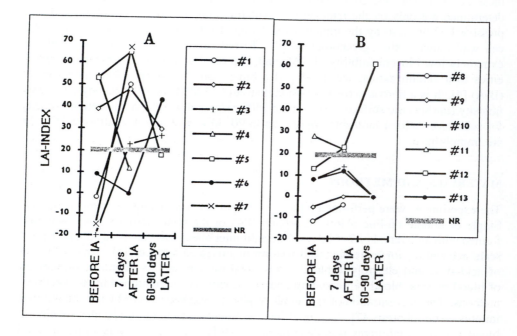

Figure 1. Kinetics of LAI index in dogs with mammary adenocarcinoma after PA: (A) on BIA and (B) on ACFM. The animal numbers correspond to the data of Table 1.

Table 2.
IgG, CIC and SMM levels in blood plasma of dogs with mammary adenocarcinoma during PA on BIA and ACFM (Mm)

Sorbate	Sorbent	Point and time of sample withdrawal (min)			
		A-pre	A-30	C-30	D-30
IgG (g/l)	ACFM	5.11 ± 0.5	5.1 ± 0.4	4.76 ± 0.4	4.15 ± 0.3
	BIA	4.13 ± 0.3	4.46 ± 0.3	4.45 ± 0.28	2.94* ± 0.21
CIC (arb. unit.)	ACFM	98.5 ± 3.5	46.9* ± 3.1	44.7* ± 3.1	20.6* ± 3.0
	BIA	120 ± 3.6	80.4* ± 2.8	77.5* ± 2.5	34.0* ± 2.4
SMM (%)	ACFM	100	98.0 ± 8.2	92.5 ± 5.1	17.7* ± 2.1
	BIA	100	98.4 ± 6.5	97.1 ± 6.2	11.4* ± 2.1

Sorbate	Sorbent	Point and time of sample withdrawal (min)				
		A-60	C-60	D-60	A post	A 7 day
IgG (g/l)	ACFM	5.18 ± 0.31	4.92 ± 0.36	4.61 ± 0.34	5.22 ± 0.51	4.9 ± 0.28
	BIA	4.52 ± 0.25	4.52 ± 0.24	3.45* ± 0.36	4.21 ± 0.25	4.33 ± 0.24
CIC (arb. unit)	ACFM	46.6* ± 2.9	50.6* ± 3.2	37.4* ± 3.5	63.3* ± 3.1	120* ± 9.9
	BIA	73.1* ± 2.5	62.1* ± 3.4	45.6* ± 3.1	61.3* ± 3.7	231* ± 15.5
SMM (%)	ACFM	91.3 ± 5.7	92.4 ± 5.8	18.1* ± 2.0	96.0 ± 5.4	—
	BIA	101.2 ± 5.5	97.7 ± 5.8	16.6* ± 2.0	77.4* ± 3.9	—

*$P < 0.05$. A, organism level; C, pre-column level; D, post-column level.

DISCUSSION

In the experiments with tumor-bearing animals we tried to model clinical advanced cancer, when the changes in homeostasis of a patient are accompanied with severe immunosuppression and various metabolic disorders. Initial LAI test results were noted to be negative (LAI < 20) in nine of 13 animals (Fig. 1). It is typical of the advanced disease stages and is determined by the excess of CIC, free tumor-associated antigens (TAA) as well as by the suppression of the system of mononuclear phagocytes of the organism. After IA the recovery of specific sensibilization of mononuclear cells for TAA is observed in all animals with initial negative index values. This process is unlikely to be determined by single limited CIC adsorption, it is rather a result of activation of the system of mononuclear phagocytes. At the same time a reduction of LAI index was observed for animals 5 and 6. This relationship enables LAI to be considered as a prognostic criterion of the therapeutic effect of IA on BIA. After IA in practically all tumor-bearing animals, as opposed to healthy dogs (9), spontaneous alleviation of side effects (fever, shiver, weakness, sometimes vomiting (dog 3)) occurred, meanwhile we observe a pronounced relation between the manifestation of antitumor and side reactions. After PA on ACFM only tumor growth stabilization (1+) was noticed in three animals. The analysis of dynamics of hematologic characteristics and proteinograms during plasmoadsorption on BIA and ACFM shows that the changes observed in dogs with mammary adenocarcinoma are similar to those in intact animals, are of transient nature and are determined by the influence of cellulose fibers in a AP-0.5H Asahi plasmaseparator (9). Analyzing Table 2, we can see that the saturation of BIA for IgG, and especially SMM, is non-existent, which is indicative of the high stability of this system.

CONCLUSION

Experimental data obtained in tumor-bearing animals show that an antitumor effect of BIA is realized through system immunomodulation, and the IA procedure on BIA does not exert any noticeable negative influence on the homeostasis of these animals.

Acknowledgment
The authors than Dr I. Krivchenko and Mrs T. Maximova for their excellent assistance in the preparation of this manuscript.

REFERENCES

1. S. C. Bansal, B. R. Bansal, H. L. Thomas *et al. Ex vivo* removal, of serum IgG in a patient with colon carcinoma. Some biochemical, immunological and histological observation. *Cancer*, **42**, 1–18 (1978).

2. G. Messerschmidt, D. H. Henry, H. W. Snyder *et al.* Protein A immonoadsorption in the treatment of malignant disease. *Clin. Oncol.*, **6**, 203–210 (1988).

3. D. S. Terman and J. H. Bertram. Antitumor effects of immobilized protein A and staphylococcal products: linkage between toxicity and efficacy, and identification of potential tumoricidal reagents. *Eur. J. Cancer. Clin. Oncol.*, **21**, 1115–1122 (1985).

4. V. A. Semernikov, V. G. Nikolaev, A. V. Sobko *et al.* Combined immunosorbents for cancer treatment. *Abstract Book: X Int. Symp. on Hermoperfusion* p. 30, Roma, 3 (1990).

5. D. S. Terman, T. Yamamoto, M. Mattiolli *et al.* Extensive necrosis of spontaneous canine mammary adenocarcinoma after extracorporeal perfusion over *Staphylococcus aureus* Cowan 1. *J. Immunol.*, **124**, 805–815 (1980).

6. V. A. Semernikov, A. V. Sobko, S. V. Khutornoy *et al.* Study of the antitumor effect of extracorporeal immunosorption of blood plasma in rats with Guerin carcinoma. *Exp. Oncol.*, **13**, 66–70 (1991).

7. L. R. Nielsen, H. H. Kisome, L. Linnet *et al.* Analysis of the decreased NK activity in lung cancer patients, using whole blood versus separated mononuclear cells. *J. Clin. Lab. Immunol.*, **29**, 71–77 (1989).

8. N. Grosser and D. M. P. Thomposon. Cell-mediated antitumor immunity in breast cancer patients evaluated by antigen induced leukocyte adherence inhibition in test tubes. *Cancer Res.*, **35**, 2571–2579 (1975).

9. V. A. Semernikov, A. V. Sobko, V. G. Nikolaev *et al.* Activated filamental charcoal material (AFCM) as a matrix for combined immunoadsorbent (CIA): *ex vivo* study. *Int. J. Artif. Organs*, **14**, 276 (1991).

Therapeutic Plasmapheresis (XII), pp. 591-594
T. Agishi *et al.* (Eds)
© VSP 1993

Therapeutic Effect of Plasma Exchange on Cellular Immunity in Lupus Nephritis

N. KIMATA, T. SANAKA, K. MURAI, W. YUMURA, H. NIHEI, K. ITO,
T. AGISHI, K. OTA and N. SUGINO

Kidney Center, Tokyo Women's Medical College, Tokyo, Japan

Key words: plasma exchange; systemic lupus erythematosus (SLE); T cell subsets; immunological abnormality; fluorescence activated cell sorter (FACS).

INTRODUCTION

Some systemic lupus erythematosus (SLE) patients are resistant to steroid or immunosuppressive treatment. Plasma exchange (PEx) is often beneficial in the treatment of these patients who do not respond to steroids or other immunosuppressive agents. However, the mechanism of its therapeutic effect is unclear. It has been reported that decreased suppressor T cell populations and increased helper/suppressor T cell ratios are implicated in the pathogenesis of SLE. Up to date, many investigators have reported that PEx is a useful modality in the treatment of SLE, and many studies have characterized the effect of PEx on humoral immunity in SLE. However, the effect of PEx on cellular immunity has not been fully understood.

The purpose of this study is to examine whether removal of autoimmune complex and other immune-related proteins by PEx improves the decreased population of suppressor T cell found in SLE patients.

MATERIALS AND METHODS

We obtained lymphocytes by venipuncture from 10 SLE patients who did not respond to prior treatment with steroids and immunosuppressive agents. The patient population consisted of eight patients with severe nephrotic syndrome and two patients with SLE-induced psychosis. For each patient, lymphocyte preparations were serially performed before PEx, immediately after PEx and 1 month later. The lymphocytes prepared were subjected to a standard fluorescence activated cell sorter (FACS) technique and divided into two groups according to Leu3a/2a ratio: a high group that had a Leu3a/2a ratio higher than 1.2 and a low group with a ratio less than 1.2.

RESULTS

Changes in IgG by PEx

Figure 1 shows serial changes in serum IgG concentration after PEx in the high Leu3a/2a group. Before PEx, the mean serum IgG level was 1290 mg/dl, which was significantly decreased to 564 mg/dl immediately after PEx. The reduction rate in IgG level was found to be 45%. Similarly, the serum levels of both immune complex and anti-DNA antibody were significantly reduced by PEx.

Changes in Leu2a by PEx

Figure 2 shows serial changes in Leu2a after PEx. Before PEx, Leu2a was $28.8 \pm 11.9\%$ in the high group and $36.6 \pm 8.4\%$ in the low group. Immediately after PEx, the Leu2a value was not changed in either group. However, 1 month after PEx, the value was significantly increased in both groups. In contrast to Leu2a, Leu3a was not affected by PEx.

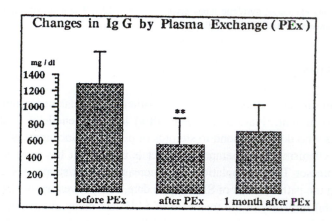

Figure 1. Serial changes in serum IgG concentration after PEx.

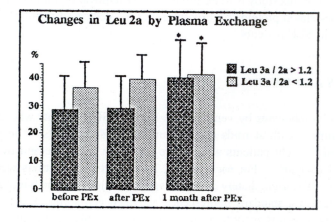

Figure 2. Serial changes in Leu2a after PEx.

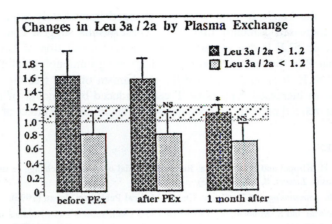

Figure 3.   Changes in Leu3a/2a ratio after PEx.

Changes in Leu3a/2a by PEx

Figure 3 shows changes in the Leu3a/2a ratio after PEx. Before PEx , the Leu3a/2a ratio was 1.64 ± 0.45 in the high group compared with 0.80 ± 0.29 in the low group, No significant change in Leu3a/2a was observed immediately after PEx in either group. One month later, the Leu3a/2a ratio was not changed in the low group. In contrast, the ratio was significantly decreased in the high group.

DISCUSSION

It has been reported that decreased suppressor T cell populations and increased helper/suppressor T cell ratios are related to the pathogenesis of SLE. Our result showed that there were not only low Leu3a/2a cases, but high Leu3a/2a cases after steroid therapy. We arbitrarily divided these to two groups by a Leu3a/2a ratio of 1.2. A Leu3a/2a ratio of more than 1.2 was classified as High group, and less than 1.2 as Low group. In general, the suppressor T cell population is increased and the helper/suppressor T cell ratio (Leu3a/2a) is decreased by steroid therapy.

Steroids directly affect cellular immunity. However, PEx does not directly affect it, because the Leu2a population and the Leu3a/2a ratio were not changed immediately after PEx therapy. Our result that the high group followed with PEx showed a similar response to the low group might be due to the removal function of humoral immunity which surrounds T cells by PEx.

It may be concluded that PEx therapy is beneficial in improving immunological abnormality in patients with SLE.

CONCLUSION

We examined whether or not PEx improves the decreased population of Leu2a and the increased ratio of Leu3a/2a that were found in steroid-resistant SLE patients. In the patients with high Leu3a/2a, the ratio was significantly decreased 1 month after PEx. In those with low Leu3a/2a, a similar decrease was observed, although it was not considered to be statistically significant. In both high and low groups, the population of Leu2a and the Leu3a/2a ratio were not changed immediately after PEx, but were significantly increased 1 month after PEx. These results suggest that the therapeutic effect of PEx on SLE is due in part to the increased population of Leu2a. It may be concluded that PEx therapy is beneficial in improving immunological abnormalities in patients with SLE. It is suggested that the mechanism of PEx treatment in SLE cases might be due to increased suppressor T cells, induced by removal of autoimmune or other immune-related protein components, not by the immediate effect of PEx treatment.

REFERENCES

1. N. Wei, J. H. Klippel and D. P. Huston. Randomized trial of plasma exchange in mild systemic lupus erythematosus. *Lancet*, **8**, 17–22 (1983).

2. O. Fujiwala. *Immunology of T cell line*. Chugai Medical Publishers, Japan (1990).

3. K. Nakabayashi and S. Minoshima. Abnormalities of T cell subsets and cytokines in the pathogenesis of primary nephrotic syndrome with MANS and other glomerular diseases. *Kidney and Dialysis*, **30**, 511–516 (1991).

4. A. N. Theoflopoulos and F. J. Dixon. Murine models of systemic lupus erythematosus. *Adv. Immunol.*, **37**, 269–390 (1985).

5. T. Sanaka, S. Wakai and S. Teraoka. Effect of therapeutic plasma exchange on immunological and renal pathological in patients with lupus nephritis. *Apheresis*, **7**, 351–353 (1990).

Therapeutic Plasmapheresis (XII), pp. 595-600
T. Agishi *et al.* (Eds)
© VSP 1993

Enhanced Macrophage Activation by Pulsed Magnetic Fields

K. FUKAYA,[1] S. MURABAYASHI,[1] A. MITO,[1] H. MIYAZAKI,[1] T. YUHTA,
T. TAKAHASHI[2] and S. SEKIGUCHI[2]

[1]*School of Engineering, University of Hokkaido, Japan*
[2]*Hokkaido Red Cross Blood Center, Sapporo, Japan*

Key words: immunomodulation; pulsed magnetic fields; macrophages; interferon-γ; lipopolysaccharide.

INTRODUCTION

Pulsed magnetic fields (PMFs), especially those of extremely low frequency (below 300 Hz), have been reported to have a profound effect on various biological systems. In the immune system the effects of PMFs have been studied from the safety point of view, and are still the subject of interest and debate. For instance, Conti showed that the blastogenic response of human peripheral blood lymphocytes was reduced by PMFs [1]. In contrast, Emilia reported enhanced effects by PMFs [2]. These contrasting results may be due to differences in the applied PMF, since Emilia used a much shorter pulse width, although the frequency and magnitude of the magnetic fields were quite similar. The detailed mechanism of such effects of PMFs are unknown; however, it is evident that PMFs modulate lymphocyte functions. If it is so, PMFs might be applicable for extracorporeal immunomodulation. Therefore, in this study, the effects of PMFs were focused on the immunomodulation point of view. Murine macrophages and human monocytes were activated by interferon (INF)-γ and lipopolysaccharide (LPS), the PMFs effects on the activation processes were studied.

MATERIALS AND METHODS

The PMFs were generated by a Helmhorz coil of diameter 22 cm. The peak magnetic field was 4.4 mT. The pulse frequency was varied from 10 to 250 Hz with the duty of 50%.

Peritoneal macrophages were prepared from pathogen-free B10 or DDY mice according to the conventional method by thioglycollate solution injection. Isolated murine macrophages were suspended to a density of 2×10^6 cells/ml in RPMI-1640 medium containing 10% FBS, 50 U/ml penicillin and 50 μg/ml streptomycin. Then, 50 ml of cell suspension was placed into each well of 24-well multidish culture plates. After incubation for 2 h at 37°C, non-adherent cells were removed by washing 3 times with Hank's balanced salt solution. The macrophages were then incubated in the RPMI-1640 medium at 37°C, and stimulated by INF-γ and/or LPS. The supernates from Con A stimulated murine spleen cell culture were used as the source of INF-γ. The macrophages were placed into two separate culture plates and cultured in the same CO_2 incubator. One was exposed to the PMF and the other was shielded to prevent PMF exposure. The degree of activation was evaluated by the measurement of glucose consumption, and expressed as the Activation Index (AI), defined as the following formula:

$$AI = \left(1 - \frac{\text{glucose concentration of the sample}}{\text{glucose concentration of the non-stimulated control}}\right) \times 100.$$

Human monocytes were prepared from peripheral venous blood of normal adults according to the conventional method of the two-step gradient centrifugation procedure using Percoll. The following experimental procedures were basically same as those used for the murine macrophages, except human recombinant INF-γ was used. The effect of PMF on Ca^{2+} influx into the monocytes was measured by a fluorescence microscope using fura-2 as a Ca^{2+} sensitive probe, which was taken in the monocytes by incubating in Hanks' solution containing 10 μM/ml fura-2 and 2 μl/ml Pluronic F-127 for 30 min at 37°C.

RESULTS AND DISCUSSION

To evaluate whether or not the PMF has any effects on the activation of murine macrophages, they were incubated at 37°C for 48 h in the presence of INF-γ alone, LPS alone, or a combination of INF-γ and LPS, and exposed to the PMF of 50 Hz. As shown in Fig. 1. glucose consumption increased with exposure of PMF when the macrophages were activated by INF-γ together with LPS, suggesting enhanced activation effects by the PMF. On the other hand, no significant effect was observed on the activation by INF-γ or LPS alone. Without stimulants, the effect of PMF was rather suppressive. It is known that the activation of macrophages by INF-γ and LPS is carried out stepwise, and INF-γ is the first signal followed by LPS activation. Therefore, the

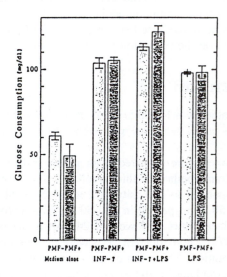

Figure 1. The effect of PMF on the glucose consumption of murine macrophages with different stimulants.

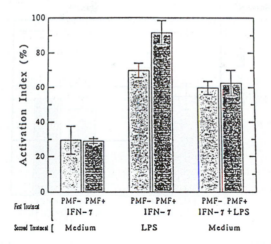

Figure 2. The effect of PMF on the two-step activation.

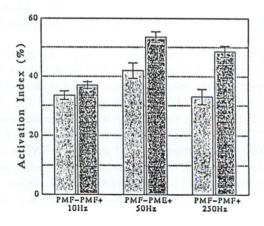

Figure 3. The frequency effect of PMF on murine macrophage activation.

effect of PMF on INF-γ activation was studied. After the macrophages were incubated and exposed to the 50 Hz PMF with INF-γ for the first 4 h, the cells were washed and incubated with 50 ng/ml LPS for the additional 60 h without PMF exposure. The AI was significantly increased by about 30% under PMF as shown in Fig. 2. There was no effect of PMF when LPS was not used as the second stimulant. These evidences suggest that the PMF affected the INF-γ activation process and enhanced the suscepti-bility to LPS. Based upon these results, the effect of PMF frequency was studied. The macrophages were subject to the two-step activation, and the first step of INF-γ was exposed to PMFs of different frequencies (10, 50 and 250 Hz). The AI was increased with the frequency as shown in Fig. 3, and the augmented effect by the PMF reached as much as 47% with 250 Hz. In addition, to evaluate the role of Ca^{2+}, the calcium channel blocker Verapamil was added in the culture medium and the PMF effect was

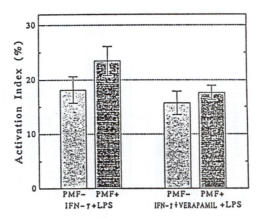

Figure 4. The effect of PMF on murine macrophage activation in the presence of Verapamil.

studied. Figure 4 shows the result and no PMF effect was observed in the presence of Verapamil. Addition of EDTA also inhibited the PMF effect. These evidences suggest that the effect of PMF on macrophage activation is probably related to the Ca^{2+} influx through the membrane.

Encouraged by these results of murine macrophages, the effect of PMF on human monocytes were studied. The monocytes were first incubated for 9 h in the presence of various concentrations of recombinant human INF-γ under 50 Hz PMF exposure, and then stimulated by 50 ng/ml LPS for 80 h. As shown in Fig. 5, the PMF induced enhanced activation of monocytes particularly at low concentrations of INF-γ. There was no significant difference in AI in the cases of INF 200 and 100 U with PMF. Probably, they reached the maximum level of activation. When monocytes obtained from another volunteer were used, as it is known human monocytes show individual differences, they were not activated by the addition of 100 U INF-γ. However, the PMF exposure could induce the activation of such monocytes in the presence of 100 U INF

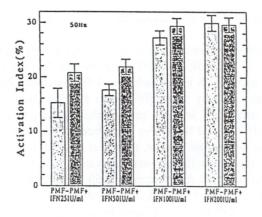

Figure 5. The effect of PMF on the activation human monocytes.

as shown in Fig. 6. Thus, the PMF affected the INF activation processes of human monocytes and enhanced the susceptibility to LPS.

In the experiments on murine macrophages, it was suggested that the effect of PMF is probably related to the Ca^{2+} influx. Therefore, Ca^{2+} ion concentration changes in the monocytes after INF stimulation were measured directly by a fluorescence microscope using fura-2 as a Ca sensitive probe, and the results are shown in Fig. 7. Compared with Fig. 7(a), which was not exposed to the PMF, the Ca ion uptake occurred more significantly and rapidly when a PMF of 100 Hz was applied during the stimulation by

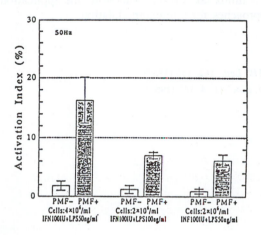

Figure 6. The effect of PMF on the activation of human monocytes.

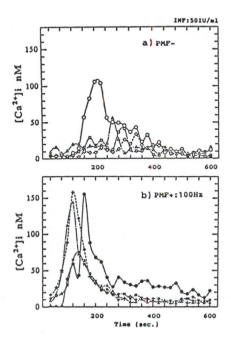

Figure 7. The time depent changes of Ca^{2+} influx in the INF-γ stimulated human monocytes.

INF as shown in Fig. 7(b). This result clearly demonstrated that the PMF enhanced the Ca^{2+} influx through the membrane. Such an effect of the PMF might be involved in the enhanced activation of monocytes. At this moment, however, it is not clear why the PMF promoted Ca^{2+} influx. In addition, it is not known how the PMF affects the process of interactions between Ca^{2+} and cellular substances such as calmodulin and protein kinase C.

Although a further study is necessary, the PMF might be useful for cellular immunomodulation, since in many cases of immunocytes activation by various stimulants, the process of Ca^{2+} influx takes place. Therefore, the application of PMF might be one of the possible approaches for immunomodulation.

REFERENCES

1. P. Conti *et al. FEBS Lett.*, **162**, 156 (1983).
2. G. Emilia *et al. J. Bioelect.*, **4**, 145 (1985).

Therapeutic Plasmapheresis (XII), pp. 601-604
T. Agishi *et al.* (Eds)
© VSP 1993

Lymphocytapheresis by using Surge System and Adoptive Immunotherapy

F. KOMATSU

Blood Transfusion Service, School of Medicine, Tokyo Medical and Dental University, Tokyo, Japan

Key words: lymphocytapheresis; haemonetics V50; surge system; adoptive immunotherapy.

INTRODUCTION

For successful adoptive immunotherapy (AI) using lymphokine activated killer (LAK) cells on cancer patients, a lot of LAK cells should be injected in to the patients. However, it is very difficult to obtain such volume of lymphocytes from the patients. An easy and suitable procedure for the collection of lymphocytes is desirable. Recently, a new procedure, the 'Surge system', on apheresis using Haemonetics V50 (Hemon-V50) was developed. It has already been shown that the surge system is useful for cytapheresis, especially platelet apheresis. In this study, the surge system was applied to lymphocytapheresis for AI in cancer patients. The usefulness of the surge system is described in this report.

MATERIALS AND METHODS

Principle of the surge system

At each cycle of cytapheresis using the Hemon-V50, plasma collected into the pheresis bag was quickly returned into the bowl. Thereafter, the platelets and white blood cells (WBC) were surged by the stream of plasma at the top of the red blood cell layer. Then, relatively pure platelets or WBC were collected separately. In lymphocytapheresis, only the WBC layer is collected. The tubing of the surge system of the Hemon-V50 is shown in Fig. 1.

Patients

Patients intended for AI were selected from cancer patients in whom cytapheresis was considered to be possible. Age, sex, body weight and the condition of anemia were not considered for the selection. Patients brain tumor, uterine cancer, melanoma and other miscellaneous cancers were included.

Collection of lymphocytes

Lymphocytapheresis was performed by using the Hemon-V50 accompanied with the surge system described above, usually once a month. The patients were administered an intravenous drip injection with saline during the donation.

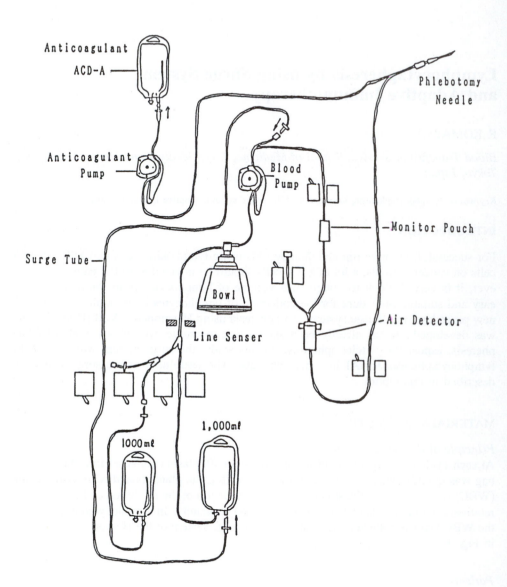

Figure 1. Tubing of the surge system on the Haemonetics V50.

Generation of LAK cells

The collected lymphocytes were cultured in Du Pont bag by incubation in 5% CO_2 at 37°C, for 7–14 days. Culture medium used was the TIL-media I (Immune-Bio Laboratory, Tokyo) plus 4% human AB serum, containing 1000 u/ml of recombinant interleukin-2. Killer activity was measured by 4 h ^{51}Cr-releasing rate. The determination of the surface marker was performed using flow cytometry.

Return of LAK cells
The generated LAK cells were washed twice with saline and returned to the patients twice a month intravenously or locally. For patients with brain tumors, the LAK cells were separated in several parts and a part was injected in once into the intracranium. The remainders were returned in turn for the next 3 weeks.

RESULTS

Donation
Each lymphocytapheresis was performed smoothly on several cancer patients. No serious problems occurred during the apheresis. Donation time was 50–70 min; 3.7–5.2 × 10⁹ WBC were obtained in one donation. Over of 90% were mononuclear cells.

LAK cell induction
By culture of the lymphocytes, 3–4 times of cell numbers were generated. Almost all cells were LAK cells. The surface marker of the cells did not differ from that of LAK cells induced from syringe donated lymphocytes. The usual killer activity in these cells was obtained. A case of patients is described.

Case: F.F. 56 year old female
She was a gastric cancer patient and gastrectomy was performed 3 years ago, followed relapse recently. AI was performed as shown in Table 1. During AI, she was not given any medication, except amino acid imbalance treatment. Six donations were performed. After the start of the therapy, her ascites disappeared. Tumor which was touched by palpation on the adbominal wall became not to be ascertained. She continued in a good state. However, the lymphocytapheresis was discontinued, because her vein was too fine for donation. She was discarded and stayed at home. She died because of general bone metastasis and emaciation after 5 months.

Table 1.
Donation and return of LAK cells in the patient (F.F.)

Donation	1992			1993		
date	12 Oct	6 Nov	20 Nov	5 Dec	16 Jan	5 Feb
cycles	8	8	6	6	8	6
volume	188 g	204 g	165 g	157 g	189 g	154 g
no. of lymphocytes	4.7×10^9	5.2×10^9	3.9×10^9	3.8×10^9	4.8×10^9	3.7×10^9
Return	1992				1993	
date	1 Nov	17 Nov	1 Dec	18 Dec	30 Jan	27 Feb
no. of LAK cells	9.3×10^9	10.9×10^9	9.8×10^9	9.4×10^9	10.6×10^9	8.9×10^9

DISCUSSION

In this experiment, the Hemon-V50 accompanied with the surge system was used for the lymphocytapheresis of cancer patients. The surge system is very useful, and a lot of lymphocytes were obtained. The advantages of the surge system are: the donation time is relatively short; the volume of extracorporeal circulation is not so much; a lot of lymphocytes are collected; and frequent lymphocytapheresis is possible, especially on patients with low body weight or anemia.

REFERENCE

1. *Haemonetics V50 Apheresis System Operation Manual*. Haemonetics Corp., Braintree, MA (1989).

Therapeutic Plasmapheresis (XII), pp. 605-609
T. Agishi *et al.* (Eds)
© VSP 1993

Preliminary Evaluation of Ultra-fine Fibers as a Substrate for Immobilizing Immunomodulators

H. MIYAZAKI, S. MURABAYASHI, A. MITO, T. YUHTA and K. ONOÉ[1]

Division of Biomedical Engineering, Faculty of Engineering, and
[1]*Institute of Immunological Science, Hokkaido University, Sapporo, Japan*

Key words: immunomodulation; fiber size effect; Con A immobilized ultra-fine fibers; lymphocyte function; IL-2 activity.

INTRODUCTION

It is well known that the adsorption behaviour of lymphocytes on fiber materials is related to the fiber size, and lymphocytes are adsorbed very efficiently only to fibers with diameters less than 10 μm [1]. In our previous study, murine lymphocytes cultured on various sizes of fibers with Concanavalin A (Con A) showed different IL-2 activity, and ultra-fine fibers of 1.5 μm showed the highest value [2]. These results suggested that fiber size affects lymphocyte functions. In the present study, to evaluate the applicability of ultra-fine fibers to the modulation of lymphocyte functions, Con A was used as a model immunomodulator and immobilized on the surface of fibers having different diameters. Murine lymphocytes were cultured on these fibers, and the fiber size effects on the cells were evaluated in terms of IL-2 production and adhesion morphology.

MATERIALS AND METHODS

Oxygen plasma treatment and Con A immobilization

Non-woven polypropylene fibers (average diameter: 1.5, 2.6, 3.3, 4.5 and 7.9 μm; Kuraray Co., Japan) were used for the substrates. To introduce reactive functional groups on the surface of fibers, O_2 plasma treatment was performed in a plasma reactor (Shimadzu, LCVD-20, Japan). The discharge conditions were as follows: O_2 pressure, 0.035 Torr; power, 25 W; treatment time, 10 min. After the treatment, the samples were reacted with 50 mg/ml 1-ethyl-3-(3-dimethylaminopropyl)-carbodiimide hydrochloride (Dojindo Laboratories, Japan) (0.1 M phosphate buffer at pH 5.8, 37°C, 3 h) followed by rinsing in distilled water, and reacted with various concentrations (1.0, 0.5 and 0.1 mg/ml) of Con A (Sigma, St Louis, MO) in distilled water (RT, 2 h). They were washed in 1% Triton X (10 min), rinsed with distilled water and dried at RT.

In vitro murine splenic lymphocyte culture and CTLL-2 assay for evaluating IL-2 activity

The samples were cut square (15 × 15 mm) and placed in the bottom of each well of a 24-well tissue culture plate (Falcon 3047, Becton–Dickinson, Oxnard CA). Surface areas of the samples were adjusted to 450–540 cm². To prevent the sample from floating in culture medium, a Teflon ring (ID = 11.8 mm) was placed on the sample. They were sterilized by gamma ray irradiation. RPMI-1640 medium (2 ml) (Gibco Laboratories, Grand Island, NY) supplemented with 10% fetal calf serum (FCS) (Granite Diagnostics, Burlington, VT), antibiotics and 2×10^{-6} M/ml 2-mercaptoethanol was poured into each well, and air bubbles were removed by pipetting and centrifugation. After removing the culture medium (CM, 1.5 ml), spleen cells from C57BL/10 (7.5×10^6 cells) suspended in CM (1 ml) were added to each well, centrifuged for 5 min at 65 g, and cultured at 37°C in 5% CO_2 for 24 h. The supernatants were stored at −70°C. CTLL-2 suspended in CM (4×10^3 cells/well, 100 μl) was added into 96-well flat-bottomed microtiter plates (Falcon 3072, Becton–Dickinson) in the presence of 1:2 dilutions of the supernatants (100 μl) and cultured for 24 h. For the final 8 h of culture, they were pulsed with 0.5 μCi/well of [³H]thymidine ([³H]Tdr), and cells were harvested onto glass fiber filters. Radioactivity was counted by liquid scintillation spectrometry. The results were expressed in c.p.m. and a stimulation index (SI) was calculated as follows:

$$SI = (S - C)/C$$

S = c.p.m. [³H]Tdr incorporated by CTLL-2 in the presence of supernatant, C = c.p.m. [³H]-Tdr incorporated by CTLL-2 in the absence of supernatant.

Evaluation of Con A dose-dependent IL-2 production

To evaluate the optimal concentration of Con A for IL-2 production, Con A was dissolved in CM (1000 μg/ml) for serial dilutions. Murine spleen cells (1.5 ml, 5×10^6 cells/ml) were added to each well of a 24-well tissue culture plate followed by serial dilutions of the Con A solution (150 μl), and cultured (37°C, 24 h). IL-2 activities of the supernatants were evaluated by the CTLL-2 assay.

Preparation of specimens for scanning electron microscopy

Each of the samples was rinsed and fixed in 0.1 M phosphate buffer (pH 7.2) containing glutaraldehyde, dehydrated through a graded series of ethanol. They were critical point dried and sputter-coated with a thin layer of gold.

RESULTS AND DISCUSSION

The IL-2 activity of lymphocytes cultured on Con A immobilized fibers of different sizes are shown in Fig. 1. The highest values were obtained by samples which were reacted with 1.0 mg/ml of Con A solution for the immobilization, and showed as much as 70–80% of the maximal activity induced by Con A solution. The activities of the samples prepared with 0.5 mg/ml of Con A solution were about 45% of those with 1.0 mg/ml solution, and the samples prepared with 0.1 mg/ml solution failed to induce significant activation. Therefore, 1.0 mg/ml was found to be appropriate among these concentrations. To evaluate the effect of fiber size on IL-2 production, the experiments were repeated and the values were averaged as shown in Fig. 2. A Con A solution of 1.0 mg/ml was used for these experiments. Statistical differences in IL-2 production were not observed among the fiber sizes, and there seems to be no fiber size effect. But probably, a fiber size effect may exist and the reason is discussed in the following. The morphology of the lymphocyte adhering on the surface of the Con A immobilized fibers is shown in Fig. 3. It was observed that the contact area of the lymphocyte with the fiber became smaller in proportion to the decrease of fiber size. Therefore, the total numbers of Con A molecules that could interact with the lymphocyte on the surface of ultra-fine fiber were expected to be much less than those on the thick fiber, if the density of immobilized Con A was equal among the fibers of different sizes. Probably, this assumption is reasonable, because the density of carboxyl groups introduced by the O_2 plasma treatment could be considered to be equal among them. It is known that IL-2 production of lymphocytes induced by Con A is dependent on the Con A concentration. It was expected, therefore, that IL-2 production of the lymphocytes adhered on the ultra-fine fibers should differ depending on the fiber size. However, no statistical differences were observed among the fiber sizes. The dose-dependence of IL-2 production on Con A concentration is shown in Fig. 4. The range of the optimal concentrations of Con A was from 0.4 to 3.0 μg/ml. The activity of Con A immobilized on the surface corresponded to the Con A concentration of 0.24 or 10 μg/ml, since the IL-2 activities induced by Con A immobilized fibers were 70–80% of the maximal value (Figs 1 and 4). Since the activity decreased by one-half when the Con A concentration was reduced to half for the immobilization (Fig. 1), it could be supposed that the activity of immobilized Con A corresponded to the 0.24 μg/ml level. Therefore, IL-2 production of the lymphocytes adhered on the ultra-fine fibers should show a lower level compared with the thicker fibers. However, there were no differences in IL-2 production among the fiber sizes. This results suggested the possibility of the fiber size effect on the functional modulation of lymphocytes.

When we think about the application of ultra-fine fibers for immunomodulation, one may be afraid that damage of the cell membrane occurs when the cells are detached and isolated from the ultra-fine fibers. However, Kayashima *et al.* reported that mitogenic

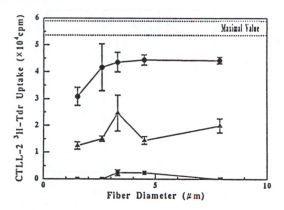

Figure 1. Effect of fiber size and concentration of Con A for immobilizing on IL-2 production by murine spleen lymphocytes adhered on Con A immobilized polypropylene fibers. Con A concentration: (•) 1.0 mg/ml, (▲) 0.5 mg/ml, (■) 0.1 mg/ml.

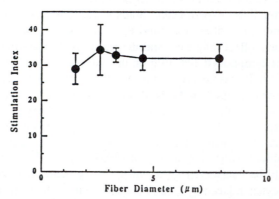

Figure 2. Effect of fiber size on IL-2 production by murine spleen lymphocytes adhered on Con A immobilized polypropylene fibers: 2.6, 7.9 μm, n = 3; 1.5, 3.3, 4.5 μm, n = 4.

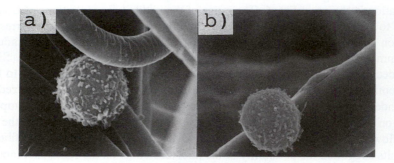

Figure 3. Scanning electron micrographs showing murine spleen lymphocytes adhering on Con A immobilized fibers of different fiber sizes; (a) 2.6 μm, (b) 7.9 μm.

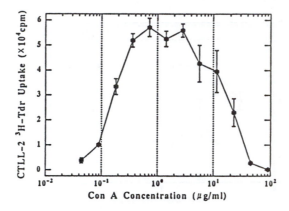

Figure 4. Dose-related murine spleen lymphocyte proliferation obtained in the presence of increasing
concentrations of Con A.

reactivity of lymphocytes obtained by fiber column separation to Con A was as high as before separation levels [3]. Their report suggests that the procedure of lymphocyte isolation from fiber materials does not affect lymphocyte function. In addition, from the viewpoint of the contact area, it might be expected that isolation of lymphocytes from ultra-fine fibers is easier than in the case of thicker ones, since the contact area is much less.

Although further studies are necessary, ultra-fine fibers might be worthwhile to consider as substrates for immobilizing immunomodulators.

REFERENCES

1. E. F. Leonard, K. Ikebe, D. Lauffenburger *et al.* Extracorporeal cellular immunotherapy. *Trans. Am. Soc. Artif. Intern. Organs*, **32**, 633–638 (1986).
2. H. Miyazaki, S. Murabayashi, A. Mitoh *et al.* Macrostructure effect of synthetic polymers on immunocyte functions. *Jpn. J. Artif. Organs*, **20**, 235–240 (1991).
3. K. Kayashima, Y. Asanuma, J. W. Smith *et al.* Simple on-line filters for the therapeutic removal of lymphocytes from blood. *Trans. Am. Soc. Artif. Intern. Organs*, **27**, 559–562 (1981).

Therapeutic Plasmapheresis (XII), pp. 611-614
T. Agishi *et al.* (Eds)
© VSP 1993

Immune Modulation Leading to Resolution of Acute and Treatment-resistant Immune Thrombocytopenic Purpura in Patients Treated with Protein A Immunoadsorption

H. W. SNYDER Jr, S. K. COCHRAN, J. P. BALINT Jr and F. R. JONES

IMRÉ Corporation, Seattle, Washington, USA

Key words: protein A; immunoadsorption; immunomodulation; immune thrombocytopenic purpura.

INTRODUCTION

Immune thrombocytopenic purpura (ITP) is an autoimmune disorder in which platelets are sensitized by association with autoantibodies and/or circulating immune complexes (CIC) making them susceptible to removal from the circulation by splenic macrophages [1–5]. Depending upon the severity of the resulting thrombocytopenia, symptoms may range from easy bruisability and petiechiae to epistaxis and gingival bleeding to anal, gastrointestinal or intracranial bleeding [1–5]. Spontaneous remissions occur in <5% of adults [6]. Steroids produce marked platelet increments in up to 75% of patients and up to 67% of those who require further therapy respond to splenectomy [6]. However, the surgery has an associated morbidity and mortality and increases the risk of overwhelming infection [7]. Patients who fail both steroids and splenectomy also tend to be resistant to other forms of treatment [6]. Recently, protein A immunoadsorption treatment columns have been developed commercially for therapeutic removal of IgG and IgG-containing CIC from patient plasma. The present study summarizes extensive multicenter experience with this new treatment modality in patients with ITP.

PATIENTS, MATERIALS AND METHODS

The therapy was evaluated in 50 adults (> 18 years of age) with acute ITP (defined as < 6 months duration with no splenectomy) and in 72 adults with treatment-resistant ITP (steroid/splenectomy failures or disease duration of greater than 6 months with failure of at least two therapies). Both groups of patients had mean pretreatment platelet counts of less than $20\,000/\mu l$. Patients received an average of six treatments of 0.25–2.0 l plasma per procedure over a 2–3 week period using PROSORBA® treatment columns (IMRÉ Corporation, Seattle, WA). A 'fair response' was defined as at least a doubling of the baseline platelet count and achievement of a count in the range of $50\,000$ to $100\,000/\mu l$. A 'good response' was defined as achievement of a count of greater than $100\,000/\mu l$. Responses maintained > 2 months were referred to as 'durable'.

Laboratory evaluations included quantitation of platelet-directed IgG (PDIgG), platelet-associated IgG (PAIgG), antibodies to purified platelet antigen GPIIb/IIIa, antibodies reactive with F(ab')$_2$ fragments from purified IgG anti-GPIIb/IIIa, total C1q-CIC and CIC containing anti-GPIIb/IIIa and anti-F(ab')$_2$ (8–10).

RESULTS

Immunologic parameters and platelet counts were evaluated before and after treatment in 22 patients with acute ITP and 42 patients with treatment-resistant ITP (Table 1). Patients presented with elevated levels of C1q-CIC, PDIgG and PAIgG as compared with normal controls ($> 10\,\mu g/ml$, $> 0.5\,\mu g/ml$ and $> 10\ ng/10^6$ platelets, respectively). The patients as a group, including both clinical responders and nonresponders, showed statistically significant decreases in these parameters after treatment, along with corresponding increases in platelet counts (Table 1). However, clinical responder patients had relatively lower pretreatment levels of CIC (averaging 31 versus $62\,\mu g/ml$ for nonresponders) and PDIgG (2.08 versus $2.73\,\mu g/ml$) and their subsequent declines were to near normal levels. This led to an absence of PAIgG in clinical responder patients which was not achieved by nonresponder patients.

Table 1.

Changes in immunologic parameters and platelet counts in ITP patients receiving immunoadsorption therapy (mean values)

	Pretreatment	Post-treatment
C1q-CIC ($\mu g/ml$)	37	22
PDIgG ($\mu g/ml$)	2.40	1.04
PAIgG ($\mu g/10^6$ platelets)	36	21
Anti-GPIIb/IIIa ($\mu g/ml$)	2.34	1.22
Anti-F(ab$'$)$_2$ ($\mu g/ml$)	1.03	2.82
Anti-GPIIb/IIIa-anti-F(ab$'$)$_2$-CIC ($\mu g/ml$)	1.16	2.44
Platelet count (x 10^{-3} per μl)	19	93

The first three tests and platelet counts were evaluated in all 64 patients. The other tests were evaluated in a subset of 40 patients who were positive in a screen for anti-GPIIb/IIIa antibodies. Data from acute and treatment-resistant ITP patients was pooled. The average of pre- and post-treatment differences exhibited by all evaluable patients in each parameter was statistically significant ($P < 0.05$) by the one-sample t-test.

Immunologic changes were examined further in terms of responses to a specific platelet antigen, GPIIb/IIIa. PDIgG in 16 acute and 24 treatment-resistant patients was comprised in part of anti-GPIIb/IIIa antibodies. The levels of anti-GPIIb/IIIa antibodies in these patients were very close to the levels of total PDIgG (Table 1) and, similarly, they became absent in clinical responders but not in nonresponders. Pretreatment levels of specific anti-F(ab$'$)$_2$ antibodies were lower than the average measured in a group of 15 normal individuals ($5.63\,\mu g/ml$). Treatment-related increases in anti-F(ab$'$)$_2$ antibodies and in CIC containing those antibodies and anti GPIIb/IIIa molecules were correlated with disappearance of the autoantibody. F(ab$'$)$_2$ isolated from post-recovery IgG molecules neutralized the binding of F(ab$'$)$_2$ isolated from affinity-purified IgG anti-GPIIb/IIIa molecules *in vitro*.

Immunoadsorption treatments were associated with good responses in 15 acute ITP patients (30%) and fair responses in 10 patients (20%). All responses occurred in 1–4 weeks. The responses were durable, making splenectomy or long-term immunosuppressive therapy unnecessary, in 21 patients (42%) followed for up to 24 months. The treatments also caused good responses in 18 patients with treatment-resistant ITP

(25%) and fair responses in 15 patients (21%). These responses were durable in 26 patients (36%) over a follow-up period of up to 26 months.

DISCUSSION

Immunoadsorption treatment causes reduction of platelet-binding IgG and CIC levels in patient plasma and thereby produces marked platelet increments in patients with ITP. However, bulk removal of these molecules cannot be the mechanism of therapy since the binding capacity of treatment columns is only approximately 1g of IgG [8]. It is possible that removal and/or changes in the character of CIC due to interaction with the protein A matrix could result in modulation of antibody responses against CIC-associated antigens [8]. However, the precise mechanism(s) remain to be established. Reported immunologic responses to protein A immunoadsorption treatment include increases in NK cell activity, monocyte IL-1 production and absolute numbers of activated T helper and B cells, a decrease in absolute numbers of activated T suppressor cells, and increases in antibodies against viral and tumor-associated antigens [8]. In the present study, increases in specific anti-F(ab')₂ antibodies, which may prove to be comprised of antiidiotypic antibodies, are described. Recently, Berchtold *et al.* [11] reported on antiidiotypic GPIIb/IIIa antibodies in therapeutic preparations of IV IgG. Inhibition of autoantibody binding ranged from 20–41% using only a concentration of 3.2% IV IgG, compatible with therapeutic concentrations *in vivo*, suggesting that small changes in concentrations of antiidiotypic antibodies induced by any therapy could have unexpectedly dramatic effects on autoantibody activity. The effects of immunoadsorption treatment on processes which may influence platelet counts in other ways, such as platelet production or availability or activity of macrophage Fc receptors, have not been evaluated.

CONCLUSIONS

CIC as well as autoantibodies may be involved in the pathophysiology of ITP. Protein A immunoadsorption is effective in reducing levels of these components, thereby causing long-term remissions in patients otherwise facing splenectomy or long-term immunosuppressive therapy. Further understanding of the mechanism of this therapy is required before its maximum effectiveness may be realized.

REFERENCES

1. C. Mueller-Eckhardt. Idiopathic thrombocytopenic purpura: clinical and immunological considerations. *Semin. Thromb. Hemost.*, **3**, 125–159 (1977).
2. R. McMillan. Idiopathic thrombocytopenic purpura. *N. Engl. J. Med.*, **304**, 1135–1147 (1981).
3. J. G. Kelton and S. Gibbons. Autoimmune platelet destruction: Idiopathic thrombocytopenic purpura. *Semin. Thromb. Hemost.*, **8**, 83–104 (1982).
4. S. Karpatkin. Autoimmune thrombocytopenic purpura. *Semin. Hematol.*, **22**, 260–288 (1985).
5. J. B. Bussel. Autoimmune thrombocytopenic purpura. *Hematol. Oncol. Clin. North Am.*, **4**, 179–191 (1990).
6. P. Berchtold and R. McMillan. Therapy of chronic idiopathic thrombocytopenic purpura. *Blood*, **74**, 2309–2317 (1989).
7. B. Styrt. Infection associated with aspenia: risks, mechanisms and prevention. *Am. J. Med.*, **88**, 5N33–5N42 (1990).

8. H. W. Snyder Jr, J. P. Balint Jr and F. R. Jones. Modulation of immunity in patients with autoimmune disease and cancer treated by extracorporeal immunoasdorption with PROSORBA® columns. *Semin. Hematol.*, **26** (Suppl. 1), 31–41 (1989).

9. H. W. Snyder Jr, J. H. Bertram, M. Channel *et al.* Reduction in platelet-binding immunoglobulins and improvement in platelet counts in patiets with HIV-associated idiopathic thrombocytopenic purpura (ITP) following extracorporeal immunoadsorption of plasma over protein A–silica. *Artif. Organs*, **13**, 71–77 (1989).

10. H. W. Snyder Jr, S. K. Cochran, J. P. Balint Jr *et al.* Experience with protein A immunoadsorption in treatment-resistant immune thrombocytopenic purpura. *Blood*, **79**, 2237–2245 (1992).

11. P. Berchtold, G. L. Dale, P. Tani and R. McMillan. Inhibition of autoantibody binding to platelet glycoprotein IIb/IIIa by anti-idiotypic antibodies in intravenous gamma globulin. *Blood*, **74**, 2414–2417 (1989).

Therapeutic Plasmapheresis (XII), pp. 615-618
T. Agishi *et al.* (Eds)
© VSP 1993

Immune Modulation and Resolution of Cancer Chemotherapy-associated Thrombotic Thrombocytopenic Purpura/Hemolytic Uremic Syndrome in Patients Treated with Protein A Immunoadsorption

H. W. SNYDER Jr, S. K. COCHRAN, J. P. BALINT Jr,
R. L. PEUGEOT and F. R. JONES

IMRÉ Corporation, Seattle, Washington, USA

Key words: protein A; immunoadsorption; immunomodulation; thrombotic thrombocytopenic purpura/hemolytic uremic syndrome.

INTRODUCTION

Thrombotic thrombocytopenic purpura/hemolytic uremic syndrome (C–TTP/HUS) is a syndrome of thrombocytopenia, microangiopathic hemolytic anemia and progressive renal dysfunction which develops in 2–10% of cancer patients who have received chemotherapeutic agents such as mitomycin-C, bleomycin or cisplatin [1]. Prior studies suggest that immunologic factors such as platelet-directed autoantibodies and circulating immune complexes (CIC) containing platelet or tumor-associated antigens may play a role in inducing or effecting platelet aggregation, a hallmark of the syndrome [2, 3]. Therapies such as corticosteroids, anti-platelet agents, immunosuppressive drugs and plasmapheresis have been generally ineffective and 75–80% of patients die within 8–12 months of diagnosis [1, 2]. However, Korec *et al.* [2] showed that adsorption of plasma over staphylococcal protein A columns caused decreases in levels of platelet-aggregating CIC and clinical responses in eight of 11 patients. In the present study, commercially-available protein A immunoadsorption treatment columns were also shown to reduce levels of disease-related immunologic factors in plasma and to induce sustained clinical remissions in C-TTP/HUS.

PATIENTS, MATERIALS AND METHODS

Fifty-five C-TTP/HUS patients were treated using columns with 200 mg protein A covalently bound to a silica matrix (PROSORBA® columns, IMRÉ Corporation, Seattle, WA). The patients received a mean total of six treatments of 1 l plasma per treatment at a frequency of 2–3 procedures per week. They were followed for up to 2 years. Response to the therapy was determined by assessing quantitative laboratory measurements of thrombocytopenia (platelet count), hemolysis (lactate dehydrogenase, hematocrit) and renal function (creatinine). Kaplan–Meyer product-limit estimates of survival were also examined and differences in survival curves were evaluated using the log rank test.

In addition, multivariate adjustment was performed using the Cox proportional hazards model for censored survival data.

Platelet-directed IgG (PDIgG), antibodies to purified platelet antigen GPIIb/IIIa, antibodies reactive with adenocarcinoma-associated antigens (fucosylated glycosphingolipid antigens containing Le^x determinants), antibodies directed against F(ab')$_2$ fragments from purified IgG anti-GPIIb/IIIa, and total C1q-CIC were all quantitated by ELISA using human IgG standards [4–6]. CIC containing GPIIb/IIIa and Le^x glycolipid antigens were isolated by adsorption to microtiter plates containing a rabbit antibody against human C1q and detected by ELISA using antigen-specific mouse monoclonal antibodies and alkaline phosphatase-conjugated anti-mouse IgG as described previously [6]. The data were reported in terms of relative units of activity (RU/ml), as compared with C1q-bound aggregated normal IgG standards. CIC comprised of anti-GPIIb/IIIa and anti-F(ab')$_2$ were detected and quantitated as described previously [4, 5]. Isolated anti-GPIIb/IIIa antibodies (affinity-purified over columns with specific antigen) and sucrose gradient-isolated antigen-specific CIC [5] were evaluated for platelet aggregating activity *in vitro* [2].

RESULTS

Patients presented with elevated PDIgG (average levels of 3.03 μg/ml) and anti-GPIIb/IIIa (2.75 μg/ml) compared with normal controls (< 0.5μ g/ml). Anti-F(ab')$_2$ levels averaged 3.43 μg/ml as compared with an average in 10 normals of 9.60 μg/ml. Anti-Le^x glycolipid antibodies were undetectable (< 0.5 μg/ml). C1q-CIC averaged 86 μg/ml, GPIIb/IIIa-CIC were 4.84 RU/ml, Le^x glycolipid CIC were 3.60 RU/ml and anti-GPIIb/IIIa-anti-F(ab')$_2$-CIC were 1.32 μg/ml.

Affinity-purified anti-GPIIb/IIIa antibodies and sucrose gradient-isolated CIC containing GPIIb/IIIa both induced aggregation of normal donor platelets *in vitro*. Aggregation was mediated by F(ab')$_2$ fragments from the purified anti-platelet antibodies. Anti-GPIIb/IIIa-anti-F(ab')$_2$-CIC did not show platelet aggregating activity, suggesting that anti-F(ab')$_2$ antibodies neutralize the autoantibody activity. Isolated Le^x glycolipid-CIC did not cause platelet aggregation *in vitro*.

Immunoadsorption treatment was associated with significant immunologic changes in 6 patients (all clinical responders) out of 15 patients evaluated (Table 1). These changes included statistically significant decreases in anti-GPIIb/IIIa antibodies and GPIIb/IIIa-CIC. In addition, there were statistically significant increases in anti-F(ab')$_2$ antibodies and anti-GPIIb/IIIa-anti-F(ab')$_2$-CIC. Cox proportional hazards regression modeling showed the association between each of these immunologic changes and prognosis (survival) to be statistically significant. Statistically significant increases in levels of anti-Le^x glycolipid antibodies and corresponding decreases in the levels of corresponding CIC were also observed (Table 1). The relevance of this finding remains to be determined.

Overall, 25 of 55 patients achieved clinical responses. Response was associated with an estimated 61% one-year survival as compared with only a 22% rate in nonresponders ($P = 0.0001$). Patients whose malignancies were in complete or partial remission had estimated 74% survival as compared with a 22% rate in historical control patients reported in the literature ($N = 70$), who received other therapies ($P = 0.0161$). Patients with stable or progressing tumors had poor prognosis regardless of therapy.

Table 1.
Quantitative changes in immunologic parameters in C-TTP/HUS patients receiving immunoadsorption therapy

	Clinical responders ($N = 6$)	Clinical non-responders ($N = 9$)
PDIgG (μg/ml)	−3.29	+1.45
Anti-GPIIb/IIIa (μg/ml)	−2.90	+0.57
Anti-F(ab')$_2$ (μg/ml)	+4.36	−0.51
Anti-Le^x gl (μg/ml)	+6.22	+0.62
Total C1q-CIC (μg/ml)	−87	+2.5
GPIIb/IIIa-CIC (RU/ml)	−3.66	−0.87
Le^x glycolipid-CIC (RU/ml)	−2.05	+0.11
Anti-GPIIb/IIIa-		
anti-F(ab')$_2$-CIC (μg/ml)	+2.85	+0.55

Differences between average changes in clinical responders and non-responders were all statistically significant ($P < 0.05$) by one sample t-test.

DISCUSSION

Protein A immunoadsorption columns have been developed commercially for therapeutic removal of IgG and IgG-containing CIC. In the United States PROSORBA® columns are marketed for the treatment of patients with the autoimmune disease immune thrombocytopenic purpura (ITP) [7]. Laboratory studies have demonstrated that treatment-related decreases in levels of CIC and platelet autoantibodies are associated with normalization of platelet counts [4, 5, 7, 8]. In experimental treatments of patients with adenocarcinoma the procedure has also been shown to remove CIC containing Le^x glycolipids, to increase levels of anti-Le^x glycolipid antibodies and to induce measurable reductions in tumor burden [6]. The present study shows that the procedure is also effective in lowering CIC and platelet-directed autoantibodies with platelet-aggregating activity from plasma of patients with C-TTP/HUS.

The precise mechanism(s) by which the observed immunomodulation is achieved is not yet resolved. It has been proposed [4] that removal and/or changes in the character of CIC due to interaction with the protein A–matrix may play a role in altering responses to CIC-associated antigens. In any case, preliminary studies have shown that all phases of the humoral antibody-based immune reactions may be affected by the treatment including the interrelated components of the phagocytic, cellular and humoral systems (reviewed in [4]). More information is also needed to completely understand the role of immunologic factors in the pathogenesis of C-TTP/HUS.

CONCLUSIONS

This study further implicates platelet-associated immunologic factors in the pathogenesis of C-TTP/HUS and establishes protein A immunoadsorption as an effective means to deplete plasma of these factors and induce long-term clinical benefit.

REFERENCES

1. J. B. Lesesne, N. Rothschild, B. Erickson *et al.* Cancer-associated hemolytic-uremic syndrome: analysis of 85 cases from a national registry. *J. Clin. Oncol.*, **78**, 781–789 (1989).

2. S. Korec, P. S. Schein, F. P. Smith *et al.* Treatment of cancer-associated hemolytic uremic syndrome with staphylococcal protein A immunoperfusion. *J. Clin. Oncol.*, **4**, 210–215 (1986).

3. S. E. Zimmerman, F. P. Smith, T. M. Phillips *et al.* Gastric carcinoma and thrombotic thrombocytopenic purpura: association with plasma immune complex concentrations. *Br. Med. J.*, **284**, 1432–1434 (1982).

4. H. W. Snyder Jr, J. P. Balint Jr and F. R. Jones. Modulation of immunity in patients with autoimmune disease and cancer treated by extracorporeal immunoadsorption with PROSORBA® columns. *Semin. Hematol.*, **26**, (Suppl. 1), 31–41 (1989).

5. H. W. Snyder, J. H. Bertram, M. Channel *et al.* Reduction in platelet-binding immunoglobulins and improvement in platelet counts in patients with HIV-associated idiopathic thrombocytopenic purpura (ITP) following extracorporeal immunoadsorption of plasma over staphylococcal protein A-silica. *Artif. Organs*, **13**, 71–77 (1989).

6. A. K. Singhal, M. C. Singhal, E. Nudelman *et al.* Presence of fucolipid antigens with mono- and dimeric X determinant (Le^x) in the circulating immune complexes of patients with adenocarcinoma. *Cancer Res.*, **47**, 5566–5571 (1987).

7. H. W. Snyder Jr, S. K. Cochran, J. P. Balint *et al.* Experience with protein A immunoadsorption in treatment-resistant immune thrombocytopenic purpura. *Blood*, **79**, 2237–2245 (1992).

8. H. W. Snyder Jr, J. H. Bertram, D. H. Henry *et al.* Use of protein A immunoadsorption as a treatment for thrombocytopenia in HIV-infected homosexual men: a retrospective evaluation of 37 cases. *AIDS*, **5**, 1257–1260 (1991).

Therapeutic Plasmapheresis (XII), pp. 619-622
T. Agishi *et al.* (Eds)
© VSP 1993

Effect of Plasmapheresis on Cytokines Production from Mononuclear Cells

I. TOMITA, H. KANAZAWA, A. SUENAGA, H. GOTO and N. SHIBUYA

Department of Neurology, Kawatana National Hospital, Nagasaki, Japan

Key words: immunoadsorption therapy; interleukins; lymphocyte subsets; neuroimmunological disorders.

INTRODUCTION

Plasmapheresis (PP) is effective for the treatment of neuroimmunological disorders such as multiple sclerosis (MS) Guillain-Barré syndrome, chronic inflammatory polyradiculoneuropathy (CIDP) and myasthenia gravis. There are many documented abnormalities of cellular immunity found in those patients. PP removes pathogenic substances and activates complement cascades in contact blood with a high molecular membrane. Activated complement fragments then influence the cellular immunity directly [1].

In order to examine how immunoadsorption therapy (IA) influences cellular immunity, we measured production of interleukins from cultured mononuclear cells *in vitro*, and lymphocyte subsets before and after a series of IA.

SUBJECTS AND METHODS

Patients

Four patients with definite MS, one with CIDP and one with HTLV-1 associated myelopathy (HAM) were included in this study.

IA

An immunocolum of tryptophan-PVA gel was used on-line with a cellulose diacetate membrane. IA was performed for a total of three times every other day. One plasma volume was treated in each IA.

Measurement of interleukin production in vitro

Mononuclear cells were collected from peripheral blood before and after IA. Peripheral blood mononuclear cells (PBMC) were isolated by cetrifugation on Ficoll-Conray gradients. PBMC were resuspended at a concentration of 10^6 cells/ml with RPMI 1640 medium supplemented with 5% fetal bovine serum and cultured for 3 days.

The concentration of IL-1α and IL-2 in culture supernatant was detected by an ELISA method.

Analysis of lymphocyte subsets
Lymphocyte subsets were analyzed by two-color FACScan.

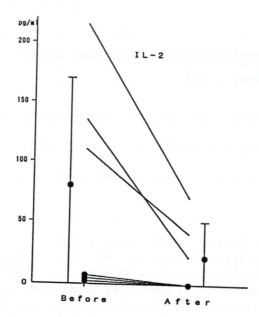

Figure 1. Effect of IA therapy on IL-2 production.

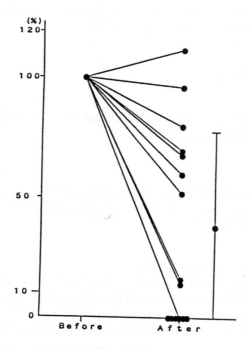

Figure 2. Changes of IL-2 production before and after IA.

RESULTS

IL-2 production from cultured PBMC was significantly reduced after a series of IA (Fig. 1). The value of IL-2 from PBMC was 80 ± 89 pg/ml (mean $\pm$ SD, $n = 6$) before IA and 22 ± 28 pg/ml after a series of IA. Its value decreased more than 70% compared with the value at pretreatment.

IL-2 production was reduced after each IA (Fig. 2). The concentration of IL-2 in cultured supernatants of PBMC after IA decreased about 40% compared with the values before IA.

IL-1α production tended to reduce after IA (Fig. 3, $51 \pm 33\%$ compared with the values before IA, $n = 15$).

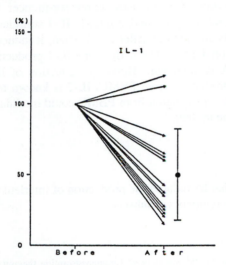

Figure 3. Effect of IA on IL-1 production.

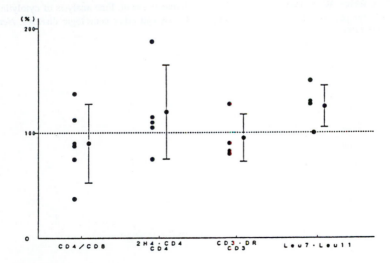

Figure 4. Effect of IA on lymphocyte subsets.

After a series of IA, the ratio of CD4/CD8 and $CD3^+DR^+/CD3^+$ was reduced to 10 ± 38 and $5 \pm 22\%$, respectively. On the other hand, the ratio of $2H4^+CD4^+/CD4^+$ and $Leu7^+Leu11^+$ increased to 18 ± 42 and $26 \pm 20\%$, respectively (Fig. 4).

DISCUSSION

A common immune abnormalities noted in neuroimmunological diseases were a loss of non-specific suppressor cell function, decreased numbers of suppressor T cells and increased CD4/CD8 ratio [2]. The complement cascade is activated during membrane PP in contact blood with a high molecular membrane leading to the cleavage of C3 and C5. The clevage fragments of C3a and C5a act as an anaphylatoxin and also have immunoregulatory properties. C3a induces suppressor-inducer lymphocytes and C5a stimulates macrophages, releasing its mediator IL-1. IL-1 stimulates many kinds of cells including B cells, T cells and natural killer cells. Then, it induces IL-2 from helper T cells and IL-2 receptors on T cells. The reason why IL-1 production from mononuclear cells is reduced after IA is unknown. However, reduction of IL-1 production might have an effect on IL-2 production from PBMC. IL-2 is known to regulate lymphocyte function. A decline of IL-2 production from PBMC could modulate lymphocyte subsets and influence the immune system.

CONCLUSION

It is strongly suggested that IA reduces the production of interleukins from mononuclear cells and then modulates lymphocyte subsets.

REFERENCES

1. H. Kanazawa, S. Fujishita, H. Takashima *et al.* Immunoadsorption therapy and cellular immunity. In: *Therapeutic plasmapheresis (VIII)*, T. Oda (Ed.), pp. 249–253, ISAO Press, Cleveland (1990).
2. W. E. J. Weber, W. A. Bauman, M. M. P. P. Vandermeeren *et al.* Fine analysis of cytolytic and natural killer T lymphocytes in the CSF in multiple sclerosis and other neurologic diseases. *Neurology*, 37, 419–425 (1987).

Therapeutic Plasmapheresis (XII), pp. 623-626
T. Agishi *et al.* (Eds)
© VSP 1993

Lymphokine Activated Killer Cell Therapy — Application of Cytokine Gene Transfer

Y. KOHGO, Y. ITOH, Y. LIU, Y. KOSHIDA, H. NEDA, M. TAKAHASHI, N. WATANABE and Y. NIITSU

Department of Internal Medicine (Section IV), Sapporo Medical College, Sapporo, Japan

Key words: IL-2 activated killer cell; TNF-α gene; retrovirus vector transfection.

INTRODUCTION

Adoptive immunotherapy using lymphokine activated killer (LAK) cells has been extensively studied. As the clinical results using LAK cells and IL-2 were not satisfactory, several attempts such as the combination use of other cytokines, use of different sources of killer cells, local transfer of killer cells to tumor tissues, etc., have been conducted. We have reported that the cytotoxicity of IL-2 activated lymphocytes derived from malignant effusion could be augmented by the transfection of the tumor necrosis factor-α (TNF) gene by the lipofection procedure [1, 2]. However, this procedure tends to lose cell viability easily and the transfection efficiency was not satisfactory for future *in vivo* use. In this paper, we present the results of retroviral gene transduction of the TNF gene to IL-2 activated killer cells derived from malignant effusions and discuss the mechanism of the augmentation.

MATERIALS AND METHODS

The lymphocytes derived from malignant effusion in the pleural or peritoneal cavity in cancer patients were used as sources of IL-2 activated killer cells. Lymphocytes from malignant effusion were separated from tumor cells by Percoll discontinuous gradient centrifugation. They were incubated with 800 JRU/ml of recombinant IL-2 (Takeda Pharm. Co. Ltd, Tokyo, Japan) for 5–7 days in RPMI 1640 medium supplemented with 10% fetal calf serum (tumor infiltrating lymphocytes, TIL). The tumor cells were stored under liquid nitrogen until use. The TNF expression vector, pcDV-TNF was derived from pSV2neo and the human TNF coding region was inserted into it [3]. pSV2neo was used as a control vector which encodes SV40 promtor and neomycin phosphotransferase, an intracellular enzyme that inactivates G418. TNF expressing retrovirus vector (pLJ-TNF) was constructed from pLJ vector by the insertion of the TNF gene (Fig. 1) [4]. The amphotropic packaging cells (ψ-CRIP, a gift from Dr Kokai, National Children Medical Center) [5] were infected with pLJ-TNF and the virus producing cells (A103) were established. By coculturing killer cells with the supernatant of A103 cells and selecting G418, stable transfectants were obtained. The cytotoxicity of transfectants against established cell lines (K562 and Daudii cells) and autologous tumor cells were examined by ^{51}Cr release assay. The concentrations of GM-CSF, IL-1, interferon-γ and lymphotoxin in the culture supernatant were determined by the enzyme-linked immunoassay procedure or bioassay. The surface phenotypes, using monoclonal antibodies, were examined by a flow cytometry.

RESULTS AND DISCUSSION

IL-2 activated killer cells from malignant effusions were incubated with culture supernatant of packaging cells (A103) and were selected with G418 addition. The integration of TNF genes to killer cell DNA was confirmed by Southern analysis. In the transfected cells, a significant amount of TNF (0.1–1.0 unit/ml) was secreted into the culture medium, whose production has persisted more than 30 days and declined at day 50. The proliferating activity of transfectants was significant and kept its growth potential for more than 50 days. Table 1 shows the TNF production and the cytotoxicity to various target cells. The killer cells in patient 1 (ovarial cancer) were only sensitive to K562 cells and the increment of cytotoxicity was observed after TNF gene transduction. In patient 2 (pancreatic carcinoma), two batches of culture and TNF gene transduction were performed. By these two experiments, different killer transfectants were obtained. Killer cells in Experiment 1 showed lower production of TNF and less cytotoxicity to all the three target cells, namely K562, Daudi and autologous cells, compared with killer cells in Experiment 2. The increment of cytotoxicity by TNF gene transduction was prominent. The magnitude of augmentation of killer activity on the basis of lytci unit per 30% killing on 10^7 lymphocytes were about 8-fold in K562 cells. 1- to 7-fold in Daudi cells and 2-fold in autologous tumor cells. It is noteworthy that the cytotoxic spectrum of obtained killer cells have no difference between the neo-gene

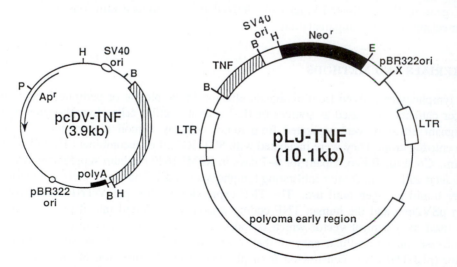

Figure 1. Physical structure of TNF-α expressing vector. Human TNF cDNA, SV40 ori, SV40 early promoter and enhancer; poly A, polyadenylation site of SV40; AP^r, amicillin resistant gene; Neo^r, neomycin resistant gene; LTR, long terminal repeat of MLV; B, *Bam*HI; E, *Eco*RI; P, *Pst*I; X, *Xho*I.

transfected control cells and TNF gene transfected cells. According to the results of surface phenotype expression by flow cytometry, the positive ratio of CD4 or CD8 antigen expression seemed to be random. This suggests that neither the periferential integration nor selection of growth of certain lymphocyte subpopulation by TNF gene transduction happened. It is noteworthy that there is no susceptibility of autologous tumor cells to exogenously added TNF from 1 to 100 unit/ml concentration, while mild cytotoxicity of K562 and Daudi cells was observed. These results suggest that the augmented cytotoxicity was not explained by the direct action of synthesized TNF from transfectants. Rather, indirect effects have to be considered.

Table 1.
The cytotoxicity of TNF-α gene transfected killer cells derived from malignant effusion

		Cytolytic activity (LU/10^7 cells)		
		K562	Daudi	Autologous tumor
Case 1	TIL/Neo	14.2	< 10	< 10
	TIL/TNF	121.2	< 10	< 10
Case 2				
Exp. 1	TIL/Neo	54.3	55.5	20.8
	TIL/TNF	120.5	75.8	45.5
Exp. 2	TIL/Neo	125.0	208.3	30.3
	TIL/TNF	800.0	1428.6	52.6

In order to examine what kind of cellular events have occurred in the killer lymphocytes transduced with the TNF gene, the expression of IL-2 receptor, the production of other cytokines and the distribution of adhesion molecules were examined. Flow cytometric analysis showed that the expression of IL-2 receptor α was not down-regulated even during the culture period in the presence of excess amounts of IL-2. This may explain the persistence of proliferating capacity during the long incubation period. By the enzyme immunoassay procedure, the increment of GM-CSF and lymphotoxin was observed, while IL-1-β was under the detection limit. The interferon-γ production confirmed by cytopathic assays was also increased. The expression of adhesion molecules such as CD2 and LFA-1 were slightly increased by transduction of the TNF gene.

Taken together, the explanation of the augmentation of killing can be drawn as follows. The TNF gene-transfected killer lymphocytes have the capability to synthesize cellular and extracellular TNF production. The increment of TNF production does not similarly affect the direct cytotoxicity to TNF sensitive tumor cells, rather it augments the indirect killing mechanisms. The indirect actions by TNF gene transduction include the proliferation capability by IL-2 through the increment of IL-2 receptor, other cytokine productions such as interferon-γ and lymphotoxin and the increase of tumor–killer cell interactions by expressing the adhesion molecules.

Acknowledgment
This work was supported by Grants-in-Aid for Cancer Research for the Ministry of Health and Welfare of Japan and for Scientific Research for the Education, Science, and Culture of Japan.

REFERENCES

1. Y. Itoh, Y. Kohgo, N. Watanabe *et al.* Human tumor-infiltrating lymphocytes transfected with tumor necrosis factor gene could augment cytotoxicity to autologous tumor cells. *Jpn. J. Cancer Res.*, **82**, 1203–1206 (1991).

2. Y. Kohgo, Y. Itoh, N. Watanabe *et al.* Antitumor properties and possible application for gene therapy with IL-2 activated killer cells. *Gann Monogr.*, in press.

3. T. Himeno, N. Watanabe, N. Yamauchi *et al.* Expression of endogenous tumor necrosis factor as a protective protein against the cytotoxicity of exogenous tumor necrosis factor. *Cancer Res.*, **50**, 4941–4945 (1990).

4. J. Price, D. Turner and C. Cepko. Lineage analysis in the vertebrate nervous system by retrovirus-mediated gene transfer. *Proc. Natl. Acad. Sci. USA*, **84**, 156–160 (1987).

5. O. Danos and R. C. Mulligan. Safe and efficient generation of recombinant retrovirus with amphotropic and ecotropic host ranges. *Proc. Natl. Acad. Sci. USA*, **85**, 6460–6464 (1988).

Therapeutic Plasmapheresis (XII), pp. 627-631
T. Agishi *et al*. (Eds)
© VSP 1993

Granulocytapheresis in *in vitro* and Animal Experiments

M. YONEKAWA, K. KUKITA, N. KAMII, K. ONODERA, M. TAKAHASHI,
H. WITMANOWSKI, J. MEGURO, A. KAWAMURA, T. KOMAI,[1]
T. MIZUTA[2] and M. ADACHI[2]

*Sapporo Hokuyu Hospital, Artificial Organ and Transplantation Hospital,
Sapporo, Japan*
[1]*Faculty of Science, Hokkaido University, Sapporo, Japan*
[2]*Japan Immunoresearch Laboratories, Takasaki, Japan*

Key words: terminal cancer; granulocyte; extracorporeal circulation; granulocytapheresis; cellulose acetate.

INTRODUCTION

It is frequently observed in patients with terminal state cancer that the granulocyte proportion in peripheral blood increases and the lymphocyte proportion decreases as their cancer progresses, which is commonly recognized as a result of a decrease of the lymphocyte defence ability against cancer. However, recent papers have revealed a strong correlation between the granulocyte count and the tumor progress. As the granulocyte and lymphocyte ratio (G/L ratio) reflects the clinical status of the host, the G/L ratio is now used as a host immunological indicator against cancer [1]. From the point of view that it might be essential to reduce the G/L ratio, we have developed the Granulocyte/Lymphocyte Regulation System [2]. In this paper we describe an experimental study of extracorporeal granulocytapheresis.

BACKGROUND

The G/L ratio was studied in three groups; group A contained 49 patients with cancer in the pre-operative period, group B contained 20 patients with terminal state cancer who died within 3 months, and group C contained 25 patients with benign diseases in the pre-operative period. The G/L ratio of group A, B and C was 1.7 ± 0.5 (mean $\pm$ SD), 2.4 ± 1.0 and 16.8 ± 23.3, respectively. The G/L ratio of terminal cancer was markedly high (Fig. 1).

IN VITRO SCREENING TEST

An *in vitro* screening test was designed using heparinized normal human blood and cancer patient blood for the selection of the most efficient material for the adsorption of granulocytes. Heparinized blood was incubated with each material (polystyrene, PETF, glass, cellulose acetate and 6-nylon) for 120 min, and the G/L ratio was determined every 30 min.

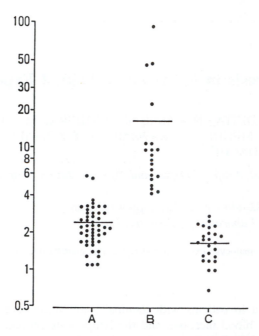

A : cancer patient, before operation (n=49)
B : cancer patient, death within 3 months (n=20)
C : benign patient, before operation (n=25)

Figure 1. G/L ratio in patients.

Among these materials, cellulose acetate and nylon beads adsorbed most granulocytes in normal human blood. However, nylon adsorbed not only granulocytes but also lymphocytes, so cellulose acetate was the most efficient material (Fig. 2). In cancer patient blood, cellulose acetate could also most efficiently reduce the G/L ratio.

EX VIVO EXPERIMENT

An *ex vivo* experiment was designed to assess cellulose acetate in a perfusion system. Heparinized blood was circulated for 180 min in an *ex vivo* perfusion system containing 500 beads of cellulose acetate. The G/L ratio was also determined each time.

The G/L ratio was gradually decreased just after perfusion and reached a minimum after 90 min (Fig. 3).

IN VIVO EXPERIMENT

An *in vivo* experiment was designed to evaluate the efficacy of granulocyte adhesion and the safety of this system using beagles. An acrylic column with a capacity of 229 ml containing 15 000 cellulose acetate beads with a 2 mm diameter was used. Changes of WBC, granulocytes, lymphocytes, the G/L ratio, platelets and fibrinogen were determined each time and the adsorption rate of the column was determined by measurement

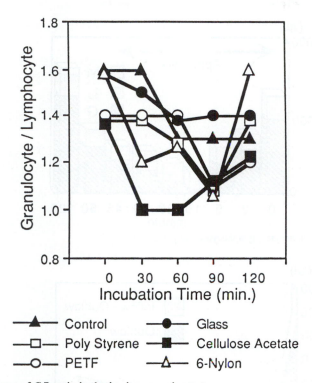

Figure 2. Changes of G/L ratio in the *in vitro* screening test.

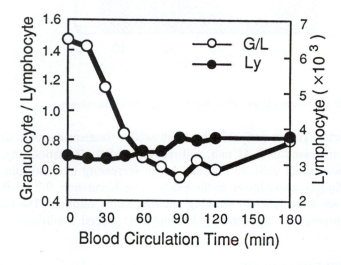

Figure 3. Changes of G/L ratio in the *ex vivo* experiment.

at the inflow and outflow points of the column. An extracorporeal circulation was set for 45 min at a rate of 100 ml/min blood flow.

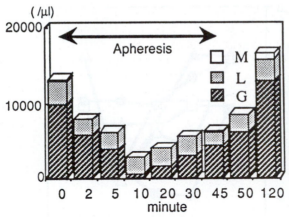

Figure 4. Changes of monocytes, lymphocytes and granulocytes.

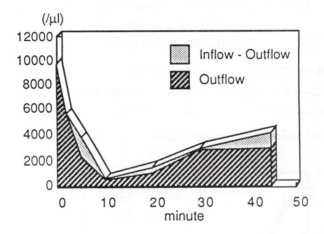

Figure 5. Changes of granulocytes at the inflow and outflow points of the column.

WBC and granulocytes in peripheral blood showed a transient decrease for 10 min and sequentially increased until 45 min, and recovered after circulation (Fig. 4). The adsorption rate was small until 30 min and began increasing after 30 min (Fig. 5). Platelets and fibrinogen also adhered to the beads. After circulation, 9.2×10^8 of WBC were obtained from the column by washing out with saline solution. The beagles did not show any abnormalities in laboratory data and their general condition.

DISCUSSION AND CONCLUSION

Many arguments have been made about the role of granulocytes in cancer [1, 3, 4]. Our clinical study, which demonstrated a marked elevation of the G/L ratio in terminal cancer, suggest that granulocytes may play a negative role in terminal cancer, so the reduction of granulocytes may bring about changes in the immunological conditions of the patient. We have developed a Granulocyte/Lymphocyte Regulation System.

In *in vitro* screening tests, of all the tested materials, cellulose acetate could most efficiently reduce the G/L ratio. In *in vivo* experiments, granulocytes showed remarkable depletion and sequential increase. This phenomenon is well known as hemodialysis leukopenia, which is recognized as the consequence of uneven distribution of granulocytes in the human body [5]. However, our data, that more than 10^8 granulocytes were obtained after circulation, indicate that granulocytes were entrapped within the column.

From the results that platelets and fibrinogen were reduced in *in vivo* studies and granulocytes were gradually reduced in *ex vivo* studies, we can estimate that platelets and some protein such as fibrinogen adhere to the surface of the beads at first, and then granulocytes adhere to the protein layer.

These results indicate that this granulocytapheresis system will become a promising method in terminal cancer therapy.

REFERENCES

1. K. Ietomi. A study on the role of granulocytes in carcinoma-bearing hosts — G/L ratio as a new host indicator. *J. Jpn. Soc. Cancer Ther.*, **25**, 662–671 (1990).

2. M. Yonekawa, N. Kamii, K. Onodera *et al.* Basic study of extracorporeal granulocyte/lymphocyte regulation system. In: *Therapeutic Plasmapheresis (X)*, ICAOT Press, Cleveland (in press).

3. H. Shau and A. Kim. Suppression of lymphokin-activated killer induction by neutrophils. *J. Immunol.*, **141**, 4395–4402 (1986).

4. H. T. Petrie, L. W. Klassen and D. Kay. Inhibition of human cytotoxic lymphocyte activity by autologous peripheral blood granulocytes. *J. Immunol.*, **134**, 230–234 (1985).

5. P. R. Craddock, J. Fehr, A. P. Dalmasso *et al.* Hemodialysis leukopenia — pulmonary vascular leukocytosis resulting from complement activation by dialyzer cellophane membranes. *J. Clin. Invest.*, **59**, 879–888 (1977).

Therapeutic Plasmapheresis (XII), pp. 633-636
T. Agishi *et al.* (Eds)
© VSP 1993

Experimental Trial of Anticancer Immunotherapy using Immobilized Pokeweed Mitogen: Immunotherapy by Extracorporeal Circulation

T. YOKOTA, K. NUMA, T. TANI, K. HANASAWA, Y. ENDO, H. AOKI,
K. MATSUDA, T. YOSHIOKA, H. ABE, H. ARAKI,
Y. TSUTAMOTO and M. KODAMA

*First Department of Surgery, Shiga University of Medical Science,
Seta Tsukinowa, Shiga, Japan*

Key words: immunomodulation; pokeweed mitogen; extracorporeal circulation.

INTRODUCTION

Recently, anticancer immunotherapy has been rapidly developed and undergoing clinical trial [1]. We have been developing new material which can enhance the immunosystem using extracorporeal circulation [2, 3]. Pokeweed mitogen (PWM), a sort of lectin, has strong potency inducing anticancer lymphocytes. It was immobilized to the beads for utilizing extracorporeal circulation.

MATERIALS AND METHODS

PWM (E. Y. Laboratories Inc., USA) was immobilized chemically at a density of 0.4 mg/ml on methyl-methacrylate-divinylbenzene copolymer beads coated with poly-hydroxyethylmethacrylatediethylaminoethyl-methacrylate (PMMA–DVB). These beads were packed into the minicolumn with a volume of 3 ml.

Human peripheral blood mononuclear cells were isolated from heparinized venous blood of normal volunteers and cancer bearing patients by centrifugation on Lymphoprep (Ficoll/Hypaque gradients). The cells concentration was adjusted to 1×10^7/ml in RPMI 1640 containing 100 U/ml penicillin, 100 μg/ml streptomycin, 0.25 M 2-mercaptoethanol and 2% heat-inactivated pooled AB human serum.

An extracorporeal circulation model was made to activate lymphocytes with columnized PWM beads. The suspension medium was injected into the circuit from three-way valve. The lymphocytes which passed through the PWM column were activated by circulatory contact stimulation for 60 min. The flow rate was 0.5 ml/min. After stimulation, lymphocytes were collected and used for effecter cells.

In order to compare with LAK cells, lymphocytes, adjusted to 5×10^6/ml, were cultured in medium containing 1 unit/ml of recombinant interleukin-2 (TPG-3; Takeda Chemical Industries Ltd., Osaka).

Cytotoxicity was measured by chromium release assay using 96-well, round-bottomed microplates (Linbro, no. 76-013-05). The target cells were labeled with 100 μCi $Na_2^{51}CrO_4$

(Japan Radioisotope Association, Tokyo) per 1×10^7 cells in RPMI-1640 medium containing 10% fetal calf serum for 90 min.

After washing three times with phosphate-buffered saline (−). The labeled cells were seeded into each well at 5×10^3 cells/well. The suspension of effecter cells was added to triplicate wells at various E/T ratios in a final volume of 200 μl. After incubation at 37°C for 4 h, the supernatant was collected and counted by a gamma counter (Packard Autogamma 5650). The percent cytoxicity was calculated by the following formula:

$$\text{cytoxicity (\%)} = \frac{\text{(experimental release} - \text{spontaneous release)}}{\text{(maximum release} - \text{spontaneous release)}} \times 100.$$

Congenital nude male Jcl:AF-*nu* mice 5–6 weeks old were inoculated 1×10^7 cells of MKN-1 (a human gastric cancer cell line) in 0.1 ml (intradermally). At 7 days after inoculation, the lymphocytes, which activated by the circulatory model with PWM column for 60 min, were administered (1×10^7) cells in 0.1 ml (intratopically) around the tumor. The control group were injected with non-activated lymphocytes in the same manner. Mean tumor diameter was measured for assessment.

Japanese white rabbits weighing about 2500 g were inoculated with 1×10^6 viable VX2 tumor cells into their left thighs. These tumor bearing rabbits were canulated into the right femoral artery and the ear vein under general anesthesia by 40 mg/kg sodium pentbarbital injection (peritoneally). Single direct hemoperfusion was carried out for 2 h using a column containing 10 ml of PWM beads 6 days after inoculation.

Then, 500 units heparin was infused into the circuit at the start of DHP. The flow rate was 2.0 ml/min. Thigh thickness and body weight were measured and survival terms were recorded for assessment.

RESULTS

The lymphocytes, which were activated by circulatory contact stimulation for 60 min, demonstrated a strong cytoxicity against both NK-sensitive K-562 cells and NK-resistant Daudi cells (Figs 1 and 2).

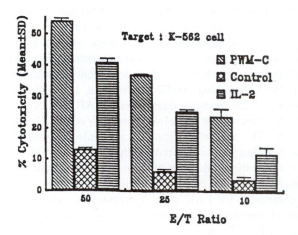

Figure 1. Cytoxicity (%) against K-562 cells using lymphocytes activated with the immobilized PWM beads.

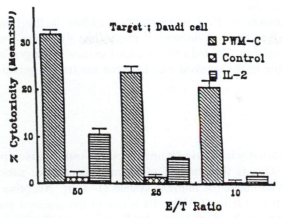

Figure 2. Cytotoxicity (%) against Daudi cells using lymphocytes activated with the immobilized PWM beads.

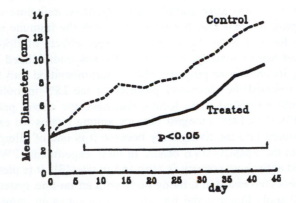

Figure 3. Comparison of MKN-1 tumor growth between the treated nude mice and the control mice.

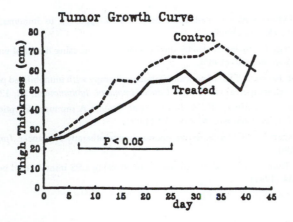

Figure 4. Comparison of VX2 tumor growth between the treated rabbits and the control rabbits.

The tumor growth of MKN-1 inoculated nude mice was significantly suppressed in the treated group (Fig. 3).

Mean tumor diameters of VX2 tumor bearing rabbits in the treated group were significantly smaller than those of the control group (Fig. 4). There were no significant differences in body weights. Treated rabbits tended to survive longer, but there was not a significant difference in the survival rate between the treated group and the control group.

DISCUSSION

There are two methods to try improving immunopotency using extracorporeal circulation or lymphapheresis. One is the removal of immunosuppressive substances in blood [4, 5]. Another is to stimulate the immune system [1-3, 6]. Adoptive immunotherapy with lymphokine activated killer (LAK) cells is one of the practical methods, although it has several problems to be performed. LAK is not so effective on clinical trials because it is difficult to induce sufficient transferable LAK cells, and relatively large amounts of IL-2 administration causes severe side effects. Moreover the method for inducing the LAK cells was very complicated, expensive and time consuming. We have been developing the new material which enhances the immune system. At first, our attention was focused upon the strong anticancer effects of lipopolysaccharides (LPS). But LPS has severe toxicity; therefore, LPS was immobilized to the fiber and beads for utilizing its anticancer property without administration into the living body. We have already reported the anticancer property of the LPS immobilized fiber and beads [2, 6]. While we found some lectins also have the strong potency to induce anticancer cells. PWM had the strongest potency among lectins we examined. PWM cannot be administered into the living body because it is one of allergens. So, PWM was immobilized to the PMMA-DVB beads. In these experiments PWM immobilized beads demonstrated anticancer potency *in vitro* and *in vivo* [3]. It is possible to activate innumerable lymphocytes easily in a living body with an on-line system. Therefore, it may be possible to apply this material for cancer treatment as an immunomodulator.

REFERENCES

1. S. A. Rosenberg. Lymphokine-activated killer cells: a new approach to immunotherapy of cancer. *J. Natl. Cancer Inst.*, **75**, 595 (1985).
2. T. Tani. A new strategy for malignancies by direct hemoperfusion using bacterial endotoxin bounding fiber. *J. Jpn. Surg. Soc.*, **86**, 148 (1985).
3. K. Numa, T. Tani, M. Kodama. Trial of anticancer immunotherapy with immobilized pokeweed mitogen: immunotherapy by extracorporeal circulation. *Cancer Immunol. Immunother.*, **32**, 125–130 (1990).
4. G. L. Messerschmidt, D. H. Henry, H. W. Snyder *et al.* Protein A immunoadsorption in treatment of malignant disease. *J. Clin. Immunol.*, **6**, 203–212 (1988).
5. S. Shiozaki, K. Sakagami and K. Orita. Extracorporeal immunotherapy for cancer. *Jpn. J. Artif. Organs*, **17**, 1561–1570 (1988).
6. H. Abe, T. Tani, K. Numa *et al.* Trial of anticancer effects using LPS immobilized beads. *Jpn. J. Artif. Organs*, **20**, 230–234 (1991).

Therapeutic Plasmapheresis (XII), pp. 637-641
T. Agishi *et al.* (Eds)
© VSP 1993

Cytotoxic T Lymphocyte Therapy as a Rational Specific Immunotherapy for Cancer

S. FUJIMOTO, K. ARAKI, S. HAMASATO and Y. NOGUCHI

Department of Immunology, Kochi Medical School, Kochi 783, Japan

Key words: tumor immunity; cytotoxic T lymphocyte; specific cancer immunotherapy; extracorporeal cell manipulation.

INTRODUCTION

Efficacy from chemotherapy against malignant tumors cannot be expected unless the specific host immune response to self-derived malignant tumors is not generated, and we are not able to overcome this disease even with any of the newly discovered anti-cancer drugs. If this fact is taken into consideration, the development of a specific immunotherapy becomes all the more essential. We elucidated that the host immune response to tumor is directly involved in both tumor growth and regression, and that T cells play a major role in the immune response to tumors in the mouse system. In particular, $CD8^+$ cytotoxic T lymphocytes (CTL) directed to tumors were shown to be one of the major effector cells which regress the corresponding tumor. However, it was found from our fundamental results that it is hard to generate CTL specific for a growing tumor in the tumor bearing host *in vivo* since immunosuppressor mechanisms to the tumor have been strongly generated *in vivo*. However, since tumor cells often manifest tumor antigens, if an *in vitro* method for activating CTL capable of destroying tumor tissue is established, it will be possible to provide a rational immunotherapy. We devised a method to activate CTL directed to autologous tumor in peripheral blood lymphoid cells (PBL) of various cancerous patients, and developed a specific immunotherapy using activated CTL designated 'CTL therapy' against cancer.

PROTOCOL OF CTL THERAPY

Our original CTL therapy procedure is illustrated in Fig. 1. First, patient's tumor cells are harvested and cultured. The tumor cells are obtained from either surgical resection or from pleural effusion or ascites. Then, PBL are separated from the peripheral blood of the patient by Ficoll–Conray gravity centrifugation followed by automatic leukopheresis. Attenuated autologous tumor cells with mitomycin C (MMC) are added to the PBL culture at the optimal ratio for tumor antigen stimulation to activate specific CTL. During 7 days of stimulation culture of PBL, 100–200 IU/ml of recombinant IL-2 is

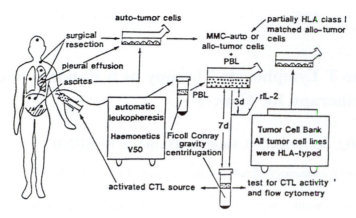

Figure 1. Protocol of human CTL therapy

added to the PBL culture on day 3 after tumor cell stimulation to propagate specific CTL. When autologous tumor cells cannot be obtained from a patient, HLA class I-partially matched allogeneic tumor cells to the patient are selected from our tumor cell bank, where tumor cell lines are all HLA typed, as stimulator cells for CTL induction. After 7 days of culture, their CTL activity is measured by cell-mediated cytotoxicity test using 16 h ^{51}Cr release assay and examined by anti-CD3 antibody blocking test. When their CTL activity is detected in PBL, activated PBL are given intravenously to the autologous patient. The number of activated PBL to be given at one time is in the range of 5×10^7 to 5×10^8 cells. This procedure is repeated once a week until tumor regression. Cyclophosphamide (200–400 mg) was given to patients prior to the activated cell transfer, to inactivate suppressor T cells generated in cancerous patients.

EFFICACY OF CTL THERAPY AND DEVIATION OF T CELL SUBSETS AND MONOCYTES IN CANCER PATIENTS

When CTL specific for tumor cells were generated in PBL from cancerous patients, flow cytometric analysis for the PBL before and after the CTL generation by 7 day culture, were performed by EPICS 752 (Coulter). PBL were stained with monoclonal antibodies to CD3, CD4, CD8 and CD14 (M3) molecules. The percentage of each positive cell was calculated from a total 10 000 cell counts. We have already treated various malignant tumor patients by the CTL therapy. However, all these patients were referred to us after tumor recurrence in spite of chemo- and/or radio-therapy. Among these cases, two of them, shown in Table 1, present effective cases by the CTL therapy. Even these advanced cases had multiple metastasis, they had enough CD3$^+$ T cells in spite of elevation of monocytes before the CTL generation. Furthermore, an increase in the total T cells and a decrease in the monocytes were observed after 7 day culture with or without tumor stimulation. CTL activity to tumor cells was augmented by tumor stimulation and further enhanced by addition of IL-2 3 days after the tumor stimulation. These two cases showed tumor regression by the original CTL therapy.

Table 1.

Effective cases: deviation of T cell subsets and monocyte in the CTL induction

CTL induction		CD3	CD4	CD8	M3	CD4/CD8	CD8/M3	% Lysis E/T=40
Case: H. O. 29 M. Epithelioid sarcoma								
1. PBL only	Day 0	46.8	16.1	18.5	8.3	0.9	2.2	—
2. PBL only	Day 7	59.9	28.7	33.4	2.1	0.9	15.9	16.0 ± 1.1
3. PBL+St.[a]	Day 7	62.6	29.8	31.2	1.5	0.8	20.8	19.6 ± 0.7
4. PBL+IL-2 (Day 3)	Day 7	67.3	26.9	34.0	0.5	0.8	68.0	77.8 ± 1.3
5. PBL+St.+IL-2 (Day 3)	Day 7	67.6	28.9	34.2	0.5	0.8	68.4	79.1 ± 1.0
Case: C. F. 33 F. Breast cancer with multiple bone metastases								
1. PBL only	Day 0	54.1	25.3	15.7	13.8	1.6	1.1	—
2. PBL only	Day 7	88.0	45.0	41.3	0.1	1.1	413.0	32.0 ± 0.8
3. PBL+St.[b]	Day 7	87.7	45.2	42.0	0.2	1.1	210.0	44.6 ± 0.9
4. PBL+IL-2 (Day 3)	Day 7	91.0	47.7	41.7	0.0	1.1	∞	44.8 ± 0.8
5. PBL+St.+IL-2 (Day 3)	Day 7	89.6	38.2	48.0	0.4	0.8	120.0	53.5 ± 0.3

R(C. F.) HLA (2, 24)(60, 61)(3, —)(6, 9, 52, 53)(1, 3).
Stimulator HLA (2, 26)(39, 46)(1, 3).
[a] Tumor cell stimulation (autologous tumor).
[b] Tumor stimulation (crossreactive allogeneic tumor).

INAPPLICABLE CASES OF ORIGINAL CTL THERAPY IN ADVANCED CANCER PATIENTS

In contrast to the former two cases, many advanced cases showed similar flow cytometric pattern of PBL as shown in Table 2. The deviation pattern of T cell subsets and

Table 2.

Unsuccessful cases: deviation of T cell subsets and monocyte in the CTL induction

CTL induction		CD3	CD4	CD8	M3	CD4/CD8	CD8/M3	% Lysis E/T=40
Case 1: H. T. 41 F. Gastric cancer terminal stage IV								
1. PBL only	Day 0	34.4	19.9	11.5	44.4	1.7	0.3	—
2. PBL only	Day 7	27.3	19.5	6.0	58.3	3.3	0.1	−7.6 ± 3.5
3. PBL+St.	Day 7	26.5	18.3	6.1	60.2	3.0	0.1	−8.1 ± 5.8
4. PBL+St.+IL-2 (Day 3)	Day 7	29.9	29.4	3.0	59.8	9.8	0.1	−7.8 ± 0.7
Case 2: M. M. 40 M. Lung cancer (Adeno. Ca.) Meta.(−)								
1. PBL only	Day 0	18.0	11.8	7.0	61.7	1.7	0.1	—
2. PBL only	Day 7	1.8	2.3	0.9	91.7	2.6	0.01	−0.1 ± 1.1
3. PBL+St.	Day 7	1.6	3.0	0.8	88.6	3.8	0.01	−1.5 ± 1.0
4. PBL+St.+IL-2 (Day 3)	Day 7	3.8	3.7	1.3	81.8	2.9	0.02	−1.6 ± 1.9

monocyte population revealed a decrease in T cell subsets and an increase in monocytes. When PBL from these patients were cultured for 7 days, this tendency became more prominent.

Moreover, addition of IL-2 3 days after tumor stimulation resulted in decreasing more T cell particularly, CD8$^+$ T cells and increasing more monocytes. It seemed that there is an inverse relationship between CD8$^+$ T cells and monocytes. Under this condition, specific CTL were unable to be generated even after tumor stimulation and addition of IL-2. These patients could not be applied for our original CTL therapy. It is suggested from these results that in the cases of advanced cancerous patients whose PBL have a high ratio of monocytes and no CTL generation, most of the increased monocytes have to be removed from PBL of these patients *in vitro* in order to generate the CTL, since we have found that monocytes of advanced cancerous patient's PBL suppress CTL generation via a soluble factor(s).

IMPROVEMENT OF THE ORIGINAL CTL THERAPY

In order to improve the original CTL generation method for the advanced cancerous patients, we have been using a nylon wool column to remove the majority of monocytes

Table 3.

An effective case by improved CTL therapy: deviation of T cell subsets and monocyte in the CTL induction (Case: M. K. 65 M. Colon cancer with liver metastases stage IV)

CTL induction		CD3	CD4	CD8	M3	CD4/CD8	CD8/M3	% Lysis E/T=40
1(6.24.'89)								
1. PBL only	Day 0	38.1	16.1	23.3	21.0	0.7	1.1	—
2. PBL only	Day 7	27.5	10.5	17.9	53.0	0.6	0.3	-0.8 ± 1.0
3. PBL+St.	Day 7	29.4	10.1	18.2	51.3	0.6	0.4	-3.6 ± 1.2
4. PBL+St.+IL-2	Day 7	32.2	11.8	24.5	45.0	1.4	0.5	-4.5 ± 1.0
(Day 3)								
5. NWP only	Day 0	71.4	30.8	39.1	0.1	0.8	391.0	—
6. NWP only	Day 7	93.3	51.4	37.0	0.4	1.4	92.5	-4.5 ± 1.0
7. NWP+St.	Day 7	94.8	47.7	40.7	0.3	1.2	135.7	2.4 ± 1.6
8. NWP+St.+IL-2	Day 7	92.5	39.3	51.0	0.3	0.8	170.0	11.3 ± 0.4
(Day 3)								
2 (8.18.'89)								
1. PBL only	Day 0	63.8	23.4	36.7	12.2	0.6	3.0	—
2. PBL only	Day 7	91.5	38.5	49.8	2.2	0.8	22.6	47.1 ± 1.2
3. PBL+St.	Day 7	90.5	39.3	47.0	2.6	0.8	18.1	40.2 ± 5.4
4. PBL+St.+IL-2	Day 7	95.7	33.4	55.9	1.0	0.6	55.9	78.6 ± 4.2
(Day 3)								
5. NWP only	Day 0	81.8	30.9	50.2	0.4	0.6	125.5	—
6. NWP only	Day 7	91.3	37.7	49.6	0.2	0.8	248.0	47.0 ± 3.2
7. NWP+St.	Day 7	88.6	36.3	49.1	1.0	0.7	49.1	54.5 ± 2.8
8. NWP+St.+IL-2	Day 7	95.4	21.3	68.5	0.2	0.3	342.5	87.7 ± 1.5
(Day 3)								

NWP: nylon wool passed lymphocytes.
St.: tumor cell stimulation.

from PBLs to generate the CTL. A typical case which was effective by the improved CTL therapy was shown in Table 3. The case is a 65 year old male colon cancer patient with liver metastasis. One year after surgery of primary tumor and liver metastasis, our improved CTL therapy was applied to this patient. At the beginning, as shown in Table 3, when the whole PBL of the patient was activated by original CTL generation protocol the CTL was not generated even after addition of IL-2, due to an increase in monocytes. However, once the majority of the monocytes were removed, CTL was weakly generated after addition of IL-2. About 2 months after continuous improved CTL therapy, CTL generation was augmented and a balance between T cell and monocyte populations in the PBL of this patient was recovered as compared to those 2 months before (Table 3). It was found when CD8/M3 ratio is more than 1, the immune state of a patient is in a good condition. This patient has been treated by the CTL therapy with very good clinical performance status for more than 3 years.

EFFICACY OF THE IMPROVED CTL THERAPY

The efficacy of our improved CTL therapy is shown in Table 4. The improved CTL therapy extended its applicability and efficacy to advanced cancer patients without any side-effects. The efficacy was determined by either tumor marker reduction in the serum and/or tumor regression.

Table 4.

Efficacy of improved CTL therapy

Type of cancer	Stage	E/T
1. Breast cancer with bone metastasis	IV	7/11
2. Hepatocellular carcinoma	IV	4/8
3. Colon cancer with liver metastasis	IV	3/5
4. Lung cancer with various metastasis	IV	1/3
5. Gastric cancer with peritoneal dissemination	IV	2/3
6. Endometrial cancer with peritoneal dissemination	IV	1/2

In conclusion, improved CTL therapy as a specific immunotherapy against malignant tumor by an extracorporeal cell manipulation is a promising strategy to suppress malignant tumor growth without any side-effects.

Therapeutic Plasmapheresis (XII), pp. 643-645
T. Agishi *et al.* (Eds)
© VSP 1993

The Effect of Photopheresis

H. YAMADA, K. TSUBAKI, A. HORIUCHI and T. TEZUKA

Department of Dermatology, Department of Internal Medicine, School of Medicine, Kinki University, Osaka, Japan

Key words: photopheresis; Sézary syndrome; cutaneous T cell lymphoma; cytokine; direct effect; indirect effect.

INTRODUCTION

Photopheresis (extracorporeal photochemotherapy) was reported by Edelson in 1986. For this treatment, after enforcing 8-MOP oral dosing, the buffy coats are collected by extracirculation, and then, after radiating UVA returned back into the body. In particular, this treatment is employed for skin T cell lymphoma (CTCL). According to the report by Edelson *et al.* [1] an improvement or complete amelioration of the anathema was observed. Its theoretical endorsement, however, is not yet clear. Photopheresis has its partial origin in that the PUVA treatment was enforced in curing CTCL by the lymphoma where CD4 was predominant. So we focused on the mechanism of photopheresis, cell viability and cytokine production have been measured.

METHODS

To start the treatment, we selected five cases with (Sézary syndrome, Mycosis Fungoides, ATL) we focused upon the mechanism of this treatment that is not clear. For this idea, we measure that WBC and atypical cells and CD4/CD8 ratio and measured a change of cytokine production in buffy coat bag before and after in Sézary syndrome.

Therakos UVAR system was used. The instrument used integrated an initial discontinuous leukapheresis step with subsequent exposure to UV in a single apparatus. The leukocyte enriched blood was collected and then irradiated by UVA. After exposure of blood to UVA, the entire amount was returned to the patient. Patient ingested those blood levels of methoxsalen at a dose determined by her body weight (0.6 mg/kg). Two hours after ingestion blood levels of the drug were determined.

To investigate the mechanism of photopheresis we measured several cytokines (IL-1-beta, IL-2, IL-6, IFN, beta, IFN-gamma) in extracorporeal serum. To investigate the selection of malignant cells, Sézary cells and CD4/CD8 ratio were calculated. The skin score was tabulated as the sum of the products of severity and surface area percentage; the highest possible total score therefore was 400.

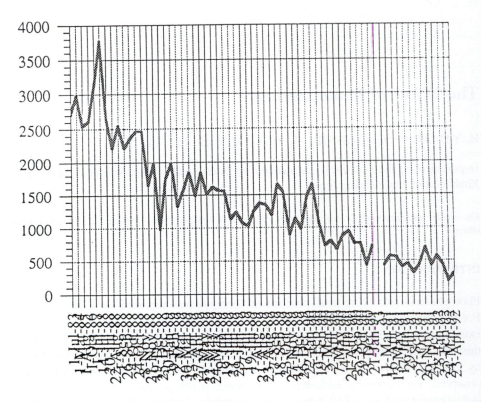

Figure 1. Time course of Sézary syndrome (June 1983–April 1992). *X* axis, time course; *Y* axis, cell number (WBC). The line shows atypical cells.

RESULTS

As seen in the Fig. 1, decreased tumor cell in the peripheral blood is apparent and is the matter of purpose. Nevertheless, the ratio of CD4/CD8 in the peripheral blood is decreased compared with the normal value. Furthermore, it is conceivable that this matter possibly reflects directly to the improvement of erythema. Sézary cells that existed at 30% in the peripheral blood in 1986 have decreased to 5% in 1992. This matter reflects not only the cell ratio but also the actual number of cells. We examined which cells among them decreased. From the fact that the ratio of CD4/CD8 decreases, the decrease of CD4 is conceivable as the selective removal of Sézary cells. Total white blood cell did not change, but CD4 positive cells decreased and an improvement of erythema was observed. Skin score was decreased from 147 to 70. When we stopped the treatment of the patient for private reason, Sézary cells and skin score were increased. They were reversible. After the findings of this phenomenon, we continued the treatment for 2 years. In 1992, atypical cells were 300–500. The skin score decreased to 60.

Cytokine response
Furthermore, to examine how the cytokines acted, the serum value was measured at the extrabody circulatory section, I, e, immediately after UVA radiation. The object was a

patient suffering from the Sézary syndrome. The measured cytokines were IL-1, IL-2, IL-6, IFN-gamma and IFN-beta. The result was that IL-1 and IFN-beta were inclined to increase. An improvement of erythema by this treatment may have some connection with this point. Mean while, IL-6 was below the sensitivity limit, while IFN-gamma did not change.

DISCUSSION

Whenever photopheresis is applied, as seen in the Sézary syndrome, irregular lymphocytes, apparently decreased. Therefore, although this treatment destroys lymphocytes non-specifically, only the clones of tumor cells remain as decreased among other things, and the normal cells proliferate to become predominant. Furthermore, the disabled tumor cells are to be returned back into the body. As a result, the antagonist of the tumor cells becomes stronger to produce anti-idiotype T cells, and thus to contain the proliferation of the tumor cells, it is conceived.

Examining its theory and practice from these observations, the decrease of tumor as the direct effect is observed at least from the Sézary syndrome. As another direct effect, the connection of the containing effect of tumor cells as the T cell vaccine effect with the cytokines was suggested.

REFERENCES

1. R. Edelson, C. Berger, F. Gasparro, B. Jegasothy, P. Heald, B. Wintroub, E. Vonderheid, R. Knobler, K. Wolff and G. Plewin. Treatment of cutaneous T cell lymphoma by extracorporeal photochemotherapy. Preliminary results. *N. Engl. J. Med.*, **316**, 297–303 (1987).

2. J. S. Wieselthier and H. K. Koh. Sézary syndrome; diagnosis, prognosis, and clinical review of treatment options. *J. Am. Acad. Dermatol.*, **22**, 381–401 (1990).

3. I. R. Cohen and H. L. Weiner. T cell vaccination. *Immunology Tod.*, **9**, 332–335 (1988).

Therapeutic Plasmapheresis (XII), pp. 647-650
T. Agishi *et al.* (Eds)
© VSP 1993

Granulocyte Apheresis for Advanced Cancer Patients by an Extracorporeal Circulating Device

H. NAKAZAWA, T. AGISHI, T. OSHIMA, H. TOMA, K. OTA,
T. MIZUTA[1] and M. ADACHI[1]

Kidney Center, Tokyo Women's Medical College, Tokyo, Japan
[1]*Japan Immunoresearch Laboratories, Japan*

Key words: granulocytapheresis; extracorporeal circulating device; immunomodulation; cancer therapy.

INTRODUCTION

Decreased host immune response in progressing cancer cases is considered as an exacerbating factor. Recent reports account for granulocytosis as one of the factors decreasing host immune response [1, 2]. Granulocytosis often occurs in terminal stage cancer patients. On this subject, Ietomi *et al.* reported that a change in the peripheral granulocyte-to-lymphocyte ratio (G/L) was strongly correlated with the prognosis of the patients [3]. Granulocytosis is known to enhance tumor growth and literature supports that NK and LAK activities are inhibited by the presence of granulocytosis. These lead to the consideration that the increase in granulocyte count would be one of the factors responsible for the patients' altered host immune response.

Recently, Tabuchi *et al.* reported that depleting granulocytes from tumor-bearing rabbits by an extracorporeal circulation device resulted in a dramatic anti-tumor effect, which leads us to consider their procedure as a potential therapeutic for cancer.

MATERIALS AND METHODS

Experimental Subjects

All patients taking part in this study (mean age 62.9 years, six males and four females) were selected according to the following criteria. (i) The disease status contraindicated surgical therapy. (ii) Non-invasive means, e.g. chemotherapy, radiation or immunotherapy, had no effect. (iii) Currently available therapeutic were inappropriate/not efficient for the case. All patients were duly informed of the purpose and extent of this study, and consented to participate. The distribution of cancer types among these patients were: five kidney cancer cases, two gastric cancer cases, one lung carcinoma case, one large intestinal cancer case and a case of prostate cancer. The performance status (PS) of each the patients included six 2 and four 3 cases. The individual data on the patients are summarized in Table 1.

Table 1.

Patient profiles

Patients	Age	Sex	Primary	Pretreatment	PS
S. Y.	64	F	kidney	IFN, IL-2	3
H. S.	57	M	kidney	IFN, UFT	3
S. T.	63	F	stomach	chemotherapy	3
T. S.	69	M	kidney	IFN, IL-2	2
H. A.	65	F	stomach	chemotherapy	2
T. K.	67	M	kidney	IFN	3
M.A.	55	M	colon	chemotherapy	2
M.A.	66	M	lung	chemo. radio.	2
R. Y.	79	M.	prostate	chemo. thermo.	3
S. E.	54	F	kidney	IFN	3

Therapeutic device

The device used in this study was an ECD equipped with a column designed for the purpose of selectively depleting circulating granulocytes. The granulocyte apheresis part of the ECD consisted of a column filled with about 22 000 cellulose acetate beads of 2 mm in diameter. The flow speed of the circulator pump was set at 50 ml/min. The patients were submitted to ECD thrice a week for a session length of 45 min each, and 15 sessions were considered as one treatment cycle.

Blood cell population and lymphocyte subset analysis

The lymphocyte and granulocyte population count on the 10th, 20th, 30th and 40th min of each ECD session was recorded. Changes over the time ourse of the EDC session were analyzed. The adsorption capacity of the column was evaluated by the inflow–outflow difference in granulocyte count.

Pre- and post-treatment lymphocyte subset frequencies were analyzed by two-color flowcytometric analysis using a FACScan flowcytometer (Becton–Dickinson USA). CD4, CD8, CD16, CD25 and HLA-DR-expressing fractions were determined using Leu-series monoclonal antibodies. Le^y expression was determined using BM-1 mono-clonal antibody (kind gift from Japan Immunnoresearch Laboratories, Takasaki, Japan).

RESULTS

Peripheral blood WBC count rapidly decreased by ECD, reaching the minimum value between the 10th to 20th min of each session. This was due to the adsorption of granulocytes by the column.

Table 2 shows the inflow–outflow granulocyte and lymphocyte counts. Granulocytes significantly decreased ($P < 0.02$). The mean granulocyte adsorption of the column per 45 min session ranged between 0.9 and 3.8×10^9 granulocytes. Lymphocytes were adsorbed at various degree, but the difference between inflow and outflow was not significant.

Changes in lymphocyte subset populations were as follows. Unchanged or slightly increased CD4- and CD25-positive fractions; unchanged or slightly increased CD8 and CD16 positive fractions. The ratio between CD4-positive and CD8-positive fractions

Table 2.
Peripheral blood cell counts

	Inlet	Outlet
Granulocyte	2772 ± 947*	1879 ± 1069*
Lymphocyte	958 ± 401	923 ± 312
G/L	3.73 ± 2.75**	2.49 ± 2.20**

Mean ± SD, $n = 12$.

Ave. ± SD, $n = 12$.

*$P < 0.01$, **$P < 0.05$.

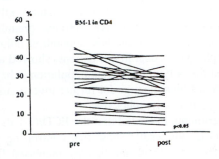

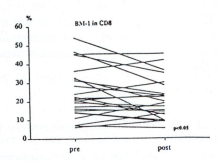

Figure 1. Changes of BM-1 expression after granulocytapheresis with G-1 column.

increased in five out of six cases. Percentage of Le^y-expressing cells in CD4-positive and CD8-positive T cells markedly decreased (Fig. 1).

Of the six patients out of the total 10, on whom the therapy could be applied for one cycle or over, three displayed improved performance status.

DISCUSSION

From the standpoint that granulocytosis could be an exacerbating factor for the cancer host, and in an attempt to improve the patient's G/L, we assessed the effect of granulocyte depletion on the host by adsorbing granulocytes with an ECD. To do so, we depleted about 20% of the patient's circulating granulocytes per session. WBC and granulocyte count decreased and G/L improved as expected. However, G/L at the end of a given session did not always match the number of granulocytes adsorbed by the column. This would owe to a re-adjustment response of the tumor host's defence system which would be supplying granulocytes from the spleen or other sources. The effect of this re-supply or re-adjustment on the tumor host immunity has yet to be clarified. This also indicates that controlling G/L by the use of ECD depletion alone requires a longitudinal therapy.

We monitored changes in lymphocyte populations by flowcytometric lymphocyte subset analysis. The common trait observed as the effect of ECD on our patients was an increase of CD4 and CD25 expressing population, and a decrease in CD8, CD16 and Le^y expressing fractions. This also resulted in an increased CD4/CD8. These changes in lymphocyte subsets would result from the application of extracorporeal circulation rather than the direct effect of granulocyte adsorption. The increase in CD4- and CD25-positive T cells implies activated helper cells, and the decreased CD16-positive population suggests a decrease of active natural killer cells (NK). Despite reports showing that granulocytes inhibit NK activity, granulocyte adsorption as we performed resulted in a decrease in active NK population rather than increasing them. The inflow–outflow lymphocyte counts in our patients showed a wide dispersion, which leads to the consideration that a lymphocyte subpopulation is being selectively adsorbed by the column. This demonstrates the urge for further investigation focused on the effect of the ECD/G-1 system on host's lymphocytes.

Although animal experiments indicated that the ECD/G-1 therapy is useful for monitoring and controlling G/L, our results show that controlling G/L in clinical practice would be difficult. On the other hand, the therapy increased IL-2 receptor expressing cells. This increase in helper T cells may contribute to the improvement of the patient's status if combined with IL-2 therapy. Although there is still much to be elucidated on the fundamental aspect of the granulocyte–immunity interaction, investigating the effect of granulocyte apheresis in cancer patients' host immunity would certainly bring novel views and further useful information.

REFERENCES

1. H. Petrie, L. W. Klassen and H. D. Kay. Inhibition of human cytotoxic T lymphocyte activity *in vitro* by autologous peripheral blood granulocytes. *J. Immunol.*, **134**, 230–234 (1985).

2. H. Shau and A. Kim. Suppression of lymphokine-activated killer induction by neutrophils. *J. Immunol.*, **141**, 4395–4402 (1988).

3. K. Ietomi. A study on the role of granulocytes in carcinoma-bearing hosts — G/L ratio as a new host indicator. *J. Jpn. Soc. Cancer Ther.*, **25**, 662–671 (1990).

Therapeutic Plasmapheresis (XII), pp. 651-654
T. Agishi *et al*. (Eds)
© VSP 1993

Immunomodulation by Pokeweed Mitogen

A. HIZUTA, K. MIYAGI, S. OHNO, N. TANAKA and K. ORITA

First Department of Surgery, Okayama University Medical School, Okayama, Japan

Key words: PWM; lymphocytes; killer cells; LGL; cancer therapy.

INTRODUCTION

Lectins such as PHA and Con A have been reported to activate lymphocytes and generate killer cells capable of lysis of natural killer resistant fresh tumor cells [1]. Among lectins pokeweed mitogen (PWM) has been demonstrated to induce activated killer (AK) cells by extremely short-term stimulation [2]. When PWM is immobilized on the surface of beads which can activate human lymphocytes to be lytic for tumor cells, PWM beads column will realize the generation of *ex vivo* AK cells by extracorporeal circulation for treatment of human malignant diseases. We thus investigated the generation and characterization of human AK cells induced by PWM-immobilized beads.

MATERIALS AND METHODS

PWM-immobilized beads, CMC-1, used were obtained from Asahi Chemical Industry Co. (Fuji, Japan). The size of the beads was $500-710 \, \mu m$ and 1 ml of the beads contained $200 \, \mu g$ of PWM on the surface [2]. For the induction of PWM-AK killer cells, 4×10^6 cells/ml of normal human peripheral blood mononuclear cells (PBMC) were mixed with 0.4 ml of CMC-1 in RPMI 1640 medium containing 10% human AB serum and incubated for 1 h at 37°C. Cells were separated from the beads by pipetting, then washed 3 times and further incubated in the medium alone for 23 h. Lymphokine-activated killer (LAK) cells were induced by incubation of human PBMC with 10^3 JRU/ml of recombinant human IL-2 for 3 days. Cytotoxicity was assessed by 4-h chromium-51 release assay.

RESULTS

Human PBMC were stimulated with CMC-1 for 5 min to 2 h, washed and incubated in medium alone for a total of 24 h. Then, cytotoxicity was assayed against K562 and Daudi tumor target cells (Fig. 1). A consistent increase in cytotoxicity against both targets was observed by as short as 5 min of stimulation, and the cytotoxicity reached a plateau at 1 h of stimulation. After 1 h stimulation with CMC-1, cytotoxicity was assayed as a function of incubation time in medium alone (Fig. 2). Killing activity against both targets had a peak at 23 h and high levels of killing activity were maintained up to 96 h without the need for exogenous cytokines.

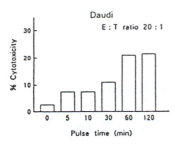
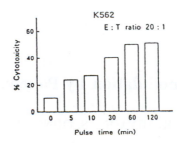

Figure 1. The cytotoxicity of human PBMC after stimulation with CMC-1 and incubation in medium alone for a total of 24 h.

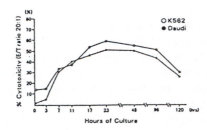

Figure 2. The cytotoxicity of human PBMC after stimulation with CMC-1 for 1 h.

Depletion of plastic adherent cells from human PBMC did not affect, rather increased the cytotoxicity of CMC-1-AK cells, indicating monocyte independence for the killer cell generation. Fresh non-adherent PBMC were fractionated by discontinuous Percoll gradient centrifugation and stimulated with CMC-1. Only low density lymphocytes which were rich in large granular lymphocytes (LGL) responded to PWM on CMC-1 to increase cytotoxicity against both targets. These results suggest that the precursors of CMC-1-AK cells reside in LGL-rich low density lymphocytes.

To determine the effect of exogenous IL-2, rIL-2 was added to culture after 1 h stimulation with CMC-1. While cytotoxicity of fresh PBMC was increased in a dose-dependent manner, that of CMC-1-stimulated cells was not influenced by addition of rIL-2, indicating independency of exogenous IL-2 for the generation of CMC-1-AK cells.

The change in surface phenotype of CMC-1-AK cells was determined up to 7 days of culture by using monoclonal antibodies and flow cytometry, and compared with that of LAK cells. The proportion of CD3, CD8, CD25 and HLA-DR positive cells in bulk culture were increased with culture time in both killer cells. Increase of CD25-positive lymphocytes in CMC-1-AK cells was more striking than that in LAK cells.

The target cell spectrum of CMC-1-AK cells was examined against K562, Daudi, RPMI 4788 colon cancer, MKN-1 gastric cancer, PC-10 lung cancer, and KB pharyngeal cancer cell line of human origin, and compared with that of LAK cells (Fig. 3). Cytotoxicity of CMC-1-AK cells was quite similar to that of LAK cells against all target cells examined.

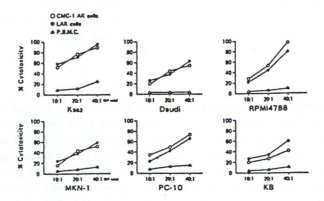

Figure 3. Target cell spectrum of CMC-1-activated killer cells.

When AK cells induced by stimulation with CMC-1 or rIL-2 were tested for proliferation, little proliferation was observed on day 1, and the highest proliferation was observed on day 3 in both AK cells. The degree of proliferation of CMC-1-AK cell culture was greater than that of LAK cell culture. IL-2, IFNγ, and TNFα in supernatant of both AK cell cultures at a starting dose of 2×10^6 cells/ml were assayed at 12–96 h of culture. While the amount of IL-2 in LAK cell culture was a reflection of IL-2 exogenously added to the culture, that in CMC-1-AK cell culture was below the assay limit from 12–96 h. The amounts of IFNγ and TNFα were greater in CMC-1-AK cell culture as compared with those of LAK cell culture throughout the culture period.

An experimental intraperitoneal carcinomatosis model in CD-1 nude mice was made by injecting 5×10^6 of RPMI 4788 human colon cancer cells. The mice developed progressive ascites and died around 40 days after tumor inoculation. Using this model, *in vivo* antitumor effect of CMC-1-AK cells was assessed. Two and 4 days after tumor inoculation, mice were treated with intraperitoneal injections of 1.5×10^6 effector cells of fresh human PBMC, CMC-1-stimulated cells with or without 23 h incubation in medium (Fig. 4). Mean survival time of mice treated with CMC-1-stimulated cells without incubation (58.6 ± 1.5 days) as well as those with incubation (71.4 ± 8.0 days) was

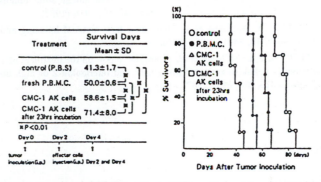

Figure 4. *In vivo* antitumor effect of CMC-1-activated killer cells in nude mice bearing RPMI 4788 human colon cancer.

significantly longer than that of mice treated with fresh PBMC (50.0 ± 0.6 days). These results indicate *in vivo* therapeutic effect of CMC-1-AK cells and *in vivo* induction of AK cells after *in vitro* stimulation with CMC-1, since cytotoxicity of cells immediately after stimulation with CMC-1 was similar to that of fresh PBMC.

DISCUSSION

The results presented in this report indicate that stimulation of normal human PBMC with PWM-immobilized beads and without exogenous IL-2 can generate killer cells with cytotoxicity similar to that of LAK cells. The characteristics of these CMC-1-activated killer cells similar to those of LAK cells include the following: (i) they are highly cytotoxic to natural killer resistant tumor target cells; (ii) the generation of the killer cells are independent of monocytes; (iii) their precursor cells resided in the LGL–rich low density fraction of lymphocytes in PBMC; (iv) they have a broad target cell spectrum; (v) they proliferate in culture with a peak at day 3; (vi) the proportion of CD3, CD8, CD25 and HLA-DR positive lymphocytes are increased in their culture; (vii) they secrete IFNγ and TNFα; and (viii) they have *in vivo* therapeutic effect in nude mice. While these observations indicate the similarity of generated effector cells between CMC-1-AK and LAK cells, the induction on these effector cells are quite different. For the generation of LAK cells, the presence of IL-2 in medium is requisite for over 3 days. CMC-1-AK cells can be inducible by as short as 5 min of stimulation with PWM on CMC-1 and 1 h is sufficient to obtain the maximal cytotoxicity. Once cells are stimulated, the presence of PWM is not required for AK cell induction, which can be proceeded *in vivo* without administration of exogenous IL-2. These characteristics for AK cell induction by CMC-1 suggest that the extracorporeal circulation using a column incorporated with CMC-1 may generate AK cells *in vivo* and provide a new strategy for therapy of human malignant diseases. Although therapy with LAK cells and IL-2 has resulted in antitumor responses against human cancer, the infusion of IL-2 has often been associated with considerable clinical toxicity [3]. Since exogenous IL-2 is not involved in the potentiation of CMC-1-AK cell activity, *ex vivo* therapy using CMC-1 without IL-2 can avoid this toxicity.

REFERENCES

1. A. Mazumder, E. A. Grimm, H. Z. Zhang *et al.* Lysis of fresh human solid tumors by autologous lymphocytes activated *in vitro* with lectins. *Cancer Res.*, **42**, 913–918 (1982).
2. T. Sugahara, K. Tsuchiya, H. Watanabe *et al.* Study on a new material inducing anti-tumor immune cells. *Jpn. J. Artif. Organs*, **18**, 1401–1405 (1989).
3. S. A. Rosenberg, M. T. Lotze, L. M. Muul *et al.* A progress report on the treatment of 157 patients with advanced cancer using lymphokine-activated killer cells and interleukin-2 or high dose interleukin-2 alone. *N. Engl. J. Med.*, **316**, 889–897 (1987).

14
Replacement Fluids

Therapeutic Plasmapheresis (XII), pp. 657-660
T. Agishi *et al.* (Eds)
© VSP 1993

Relationship Between Albumin Concentration in Supplementation Fluid and Change of Total Plasma Protein Level in Double Filtration Plasmapheresis

M. MINESHIMA, T. AGISHI, K. ERA, T. SANAKA,
S. TERAOKA and K. OTA

Kidney Center, Tokyo Women's Medical College, Tokyo, Japan

Key words: plasma exchange; double filtration plasmapheresis; supplementation fluid; albumin concentration; kinetic modeling.

INTRODUCTION

In 1980, double filtration plasmapheresis (DFPP) was introduced in order to cut down the amount of supplementation fluid under the same therapeutic effectiveness as single filtration plasmapheresis [1]. There is, however, a limit in plasma fractionation between albumin and immunoglobulins which involves some kind of toxins related to auto-immune diseases, because the currently available plasma fractionators do not have a clear cut-off property between these proteins [2].

As a result, a certain amount of condensed albumin is also discarded together with a large amount of immunoglobulins during the treatment. A higher concentration of albumin in supplementation fluid is needed to avoid a decrease of total plasma protein level of the patient. Albumin concentration of the supplementation fluid, however, has been empirically determined until recently. Inadequate albumin infusion often leads to hypoproteinemic symptoms such edema.

In this study, a characterization parameter, aimed condensation coefficient (CC_{aimed}), is newly introduced in an attempt to estimate appropriate serum albumin and total plasma protein levels for each patient.

DFPP

In DFPP, two types of filters with different pore sizes are utilized. After the extracorporeal patient's blood into the plasma separator (PS), filtrated plasma is also introduced to the plasma fractionator (PF). In this secondary filter, the condensed plasma fraction, containing relatively higher molecular weight proteins such as immunoglobulins, is partially discarded, while the albumin-rich plasma is returned to the patient with the necessary volume of supplementation fluid. In a typical condition of DFPP, nearly five times condensed immunoglobulins are discarded and one-fifth of the volume of supplementation fluid is used in comparison with single filtration plasma exchange.

KINETIC MODELING

Kinetic modeling using a one-compartment model for albumin transport during DFPP treatment was introduced to determine the optimum concentration of the supplementation fluid as shown in Fig. 1. In this model, the albumin transfer rate between the patient's total plasma and the DFPP circuit is considered as a rate-determining stage in comparison with other albumin transfer rates. A time-averaged value of an albumin sieving coefficient is applied to the modeling because of a degree of albumin plugging to the membrane and a change of serum albumin level are much smaller than other proteins. Furthermore, total plasma volume of the patient is assumed to be constant during a single DFPP treatment because an albumin amount in the changed volume is extremely small compared with the initial value of patient's total plasma.

Several parameters for DFPP can be theoretically introduced by material balance equations. At first, the condensation coefficient (CC) of DFPP can be described:

$$CC = \frac{C_D}{C_P} = \frac{C_D}{C_{F1}} \cdot \frac{C_{F1}}{C_P} = \frac{Q_{F1} \cdot C_{F1} - Q_{F2} \cdot C_{F2}}{Q_D \cdot C_{F1}} \cdot \frac{C_{F1}}{C_P}$$
$$= \frac{1 - FF_{PF} \cdot SC_{PF}}{1 - FF_{PF}} SC_{PS} \qquad (1)$$

where SC_{PS} and SC_{PF} are sieving coefficients of the plasma separator and plasma fractionator, and FF_{PF} denotes the filtration fraction in the plasma fractionator.

A value of CC means a degree of albumin condensation in the DFPP treatment. When both SC_{PS} and SC_{PF} are equal to unity, no albumin condensation can be found because CC is also equal to unity. A combination between higher values of CC for immunoglobulins and lower values for albumin leads to better separation between these proteins. If we take only this CC value into consideration for the determination of the optimum concentration, the amount of total plasma protein decreases because some kinds of plasma proteins are removed during DFPP treatment.

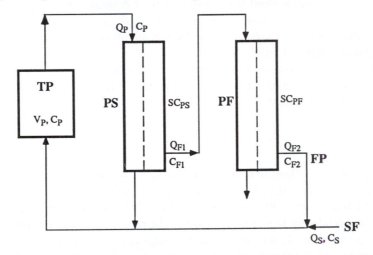

Figure 1. A schematic diagram of the one-compartment model for protein transport in a DFPP treatment: TP, patient's total plasma; PS, plasma separator; PF, plasma fractionator; FP, filtrated plasma; DP, discarded plasma; SF, supplementation fluid.

On the other hand, a newly introduced parameter, aimed condensation coefficient, (CC_{aimed}), can be described as follows:

$$CC_{aimed} = \frac{C_S}{C_D} = \frac{C_S}{CC \cdot C_P} = 1 - \frac{1 - CR}{1 - \exp(-CC \cdot VR)} \qquad (2)$$

Where CR denotes a change ratio of albumin concentration during the treatment and VR is the volume ratio of the supplementation fluid (V_S) to the patient's total plasma (V_P). These are defined as follows:

$$CR = C_P(t)/C_P(0) \qquad (3)$$
$$VR = Q_S \cdot t/V_P = V_S/V_P \qquad (4)$$

Finally, the optimum albumin concentration in the supplementation fluid (C_S) can be determined using CC and CC_{aimed} values, and the patient's serum albumin concentration (C_P):

$$C_S = CC \cdot CC_{aimed} \cdot C_P \qquad (5)$$

IN VIVO STUDY

In order to determine an appropriate value of albumin concentration in the supplementation fluid, a change of total plasma protein level in single DFPP treatment was examined during an *in vivo* study of eight patients with autoimmune disease. Figure 2 shows a relationship between CR(T.P.) and CC_{aimed}. A good correlation was obtained for a wide range of CC_{aimed} values during 19 DFPP treatments. From this result, the empirical equation was obtained as follows:

$$CR(T.P.) = 0.653 + 0.183 \times CC_{aimed}(alb) \quad (r = 0.730) \qquad (6)$$

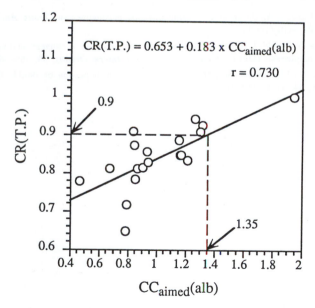

Figure 2. Relationship between CC_{aimed} and CR(T.P.).

OPTIMUM ALBUMIN CONCENTRATION IN SUPPLEMENTATION FLUID

For an example, it is supposed that a patient having body weight of 50 kg, hematocrit of 30% and serum albumin concentration of 3.0 g/dl receives a DFPP treatment using ASAHI AP-05H having an SC_{PS}(alb) of 0.970 as a plasma separator and Kawasumi Evaflux 2A having SC_{PF}(alb) of 0.526 under FF_{PF} of 0.8 with V_S of 500 ml. These SC values are obtained in a previous paper [3].

The condensation coefficient of albumin, CC(alb), can be calculated by substituting SC and FF values into Equation (1) and obtained as 2.81. If 10% reduction for T.P. level during a DFPP treatment, namely CR(T.P.) of 0.9, is allowed, the CC_{aimed} value can be estimated as 1.35 from Equation (6). It means that more than a 35% increase in albumin concentration of the supplementation fluid is needed in order to not induce some kind of complication such as hypoproteinemia. Finally, optimum albumin concentration in supplementation fluid can be determined as 11.4 g/dl for this patient by Equation (5).

CONCLUSIONS

In this paper, optimum albumin concentration in the supplementation fluid during a DFPP treatment can be determined by kinetic modeling using a one-compartment model. The aimed condensation coefficient, which was newly introduced in this study, is valid for determining the optimum albumin concentration in the supplementation fluid and maintaining appropriate plasma protein levels of the patient. A good correlation between aimed condensation coefficient and change of total plasma protein level can be obtained from an *in vivo* study.

REFERENCES

1. T. Agishi, I. Kaneko, Y. Hasuo *et al.* Double filtration plasmapheresis. *Trans. Am. Soc. Artif. Intern. Organs,* **26**, 406–410 (1980).
2. M. Mineshima, T. Agishi, I. Kaneko *et al.* Performance evaluation of conventional and modified double filtration plasmapheresis (DFPP). *Trans. Am. Soc. Artif. Intern. Organs,* **30**, 665–669 (1984).
3. T. Agishi and M. Mineshima. Separation and fractionation of plasma by double filtration technique. *J. Memb. Sci.,* **44**, 47–54 (1989).

Therapeutic Plasmapheresis (XII), pp. 661-666
T. Agishi *et al.* (Eds)
© VSP 1993

Internal Dynamics of Aluminum Contained in Albumin Solutions — Fluid Replacement for Plasmapheresis

Y. MASAKAZU, Y. KEN, K. YOSHINORI, K. TOSHIAKI, T. MASAYUKI,
F. SHIN, T. HIROSHI, H. HIROSHI and H. SHUNICHI

Department of Internal Medicine, Juntendo University, Tokyo, Japan

Key words: double filtration plasmapheresis; fluid replacement; albumin preparations; aluminum.

INTRODUCTION

Recent reports show aluminum toxicity to be an etiologic factor in the development of conditions such as osteomalacia, multiple bone fractures and encephalopathy. Since 1970, aluminum toxicity has been observed in patients on dialysis for chronic renal failure. Lately, double filtration plasmapheresis (DFPP) has become the mainstay for this form of treatment. Consequently, albumin preparations are now frequently used as displacement fluids. Aluminum contamination of these albumin-preparation based displacement fluids directly increases the plasma aluminum concentration of the blood. This increases the risk of the possible future development of clinical symptoms of aluminum toxicity. Since we obtained an albumin preparation low in aluminum for the present study, we report here the results of a comparison of aluminum dynamics during DFPP between this and commercial preparations.

MATERIALS AND METHODS

We examined 10 patients, one man and nine women, with rheumatoid arthritis (RA). According to the criteria of the American Rheumatism Association, all patients were classified as Stage II or III and Class 1 or 3. The patients' ages ranged between 41 and 67 years, the mean age being 51.5 years. The mean duration of the disease was 10.4 years. Duration of treatment with DFPP varied from 27 to 64 months and the mean was 41.5 months (Table 1).

Regarding renal function, six of the 10 patients were negative for proteinuria and four patients had continuous proteinuria. Creatinine levels were elevated in three patients and BUN in five patients (Table 2).

Moreover, during the observation period, none of the patients received any aluminum preparations for peptic ulcers. They were also instructed to refrain from drinking soft drinks from aluminum cans.

DFPP was performed according to the common method applying membrane separation (Fig. 1). We used a filter with a pore size of 0.03 microns for the secondary membrane. In each cycle of the DFPP, 2000 ml of plasma was processed. Of this

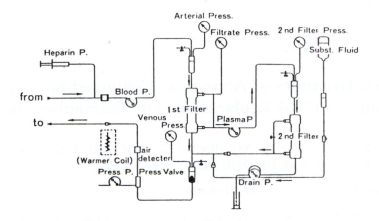

Figure 1. Double filtration plasmapheresis.

Table 1.
Patients' profile

Case	Age	Sex	Diagnosis	Duration of disease (years)	Duration of plasmapheresis (months)
1	48	F	RA	12	38
2	67	F	RA	6	27
3	43	F	RA	15	60
4	62	M	RA	8	64
5	58	F	RA	7	48
6	52	F	RA	20	30
7	50	F	RA	4	33
8	41	F	RA	4	42
9	45	F	RA	10	32
10	49	F	RA	18	43

amount, 20% was evacuated, which we replaced with an equivalent amount of albumin solution. We dissolved 100 ml of a 25% albumin preparation in 500 ml of an electrolyte solution. An ordinary aluminum preparation and one low in aluminum were used for the 25% albumin preparations. The different preparations were each given to five patients. After an interval of 2 weeks, an albumin preparation low in aluminum was given to the group that had received the ordinary albumin preparation first and then underwent DFPP. On the other hand, the group that received the albumin preparation low in aluminum first received the ordinary albumin preparation after an interval of 2 weeks.

Blood samples were drawn before, immediately after and 24 h after DFPP treatment to measure the aluminum concentration in both 25% albumin and solutions with added electrolytes.

Table 2.
Renal function

Case	BUN (mg/dl)	Creatinine (mg/dl)	Proteinuria (g/day)
1	13	0.5	0
2	14	0.4	0
3	13	0.5	1.5
4	23	1.2	0
5	21	0.7	0
6	39	3.3	1.0
7	49	2.8	0
8	13	0.6	0
9	27	0.7	0.4
10	14	0.6	1.6

Table 3.
Aluminum concentration of albumin preparation

Albumin preparation	Albumin concentration (%)	Aluminum volume (μg/dl)
A	25	4
B	25	33
C	25	79
D	25	33
E	25	124
F	20	100
G	20	59

Aluminum concentration in common albumin preparations varied widely from 33 to 124μg/dl (Table 3). For the present study, we used an albumin preparation low in aluminum 'A' and an ordinary commercial albumin preparation 'B'.

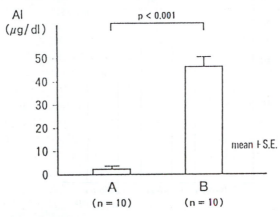

Figure 2. Comparison of aluminum concentration in albumin preparations.

RESULTS

The electrolyte-added solution did not contain aluminum. Albumin preparation 'A'
had an aluminum concentration of 2.5 ± 0.17 μg/dl, and 'B' had a concentration of
40.3 ± 12.5 μg/dl (Fig. 2). Thus, we observed a significant difference of less than
$P < 0.001$.

The plasma aluminum concentration increased slightly after DFPP when 'A' was
used as the displacement fluid, but the difference, was not significant (Fig. 3).

When 'B' was used as the displacement fluid, the plasma aluminum concentration
increased significantly after DFPP, but returned to the original value after 24 h (Fig. 4).

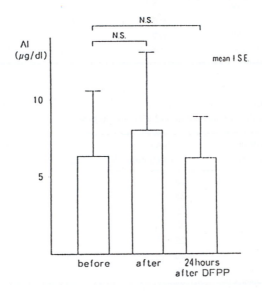

Figure 3. Changes of plasma aluminum concentration: A preparation ($n = 10$).

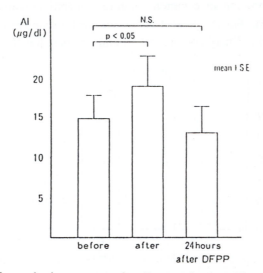

Figure 4. Changes of plasma aluminum concentration: B preparation ($n = 10$).

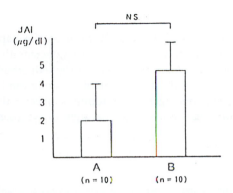

Figure 5. Changes of plasma aluminum concentration before and after DFPP: comparison of A and B preparations.

We calculated the difference between the plasma aluminum concentration immediately after treatment and before treatment to determine the rate of elevation. Although 'B' showed a strong tendency to increase the aluminum concentration, the difference was not significant.

DISCUSSION

Aluminum toxicity following long periods of dialysis has been known since the end of the 1960s in the Newcastle district of England as a factor that increases the incidence of myopathy, ostalgia and osteomalacia associated with multiple bone fractures. High aluminum concentrations are suspected as the cause of progressive encephalopathy, microcytic hypochromic anemia, Alzheimer's disease, porphyria and amyotrophic lateral sclerosis besides pathological bone lesions.

Usually, orally ingested aluminum is derived from food or drugs or is inhaled as dust. It is also absorbed from the intestinal tract, but as long as there is no renal dysfunction, most is excreted. However, when aluminum is administered parenterally into the vessels, its concentration may exceed the level excreted, thus leading to symptoms of toxicity. Albumin preparations are widely used in dialysis patients to increase the plasma volume and in patients with severe nephrosis to increase their urine output. These preparations are frequently used for patients with renal dysfunction.

Large amounts of albumin preparations are further used as displacement fluids during plasmapheresis for patients with RA, SLE, cryoglobulinemia, Good Pasture syndrome, rapidly progressive glomerulonephritis, TTP, multiple myeloma, renal transplant rejection and similar pathologic conditions.

It is, of course, essential to consider aluminum toxicity due to albumin administrations in patients with renal failure, even when monitoring their renal function.

The 25% albumin preparation that we used in the present study was prepared using a new purification method. Compared with conventional products, it had a low aluminum concentration of 2.5 μg/dl.

Thus, aluminum toxicity can be regarded as low, but repeated administration requires regular monitoring of plasma aluminum levels. Detection of even the slightest indication in clinical signs or symptoms warrants a thorough examination.

CONCLUSION

When 10 patients with RA were given double filtration plasmapheresis, we used albumin preparations as displacement fluids. Aluminum concentration in common albumin preparations varied widely, but their differences using both albumin preparations as the displacement fluid were not significant. Aluminum toxicity can be regarded as low, but repeated administration requires regular monitoring of plasma aluminum levels and detection of even the slightest indication in clinical signs or symptoms warrants a thorough examination.

REFERENCES

1. S. Hosokawa, A. Oyamaguchi and O. Yoshida. Trace elements and plasmapheresis. *Int. J. Artif. Organs*, **14**, 242–245 (1991).
2. C. Koppel, H. Baudisch and K. Ibe. Inadvertent metal loading of critically ill patients with renal failure by human albumin solution infusion therapy. *Clin. Toxicol.*, **26**, 337–356 (1988).
3. E. R. Maher, E. A. Brown, J. R. Curtis, M. E. Phillips and B. Sampson. Accumulation of aluminum in chronic renal failure due to administration of albumin replacement solutions. *Br. Med. J.*, 292–306 (1986).
4. G. S. Fell and D. Maharaj. Trace metal contamination of albumin solutions used for plasma exchange. *Lancet*, Aug, 467–468 (1986).
5. D. S. Milliner, J. H. Shinaberger, P. Shuman and J. W. Coburn. Inadvertent aluminum administration during plasma exchange due to aluminum contamination of albumin replacement solutions. *N. Engl. J. Med.*, **312**, 165–167 (1985).
6. E. A. Loeliger and F. A. Wolff. Aluminum contamination of albumin replacement solutions. *N. Engl. J. Med.*, **312**, 1389–1390 (1985).
7. A. B. Sedman, G. L. Klein, R. J. Merritt, N. L. Miller, K. O. Weber, W. L. Gill, H. Anand and A. C. Alfrey. Evidence of aluminum in infants receiving intravenous therapy. *N. Engl. J. Med.*, **312**, 1337–1343 (1985).
8. G. L. Klein, A. C. Alfrey, N. L. Miller, D. J. Sherraer, T. K. Hazlet, M. E. Ament and J. W. Coburn. Aluminum loading during total parenteral nutrition. *Am. J. Clin. Nutr.*, **35**, 1425–1429 (1982).
9. M. K. Ward. Evidence for a water-borne etiological agent, probably aluminum. *Lancet*, **1**, 1841 (1978).
10. A. C. Alfrey. Aluminum metabolism. *Kidney Int.*, **29**, S8–S11 (1986).

15
Adverse Effects

Therapeutic Plasmapheresis (XII), pp. 669-670
T. Agishi *et al.* (Eds)
© VSP 1993

Influence of Plasmapheresis on Trace Elements: Long-term Follow Up

S. HOSOKAWA

Utano National Hospital, Kyoto, Japan

Key words: plasmapheresis; trace elements; iron; aluminum; zinc; copper.

INTRODUCTION

Recently, plasmapheresis (PP) has been used clinically for the treatment of patients with various kinds of diseases. Several side effects such as hypotension, chest pain, and nausea, etc., have been well-known in PP treatment. Solutions used as replacement fluids for PP, particularly albumin solution, are contaminated with trace elements [1]. Mousson *et al.* [2] reported that aluminum (Al) accumulation contributed to Al bone deposition in patients with long-term maintenance of PP. Herein, I describe the change in the levels of serum trace elements such as Al, zinc (Zn), iron (Fe) and copper (Cu) with PP therapy for 3 years.

MATERIALS AND METHODS

The changes of serum Al, Fe, Zn and Cu levels of 12 patients (six with myasthenia gravis, two with multiple sclerosis, two with rheumatoid arthritis, two with CIPD) undergoing plasmapheresis treatment were examined for 3 years. A plasma separator was used as a first filter and a separator of plasma components was used as a second filter. Two liters of plasma were treated in each PP therapy. Blood flow was 60–70 ml/min and plasma flow was 20 ml/min. Twenty five percent albumin solution (Green Cross Co., Japan) and electrolyte solution were used as replacement fluids for PP. Serum Al, Zn, Cu and Fe were measured with a flameless atomic absorption spectrophotometer (Hitachi, KK, Japan) as described previously [3]. Calculations were performed with computers. All data are given as mean and standard deviation (SD). Student's t-test, with separate estimates of variance in each group, was used to calculate statistical significance. P values less than 0.05 were considered as indicating significant differences.

RESULTS

A 200 ml 25% albumin solution was used in each PP session. The concentrations of trace elements in the 25% albumin solution were (μg/dl): Al, 10.4; Zn, 79; Cu, 70; and Fe, 330 (average values). Total protein (TP) removed was $20 \pm 5\%$, serum albumin removed was $24 \pm 6\%$ with each PP treatment.

Serum Al levels increased significantly ($P < 0.01$) from $1.1 \pm 0.3\,\mu g/dl$ pre-PP to $2.4 \pm 0.7\,\mu g/dl$ post PP. Serum Zn, Cu and Fe values decreased significantly ($P < 0.01$) from 89.4 ± 6.6, 120 ± 14 and $118 \pm 16\,\mu g/dl$, respectively, post-PP therapy.

At 3 days after the end of 3 years PP treatment, serum Al levels increased significantly ($P < 0.01$) from 1.1 ± 0.3 to $4.0 \pm 0.5\,\mu g/dl$.

Total protein was not significantly changed from 6.9 ± 0.4 to $7.0 \pm 0.5\,g/dl$ for 3 years. Serum albumin levels were not significantly changed from $4.6 \pm 0.3\,g/dl$ for 3 years. Serum Zn levels and serum Cu levels were not significantly changed from 89.4 ± 6.6 and $120 \pm 14\,\mu g/dl$ to 90.2 ± 7.1 and $122 \pm 18\,\mu g/dl$, respectively, for 3 years during PP therapy. No significant change of serum Fe values was found from $118 \pm 16\,\mu g/dl$ to $120 \pm 21\,\mu g/dl$ for 3 years.

DISCUSSION

Serum Al concentrations significantly increased as reported by others [4, 5], but serum Zn, Cu and Fe levels significantly ($P < 0.01$) decreased after each PP session. Serum Al levels significantly rose 3 days after the end of 3 years PP treatment as more Al entered from the albumin solution used as a replacement solution for PP than was removed with PP and accumulated in the body, particularly bone, plasma and other organs. The massive Al accumulation may contribute to pathological effects such as severe encephalopathy and osteomalasia [6]. These results suggest that Al should be removed with desferoxamine in long-term PP. Al of albumin solution should be reduced with industry levels in near future. There were no significant changes of serum Zn, Cu and Fe levels between before the start of PP and at 3 days after the end of 3 years PP treatment. These facts suggest there are no biological and physiological problems with Zn, Cu and Fe for long-term PP therapy.

CONCLUSION

Serum Al levels significantly increased during each PP treatment and also 3 days after the end of 3 years PP treatment. Al accumulation should be treated with desferooxamine (DFO) or with low Al solution as replacement fluid. Serum Zn, Cu and Fe significantly decreased after each PP; however, serum Zn, Cu and Fe levels did not significantly change at 3 days after the end of 3 years PP treatment.

REFERENCES

1. F. Monteagudo, L. Wood, P. Jacob et al. Aluminum loading during therapeutic plasma exchange. J. Clin. Apheresis, 3, 161–163 (1987).
2. C. Mousson, S. A. Charon, M. Ammar et al. Aluminum bone deposits in normal renal function patients after long-term treatment by plasma exchange. Int. J. Artif. Organs, 12, 664–667 (1989).
3. S. Hosokawa, A. Oyamaguchi and O. Yoshida. Trace elements and complications in patients undergoing chronic hemodialysis. Nephron, 55, 357–379 (1990).
4. E. A. Loeliger and F. A. Wolf. Aluminum concentration of albumin replacement solutions. N. Engl. J. Med., 312, 1389 (1985).
5. G. S. Fell and D. Maharaj. Trace metal contamination of albumin solutions used for plasma exchange. Lancet, i, 467–468 (1986).
6. D. Maharaj, G. S. Fell and B. F. Boyce. Aluminum bone disease in patients receiving plasma exchange with contaminated albumin. Br. Med. J., 295, 693–696 (1987).

Therapeutic Plasmapheresis (XII), pp. 671-672
T. Agishi *et al.* (Eds)
© VSP 1993

Liver Function during Long-term Plasmapheresis

S. HOSOKAWA

Utano National Hospital, Kyoto, Japan

Key words: plasmapheresis (PP); liver function; long-term PP; maintenance PP; side effects.

INTRODUCTION

Plasmapheresis (PP) has been developed as one kind of therapy for various sorts of autoimmune diseases. PP therapy has become popular due to easy to operate apparatus [1–4]. Several side effects with PP [1] treatment are known. However, many other side effects are not well known, especially in long-term maintenance PP therapy. Therefore, I describe the influence of PP therapy on liver function in patients with long-term PP treatment.

MATERIALS AND METHODS

The liver function in 15 patients (six patients with myasthenia gravis, four patients with multiple sclerosis, three patients with chronic inflammatory demyelinating polyradicaloneuropathy, two patients with rheumatoid arthritis) treated with PP was examined for 2 years. GOT, GPT, alkalinphosphatase, γ-GTP, total bilirubin, direct bilirubin, indirect bilirubin and ZTT values were measured. Liver imaging studies, such as CT scanning and echogram, were also performed for 2 years. A Plasouto 1000 was used and plasma separator was used as the first filter. A separator of plasma component was used as the second filter. Twenty five percent albumin solution and electrolytes solutions were used for replacement fluid in PP therapy. Two liters of plasma were treated during each PP therapy. Blood flow was 60–70 ml/min and plasma flow was 20 ml/min. All data are given as mean and standard deviation (SD). Student's t-test was used and $P < 0.05$ was considered as significant.

RESULTS

Values of GOT, GPT, ALP in serum and γ-GTP were 22 ± 6 IU/l and 22 ± 4 mU/ml before PP and 21 ± 7, 21 ± 9, 158 ± 68 and 21 ± 6 at 2 years after the start of PP. Differences in these values between before and at 2 years after the beginning of PP were not found. Total bilirubin, direct bilirubin, indirect bilirubin and ZTT levels in serum were 0.6 ± 0.3 mg/dl, 0.3 ± 0.2 mg/dl, 0.3 ± 0.1 mg/dl and 7 ± 3 K-U before the beginning of PP and 0.7 ± 0.4, 0.3 ± 0.2, 0.3 ± 0.1 and 6 ± 4 at 2 years after the start of PP. No significant difference in these values between before the beginning of

PP and at 2 years after the start of PP were found. In liver CT imaging studies, almost normal findings in 15 patients were obtained before PP and at 2 years after the start of PP. Also, echograms in the 15 patients were almost normal before and after PP for 2 years.

DISCUSSION

To perform PP therapy, heparin has been used as an anticogulant which may cause bleeding [5]. It is well known that replacement fluid [particularly fresh frozen plasma (FFP)] sometimes contributes to side effects in PP treatment [6, 7]. Also, several biological and physiological changes were found during PP. However, this paper describes a preliminary follow up of liver function in PP therapy for long periods. None of 15 patients received blood transfusion or FFP during PP therapy for 2 years. No hepatotoxic substances were used in the 15 patients for the PP therapy for 2 years. Liver function of the 15 patients was normal before and after PP treatment for 2 years. Liver imaging studies were almost normal before and after PP for 2 years. These facts indicate that long-term PP therapy does not impare liver function. None of the 15 patients had any severe side effects. Thus, for the 15 patients, PP was an effective and safe therapy in a clinical setting.

CONCLUSION

Long-term PP did produce any kind of damage to liver in patients.

REFERENCES

1. S. Hosokawa and O. Yoshida. Prevention of side effects and problems in double filtration plasma-pheresis. In: *Therapeutic plasmapheresis (VII)*, T. Oda (Ed.), pp. 261–263, ISAO Press, Cleveland (1988).
2. S. Hosokawa, A. Kawazi, T. Imai *et al.* Plasma exchange treatment for fulminant hepatic failure. In: *Therapeutic plasmapheresis (IV)*, T. Oda (Ed.), pp. 317–321, Schattauer Verlag, Berlin (1984).
3. S. Hosokawa, H. Mizuno and R. Abe. Effective treatment for cancer by double filtration plasmapheresis. *Curr. Therapeut. Res.*, **45**, 152–161 (1989).
4. S. Hosokawa, H. Mizuno, R. Abe *et al.* Kinetics of cisdichlorodiammine platinum during plasmaphere-sis. *Artif. Organs*, **14**, 442–446 (1989).
5. S. Hosokawa, A. Oyamaguchi and O. Yoshida. Optimization of heparinization in clinical double filtration plasmapheresis. *Int. J. Artif. Organs*, **12**, 544–548 (1989).
6. Y. Shinoda, T. Matsubuchi and H. Kawagoe. Post-transfusion hepatitis after plasma exchange. In: *Therapeutic Plasmapheresis (II)*, T. Oda (Ed.), pp. 143–148, Schattauer Verlag, Berlin (1982).
7. T. Sanada, K. Kubo, T. Suzuki *et al.* Complications associated with plasma exchange. In: *Therapeutic Plasmapheresis (II)*, T. Oda (Ed.), pp. 586–589, Schattauer Verlag, Berlin (1982).

Therapeutic Plasmapheresis (XII), pp. 673-677
T. Agishi *et al.* (Eds)
© VSP 1993

Side Effects and Complications in Therapeutic Plasma Exchange

R. BAMBAUER and M. SCHÄTZLE

University of Saarland, D-6650 Homburg/Saar, Germany

Key words: side-effects; complications; therapeutic plasma exchange.

INTRODUCTION

Since hollow fibre membrane separators have become available the therapeutic plasma exchange (TPE) method has been used in the treatment of a variety of diseases. The advantages of membrane plasma separation are, in addition to a complete separation of corpuscular components from plasma, a simple elimination of macromolecules and plasma components, and no carry over of cells into the separated plasma. Cell damage is much less than by using centrifuges as separation methods [1]. Only a small number of controlled studies have been carried out for different diseases in the last years. Therefore a final conclusion of effects of these separation methods is not yet possible on most of the treated diseases.

In agreement with Wiliams and his hypothesis about the life cycle of medical technologies, TPE appears to rest between no acceptance and decay, and it might hopefully reach a steady state in the next years [2]. We can confirm this hypothesis with our own observations of TPE treatments over 11 years. In a retrospective study the hazards and side effects of TPE treatments which were performed over the last 11 years in our department were investigated.

METHOD AND PATIENTS

From 1979 to 1990 a total of 7729 TPE treatments in 735 patients were performed. The complete data of 658 out of 735 patients were available, therefore only 6195 TPE treatments could be used for this investigation. The data of the selective plasma separation methods e.g. immunoadsorption, plasmaperfusion and LDL apheresis treatments were not complete, and therefore excluded. TPE was performed in 348 female patients and 310 male patients (1–244 TPE/patient). The average age of the patients was 42.8 years (1 day–82 years). Table 1 summarizes all treated diseases. The side-effects are expressed as percentages of the total treatment number. In 318 patients (48.3%), between one and 23 side-effects were observed in a total of 701 side-effects (11.3%). The other 340 patients (51.7%) showed no side-effects during or after TPE treatment.

Blood pressure was measured before, during and after treatment, and in all situations when side-effects were observed. All side-effects during or after TPE were documented

Table 1.
Diseases, side-effects in TPE

Diseases	Patients	TPE		Exchange volume	Side-effects	
	n	n	%	mean (l/TPE)	n	%
Nephrology	56	648	11.6	2.24	76	11.7
Gastroenterology	164	1079	6.6	2.63	203	18.8
Hematology	169	1305	6.7	2.20	137	10.5
Neurology	61	605	9.9	2.57	72	11.8
Metabolism	28	470	16.8	2.28	31	6.5
Dermatology	38	363	9.6	2.51	40	10.9
Connective tissue	39	1351	34.7	2.41	84	6.2
Miscellany	76	374	4.9	3.19	58	15.5

in special hemodialysis records. The side-effects were divided as mild, moderate and severe. As vascular access, large bore catheters were inserted in the internal jugular or subclavian vein or in newborns smaller catheters were inserted in the femoral or umbilical veins. In other patients peripheral veins were used. In patients with acute hepatic failure an additional large bore catheter was inserted in the femoral artery to infuse the substitution solution, especially fresh frozen plasma. Heparin was used for anticoagulation for the extracorporeal circuit at a dosage between 500 and 8000 U/treatment.

The substitution solutions used were human albumin with isotonic electrolytes 3–6% in 57.4% of the treatments, serum protein solution 5% Biseko (Biotest, Frankfurt, Germany) in 14.1%, lyophilized plasma (Lyoplasma, Immuno, Heidelberg, Germany) in 6.1% and fresh frozen plasma in 22.4%. Only in severe acute hepatic failure or coagulation disturbances was fresh frozen plasma and/or lyoplasma used.

RESULTS

In 43 different diseases, plasmapheresis was performed as a supportive therapy. In 1939 treatments no side effects were observed, only one complication was seen in 1258 treatments, two to five side-effects were documented in 1771 treatments, and more than six side-effects were seen in 1227 TPE treatments. Nine patients died as a result of their primary diseases and two patients under TPE. The side-effects in dependence of the substitution solution can be summarized as nausea, dyspnea, prurigo, fever, shivers, blood pressure decrease and allergic reactions until anaphylactic shock (Table 2). The

Table 2.
Side-effects depending on substitution solution

	Patients	TPE	Side-effects	
	n	n	n	%
Human albumin	457	5175	52	1.0
Serum protein solution	265	3595	60	2.4
Lyo-plasma	90	600	29	4.8
Fresh frozen plasma	242	1784	44	2.4

Table 3.
Side-effects in different diseases under TPE in 658 patients with 6195 treatments

Diseases	Patients	TPE		Side-effects	
	n	n	per patient	n	%
RPGN	30/650	403	13.4	37	9.2
Acute hepatic failure	126/164	923	7.3	268	18.2
Plasmocytoma	64/194	651	10.2	50	7.7
Polyradiculitis	29/ 57	328	11.3	36	11.0
Hypercholesterolemia	11/ 28	173	15.7	13	7.5
Drug intoxiation	27/ 76	59	2.2	12	20.3
Prurgo of unknown origin	9/ 9	67	7.4	13	19.4
SLE	24/ 39	1132	47.2	77	6.8
Total	318/658	3736	11.7	406	12.5

Table 4.
Severe side-effects under TPE ($n = 18/658$ patients)

Mayor cause	Diagnosis	Patients	Age	Sex	TPE	Course
		n	(years)		n	
Cardiovascular	Plasmocytoma	1	71	m	1	improved
(reanimation)	Hemolysis postoperative	2	52/67	f	1/1	improved
	Acute hepatic failure, postoperative	1	54	m	1	worsening
Respiratory	Asthma bronchiale	1	52	f	2	worsening
	Thrombopenia	1	28	f	16	improved
	Rh-erythroblastosis	1	1 day	m	2	worsening
Death due to primary disease	Thyroid storm	1	71	f	1	died
	Acute hepatic failure, postoperative	2	20/37	f	10/1	died
	Sepsis	2	9/64	f	1/1	died
	Severe hemolysis	1	68	f	1	died
	Moschkowitz–syndrome	1	20	f	8	died
	EPH-gestosis	1	28	f	2	died
	Polyradiculitis	1	55	m	3	died
TPE	Acute hepatic failure (Budd–Chiari syndrome) blood pressure decrease	1	20	f	4	died
	Sepsis, postoperative anaphylactic shock	1	1	m	1	died

most severe complications of allergic reactions to anaphylactic shock were seen only when fresh frozen plasma was used for substitution. TPE must be stopped due to severe side-effects in patients, coagulation in the extracorporeal system due to insufficient heparinization and or due to insufficient blood flow in 172 treatments in 133 patients.

Side-effects in dependence of the vascular access were documented in 0.09% of all treatments. The most important side-effects in vascular accesses were with 48.3% infections, abscess, bacteriemia and septicemia. In 10.1%, a faulty puncture-like puncture of a artery was observed. Thrombosis of the subclavian or upper cava vein was seen in 5.2%. Bleedings and hematoma were documented in 3.7% and in the same range pneumothorax or hematothorax were observed after puncturing of large vessels. In 29.1% fault in the catheter materials were found and the catheter had to be changed.

In Table 3 the diseases with the highest complication rates are shown. The largest complication rate, 20.3%, was observed in exogenous intoxication. All patients suffered from severe intoxication with lethal drug concentrations in the blood. The side-effects in the treatment of acute hepatic failure with 18.2% are following and prurigo of unknown origin with 19.4%.

In Table 4 the most severe side-effects and complications which were documented are summarized. The incidence of severe side-effects was low (0.29%). All patients mentioned in this table suffered a very severe course of their primary disease. At the start of TPE most of them were in a bad condition and conservative therapy had failed in all of them. Inclosed are the nine patients (0.15%) who died due to their primary disease. The TPE treatment had also failed in these patients. They died after the TPE treatments. Two patients died under TPE, one in a anaphylactic shock due to fresh frozen plasma as substitution solution, the other one due to an irreversible blood pressure decrease.

DISCUSSION

Despite all in the impressive results achieved with plasmapheresis in recent years, this therapy can be associated with considerable side-effects [3]. These comprise infections inflicted through the vascular accesses or because of the removal of immunoglobulins and allergic reactions up to anaphylactic shock caused by the substitution solution [4].

Two of 11 patients died during TPE treatment. The other nine patients died after plasmapheresis due to a severe course of their primary disease and are not related directly to TPE.

In 1989, the Canadian Apheresis Study Group reported 5235 plasmapheresis treatments with seven deaths, five were not related directly to TPE. The total side-effects, 12%, were in the same range as in our retrospective study.

Severe side-effects were seen there when using fresh frozen plasma as substitution solution [5]. This means that one has to consider very carefully which substitution solution should be applied. In contrast to other authors, we observed a lower incidence of side-effects in patients who received a combination therapy of immunosuppressive drugs and TPE against patients who received only TPE (Table 5). In patients with autoimmune diseases like SLE, who were treated with TPE and immunosuppressive drugs very intensively, the incidence of side effects was, at 6.8%, very low in our investigation also.

The highest complication rates showed in patients with drug intoxication and acute hepatic failure. Most of them were in a very bad condition with additional diseases like acute renal failure, coagulation disturbances and/or artificial respiration. TPE caused severe immunodeficiency, worsening the primary disease in a higher percentage of these patients, and was responsible for a higher complication rate.

Table 5.
Side-effects depending on drugs and TPE

	Patients		TPE	Side-effects	
	n	%	*n*	*n*	%
No drugs	464	70.5	2782	418	15.8
Steroids	82	12.5	1365	113	8.3
Cytotoxics	112	17.0	2048	170	8.3

Most patients treated with TPE had very bad prognosis of their diseases, and in most of these patients the available conservative therapies had failed. A final conclusion cannot be given. For the most treated diseases no results from controlled studies are available, there is no convenience about the system, the anticoagulation, the exchange volume and the substitution solution. Therefore most reported results from other authors are not comparable.

Plasmapheresis is a very effective therapy method but in view of the side-effects and complications observed, it must be concluded that it is compulsory to balance the possible risk against the expected beneficial results. The type of substitution solution should meet clinical requirements. The indications for TPE should be narrowly defined. The plasmapheresis technique must be made transparent and comparable. For all accepted plasmapheresis indications, compulsory drugs must be defined and protocols must be available. Finally, more controlled multicenter studies must begin to prove the effectiveness of plasmapheresis.

REFERENCES

1. R. Bambauer. *Therapeutischer Plasmaaustausch und verwandte Plasmaseparationsverfahren.* Schattauer, Stuttgart (1988).
2. A. Williams. The role of economics in the evaluations of health care technologies. In: *Economic and Medical Evaluation of Health Care Technologies*, A. J. Culyer and B. Horisberger (Eds), pp. 38–68, Springer, Berlin (1983).
3. H. G. Klein, J. E. Balow, P. C. Dau, M. J. Hamburger, S. F. Leitman, A. A. Pineda and R. S. A. Tindall. Clinical applications. *J. Clin. Apheresis*, 3, 4 (1986).
4. K. H. Shumak and G. A. Rock. Therapeutic Plasma Exchange. *N. Engl. J. Med.*, **310**, 762–771 (1984).
5. Canadian Apheresis Study Group.

Therapeutic Plasmapheresis (XII), pp. 679-681
T. Agishi *et al.* (Eds)
© VSP 1993

Adverse Effects of Platelet Donation by Apheresis

M. A. MOTA, A. MENDRONE Jr, A. M. SAKASHITA, A. M. ARRIFANO,
P. E. DORLHIAC-LLACER, J. M. KUTNER and D. A. F. CHAMONE

*Fundação Pró-Sangue Hemocentro de São Paulo and Hematology Department,
University of São Paulo, São Paulo, Brazil*

Key words: apheresis; blood donation; paresthesia; thrombocytopenia; citrate toxicity.

INTRODUCTION

As more aggressive chemotherapy protocols are used for cancer treatment, resulting in longer thrombocytopenia, platelet transfusion needs have greatly increased. In this way, the development of more efficient platelet harvesting techniques from single donors has made platelet transfusions available on a large scale. Transfusion of large amounts of platelets from single donors, instead of multiple donors, reduces the patient's exposure to blood transmitted diseases and to donor antigens. Single donor platelets collected from histocompatible individuals by apheresis have become the mainstay of transfusion therapy for allommunized patients [1]. The increased use of platelet transfusions resulted in more donors being subjected to repeated plateletpheresis.

Studies of platelet donors indicate a low rate of complications [2]. Modest decreases in donor's platelet count (around $60 \times 10^9/l$) occur with each procedure [3]. Problems such as citrate toxicity, hypovolemia and anxiety, often attributed to citrate anticoagulant concentration and individual idiosyncratic reactions, have been reported [4].

In order to evaluate the frequency of adverse reactions in plateletpheresis donors in our hospital, we retrospectively analyzed 626 donations.

MATERIAL AND METHODS

Between April 1990 and April 1991, 626 plateletpheresis procedures were performed in 289 donors using continuous flow equipment (Vivacell CE-798, Dideco, Italy) and the adverse effects registered.

In 469 (74.9%) donations the total volume processed was in the range 3000–4000 ml (group I) and in 157 (25.1%) it was 4000–5000 ml (group II). The mean processing time was 64.9 min (range 40–90 min) with an outflow range from 50 to 80 ml/min.

RESULTS

Adverse effects were observed in 85 procedures (13.6%; 65 donors), 41 in group I (8.7%; 32 donors) and 44 in group II (28.0%; 37 donors); $P < 0.05$.

Symptoms are described in Table 1.

Table 1.
Adverse effects observed in plateletpheresis donors

Symptoms	Group I	Group II	Total (%)	
Circumoral paresthesia	26	38	64	(69.6)
Hypotension	6	2	8	(8.7)
Chills	2	4	6	(6.5)
Chest discomfort	3	2	5	(5.4)
Facial rash + eye irritation	4	0	4	(4.3)
Nausea	1	1	2	(2.2)
Dizziness	2	0	2	(2.2)
Generalized paresthesia	0	1	1	(1.1)
Total	44	48	92	(100)

Except for one procedure, where the donation had to be interrupted because of a supraventricular tachycardia (in Table 1, this donor is included in 'Chest discomfort', Group II), all others had the adverse effects easily controlled and needed no interruption.

DISCUSSION

Plateletpheresis is considered to be generally uneventful for the donor. However, adverse effects have been reported. Mild paresthesias are most common side-effects, reported to occur in one-third to one-half of all donors. It is caused by the citrate anticoagulant, and attributed to a decrease in the level of ionized calcium, which can drop by an average of 32.4%, leading to neuromuscular hyperactivity [5–7].

In this study, mild paresthesia was also the most frequent adverse effect verified. This symptom was more frequent in Group II (in 24.2% of donations), and this can be attributed to the fact that the total volume processed was higher than in Group I (paresthesia in 5.5% of donations), but in a similar period of time. Other symptoms occurred less often, some caused also by citrate (chest pain, nausea, vomiting and chills, secondary to increased muscular tension) and others probably caused by circulatory effects, as a consequence of the removal of blood in large volumes and/or to shifts in body fluids. Anxiety, alone or in association with other factors, must also be considered as a possible cause.

Ethylene oxide gas, used for sterilization of the disposable material, has been reported to be responsible for allergic type reactions, including facial rash and eye irritation [8].

Because of the undesirable effects of citrate, some authors have suggested the use of a 'half-strength' ACD solution as anticoagulant [6].

CONCLUSIONS

Plateletpheresis is a safe procedure, but not exempt from adverse effects, some of them common (as for circumoral paresthesias). These are usually mild and easily reversed with simple measures. However, staff must be aware of the fact that more severe reactions can rarely occur and be ready to manage the situation.

Acknowledgments
Supported in part by a grant from Fundação Banco do Brasil.

REFERENCES

1. D. G. Ross, S. Holme and W. A. L. Heaton. *In vitro* and *in vivo* comparison of platelet concentrates collected by automated versus manual apheresis. *Vox. Sang.*, **57**, 25–28 (1989).

2. J. A. Koepke, W. M. Parks, J. A. Goeken *et al.* The safety of weekly plateletpheresis: Effect on the donor's lymphocyte population. *Transfusion*, **21**, 59–63 (1981).

3. J. A. Koepke, K. K. Wu, J. C. Hoak *et al.* A comparison of platelet production methods suitable for a service-oriented blood donor center. *Transfusion*, **15**, 39–42 (1975).

4. J. Nusbacher, M. L. Scher, J. L. MacPherson. Plateletpheresis using the Haemonetics Model 30 cell seperator. *Vox. Sang.*, **33**, 9–15 (1977).

5. T. H. Price. Plateletpheresis and leukapheresis. In: *Principles of Transfusion Medicine*, E. C. Rossi, T. L. Simon and G. S. Moss (Eds), Williams and Wilkins, Baltimore (1991).

6. P. R. Olson, C. Cox and J. McCullough. Laboratory and clinical effects of the infusion of ACD solution during plateletpheresis. *Vox. Sang.*, **33**, 79–87 (1977).

7. T. L. Simon. Apheresis: principles and practices. In: *Principles of Transfusion Medicine*, E. C. Rossi, T. L. Simon and G. S. Moss (Eds), Williams and Wilkins, Baltimore (1991).

8. J. Dolovich, M. Sagona, F. Pearson *et al.* Sensitization of repeat plasmapheresis donors to ethylene oxide gas. *Transfusion*, **27**, 90–93 (1987).

Therapeutic Plasmapheresis (XII), pp. 683-684
T. Agishi *et al.* (Eds)
© VSP 1993

Significant Complications of Therapeutic Plasma Exchange

D. SUTTON, G. ROCK and MEMBERS OF THE CASG*

Canadian Apheresis Study Group, Ottawa, Ontario, Canada

Key words: plasma exchange; severe reactions.

INTRODUCTION

The Canadian Apheresis Study Group (CASG) has collected data on reactions to plasma exchange (PE) since 1985. Reactions are classified as mild, moderate or severe, with a severe reaction being one in which a patient becomes clinically unstable requiring intervention by a physician and early termination of the procedure.

METHODS

The incidence of severe reactions associated with therapeutic PE was examined by reviewing information on all PEs performed across Canada during the years 1988, 1989 and 1990. Data sheets were submitted on each procedure detailing the diagnosis, the specific indication for PE, the clinical status of the patient before exchange, the type of machine, the type of anticoagulant, the method of vascular access, the type of replacement fluid, and a description of any reaction judged by the nurse or physician to be severe.

RESULTS

Severe reactions occurred during 109 (0.6%) of 18 129 PEs involving 83 (4.5%) of 1876 patients treated during the three year period (Table 1).

Reactions were characterized by several different symptom complexes, the most common being fever and rigors (usually associated with the use of plasma as replacement fluid), hypotension, dyspnea, bronchospasm and chest pain. Several neurologic events, including grand mal seizures, occurred in patients with thrombotic thrombocytopenic purpura (TTP). There were three deaths, two of which were thought to be due, primarily,

---

*The members of the CASG are as follows: Grenfell Adams, MD, Barrett Benny, MD, Noel A. Buskard, MD, Stephen N. Caplan, MD, Robert Card, MD, William F. Clark, MD, Peter Ford, MD, John J. L. Freedman, MD, Philip Gordon, MD, John Klassen, MD, Max M. Gorelick, MD, Pierre Leblond, MD, Mariette Lepine-Martin, MD, Jack McBride, MD, Marc P. Monté, MD, Rama C. Nair, PhD, Gail A. Rock, PhD, MD, Tsiporah Shore, MD, Kenneth H. Shumak, MD, and David M. C. Sutton, MD.

to the PE as well as several alarming events, including transient cardiac arrhythmias and a cardiac arrest.

Table 1.
Incidence of severe reactions

Year	Total		Reactions		%	
	PE	(patients)	PE	(patients)	PE	(patients)
1990	6016	(754)	25	(21)	0.4	(2.8)
1989	6026	(701)	46	(33)	0.8	(4.7)
1988	6087	(695)	38	(29)	0.6	(4.2)
Total	18,129	(1876)	109	(83)	0.6	(4.5)

CONCLUSIONS

Although PE is, generally, a safe and well tolerated procedure, serious side effects do sometimes occur. Severe reactions are encountered more frequently in patients with TTP ($P < 0.01$) and when whole plasma is used as the replacement fluid. Proper assessment of patients before and during treatment is essential and apheresis personnel must be prepared to deal with life-threatening complications.

16
Vascular Access

Therapeutic Plasmapheresis (XII), pp. 687-691
T. Agishi *et al.* (Eds)
© VSP 1993

Recirculation in Single-needle Plasmapheresis and Single-needle Hemodialysis

R. BAMBAUER and G. JACOBS

Institute for Blood Purification, D-6650 Hamburg/Saar, Germany

Key words: single-needle plasmapheresis; single-needle hemodialysis.

INTRODUCTION

The use of the single-needle method in hemodialysis was first described by Kopp in 1972 [1]. Since then various pumps and clamp devices have been developed enabling, through the use of time or pressure control, an alternating blood flow through one needle. A so-called double-headed pump, first mentioned by Ringoir *et al.* in 1973, has proven of particular merit [2].

As, due to the method of functioning of this single-needle system, a recirculation of suctioned and re-pumped blood occurs, the effectiveness of dialysis compared with the two-needle method may be reduced.

Therefore, the recirculation volume was measured in an experiment and compared with data compiled during routine hemodialysis and plasmapheresis treatment. Furthermore, the recirculation values indicated in the literature and by the manufacturers were compared with our own data.

METHODS AND PATIENTS

The principle is basically a closed extracorporeal circulation system, which is connected up to the patient's circulation via a needle or large bore catheter. This system for the carrying out of plasmapheresis comprises not only the double pump but also a balancing pump and a heating unit [3]. For hemodialysis treatment an additional dialysate proportioner is required.

The double pump, as first described by Ringoir *et al.* [2] functions according to the principle of pressure–pressure and volume control. The system safety precautions comprise a combined air and level detector as a volume control. As both pumps function intermittently, this method provides a constant change in flow and pressure. The venous return flow is regulated by a pump. Thus, the inevitable high blood pressure subsequent to passage through the plasma filters which occurs in other single-needle systems with only one blood pump is avoided. Essential advantages of the double-pump system are considered to be:

(i) A relatively large phase volume reaches the hollow fibre membrane, without maximum pressure exceeding the safety limits.

(ii) The maximum pressure in the membrane separator can be adapted as required. This is of importance in the case of several plasmapheresis membranes due to the danger of hemolysis after a certain maximum pressure (> 150 mm Hg) is exceeded.

(iii) Due to the constant change in flow and pressure, only a delayed protein concentration polarization occurs.

Heparin in the usual dosage was used to achieve anticoagulation in the extracorporeal circulation system. The recirculation volume of the single-needle method was first of all examined using a model shunt and a large bore catheter, and subsequently with various vascular accesses in 25 patients receiving chronic hemodialysis or plasmapheresis treatment. Nine patients were suffering from end-stage renal failure. Six patients had rapid progressive glomerulonephritis, acute hepatic failure or plasmocytoma. In these cases, not only hemodialysis but also plasmpaheresis treatment was given. Four further patients with various illnesses were only treated with plasmapheresis.

In a total of 15 patients, five with acute shunt closure and 10 with acute commencing illnesses, large bore catheters had to be inserted into the internal jugular vein or subclavian vein.

Recirculation

In single-needle dialysis recirculation is the extent of the mingling of dialyzed and non-dialyzed blood in the extracorporeal circulation system, resulting in a reduction of clearance effectiveness. The recirculation phenomena can be divided into three groups:

(i) *First recirculation effect.* This is generally understood as the mingling of cleansed and non-cleansed blood in the vessel and fistula. In the case of the double-needle system recirculation is dependent on the distance to the second puncture.

(ii) *Second recirculation effect.* This is generally understood to mean the mingling of cleansed and non-cleansed blood in the needle and catheter, caused by the dead space volume. This mingling effect arises when the system switches over.

(iii) *Third recirculation effect.* This relates to the recirculation phenomena caused by tube compliance. A part of the cleansed blood flowing back to the patient is retained in the venous tube due to the elasticity of the tube system and mingles with the non-cleansed blood during the aspiration phase.

As the recirculation volume cannot be separated into the three different recirculation phenomena either *in vitro* or *in vivo*, the total recirculation volume was calculated, both for single-needle dialysis and for single-needle plasmapheresis, according to the following simplified formula:

$$RV = \frac{(C_B - C_A)}{(C_B - C_V)} \times 100 \, (\%)$$

where

RV is the recirculation volume (%),

C_B is the concentration of a substance x in the peripheral venous blood (mg/dl),

C_A is the concentration of a substance x in the arterial tube just in front of the dialysator/ membrane separator (mg/dl) and

C_V is the concentration of a substance x in the venous tube just in front of the Y-piece behind the dialysator/membrane separator (mg/dl).

The extracorporeal treatment was carried out using punctuation needles and tube systems commonly available on the market. The hemodialysis session lasted for 2–3.5 h, plasmapheresis for 2–2.5 h. The blood extractions were performed as indicated in the above formula for RV. The first extraction (C_B) was prior to commencement of hemodialysis or TPE, C_A, C_V 5 min after commencement of hemodialysis or TPE. C_A was only extracted during the aspiration phase and C_B only during the venous return flow phase. The pre-determined blood flow and pressure rates were kept constant as far as possible during all treatment sessions.

RESULTS

Table 1 shows a summary of the results of the most important parameters (RV, percentual and absolute), blood flow per stroke, Q_B(ml/min) and volume V_B (ml/stroke) transported per stroke. The highest RV was in the plasmpaheresis using large bore catheters with 25.6%, followed by dialysis with Gore–Tex protheses with 21.2%. The flow conditions are expressed in: flow/min (Q_B) and stroke per cycle V_n). Here high blood flows are to be found in dialysis and low ones in plasmapheresis. The percent recirculation volumes have been compiled once again in Fig. 1.

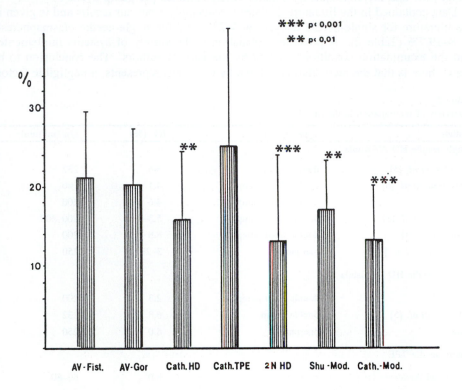

Figure 1. Percentual recirculation volumes in single-needle techniques.

Table 1.
Recirculation volume in single-needle techniques

Vascular access	n	RV (%)	RV (ml)	Q_B (ml/min)	V (ml/cycle)
AV-Fistula	115	20.8 ± 8.2	9.1 ± 3	215 ± 31	43.7 ± 9.2
AV-Goretex	15	21.2 ± 9.6	7.8 ± 2.2	98 ± 40	38.0 ± 8.8
Cath. HD	47	14.9 ± 8.3	7.3 ± 4	215 ± 22	51.8 ± 11.2
Cath. TPE	28	25.6 ± 15.8	6.0 ± 4.1	108 ± 22	24.0 ± 7.1
Two-needle HD	11	12.6 ± 10.9	—	254 ± 10	—
Shunt model	15	17.8 ± 6.1	5.8 ± 6.1	227 ± 1	47.1 ± 5.4
Cath. model	44	13.3 ± 7.4	5.8 ± 6.1	227 ± 1	42.1 ± 5.4

DISCUSSION

The recirculation effect is one of the most important factors influencing the efficacy of the single-needle method. Thus the flow conditions in the vessel, the compliance of vessel and tube systems, the dead space and the flow resistance as well as the setting of the pump all exercise a considerable influence on the extent of recirculation [4].

We can conclude from our results that the smaller the blood flow in the vessel which serves as the entry point for the treatment, the higher will be the proportion of recirculating volume. We found the lowest absolute recirculation volume in single-needle plasmapheresis using large bore catheters, which can be explained by slower blood flow and the consequently smaller volume strokes per pump cycle.

Data contained in the literature deviates considerably from our results and is given in the literature for single-needle dialysis as 3–29% and for single-needle plasmapheresis as 8–19.7% (Table 2). A possible explanation is the variety of systems implemented and the examination conditions applied by the various authors. The conclusion to be drawn here is that the recirculation volume by no means represents, a negligible factors

Table 2.
Overview of recirculation in the literature

Author	Type of pump	RV (%)	Q_B (ml/min)
Single-needle HD AV-fistula			
Virgillis et al. [5]	double pump	3.6	232
Weinstein et al. [6]	double head pump	4.1	140
Koch [7]	double head pump	4.6	200
Hilderson et al. [8]	double head pump	5.3–8.6	200–300
Kopp et al. [9]	double head pump	8.8	200
Blumenthal et al. [4]	one pump	3–29	250
Double-needle HD AV-fistula			
Koch [7]	double head pump	2.3	200
Virgillis et al. [5]	double pump	6.8	232
Nardi	one pump	6.0	250
Single-needle TPE			
Cunio and Anderson [10]	centrifuge	8.0	60–80
Sprenger et al. [11]	double head pump	19.7	100

either in single-needle dialysis or in single-needle plasmapheresis. The reduction in efficacy resulting therefrom far exceeds the advantages of the single-needle method and must, therefore, be taken into consideration in the choice of method to be implemented.

REFERENCES

1. K. Kopp, C. Gutch and W. Kolff. Single needle dialysis. *Trans. Am. Soc. Artif. Intern. Organs*, **18**, 75–81 (1972).

2. S. Ringoir, M. De Broe, M. Carclon and J. P. van Walleghem. New pump system for one needle hemodialysis (abstract). *Eur. Dial. Transpl. Ass.*, **10**, 200 (1973).

3. R. Bambauer. Therapeutischer plasmaaustausch und verwandte separationsverfahren. In: *Technische Grundlagen, Pathophysiologie und klinische Ergebnisse*, Schattauer Verlag, Stuttgart (1988).

4. S. Blumenthal, M. Ortiz, J. Kleinmann and W. Piering. Inflow time and recirculation in single-needle hemodialysis. *Am. J. Kidney Dis.*, **8**, 202–206 (1986).

5. G. de Virgillis, M. Vanin, U. Buoncristiani. A new single needle dialysis system. *Trans. Am. Soc. Artif. Intern. Organs*, **31**, 116–119 (1985).

6. A. Weinstein, P. Frederick and J. Sullivan. Single needle venous dialysis: a comparison of three systems. *Uremia*, **8**, 69–77 (1985).

7. G. Koch. Quantitative Aussagen zur hämodialyse und untersuchungen über die rezirkkulation beim Single-Needle-Verfahren. *Nieren- und Hochdruckkrankh.*, **12**, 495–500 (1983).

8. J. Hilderson, S. Ringoir, J. van Waeleghem, J. van Egmond and K. Schelstraete. *Die Doppelkopfpumpe.* (1985).

9. K. Kopp, R. Pfab, G. Wochner, G. Schätze and M. Mohlzahn. Toward automation of single needle vascular access. *Trans. Am. Soc. Artif. Intern. Organs*, **30**, 463–467 (1984).

10. J. Cunio and W. Anderson. Continous flow plasma exchange utilizing 'single needle' technique. *Trans. Am. Soc. Artif. Intern. Organs*, **27**, 650–653 (1981).

11. K. Sprenger, W. Kratz, K. Huber and H. Franz. Single-needle membrane plasma separation: costs and kinetic modeling. In: *First Int. Symp. Single Needle Dialysis*, pp. 244–249, ISAO Press, Cleveland (1984).

Therapeutic Plasmapheresis (XII), pp. 693-697
T. Agishi *et al*. (Eds)
© VSP 1993

Optimizing Superficial Vein Blood Extraction

P. R. PRINCE

*Baxter Healthcare Corporation, BIOTECH GROUP, Fenwal Division,
Santa Ana, California, USA*

Key words: access; extraction; flow; occlusion; vein.

INTRODUCTION

Much work has been to minimize blood trauma and stress in extracorporeal blood processing systems. An integral part of these systems is the vein itself. Blood exposed to stress within the vein and needle prior to anticoagulation can lead to platelet activation, hemolysis and initiation of clotting processes. Methods used to minimize this stress, yet extract blood at the maximum flow rate possible, are presented.

MODEL

Figure 1 models a superficial vein in the arm, illustrating a typical intravenous pressure of about 10 mm Hg with respect to extravascular pressure in that region. This small positive pressure is sufficient to expand the vein. If the vessel internal pressure drops below local external venous pressure it will collapse and flatten. Placing and inflating a pressure cuff on the arm down-stream from the venepuncture site creates pressure within the arm that acts as a pinching valve and restricts the flow of blood under the pressure cuff.

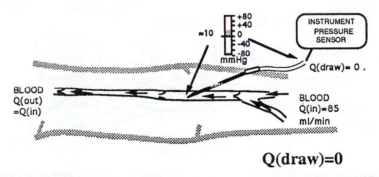

Figure 1. Model of superficial vein, showing typical internal vein pressure that is monitored with the needle and pressure sensor.

Generally the pressure internal to the vein must approach the pressure in the pressure cuff in order for blood to escape freely under the cuff and return to the heart (see Fig. 2). As blood is drawn through the needle, a pressure drop across the needle is algebraically added to the internal vein pressure. Since the needle pressure drop is negative as seen at the pressure sensor, the actual pressure seen (neglecting gravity terms as though the pressure sensor is at arm level) is equal to the internal vein pressure minus the magnitude of pressure developed across the needle.

As long as the flow rate drawn through the needle, Q(draw), is less than that of Q(in), which is the blood flow rate into the vein, there is blood returned to the heart, and lost with respect to the apheresis procedure. If Q(draw) exceeds the vein input flow the vein will become depleted of blood locally, and will collapse. When the vein collapses, the needle becomes occluded against the vein wall, and the vein flattens and creates additional resistance to flow. If the pump is allowed to continue, unrestricted, a high negative pressure will develop. There is ultimately a balance achieved between the pump flow efficiency due to the high negative input pressure, and a corresponding high pressure drop created within the vein and against the needle tip.

This pressure may be several multiples of the normal pressure drop across the needle, and creates a high fluid shear in the blood as it passes through the constrictions.

Many extracorporeal blood processing systems employ an absolute pressure limit (such as −200 mm Hg), beyond which the blood pump is controlled to slow down.

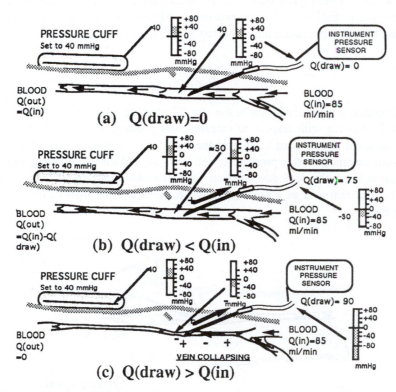

Figure 2. Superficial vein model in which (a) Q(draw) = 0; Q(out) = Q(in), (b) Q(draw) < Q(in); Q(out) = remaining flow not drawn, and internal vein pressure ≈ 40 mm Hg, and (c) Q(draw) > Q(in) causing vein collapse and needle occlusion.

Others attempt to operate at the onset of occlusion (identified by the first time derivative of pressure. This is very difficult to control when $Q(in)$ is continuously changing). If there is no means to control internal vein pressure above external pressure, the vein will collapse, and unnecessary blood shear will result (depicted in Fig. 2(c), and in the pressure–flow diagram of Fig. 4(b), showing the 'trajectory of an occlusion').

In externally anticoagulated procedures this shear occurs prior to anticoagulation and can cause platelet activation. If the shear is sufficiently high it can cause hemolysis. Under these conditions, or if the endothelial cell layer within the vein becomes damaged at the needle tip, clotting cascade can be initiated.

Depending upon the vessel size and elasticity (vein draw rate minus input blood flow rate), the time it takes to collapse a typical vein can vary from a *a fraction of a second to about a minute*. Refill time is in the same range. Figure 3 was generated (by assuming L/D of 5–20, where L is the length of the section of vessel that actually collapses and D is the diameter of the vessel) for extremes of diameter in typical peripheral veins of use in apheresis.

REQUIREMENTS

To avoid vein collapse it is necessary to maintain pressure within the vein somewhat above atmospheric pressure. Yet to capture substantially all of the blood flowing into the vein it is necessary to maintain the internal vein pressure somewhat below the cuff pressure. It is therefore required to know the internal vein pressure with sufficient accuracy to insure that these two conditions are always met. This condition is illustrated in Fig. 4(a) showing, for example, internal vein pressure maintained between about 10 and 30 mm Hg.

Additionally, to adapt to varying vessel size and input flow values, it is necessary to control blood pump acceleration, and helpful to deduce input vein flow rate, setting a transient protective flow rate ceiling. Plotting pressure vs blood flow graphically illustrates the relationship between internal vein pressure (shown along the zero blood-flow axis), and the pressure measured down-stream from the needle. The parallel

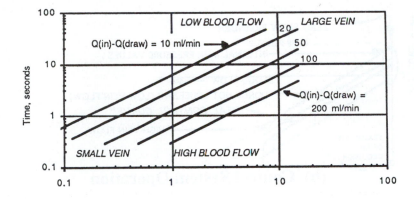

Figure 3. Vein depletion time vs local vein volume for various net flow rates.

lines in Fig. 4(b) represent pressure-flow relationships for various values of internal
vein pressure. Note that along the 'Ideal Control Curve', *low vein flow values* (the
donor is not squeezing the hand) and *high vein flow values* each stabilize at similar
internal vein pressure values. It is clear from the diagram that the instant needle–
blood viscosity relationship must be calibrated in order to extrapolate accurately from
pressure measurement values at finite flow back to the zero-flow internal vein pressure.
Various needle diameters and blood viscosity's yield large variations in the slope of the
pressure-flow lines in Fig. 4(b).

RESULTS AND DISCUSSION

The Autopheresis-C® plasmapheresis instrument has employed this control system for
several years, performing more than 18 000 000 procedures to date. Recently, further
advances in the control system and calibration system have extended operation from
about 20 to 150 ml/min blood flow rates.

Figure 5 illustrates data collected during a donor procedure (one extraction cycle
of an Auto-C procedure). Following calibration, pressure-flow data was sampled each
second.

The measured pressure points, the calculated 'Control Curve' values, and the calculated internal vein pressure values are plotted. Note that despite large variation in Q (in)
(donor not squeezing, then later squeezing), the system stabilizes along the control curve
and extracts substantially all blood entering the vein, without vein collapse.

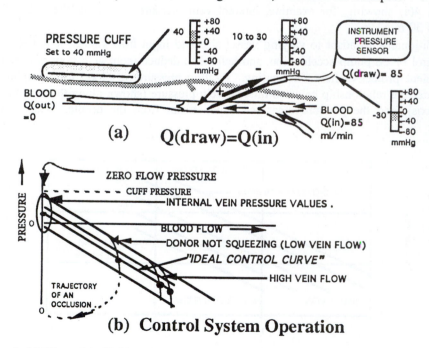

Figure 4. (a) Vein model with blood drawn at a flow rate equal to Q(in) and (b) pressure–flow relationship
for optimum control.

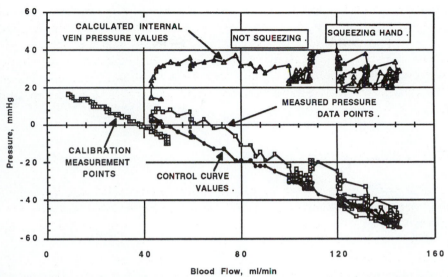

Figure 5. Pressure vs flow data for a donor initially not squeezing, then squeezing to stimulate increased vein input flow.

CONCLUSIONS

Substantially all blood flowing into a superficial vein can be extracted without creating the condition of vein collapse, needle occlusion, and increased blood shear. It is only necessary to insure that the internal vein pressure is continuously maintained between two bounds, and can be accomplished by accurately calibrating the needle–blood characteristics, extrapolating back to determine internal vein pressure, and controlling blood flow accordingly.

REFERENCES

1. J. D. Hellums, D. M. Peterson, Stathopoulos *et al. Studies on the Mechanisms of Shear-Induced Platelet Activation; Cerebral Ischemia and Hemorheology.* Springer-Verlag, Berlin (1987).
2. J. D. Hellums and C. H. Brown, III. Blood cell damage by mechanical forces. In: *Cardiovascular Flow Dynamics and Measurements,* University Park Press, Baltimore (1977).
3. N. S. Green and D. Steckler. *Donor Room Policies and Procedures.* American Association of Blood Banks, Arlington, Virginia (1985).
4. R. W. Colman, J. Hirsh, V. J. Marder *et al. Hemostasis and Thrombosis Basic Principles and Clinical Practice.* 2nd ed. J. B. Lippincott Company, Philadelphia (1987).
5. D. W. Schoendorfer. Automation in apheresis. In: *Proc. 13th Int. Symp. on Blood Transfusion,* Groningen (1988).

Storage for vein blood transfer

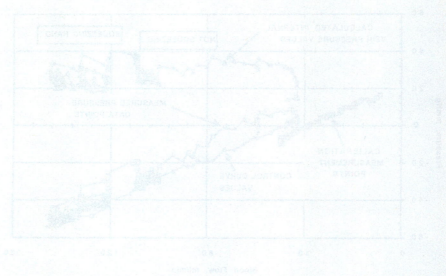

Figure 5. Pressure vs flow data for a shunt subunit and apparatus, thus equating to a stimulus increased vein input flow.

CONCLUSIONS

Substantially all blood flowing into a superficial vein can be extracted without creating the condition of vein collapse, needle occlusion, and increased blood shunt, if it is only necessary to insure that the internal vein pressure is continuously maintained between two bounds, and can be accomplished by accurately calibrating the needle-blood characteristics, extrapolating back to intraunit internal vein pressure, and controlling blood flow accordingly.

REFERENCES

1. S. D. Bellman, D. M. Iverson, Semiquantitative et al. Studies on the Measurement of Near-Infrared Plasma, Anesthesia, Cerebral Ischemia and Hemodynamics, Springer-Verlag, Berlin (1963).

2. J. D. Bellman and C.M. Davis, III, Grose cell Energy of Anesthetics on Hemodynamics: Their Dynamics and Measurement, University Park Press, Baltimore (1977).

3. S. Green and D. Von Ette-Cotter, Room Physics and Peripheral Anesthetic, Association of Blood Banks, Arlington, Virginia (1983).

4. E. W. Cotman, J. Bush, V.J., Studies et al. Physicians and Blood Cells Blood Physiology and Circle Practice 2nd ed. J. B. Lippincott Company, Philadelphia (1977).

5. D. W. Schneidman, Automation in apheresis. In Proc. Uses of Study on Blood Transfusion Techniques (1980).

17
Rheology

Therapeutic Plasmapheresis (XII), pp. 701-704
T. Agishi *et al.* (Eds)
© VSP 1993

Effect of 50 Gy Irradiation on the Rheology of Fresh and Stored Blood

N. MAEDA, Y. SUZUKI, A. SEIYAMA and N. TATEISHI

Department of Physiology, School of Medicine, Ehime University, Shigenobu, Onsen-gun, Ehime, Japan

Key words: X-ray irradiation; blood viscosity; CPD blood; red cell deformability; red blood cells.

INTRODUCTION

X-ray irradiation of blood has a preventive effect to the induction of graft-versus-host disease [1, 2]. However, the adverse effects for transfusion of irradiated blood relates to hemorheological aspects. In particular, rheological properties of red cells, a major constituent of blood, are important in controlling blood flow [3].

This paper describes the rheological properties of CPD blood (especially red cells) irradiated by X-rays at 50 Gy in polyvinyl chloride (PVC) bags and glass containers, and the rheological changes of the subsequently stored blood, dealing with the hematological and biochemical changes of red cells.

MATERIALS AND METHODS

X-ray irradiation
Each 14 ml of CPD blood in glass containers and small PVC bags was irradiated by X-ray 50 Gy (for 30 min with 10 000 rad) using an X-ray generator. Irradiated and non-irradiated (control) blood was stored at 4 °C up to 4 weeks.

Rheological properties
Blood viscosity was measured at various shear rates at 25 °C with a cone-plate viscometer.

Red cell deformability was measured in isotonic HEPES-buffered saline containing 20 g/dl Dextran T-40 at shear rates of 90–890 s^{-1} at 25 °C using a high-shear rheoscope [3, 4]. The long (L) and short (S) radii of more than 50 ellipsoidally deformed cells videotaped under a flash light were determined on video images using a computer, and the 'deformability' was expressed by the deformation index, $(L - S)/(L + S)$.

Hematological and biochemical properties of red cells
Hematological parameters were determined by a standard method. Cell shape was observed with a scanning electron microscope and the degree of echinocytic transfor-

mation was expressed by the morphological index (MI): discocyte (MI = 0), echinocyte I (MI = 0.5), echinocyte II (MI = 1), echinocyte III (MI = 2) and spheroechinocyte (MI = 3), on the basis of Bessis' classification [3].

The 2,3-DPG content was determined by an enzymatic method [5]. Contents of purine nucleotides in acid extracts were determined by high performance liquid chromatography [5]. The energy charge of adenylates was calculated by $(2[ATP] + [ADP])/2 \times ([ATP] + [ADP] + [AMP])$.

Membrane proteins of red cells were analyzed by electrophoresis on a slab gel containing 5.6% polyacrylamide and 0.1% SDS (without disulfide reducing agent) [6].

RESULTS AND DISCUSSION

Viscosity of fresh and subsequently stored CPD blood

Slight increase of the viscosity of CPD blood during storage was observed. However, X-ray irradiation did not significantly affect the change of blood viscosity during storage, in both glass containers and PVC bags (the blood viscosity was lower in PVC bags than in glass containers, especially at 2 weeks of storage; Table 1).

Table 1.
Effect of X-ray irradiation on the rheological, hematological and biochemical properties of CPD blood in glass containers and PVC bags: changes after 2 weeks of storage (a representative result)

	Glass container		PVC bag	
	control	irradiated	control	irradiated
η (cP) at 18.8/s	13.0	11.8	8.3	8.7
at 150/s	6.0	5.9	5.2	5.2
DI at 25 dyn/cm^2	—	—	0.24	0.26
at 98 dyn/cm^2	—	—	0.43	0.44
MI	1.23	1.47	0.42	0.51
MCHC (g/dl RBC)	33.2	33.0	34.1	34.2
2, 3-DPG (mM/l RBC)	4.90	5.14	5.41	4.85
AMP (mM/l RBC)	0.027	0.025	0.025	0.024
ADP (mM/l RBC)	0.130	0.158	0.191	0.146
ATP (mM/l RBC)	0.490	0.443	0.748	0.653
EC	0.858	0.835	0.875	0.883
GTP (mM/l RBC)	0.040	0.039	0.048	0.043

η, blood viscosity; DI, deformation index of red cells; MI, morphological index; EC, energy charge of adenylates.

Red cell deformability

Red cell deformability is a factor influencing blood viscosity [3]. The deformation index slightly decreased during storage. However, X-ray irradiation did not affect the deformation index of fresh red cells and the change of deformability during the storage of blood (Table 1).

Factors influencing red cell deformability

Red cell deformability is affected by red cell shape, intracellular viscosity (mainly MCHC) and membrane viscoelasticity (in particular oxidative crosslinking of cytoskeletal membrane proteins) [3].

(i) Discocytes progressively transformed to echinocytes (i.e. MI increased) during storage, but the shape change was not altered by X-ray irradiation (the biconcave disc shape was reserved much better in PVC bags than in glass containers; Table 1).

(ii) MCHC was not modified by X-ray irradiation (Table 1). Potassium leakage from red cells by X-ray irradiation [7] may induce the dehydration of red cells. However, it did not affect the deformability in the present results.

(iii) Crosslinked and/or abnormal proteins were not detected during storage up to 4 weeks after X-ray irradiation to CPD blood in both glass containers and PVC bags. Probably, the irradiation does not alter the membrane viscoelasticity of red cells.

In short, the decreased deformability of red cells during storage is mainly induced by the echinocytic shape change [3, 8], which increases the hydrodynamic effective volume of red cells [9]. X-ray irradiation does not alter the deformability change, thus the viscosity of blood.

Organic phosphates in red cells

During storage, ATP, GTP and 2,3-DPG decreased gradually, while AMP, ADP and IMP increased (ATP and 2,3-DPG contents were reserved at higher levels in PVC bags than in glass containers). Energy charge of adenylates decreased during storage, as ATP decreased. These changes of organic phosphates during storage were not altered by X-ray irradiation, as reported in part previously [10, 11].

CONCLUSION

X-ray irradiation at 50 Gy of fresh CPD blood and the subsequent storage of the irradiated blood up to 4 weeks do not cause significant deterioration in rheological, biochemical and hematological properties of red cells. Furthermore, the irradiation of PVC bags does not affect the properties of red cells through any alteration of bag constituents such as the plasticizer.

Acknowledgments
We thank to Mr K. Takaoka for this technical assistance in irradiating CPD blood. The work was supported in part by grants from the Ministry of Education, Science and Culture of Japan and from the Ehime Health Foundation.

REFERENCES

1. S. F. Leitman. Use of blood cell irradiation in the prevention of posttransfusion graft-vs-host disease. *Transfus. Sci.*, **10**, 219–232 (1989).
2. K. C. Anderson and H. J. Weinstein. Transfusion-associated graft-versus-host disease. *New Engl. J. Med.*, **323**, 315–321 (1990).
3. T. Shiga, N. Maeda and K. Kon. Erythrocyte rheology. *Crit. Rev. Oncol. Hematol.*, **10**, 9–48 (1990).
4. K. Kon, N. Maeda and T. Shiga. Erythrocyte deformation in shear flow: influences of internal viscosity, membrane stiffness, and hematocrit. *Blood*, **69**, 727–734 (1987).

5. Y. Suzuki, T. Nakajima, T. Shiga *et al.* Influence of 2,3-diphosphoglycerate on the deformability of human erythrocytes. *Biochim. Biophys. Acta*, **1029**, 85–90 (1990).

6. G. Fairbanks, T. L. Steck and D. F. H. Wallach. Electrophoretic analysis of the major polypeptides of the human erythrocyte membrane. *Biochemistry*, **10**, 2606–2617 (1971).

7. R. G. Strauss. Routinely washing irradiated red cells before transfusion seems unwarranted. *Transfusion*, **30**, 675–677 (1990).

8. K. Kon, N. Maeda and T. Shiga. Functional impairments of human red cells, induced by dehydroepiandrosterone sulfate. *Pflugers Arch. Eur. J. Physiol.*, **394**, 279–286 (1982).

9. S. Chien. Shear dependence of effective cell volume as a determinant of blood viscosity. *Science*, **168**, 977–979 (1970).

10. L. N. Button, W. C. DeWolf, P. E. Newberger *et al.* The effects of irradiation on blood components. *Transfusion*, **21**, 419–426 (1981).

11. G. L. Moore and M. E. Ledford. Effects of 4000 rad irradiation on the *in vitro* storage properties of packed cells. *Transfusion*, **25**, 583–585 (1985).

Therapeutic Plasmapheresis (XII), pp. 705-710
T. Agishi *et al*. (Eds)
© VSP 1993

Efficiency Control in Therapeutic Hemapheresis

H. ULLRICH,[1] M. MICHELS,[2] Y. WAXENBERGER,[1] K. V. TOYKA,[2]
D. WIEBECKE[1] and E. FUCHS[1]

*Departments of [1]Transfusion Medicine and Immunohematology, and [2]Neurology,
University of Würzburg, Germany*

Key words: viscosity; plasma exchange; anti-acetylcholine receptor antibodies; efficiency control.

INTRODUCTION

Since December 1977 we have carried out 1752 therapeutic, cytaphereses to treat patients suffering from myeloproliferative disorders, acute myelogenous leukemia and chronic lymphocytic leukemia.

A total of 2899 plasma exchanges were carried out with the frequencies indicated in parenthesis. We treated patients with Guillain–Barré syndrome (GBS) (709), plasmocytoma (455), myasthenia gravis (MG) (298), polymyositis (162), polyneuropathy (148), Waldenström's macroglobulinaemia (30) autoimmune hemolytic anemia (22), hyperlipoproteinemia IIb (34), disseminated encephalomyelitis (34), Lambert Eaton syndrome (28), thrombotic thrombocytopenic purpura (19), lupus erythematosus (16), scleroderma (11) and various other diseases.

A total of 105 immunoadsorption treatments with disposable tryptophane–polyvinyl-alcohol–columns (IMT 350) were carried out to treat MG.

In addition, since 1987 five patients with familial hypercholesterolemia IIa were treated by weekly LDL apheresis for up to 4 years using sepharose-bound anti-Apo-B columns.

MATERIALS, METHODS AND RESULTS

To compare plasma exchange and plasma adsorption with IMT 350 columns, anti-acetylcholine receptor antibodies (AChR-AB) were examined daily in all patients with severe MG.

The typical decrease of immunoglobulins is shown in Fig. 1, whereas albumin stays constant due to the exact substitution of 5% human albumin solutions.

No problems, especially no allergic reactions or electrolyte disturbances, were caused by the albumin solutions used throughout the last 5 years, even when the patients received several treatment cycles.

Three courses of plasma exchange are shown in Fig. 2, demonstrating the typical decline of AChR-AB induced by plasma exchange and the combined reduction of IgG in a patient with respirator-dependent MG.

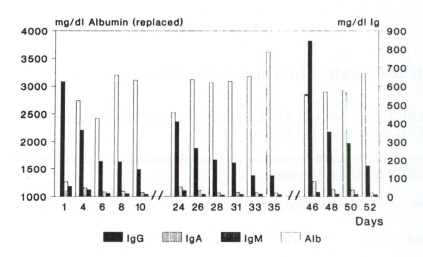

Figure 1. Treatment with plasma exchange in MG: serum levels of immunoglobulins.

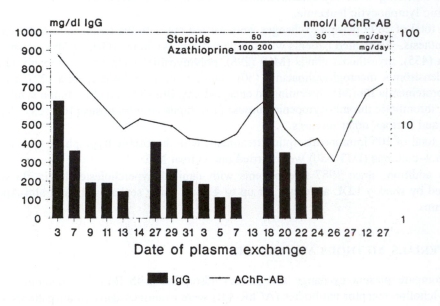

Figure 2. Serum levels of IgG and AChR-AB.

In all plasma exchange patients a continuous drop in AChR-AB was seen, as represented in Fig. 3 by antibody levels determined directly before plasma exchange.

An efficient reduction of AChR-AB can also be achieved by immunoadsorption (IA) with IMT 350 columns (Fig. 4). The accompanying immunosuppressive medication is indicated on the upper part. AChR-AB removal by IA was comparable to plasma exchange-induced changes. However, the rate of severe side effects (always reversible, e.g. respiratory distress, cardiac arrest) was significantly higher during IAs (plasma

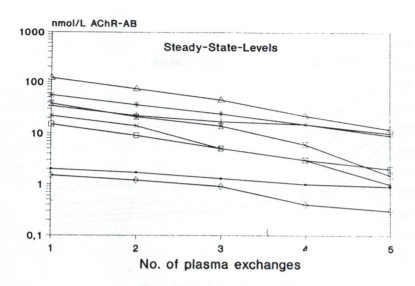

Figure 3. Serum levels of AChR-AB.

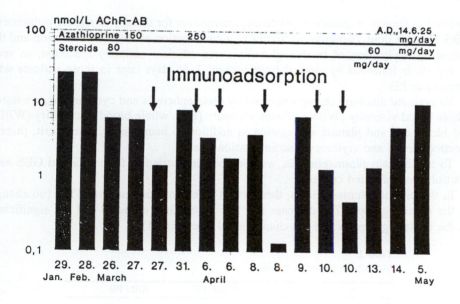

Figure 4. Immunoadsorption by IMT 350 columns.

exchange: 0.1%, IA: 0.7%).

In MG, one of the best characterized human autoimmune disorders, efficiency control can be quantified by a specific protein.

In contrast, in GBS several protein abnormalities are seen, but so far only IgG levels can be determined to quantify successful treatment. Early plasmapheresis is recom-

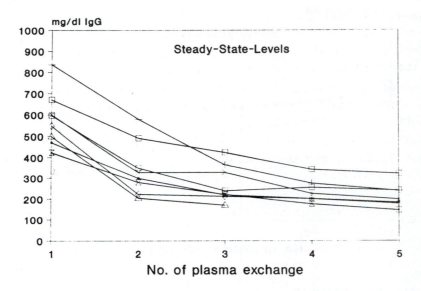

Figure 5. Serum levels of IgG in patients with GBS.

mended to prevent respirator dependency, alternatives for therapy in rapidly progressive GBS are high dose 7s-immunoglobulins or a combination of antibody reduction and the following application of immunoglobulins. An efficient antibody reduction, as seen in Fig. 5, is followed by clinical improvement 1–15 days later in those patients who respond to PE.

To evaluate rheology changes induced by plasmapheresis and cytapheresis, we tested whole blood viscosity (WBV), plasma viscosity (PV), whole blood filterability (WBF), red blood cell and platelet aggregation in addition to hemoglobin, hematocrit, protein electrophoresis and erythrocyte sedimentation rate.

To avoid sham plasmapheresis, we used patients suffering from MG and GBS as a control after informed consent.

In the plasmocytoma patients, there was a significant decrease in WBV (no change in the control group). The decrease in PV was less than expected and not significant. In the control group PV did not change at all (see Table 1).

Table 1.
Viscosity in plasma exchange

	Before PE	After PE
Whole blood viscosity (mPas)		
therapy group	2.53 ± 0.42	2.09 ± 0.47
control group	2.85 ± 0.71	2.30 ± 0.54
Plasma viscosity (mPas)		
therapy group	1.34 ± 0.50	0.94 ± 0.28
control group	1.42 ± 0.54	1.46 ± 0.74

High fibrinogen levels are a main cause for increased PV. Their well-known decrease in the course of PE was significant and comparable in both groups.

Filterability did not show any changes, neither in the plasmapheresis nor in the cytapheresis groups (RCTT before treatment: 6.74 ± 1.39 s, after treatment: 7.05 ± 1.42 s), indicating that no cell damage occurred during PE and cytapheresis

Therapeutic thrombocytapheresis (TA) was either carried out selectively or in combination with leucocytapheresis or bloodletting, depending on the patients' disease and cell counts.

Two cell separators (Fresenius As 104 and Cobe Spectra) were compared for these indications. Platelet count was reduced significantly in a short time (AS 104: before TA: 1232 ± 459/nl, after TA: 864 ± 267/nl; Spectra: before TA: 1011 ± 267/nl, after TA: 685 ± 131/nl).

In some patients, there are more platelets in the concentrate than expected, due to platelet release from the marginal pool during TA.

TAs with AS 104 were mainly done by manual program, which resulted in greater platelet yields, but required closer survey. The Spectra automatic program had to be changed, so that the platelet draw speed was increased to avoid clogging in the cell concentrate line.

In cytaphereses (CA) no difference in viscosity was observed between the control group of platelet donors and the treatment group. A slight decrease in WBV and PV was only seen after several treatments (Table 2).

In therapeutic cytaphereses significant changes in rheology can only be expected in patients with high granulocyte or blast cell counts.

Table 2.
Viscosity in cytaphereses

	Before CA	After CA
Whole blood viscosity (mPas)		
therapy group	2.40 ± 0.13	2.33 ± 0.09
control group	2.28 ± 0.07	2.18 ± 0.08
Plasma viscosity (mPas)		
therapy group	1.42 ± 0.14	1.17 ± 0.05
control group	1.16 ± 0.03	1.12 ± 0.03

CONCLUSION

During the few last years, considerable progress in the field of efficiency control in hemapheresis had been achieved. However, clinical outcome can still not be predicted safety by any of the following parameters: anti-acetylcholine receptor antibodies, IgG, whole blood viscosity, plasma viscosity and blood cell count.

REFERENCES

1. M. Michels, R. Hohlfeld, H. P. Hartung, K. Heininger, U. Besinger and K. V. Toyka. Myasthenia gravis: discontinuation of long-term azathioprine. *Ann. Neurol.*, **24**, 798 (1988).

2. U. Besinger, K. V. Toyka, M. Hömberg, K. Heininger, R. Hohlfeld and A. Fateh-Moghadam. Myasthenia gravis: long-term correlation of binding and bungarotoxin blocking antibodies against acetylcholine receptors with changes in disease severity. *Neurology*, **33**, 1316–1321 (1983).

3. K. V. Toyka, U. A. Besinger, K. Heininger, W. Samtleben, D. Hein, A. Fateh-Moghadam, H. J. Gurland and B. Grabensee. Myasthenia gravis: the pathogenic role of antibodies to acetylcholine receptors and the effects of antibody depletion. In: *Plasma Exchange Therapy*, H. Borland and P. Reuther (Eds), pp. 172–179, Thieme Verlag Stuttgart (1981).

4. H. Ullrich, D. Wiebecke, R. Hohe, U. Gunzer and B. Mansouri-Taleghani. Plasma exchange with cell separators in various diseases. In: *Therapeutic Plasmapheresis (VI)*, T. Oda, Y. Shiokawa and N. Inoue (Eds), ISAO Press, Cleveland (1987).

5. G. D. O. Lowe. Blood rheology *in vitro* and *in vivo*. *Baillière's Clin. Haematol.*, **1**, 597–665 (1987).

6. H. A. Henrich. *Personal communication* (1991).

7. H. Borberg and R. Böhm. The safety of blood component preparation with blood cell separators. *Infusions Ther.*, **16** (Suppl. 2), 21–29 (1984).

8. V. Kretschmer, D. Söhngen, W. Göddecke, J. Kadar, H. Pelzer, H. Prinz and R. Eckle. Biocompatibility and safety of cytapheresis. *Infusions Ther.*, **16** (Suppl. 2), 10–20 (1989).

Therapeutic Plasmapheresis (XII), pp. 711-718
T. Agishi *et al.* (Eds)
© VSP 1993

Changes in Blood and Plasma Viscosities after Plasmapheresis Therapy

S. FUJITA, K. YAMAJI, Y. KANAI, T. KAWANISHI, M. TOUMYO,
M. YOKOYAMA, H. TSUDA, H. HASHIMOTO and S.-I. HIROSE

*Department of Internal Medicine, Juntendo University School of Medicine,
Tokyo, Japan*

INTRODUCTION

It is thought that an increased plasma viscosity is involved in the etiology of Raynaud's phenomenon with recurrent skin ulcers in patients with connective tissue diseases such as systemic lupus erythematosus (SLE) and mixed connective tissue disease (MCTD), and the plasmapheresis therapy is expected to improve their symptoms [1, 2] because plasmapheresis therapy is considered to decrease plasma viscosity. So we planned to study the efficacy of plasmapheresis therapy on patients with Raynaud's phenomenon. Before this study, we had to know what is the most effective plasmapheresis method to decrease blood and plasma viscosities. However, there have been few reports about the differences in blood and plasma viscosities after various methods of plasmapheresis. We thus investigated the differences in the blood and plasma viscosities after four methods of plasmapheresis therapy were performed on patients with SLE, MCTD and rheumatoid arthritis.

MATERIALS AND METHODS

Twenty six RA, nine SLE and three MCTD patients were randomly selected from among patients who were diagnosed as having SLE and RA on the basis of the American Rheumatism Association criteria and diagnosed as having MCTD using the criteria of the Japanese Ministry of Health and Welfare (Table 1). We performed plasmapheresis therapy because their clinical symptoms and signs, including arthralgia, erythema, proteinuria and Raynaud's phenomenon had not responded to conventional drug therapies such as steroids, non-steroidal anti-inflammatory drugs, D-penicillamine and/or other immunosuppressive drugs. We allocated these patients into four groups according to the method of plasmapheresis. We performed plasmapheresis by four methods, i.e. double-filtration plasmapheresis (DFPP) using hollow fibers [3] and adsorption therapies using dextran sulfate (DS), phenylalanine (IMP) and tryptophan (IMT). The DFPP group included nine RA, five SLE and three MCTD patients. The DS group included four SLE patients. The IMP and IMT groups included nine and eight RA patients, respectively.

Table 1.

Patient profile

	DFPP	DS	IMP	IMT
Patients	17	4	9	8
Age (mean±SD)	48 ± 13	45 ± 18	57 ± 11	58 ± 13
Sex				
M	3	1	3	3
F	14	3	6	5
Disease				
RA	9	0	9	8
SLE	5	4	0	0
MCTD	3	0	0	0

Blood access was made by puncture of veins in all the patients. In the system, blood was obtained continuously from the patients at 50–80 ml/min and passed into the first filter, which was made of hollow fibers. The plasma separated from the blood in the first filter passed into the second filter or adsorption columns.

In DFPP, the plasma was filtered through hollow fiber membranes that had 0.02 μm pores. We discarded 20% of plasma that did not pass through the second filter and replaced it with a 5% albumin solution.

In adsorption therapies, the plasma is passed through adsorption columns made of DS, IMP or IMT. Rheumatoid factors and circulating immune complexes are adsorbed to IMP and IMT columns.

The DS column is made by modifying the column used in LDL apheresis. This column adsorbs anti-DNA antibodies due to the negative charge of DS.

In all methods, 2000 ml of plasma was processed in each treatment. We injected 2000 units of heparin at the beginning and 1000 units/h continuously during each treatment as an anticoagulant.

We determined the blood and plasma viscosities and performed other laboratory tests before and after the first treatment and before and after the second filter and adsorption columns. In seven DFPP group cases, we performed plasmapheresis three times every 2 weeks and determined the blood and plasma viscosities and other laboratory test values at 2 weeks after the final DFPP treatment.

The plasma viscosity was measured with a capillary viscometer at 37 °C and expressed as the relative viscosity against distilled water. The blood viscosity was measured with a cone and plate type rotational viscometer (Wells-Brookfield Inc.) at 37 °C and at shear rates of 230, 115, 46, 23 and 11.5 s^{-1}. The hematocrit was adjusted to 35%.

Statistical analysis was performed by Student's t-test and the paired t-test.

RESULTS

The blood viscosity after DFPP was significantly decreased at all shear rates (Fig. 1).

The blood viscosity after DS was significantly decreased at shear rates of 11.5 to 115 s^{-1} (Fig. 2).

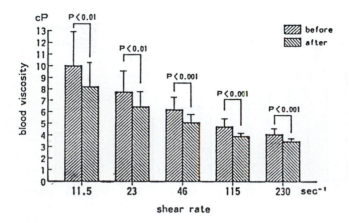

Figure 1. Changes in whole blood viscosity after DFPP.

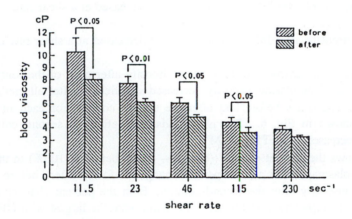

Figure 2. Changes in whole blood viscosity after DS.

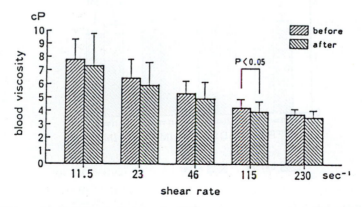

Figure 3. Changes in whole blood viscosity after IMP.

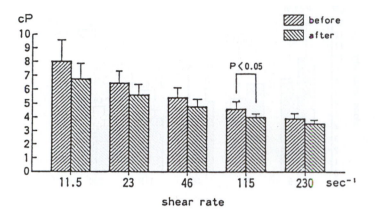

Figure 4. Changes in whole blood viscosity after IMT.

The blood viscosity after IMP was significantly decreased at a shear rate of 115 s^{-1} (Fig. 3).

The blood viscosity after IMT was significantly decreased at a shear rate of 115s^{-1} (Fig. 4).

Figure 5 shows the changes in the plasma viscosity after each of the four methods of plasmapheresis. The plasma viscosity decreased significantly after all methods.

The plasma viscosities before and after the second columns of each of the four methods are shown in Fig. 6. The plasma viscosity after the second column was significantly decreased in DFPP and IMT.

Figure 7 shows the percent change ((before − after)/ before × 100%) in the plasma viscosity after plasmapheresis and the percent change ((before − after)/ before × 100%) in the plasma viscosity after the second column. Both the percent changes after one plasmapheresis therapy and after the second column were the largest with DFPP.

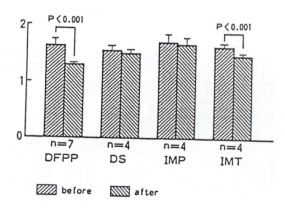

Figure 5. Plasma viscosity before and after each column.

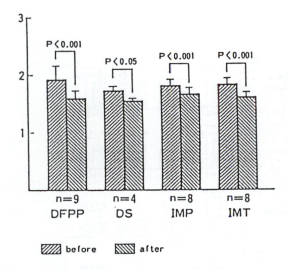

Figure 6. Changes in plasma viscosity after plasmapheresis therapy.

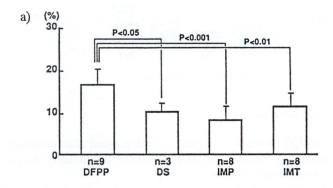

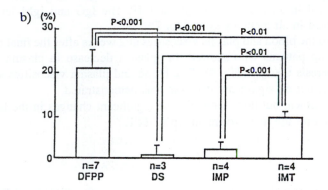

Figure 7. a) Percent change in the plasma viscosity after plasmapheresis therapy; b) Percent change in the plasma viscosity after the second column.

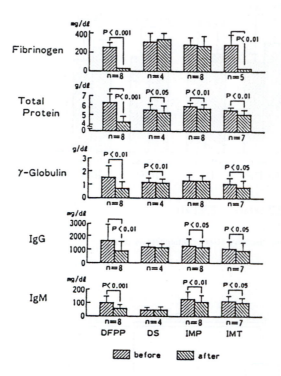

Figure 8. Laboratory findings before and after each column.

The total protein and IgG levels were significantly decreased after plasmapheresis by each method. The gamma-globulin and IgM levels were significantly decreased after three of the plasmapheresis methods, excluding DS.

Figure 8 shows the laboratory findings before and after the second columns. The total protein level was significantly decreased in all methods. The gamma-globulin level was significantly decreased in all methods except for IMP. The IgG and IgM levels were significantly decreased in all methods except for DS.

We also examined the blood and plasma viscosities at 2 weeks after the final treatment in seven DFPP group patients who showed the greatest decrease in plasma viscosity after one plasmapheresis therapy (Fig. 9). The blood and plasma viscosities showed a decreasing tendency, but no significant decrease was demonstrated.

The data are not shown, but there were also no significant changes in the laboratory findings at 2 weeks after the final treatment with DFPP.

DISCUSSION

It is thought that an increased plasma viscosity is involved in the etiology of Raynaud's phenomenon. Plasmapheresis therapy is considered to decrease the plasma viscosity and thus expected to alleviate Raynaud's phenomenon with recurrent skin ulcers. There

a) CP

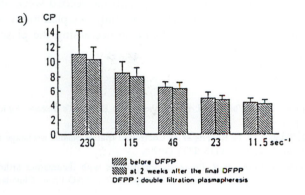

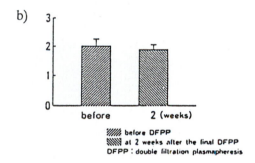

WWA before DFPP
NNN at 2 weeks after the final DFPP
DFPP : double filtration plasmapheresis

Figure 9. a) Changes in blood viscosity at 2 weeks after the final DFPP; b) Changes in plasma viscosity at 2 weeks after the final DFPP.

have been many reports regarding the efficacy of plasmapheresis therapy for connective tissue diseases. However, there have been only a few reports about the changes in the blood and plasma viscosities as a result of plasmapheresis therapy. In this study, we investigated the changes in the blood and plasma viscosities after four methods of plasmapheresis therapy together with other laboratory test findings and compared them with each other.

As we have shown in Figs 1–9, the blood and plasma viscosities were significantly decreased after each of the four plasmapheresis methods. Especially after DFPP, the blood viscosity was significantly decreased at all shear rates and the percent change in the plasma viscosity after plasmapheresis was the largest. Based on these results, DFPP is thought to be the most effective method for decreasing the blood and plasma viscosities among the four plasmapheresis methods.

Examination of other laboratory test parameters showed significant decreases in the total protein, gamma-globulin, IgG and IgM levels after DFPP. These results suggest that the decrease in plasma viscosity is associated with these laboratory findings.

The blood and plasma viscosities at 2 weeks after the final treatment by DFPP group showed a decreasing tendency, but no statistical significance was demonstrated. The laboratory findings also showed no significant changes.

In this study, the number of cases followed up until the second week after the final treatment by DFPP was small. Therefore, in the next study, we plan to investigate more cases and determine how long the effect of DFPP in decreasing the plasma viscosity continues.

REFERENCES

1. G. Talopos, M. Horrocks, J. M. While *et al.* Plasmapheresis in Raynaud's disease. *Lancet*, i, 416–417 (1978).
2. M. J. G. O'Reilly, G. Talopos, V. C. Roberts *et al.* Controlled trial of plasma exchange in treatment of Raynaud's syndrome. *Br. Med. J.*, 1, 1113–1115 (1979).
3. Y. Kanai, T. Kawanishi, S. Fujita *et al.* Prognosis for patients with rheumatoid arthritis treated by plasmapheresis. In: *Therapeutic plasmapheresis (VIII)*, pp. 69–73, ISAO Press, Cleveland (1989).

18
Rehabilitation

Therapeutic Plasmapheresis (XII), pp. 721-724
T. Agishi *et al.* (Eds)
© VSP 1993

Rehabilitation of Patients with Renal Disorders after Plasmapheresis

R. SRIVASTAVA, R. HOTCHANDANI and A. DAR

Nephrology Department, Safdarjang Hospital, New Delhi, India

Key words: rehabilitation; renal disorders; plasmapheresis.

INTRODUCTION

Rehabilitation in an End Stage Renal Disease (ESRD) patient is the need and right of the patient. It is medically and ethically a part of the management of ESRD. In the way that it is useful for other catastrophic illnesses it should also be economically sound for ESRD patients. It was seen that despite regular maintenance hemodialysis in patients with renal disorders, patients did not return to a full functional capacity or returned after a prolonged duration. Double filtration plasmapheresis (DFPP) was attempted to bring about an earlier return to a full working ability. It was observed by the Director of Rehabilitation of the University of Emory. Dr. Samuel, who himself suffered from ESRD and was on maintenance hemodialysis (MHD) for the last 3 years of his life.

MATERIALS AND METHODS

Fifteen patients with various nephrology conditions (six acute renal failure; six chronic renal failure; one RPGN; and two renal transplants) were taken up for weekly DFPP with PP-20, with Albusave of Dideco for six sittings. Post renal transplant required only three sittings. Hemodialysis was discontinued during this period.

Fifteen cases of comparable age and sex, were continued on hemodialysis.

The two groups were compared at weekly intervals on a functional scale of

Occupational ability.
Social rehabilitation.
Sexual rehabilitation.
Biochemical parameters.

The details are shown in Tables 1–5.

Table 1.
Sex distribution

Sex	No. of patients
Females	6
Males	9
Total no. of patients =	15

Table 2.
Age distribution

Age group	No. of patients
0–10	1
11–20	5
21–30	1
31–40	4
41–50	2
51–60	1
61–70	1
Total no. of patients =	15

Table 3.
Geographical distribution

State	No. of patients
Delhi	13
Thailand	1
UP	1
Total no. of patients =	15

Table 4.
No. of sittings

Sittings	No. of patients
3	2
6	13
Total no. of sittings =	15

Table 5.
Diagnosis

Diagnosis	No. of patients
RPGN	1
ARF	6
CGN with CRF	4
SLE with CRF	2
R. Tx. Rej.	2
Total no. of patients =	15

DISCUSSION

Evaluation of rehabilitation is done by: (i) muscle charting and (ii) cardio-vascular capacity.

The degree of successful rehabilitation depends/varied with the following factors

(i) Age. The younger the age, the better is the rehabilitation and return to employment.
(ii) Sex. Males above 51 showed poor response compared with females.
(iii) Disease. If the primary disease is diabetes then the success of rehabilitation is low.
(iv) Treatment method. Low in peritoneal dialysis (PD) high in HD, renal transplant, DFPP, but in this study we have compared only DFPP cases with/without HD in which DFPP was superior.
(v) Method of rehabilitation/exercise. It was found that patients with active physio-therapy and exercise regimen showed drastically better results.

Even two decades ago the psychological adjustments in the patients under MHD was considered necessary [1]. Many changes occur in the family relationship of the patients of dialysis and transplant during the procedure [2]. Renal rehabilitation in CRF and MHD cases was studied by Laidlaw Foundation, Toronto [3] and Williams *et al.* in Baltimore [4]. Gradually the trend is changing; recently, by rendering vocational placement services to the renal patients for providing rehabilitation [5]. Effective social environment and hemodialysis adaptation are vital for renal rehabilitation [6]. By providing plasmapheresis as a better treatment for renal failure of immune complex nature, supported by positive physiotherapy and proper rehabilitation in ESRD patients improves the quality of life [8, 9].

CONCLUSION

Normally a functioning renal transplant offers superior rehabilitation to peritoneal dialysis but is equivalent to hemodialysis and plasmapheresis.

Participation in self-care improves self-image and life quality.

This is a unique kind of study done for the first time in our country and, since the study comprises a smaller group of patients, it is suggested that more studies should be done on a larger patient population and the maximum number of patients must be provided with the benefit of the treatment regime. Thus plasmapheresis as an adjunct to a adequate renal replacement therapy and proper renal rehabilitation will usher in a new era of hope for these patients.

REFERENCES

1. E. A. Friedman, N. J. Goodwin and L. Chaudhry. Psychosocial adjustment to maintainance hemodialysis. *NY J. Med.*, **70**, 629 (1970).

2. M. P. Beard. Changing family relationship. *Dialysis Transplant*, **4**, 35 (1975).

3. S. F. Hagarty and L. M. Hagarty. *Beyond Survival: A Study of the Rehabilitation of Kidney Dialysis and Transplant Patients.* Laidlaw Foundation, Toronto (1977).

4. S. B. Chyatte (Ed.). *Rehabilitation in Chronic Renal Failure.* Williams and Wilkins, Baltimore (1978).

5. R. S. Decker. Vocational placement services for the renal disease. *Clin. Dial. Transplant.*, **7**, 561 (1978).

6. M. E. Obrien. Effective social environment and hemodialysis adaptation. A panel analysis. *J. Health Soc. Behav.*, **21**, 360 (1980).

7. S. Palmer, L. Canzona, J. Conley *et al.* Vocational adaptation of patients on home dialysis: its relation ship to personality, activities and support received. *J. Psychosom. Res.*, **27**, 201 (1983).

8. R. Srivastava, A. Dar and A. Pasricha. Renal rehabilitation with DFPP in India. *Indian J. Apheresis*, in press.

9. E. A. Friedman. Variables in selecting long-term therapy for uremic patients. In: *The Kidney*, 4th edn., B. M. Brenner and F. C. Rector (Eds), pp. 2413–2415. W. B. Saunders, Philadelphia (1991).

Therapeutic Plasmapheresis (XII), pp. 725-727
T. Agishi *et al.* (Eds)
© VSP 1993

Orthopaedic and Vocational Rehabilitation in Rheumatoid Arthritis after Plasmapheresis

R. SRIVASTAVA, R. HOTCHANDANI and A. DAR

Nephrology Department, Safdarjang Hospital, New Delhi, India

Key words: rehabilitation; rheumatoid arthritis; single and double filtration plasmapheresis.

INTRODUCTION

Despite advances in the treatment of RA many patients are left with sequelae which lead to a compromise in their vocational abilities. This handicap may be in the form of being able to work for shorter durations, changing over to less strenuous and lower paying professions, taking frequent holidays and often long absences from work during periods of acute exacerbations. All these lead to a decreased earning capacity and, if the patient is the bread earner for the family, repercussions are left in all spheres.

Plasmapheresis (PP) was tried as a mean for treating these patients to achieve an early and more complete work capacity.

MATERIALS AND METHODS

Twenty patients with crippling arthritis were taken for the study and followed up regularly at monthly interval. The patients undergoing PP were given five to nine sittings of 80–120 min duration each (PF-20, Albusave and Toray filter).

After completion of DFPP the patients were followed up at 2 monthly intervals.

RESULTS

It was found that the patients who had undergone DFPP returned to their full vocational capacity earlier than patients undergoing conventional treatment. Also, the incidence of acute exacerbations and recurrences were less in patients undergoing DFPP.

The results were consistent with the use of PP in all the cases, while most of the cases, not under DFPP, could not return to their previous occupations and only a few were able to take less strenuous jobs. See Table 1.

Table 1.
Rehabilitation of patients

Total no. of patients	Returned to previous occupation	Returned to less strenuous occupation
20	15	5

DISCUSSION

In view of the crippling nature of rheumatoid arthritis (RA) more and more treatment modalities are being used for long-lasting successful result. Successful treatment means a method which provides remission for longer periods, minimizes the relapses and maximizes the functional capacity, so that the patient can return back to his earlier normal work/occupation. This, when achieved, is real orthopaedic and vocational rehabilitation. From the past many old and new drugs from the category of anti-inflammatory agents of non-steroidal nature have been tried by various workers; however, these proved to be only limited in nature, relieving pain and inflammation temporarily with no significant control of remission of relapses. In the last few years there has been an increasing practice of using cytotoxic drugs for the treatment of RA, which has shown some results but the ill effects of immunosuppression are also accompanied with this. Research has been an on-going process in this field and immunomodulation techniques which cause least side-effects are being preferred [1]. DFPP is one such remarkable technique where qualitative and quantitative control of the treatment is also possible by virtue of direct removal of immune complex (globulin) [2]. In our centre also, DFPP was tried with these aims and objectives only in cases who failed on long standing drug therapy and who where compared to those who received only drugs. The results obtained are so remarkable to be self-explanatory of the efficacy and value of this treatment. The pre- and post-treatment immunological parameters of the patients suggested that this treatment is much better than other treatments.

The auto immuno nature of RA is well known. Recent trends in the treatment include mainly PP. There have been many studies across the world, of the same nature [3, 4]. In India, plasmapheresis (SFPP or DFPP) is also now being used extensively for the treatment of RA [5]. Evaluation of the treatment shows remarkable improvement in these patients after DFPP [6]. When combined with proper physiotherapy and exercise this treatment has by far proved to be the best rehabilitation method for these patients [7].

CONCLUSION

The treatment is better because PP removes the causative pathogens, namely circulating immune complexes, from the blood, which no drug is capable of. Thus it has a better significance in treatment, providing relief in acute exacerbations, minimizing relapses and a long standing remission leading to better orthopaedic and vocational rehabilitation. This is very important for total physical, mental, social, domestic, sexual and functional rehabilitation of the patients, which is the ultimate goal of the physician.

REFERENCES

1. M. Ziff. Auto-immune process in rheumatoid arthritis. *Progr. Immunol. II*, **5**, 37–46 (1974).
2. D. J. Wallace, D. Goldfinger, R. Gatti *et al.* Plasmapheresis and lymphoplasmapheresis in the management of rheumatoid arthritis. *Arthritis Rheum.*, **22**, 703–710 (1979).
3. A. J. Wysenbeek, W. J. Smith and R. S. Krakauer. Plasmapheresis review of clinical experience. *Plasma Ther.*, **23**, 785–790 (1981).
4. H. Sakamoto, T. Takaoka, M. Usami *et al.* Apheresis: clinical response to patients unresponsive to conventional therapy. *Trans. Am. Soc. Artif. Intern. Organs*, **31**, 704–708 (1985).
5. R. Srivastava, G. K. Vishwakarma and S. Tyagi. Plasmapheresis therapy in rheumatoid arthritis in Indian patients. *JAPI*, **35**, 133–135 (1987).

6. R. Srivastava, G. K. Vishwakarma and S. Tyagi. Use of a new hollow fibre cellulose, diacetate plasma filter in rheumatoid arthritis in India. *IJN*, **3**, 127–131 (1987).

7. R. Srivastava, A. Dar and A. Pasricha. Rehabilitation of rheumatoid arthritis patients after DFPP. *Indian J. Apheresis*, in press.

19
Management

Therapeutic Plasmapheresis (XII), pp. 731-733
T. Agishi *et al.* (Eds)
© VSP 1993

A Case of Intractable Sepsis Treated by a Multidisciplinary Approach with Special Reference to the Cost and Benefit

Y. ASANUMA, K. KOMATSU,[1] W. SATO,[1] J. TANAKA, S. OMOKAWA, H. ANDO, M. ITO and K. KOYAMA

Departments of Surgery and [1]Pediatrics, Akita University, Akita, Japan

Key words: sepsis; plasma exchange; cost and benefit.

INTRODUCTION

To assess the information on costs and benefits of aggressive therapy including blood purification treatment, the hospital costs were analyzed in a patient who suffered from intractable sepsis caused by severe enteritis.

CASE REPORT

A 3 year old boy suffered from prolonged diarrhea, high fever and cellular immune insufficiency, and was transferred to our university 1.5 years ago. He developed sepsis and candidiasis due to severe enteritis and suffered from high fever (around 42 °C) every day. Since ordinary treatments such as fasting, antibiotics and γ-globulin were ineffective, exchange transfusion was initiated for a total of four times, then plasma exchange using a miniature plasma separator (polyvinyl alcohol, 0.09 m^2 effective surface area) and fresh plasma was introduced [1]. Furthermore, granulocyte transfusion, interferon and transfer factor were administered concomitantly. Among these treatments, the most effective one was plasma exchange plus granulocytes transfusion carried out for 5 days consecutively. During these 5 days, maximum body temperature decreased below 40 °C on 2 days for the first time in these 6 months (Fig. 1). There were no shaking chills on these 2 days; however, the temperature increased to 42.8 °C on the following day and, finally, the patient died of multiple organ failure.

COST ANALYSIS

Of the cost during 19 months hospitalization, the monthly cost was about 3000 dollars during the first 13 month after admission. However, when the patient became septic and antibiotics began to be administered, the cost increased rapidly and reached 53 000 dollars when DIC developed and platelet had to be administered (Fig. 2). Thereafter, plasma exchange was initiated and the monthly cost decreased to 41 000 dollars including 5 times exchange transfusion and plasma exchange as well, administration of

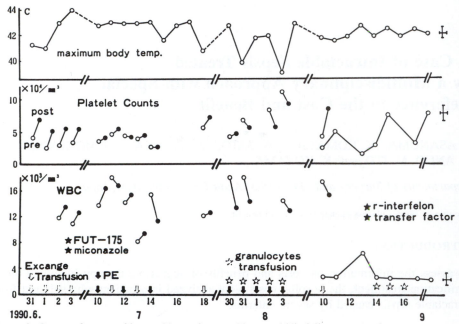

Figure 1. Course of a case of intractable sepsis treated by a multidisciplinary approach.

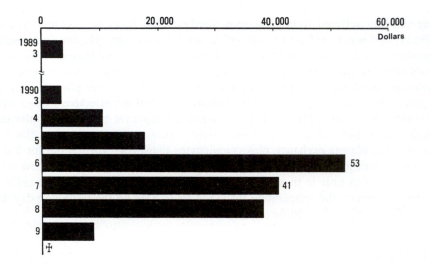

Figure 2. Changes of monthly costs.

260 units of concentrated platelet and other blood products. One unit of platelet costs 53 dollars, so that 260 units cost 14 000 dollars and occupy 34% of the total expense of this month. Finally, 63% of the total amount is occupied by various blood products (Fig. 3).

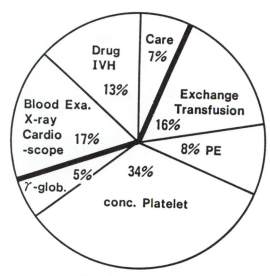

Figure 3. Details of the 41 000 dollar monthly cost for July, 1991.

DISCUSSION

With regard to the costs for patients dying of hepatic failure without liver transplantation, the mean cost of hospitalization for the last 12 months averaged 45 000 dollars [2] among 20 patients without extracorporeal hepatic support. Compared with an average cost of 92 000 dollars per liver transplantation and considering a rehabilitation rate of 82% in those patients surviving the first year, this figure places the cost of transplantation in a favorable perspective. With regard to human small intestine transplantation [3], this has not become a reality yet because of the difficulties in immunosuppression, graft preservation and diagnosis of graft rejection, and economic issues has not been analyzed. For the patient discussed in this paper, small intestine transplantation could have been the single treatment modality to save his life and to restore useful life in a cost-effective manner.

REFERENCES

1. Y. Asanuma, J. Tanaka, T. Takahashi *et al*. Preclinical evaluation of plasma cross circulation for infants. In: *Therapeutic Plasmapheresis (VI)*, T. Oda (Ed.), pp. 359–364, ISAO Press, Cleveland (1987).
2. J. W. Williams, S. Vera and L. S. Evans. Socioeconomic aspects of hepatic transplantation. *Am. J. Gastroenter.*, **82**, 1115–1119 (1987).
3. M. Z. Schwartz. Small intestine transplantation. In: *Principles of Organ Transplantation*, M. W. Flye (Ed.), pp. 500–515, Saunders, Philadelphia (1989).

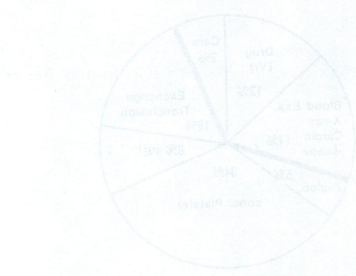

Figure 3. Details of the $4200 dollar monthly cost for July, 1991.

DISCUSSION

With regard to the costs for patients dying of hepatic failure without liver transplantation, the mean cost of hospitalization for the last 12 months averaged 45 000 dollars [2] among 20 patients without extracorporeal hepatic support. Compared with an average cost of 92000 dollars per liver transplantation and considering a rehabilitation rate of 85% to those patients surviving the first year, this figure makes the cost of transplantation in a favorable perspective. With regard to human small intestine transplantation [3] this has not become a reality yet because of the difficulties in immunosuppression, graft preservation and diagnosis of graft rejection, and economic issues have not been analyzed. For the patient discussed in this paper, small intestine transplantation could have been the single treatment modality to save his life and to restore useful life in a cost-effective manner.

REFERENCES

1. Y. Vanrenterghem J. Tricot J. Thielemans et al. Prognostic evaluation of patients with cirrhosis. In: J.M. The Prognosis of Hospital survival (Ed.: T. Oaks (Ed.), pp. 258–364, CRC Press, Cleveland (1987).

2. J. W. Williams S. Vera and L. S. Evans. Socioeconomic aspects of hepatic transplantation. Am. J. Gastroenterol. 82, 1115–1119 (1987).

3. M. Z. Schwartz. Small intestine transplantation. In: Principles of Organ Transplant. Ann. M. W. Fine (Ed.), pp. 601–615. Saunders, Philadelphia (1989).

Therapeutic Plasmapheresis (XII), pp. 735-738
T. Agishi *et al.* (Eds)
© VSP 1993

A Quality Assurance Programme for a Hospital-Based Apheresis Unit

D. L. THORP, G. W. DART, A. CANTY and G. CHEETHAM

*Apheresis Unit, Institute of Medical and Veterinary Science,
Adelaide, Australia*

Key words: apheresis; quality assurance programme.

INTRODUCTION

The Institute of Medical and Veterinary Science (IMVS) Transfusion Service (TS) decided in 1986 to seek American Association of Blood Bank (AABB) accreditation. As part of the TS, the Apheresis Unit set up its Quality Assurance Programme (QAP).

This programme embraces: the management and organization of the unit; staffing matters; documentation; schedules for machine and equipment calibration and maintenance; standards to safeguard donors and patients; and standards for apheresis derived blood products.

MANAGEMENT AND ORGANIZATION

Staff structure is defined. Our unit is directed by a Consulting Haematologist and all operators are experienced Registered Nurses. Operator/patient ratios are defined and lines of communication are clearly spelled out.

The attributes of the physical work area are also detailed: number of beds/chairs; machine space; type of electrical supply and how to access emergency power; and oxygen, suction and resuscitation facilities.

STAFFING MATTERS

Staff selection, training and performance are fully defined. There is an orientation and training package for the new operator. Staff appraisal and peer reviews are conducted regularly, identifying learning goals and areas for staff development. Further education is encouraged.

DOCUMENTATION

Detailed records are kept of all aspects of the unit's operation, including:
- Policy and procedure manuals including standard operating procedure for emergencies and infection control strategies.
- Individual patient care plans.
- Patient-specific directed donor lists.
- Random donor panel, including HLA typed donors.
- Records for each procedure performed.
- Machine and equipment purchase and maintenance history.
- Incident reports.
- Statistics.
- Stores inventory.
- Blood product QC protocols and results.

Computer protocols define who has access to the unit's computers containing patient and donor data and incorporates security measures to safeguard data.

MACHINES AND EQUIPMENT

A history is kept for each machine. This includes purchase, maintenance, parts history and calibration records, as well as maintenance schedules with a reminder method.

Records for other equipment such as scales, interval timers, blood pressure monitors and blood warmers include calibration methods and results.

Cleaning procedures for all equipment and methods for disposal of used equipment and other hazardous waste are documented.

STANDARDS TO SAFEGUARD DONORS

Standards for donors detail acceptable donation criteria including age, weight, blood pressure, temperature, general health assessment and the blood picture parameters which are acceptable for donation.

Also covered are:
- For plasma donors the total protein level.
- The number of donations which can be given in any year.
- Time interval between donations.
- Maximum extracorporeal volume allowed.
- Medications which exclude donors and those which can be used to enhance donation.
- A means by which a donor who does not meet criteria can be accepted as an apheresis donor.
- Donor consent requirements, including a donor self exclusion form.
- Pre-donation medical check requirements.
- Donor monitoring during the procedure.

An instruction card is given to the donor post-procedure detailing where the donor can access medical treatment in the event of complications or reactions.

STANDARDS TO PROTECT PATIENTS

Standards for patients include a *referral mechanism*. The apheresis physician in consultation with the referring physician decide on the type and duration of therapy.

Consideration is given to:

- The patient's current clinical status.
- Expected prognosis and the therapeutic goals.
- The patient's ability to withstand the procedure.
- Adequacy of vascular access.
- Concurrent drug therapy.
- Cost justification.

This information is incorporated on a referral form which is signed by the referring physician.

A *treatment plan* is produced. This includes:

- Patient identification details.
- Diagnosis, other pertinent medical information, and current medical status.
- Procedure to be performed.
- Amount and component to be removed.
- Replacement solutions, and quantities to use.
- Frequency and duration of procedures.
- Provision for emergency treatment, including written orders in the event of complications.
- Specific laboratory tests required.

Written information and a contact number for the patient and his home ward is provided.

Provision is made for periodic review of the efficacy of the procedure by the apheresis physician and the referring physician.

Procedure records are kept detailing:

- Donor/patient identifier.
- Pre-donation/treatment laboratory findings.
- Operator and machine identifiers.
- Batch/lot numbers for infusion fluids and software.
- Procedure details including duration, volumes and progress notes.
- Laboratory findings on products collected.
- Any adverse reaction and treatment given or action taken.
- Type of vascular access.

All this is accomplished by the operator filling in the individual run sheet, which is then stored in the patient's notes.

STANDARDS FOR THE PRODUCTS PRODUCED BY APHERESIS

Methods to calculate yields and collection efficiency are detailed and calculated for each collection.

There is a product integrity testing schedule covering sterility, pH, lactate and number of platelets.

Methods for storage, manipulation of the product (e.g. plasma depletion) and infusion are detailed.

Clinical evaluation is performed by calculating the post-infusion increment. A mechanism to initiate 1 h increment calculations, if the 24 h increment is unsatisfactory, has increased the efficiency of the service provided.

By keeping all records current and updated, yearly revisions are easily accomplished. Initiation of the QAP has enabled the TS to achieve AABB accreditation and to assure the quality of the work performed by the unit.

REFERENCES

1. American Association of Blood Banks, *Standards for Blood Banks and Transfusion Services*, 14th edn. AABB (1991).
2. Australian Guidelines, *National Blood Transfusion Committee of Australian Red Cross*. Sydney, (1978).
3. British Clinical Haematology Task Force, *Guidelines for the Use of Cell Separators*. BCHTF (1990).
4. Haemonetics Corporation, *Guidelines for Therapeutic Apheresis*. HC (1980).
5. Hemopheresis Specialists Standards Committee, *Guidelines for Apheresis Specialists*. HSSC (1987).
6. International Society of Blood Transfusion, *Standards in Haemapheresis*. ISBT (1986).

20
Technology and Materialology

Therapeutic Plasmapheresis (XII), pp. 741-745
T. Agishi *et al.* (Eds)
© VSP 1993

Routine Thrombocytapheresis with the Excel

M. VALBONESI, G. LERCARI, R. FRISONI, G. FLORIO, L. MALFANTI,
C. CAPRA, G. GIANNINI and P. CARLIER

Immunohematology Services, San Martino Hospital, Genova, Italy

Key words: plateletapheresis; thrombocytapheresis; donor apheresis; platelet concentrates; platelet yields.

INTRODUCTION

With the Dideco S.r.l. Excel another third generation apparatus for apheresis has been introduced in the international market. The very first presentation, at the ESFH Meeting held in September 1991 [1], was limited to the presentation of 13 thrombocytapheresis procedures which gave an average yield of 4.7×10^{11} in a needle to needle time of 72 min with a platelet efficiency per minute of 6.5×10^9. The leukocyte contamination was of 0.8×10^6 and that of erythrocytes of 0.4×10^7. Since then the very first apparatus has undergone several hardware and software modifications, which are going to be introduced into the definitive, commercial model. As a consequence, it is worthy to report the effect of these modifications in the production of platelet concentrates for clinical use.

THE SYSTEM AND THE MACHINE

The Excel is the latest evolution of the original Dideco continuous flow Vivacell machine. In fact, the Excel is a two stage eccentric plate apparatus with automated priming and procedure, in which platelets are collected out of the belt. Single-needle procedures are possible but presently only in the manual mode and the normal protocol remains with double-needle blood access for continuous flow thrombocytapheresis. The machine, as all Vivacell apparatuses, is equipped with five peristaltic pumps for whole blood, anti-coagulant (ACD-A from 1/8 to 1/16 to blood), packed red blood cells (RBC), plasma and cell product. The eccentric plate contains a slot, in which a PVC separation belt is allocated, very similar to the one that is employed in the Vivacell DE model. Blood separation is obtained in a dual-stage system in which, during centrifugation, the separation between the primary chamber (for PRP separation) and the secondary one (for platelet separation from PRP) is maintained by the difference in their radii. When centrifugation is over (or at less than 500 r.p.m.), the separation between the two chambers is determined by the extrusion of a spring-loaded eccentric that works from the inner part of the plate. This prevents contamination of the platelet product. What is totally new for the machine, and in general for Dideco, is the application of the 'Adam's rope' principle, which is necessary to keep the separation systems closed. Sterility is also maintained with the use of filters for all the solutions employed during the priming and

procedural phases. Priming is totally automated and takes approximately 7 min. After
needle insertion, thrombocytapheresis is automatically carried out. The platelets which
arrive in the second secondary separation chamber are forced to get out of the belt under
the action of a specific pristaltic pump. Contemporary platelet poor plasma collection
can be carried out. The separation of PRP is controlled by a peculiar sensor based
on CCD technology, aimed at stabilizing the buffy-coat and preventing the spillover of
white and red blood cells into the secondary separation chamber. If during any procedural phase something unusual or wrong takes place, the procedure is automatically halted
and a warning is given. By asking the apparatus computer, the necessary countermeasures are indicated to overcome that peculiar problem. When the procedure end point
is reached, the residual platelets which remain in the secondary separation chamber are
washed out of the belt with saline flushing (80 ml) and the residual blood remaining
in the primary chamber is given back to the donor. The reinfusion phase takes another
4 min. Blood flow rates from 25 to 80 ml/min have been employed safely during our
studies. The automation that assists the procedure is total, even if at any moment the
necessary manual adjustments can substitute for computer guided programs. After the
initial learning phase, in which the blood flow rates were progressively increased, the
procedure has been standardized for routine application. ACD-A to blood ratio was
1/12 and the blood flow rate (BFR) was 60 ml/min. The end point was set at 3.5 l
of blood processed in the double-vein procedures. The average PRP collection was
4 ml/min. The r.p.m.s were from 1500 (donor's hematocrit 38–40%) to 1650 (donor's
hematocrit > 43%). All procedures were of the plasma-thrombocytapheresis type, with
250 ml of PPP collected along with the platelet concentrate.

MATERIALS AND METHODS

Thirty six voluntary donors were enrolled. They gave written informed consent both
to platelet donation and to studies necessary to validate the new Dideco cell separator.
Their characteristics are summarized in Table 1. They satisfied the Italian regulations
for platelet collection [2]. Pre- and post-apheresis cell counts were carried out by
means of phase microscopy and automated counting; a CK 618 (Kontron Instruments,
Milano, Italy) apparatus was used for automated countings. Cell counts in the platelet

Table 1.
The donor population

Number of procedures	36
Male/female ratio	23/13
Mean age (years)	37.4
Mean body weight (kg)	69.5
Platelet precount ($\times 10^3/\mu l$)	47 ± 51
Leukocyte precount ($\times 10^3/\mu l$)	6.7 ± 4.8
Hematocrit (%)	42.7 ± 3.2
Calculated blood volemia (ml)	5198.8 ± 208

concentrates were done by applying phase microscopy and confirmed by flow cytometry counting, employing a Cytoron apparatus (Ortho Diagnostics, Raritan, NJ, USA). The presence of platelet aggregates in the platelet concentrates was measured according to Wu and Hoak [3]. To determine the expression of membrane glycoproteins and markers of activation on the platelet membrane, a flow cytometry technique was used [4]. The necessary antibodies against GMP-140 and markers of platelet activation were obtained commercially from Immunotech International (anti-CD62 and anti-CD63, Immunotech International, Luminy, Marseille, France) and used with a Cytoron Instrument. Platelet morphology was evaluated according to Kunicki [5]. Platelet aggregation induced by ADP (10 μM), collagen (10 μg/ml) and ristocetin (1.5 mg/ml) was measured with an Aggregocoder PA-3210 (Menarini Diagnostici, Firenze, Italia). These studies were carried out prior to apheresis and in the platelet concentrate at 1 h of collection and 24 h later. The platelet concentrates were used clinically and their post-transfusion survival was evaluated as corrected count increments in eight patients with no anti-HLA or platelet specific antibodies [6].

RESULTS

In routine application the platelet product of Excel was very satisfactory in terms of yields and WBC contamination, as summarized in Table 2. In no concentrate was the yield less than 4×10^{11} platelets, even when difficult veins created technical problems.

Table 2.
The platelet product

Needle to needle time (min)	61 ± 8
Platelet yield ($\times 10^{11}$)	5.2 ± 1.1
Platelet efficiency/min ($\times 10^9$)	8.7 ± 1.9
Blood flow rate (ml/min)	61 ± 10
Volume of blood processed (ml)	3537 ± 223
Leukocyte contamination ($\times 10^7$)	0.43 ± 0.4
Platelet concentrate extraction (ml/min)	4.4 ± 0.5
Platelet concentrate volume (ml)	331 ± 51

The average volume of blood that was processed was 3.55 l, in an average time of 61 min. The blood flow rate averaged 61 ml/min and the platelet efficiency per minute was 8.7×10^9. The mean yield was 5.2×10^{11} and the leukocyte contamination was 0.4×10^7. These results may be considered very interesting for a machine which has carried out no more than 150 procedures with different configurations of the plate, different approaches for cell collection, and any kind of modification which is necessary to bring a prototype machine to routine. Equally promising is the fact that the quality of the cell product, as measured by aggregation studies, morphology of the platelets, presence of aggregates, absence of surface markers of platelet activation and post-transfusion survival studies, is among the best we have seen with different kinds of cell separators. These preliminary data are summarized in Table 3. Table 4 shows standard collection procedures.

Table 3.
The quality of the platelet product

Wu–Hoak ratio (N.V. 0.9–1)		0.93	
Aggregation (% relative to pre-apheresis):			
	ADP 10 μM	83	65 (at 24 h)
	collagen 10 μg/ml	98	60 (at 24 h)
	ristocetin 1.5 mg/ml	88	62 (at 24 h)
pH		7.2	7.1 (at 24 h)
Platelet morphology	practically unchanged		
Anti-GPM-140 binding (CD62)	practically unchanged		
Anti-CD63 binding	practically unchanged		
Post-transfusion corrected count increments		18.3 ± 5.1 (at 24 h)	

Table 4.
The standardized procedure for platelet collection (two vein procedure)

ACD-A to blood flow ratio	1/12
Blood flow rate (ml/min)	60
Centrifuge speed (r.p.m.)	from 1500 (Hct < 38%)
	to 1650 (Hct > 43%)
Buffy-coat level (mm)	15
Volume of blood to be processed (l)	3.5
Cell collection (ml/min)	4.5

COMMENT

This is the very first report on the routine application of the new Dideco cell separator. The report is limited to thrombocytapheresis. As a consequence, these data may soon become obsolete, since further improvements are expected. Nonetheless our presentation confirms that another third generation machine will soon be marketed. As to our experience, Excel offers the most advantageous combination of positive features compared with the other thrombocytapheresis machine we have in use at our hemapheresis unit. So far, we have not tested the validity of the bags for long-term preservation of the platelet product.

REFERENCES

1. M. Valbonesi, R. Frisoni, L. Malfanti *et al.* Excel: a very new cell separator in its very first clinical application. Presentation at the *European Society for Hemapheresis Meeting*, 8–14 Sept., Wurzburg 1991.
2. Italian Health Ministry Decree–January 15. Protocols for establishing the identity of the donors of blood and components, in execution of the law no. 107, May 4, 1990 on the collection, preservation and distribution of human blood.

3. K. K. Wu and J. C. Hoak. A new method for the quantitative detection of platelet aggregates in patients with arterial insufficiency. *Lancet*, **2**, 924 (1974).

4. R. Fijnheer, P. W. Moddermann, H. Veldman *et al.* Detection of platelet activation with monoclonal antibodies and flow cytometry. *Transfusion*, **30**, 20 (1990).

5. T. G. J. Kunicki, M. Tucelli, G. A. Becker *et al.* A study of variables affecting the quality of platelets stored at room temperature. *Transfusion*, **15**, 414 (1975).

6. L. A. Warfolk and B. R. Macpherson. The detection of platelet allo-antibodies by flow cytometry. *Transfusion*, **31**, 340 (1991).

Therapeutic Plasmapheresis (XII), pp. 747-751
T. Agishi *et al.* (Eds)
© VSP 1993

Plasma Protein Fractionation by Inorganic Microporous Membranes

T. TOMONO,[1] T. SUZUKI,[1] T. IDE,[1] T. SATA[2] and S. SEKIGUCHI[1]

[1]*Japanese Red Cross Plasma Fractionation Center, Tokyo, Japan*
[2]*Tokuyama Research Lab., Tokuyama Soda Co. Ltd, Yamaguchi, Japan*

Key words: albumin; immunoglobulin; fractionation; inorganic membrane; porous glass.

INTRODUCTION

Porous glass membranes have such advantageous characteristics for membrane separation technique as having very limited pore size distribution [1, 2], and the capability of complete and repeated regeneration of fouled membranes by rinsing with chemicals [2].

The purpose of this study is to clarify the filtration characteristics of tubular or hollow-fiber porous glass membranes for plasma protein fractionation.

MATERIALS AND METHODS

The specifications of tubular or hollow-fiber porous glass membranes tested are summarized in Table 1. TS membranes (Tokuyama Soda Co. Ltd, Yamaguchi, Japan) prepared from SiO_2–Al_2O_3–CaO glass by phase separation were used in the present study. Mean pore diameters were calculated by the equation for the porous glass membranes according to Nakashima *et al.* [1].

$$D_p = 2(8\mu d\text{PWP}/0.574/H)^{0.5} \qquad (1)$$

where D_p is the pore diameter, μ the viscosity of water, d the wall thickness, PWP the pure water permeability and H the porosity, respectively.

Figure 1 shows the schematic diagram of the experimental apparatus. Plasma proteins prepared by the Japanese Red Cross Society, albumin and intramuscular immunoglobulin G (IgG) were dialyzed against saline to remove the stabilizers. The feed solution, consisting of 0.3% of albumin, 0.3% of IgG and 150 mM NaCl (pH 7.0), was filtered through membrane at a flow-rate of 606 cm/min under a constant transmembrane pressure of 100 mm Hg at 25 °C.

Transmembrane pressure (TMP) and sieving coefficient (SC) were calculated by using the following equations

$$\text{TMP} = (P_{Bi} + P_{Bo})/2 - P_F \qquad (2)$$

and

$$\text{SC} = C_F/C_B \qquad (3)$$

where P_{Bi} and P_{Bo} are the feed pressures of inlet and outlet, P_F the filtrate pressure, C_F and C_B the protein concentrations of feed and filtrate.

Table 1.
Specification of porous glass membranes

Module	Membrane area (cm²)	Inner diameter (mm)	Wall thickness (mm)	Porosity (—)	PWP[a] × 10⁵ (ml cm⁻²min⁻¹ mm Hg⁻¹)	Pore diameter (nm)
TS15	71.0	2.15	0.43	0.51	0.35	15.3
TS32	69.3	2.10	0.40	0.55	1.56	31.5
TS36	73.0	2.21	0.33	0.57	2.75	35.6
TS51	68.0	2.06	0.30	0.44	4.65	50.5
TS59	68.0	2.06	0.30	0.44	6.37	59.0
TS65	62.6	1.90	0.28	0.51	9.75	65.4
TS89	66.9	2.03	0.33	0.40	11.9	88.8
TS60H	49.0	0.80	0.13	0.65	22.3	59.6

[a] PWP = pure water permeability.

RESULTS AND DISCUSSION

Figure 2 shows the dependence of sieving coefficient of albumin and IgG on pore diameter. The sieving coefficient of albumin (molecular size; 15 × 3.8 nm [3]) drastically changed in the range of the pore diameters from 20 to 50 nm, and also SC for IgG (25 × 5 nm [4]) changed from 30 to 60 nm. These ranges are very limited. This may be due to the sharp pore size distribution of porous glass membranes. Further-

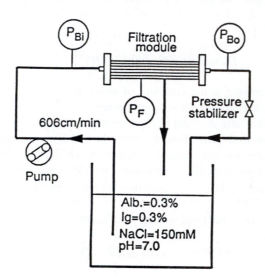

Figure 1. Schematic diagram of experimental apparatus.

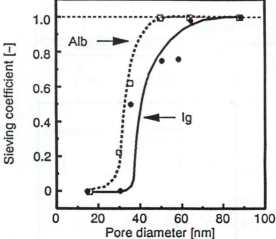

Figure 2. Dependence of sieving coefficient of albumin and immunoglobulin on pore diameter.

more the minimal pore diameters for both proteins to permeate are very similar to each molecular size.

Figure 3 shows the sieving coefficients of plasma proteins for each membrane. Aggregated IgG was rejected by any porous glass membranes with pore diameters ranging from 32 to 89 nm, although it was not the case with synthetic polymer membranes. These results indicated that plasma proteins were fractionated much more sharply by using porous glass membranes than by the use of synthetic polymer membranes.

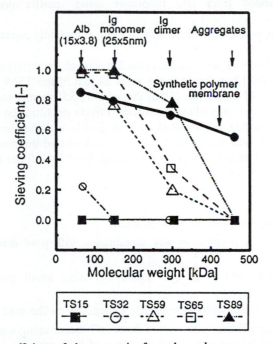

Figure 3. Sieving coefficients of plasma proteins for each membrane.

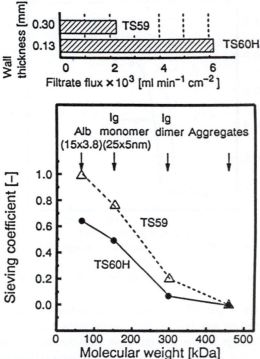

Figure 4. Effect of wall thickness on filtration characteristics.

Albumin was separated from IgG monomer using smaller pore-sized membranes (32 nm).

The TS15 membrane, with a pore diameter of 15 nm, completely rejected any proteins larger than albumin.

Figure 4 shows the effects of wall thickness on filtration characteristics. Although the pore diameter of the TS60H membrane is the same as that of the TS59 membrane, the wall thickness of the TS60H membrane is half that of the TS59 membrane (see Table 1). Reduction of the wall thickness yielded significant effects on filtration characteristics. Accordingly, the filtration flux increased more than double and the sieving coefficient of any proteins decreased with the decrease of wall thickness of the membrane.

In addition, IgG monomer was efficiently separated from IgG dimer using TS60H.

CONCLUSION

The following facts were found in the present study.

(i) Aggregated IgG was rejected by any membranes with pore diameters ranging from 32 to 89 nm.

(ii) Albumin was separated from IgG monomer using small pore-sized membranes (32 nm).

(iii) Filtration characteristics were significantly dependent on the wall thickness.

(iv) IgG monomer was efficiently separated from IgG dimer using a membrane with a pore diameter of 60 nm and a wall thickness of 0.13 mm.

REFERENCES

1. T. Nakashima and M. Shimizu. Liquid permeability of porous glass membrane and its surface conditions. In: *SPG Kenkyu Ronbunshyu*, K. Kusano, K. Imada and T. Nakashima (Eds), pp. 89–95, SPG Ouyou Gijyutsu Kenkyukai, Miyazaki (1989).

2. K. Ozawa, K. Ohashi, T. Ide *et al.* Technical evaluation of newly-developed inorganic membranes for plasma fractionation. *Int. J. Artif. Organs*, **12**, 195–198 (1989).

3. T. Peters. Serum albumin. In: *Plasma Proteins 3*, W. F. Putnam (Ed.), pp. 147–149, Academic Press, New York (1975).

4. T. Kuroyagi, Y. Otaka and T. Matsuhashi (Eds). pp. 7–22, *Immunoglobulin*, Igaku Shoin, Tokyo (1970)

Therapeutic Plasmapheresis (XII), pp. 753-756
T. Agishi *et al*. (Eds)
© VSP 1993

Hemodynamics and Security during Low Density Lipoprotein Apheresis

T. FUJIWARA, M. SEKIGUCHI, T. SHINODA,[1] H. ARAKURA,[1]
M. HARADA[2] and S. TANI[3]

First Department of Internal Medicine and [1]*Department of Artificial Organs,*
Shinshu University School of Medicine, Matsumoto, Japan
[2]*Gunma Cardiovascular Hospital, Takasaki, Japan*
[3]*Kaneka Corporation, Tokyo, Japan*

Key words: LDL apheresis; security; hemodynamics; hypovolemia; small plasma separator.

INTRODUCTION

Low density lipoprotein (LDL) apheresis has been established as an effective method of lowering plasma cholesterol levels in both homo- and heterozygous patients with familial hypercholesterolemia (FH). No progression or regression of arteriographically determined coronary artery lesions by means of this therapy were reported [1–4]. Recently, indication of this therapy for arteriosclerotic obliterans has been approved [5]. Although LDL apheresis has become a common therapy in Japan, security with regard to the development of symptoms and signs of ischemic heart disease has not been clarified. We investigated hemodynamic changes during or after apheresis.

MATERIALS AND METHODS

Six patients with hetero-FH, including two patients who had undergone coronary artery bypass graft surgery (CABG), were studied. The LDL apheresis system and its priming volume are shown in Fig. 1. A circuit was mounted on a MA-01 system (Kaneka Corp., Tokyo, Japan). Sulflux, as a plasma separator, and Liposover (LA-15), a specific adsorbent of LDL (Kaneka Corp.), were used. An optic catheter (Baxter, Tokyo, Japan) was inserted in the left subclavian vein before apheresis in all patients. Pulmonary capillary wedge pressure (WP), central venous pressure (CVP), cardiac output (CO), O_2 saturation of central vein (SVO_2), systolic blood pressure (SBP) and heart rate (HR) were measured every 30 min. All data are presented as the mean $\pm$ SD. Statistical analysis was carried out with the paired Student's *t*-test.

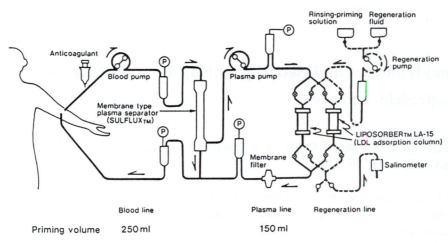

Figure 1. Priming volume in the LDL apheresis system.

RESULTS

One patient complained of nasal obstruction and slight chest discomfort at 90 min after starting the apheresis and two patients felt anginal chest pain at the ending. PA, WP and CVP decreased by 3.4, 3.6 and 2.8 mm Hg, respectively, 90 min later ($P < 0.05$). The decreases of PA, WP and CVP remained before the end, and rapidly increased by 6.1, 4.8 and 6.0 mm Hg for a short time at the end, respectively. Although CO and SVO_2 decreased similarly by 1.30 l/min and 6% 90 min later, the decreases of SVO_2, which occurred from 60 min later, were seen earlier than those of CO. SVO_2 also increased at the end in patients who complaining of anginal chest pain (Fig. 2). SBP also decreased in a similar manner at 90 min, but increased gradually until the end. So there were no differences between the pre-ending and the ending stage. On the other hand, HR did not change throughout the procedure (data not shown). The use of a small plasma separator (FS-03) and returning blood without plasma at a speed of 20 ml/min were effective in reducing the priming volume in half as the countermeasure in patients who complained of anginal chest pain.

DISCUSSION

Hombach *et al.* [3] reported that there were no hemodynamic changes during LDL apheresis, but anginal attacks occurred in two out of the six patients. In this study, we observed two patterns of chest pain: one occurred at 90 min after starting the apheresis and the other at the end. The former might be due to hypovolemia and the latter due to rapid increases in preload. The nasal obstruction which was observed in one patient might result from nasal congestion. In fact, hypovolemia occurred at 60 min in the light of SVO_2 data. Adding 100 ml of saline at 60 min after starting was effective for relieving the symptoms. The anginal chest pain at the end can be prevented by using the methods mentioned above. On the other hand, if SVO_2 did not increase at the end, cardiac dysfunction should be considered. Actually, if we should meet patients with

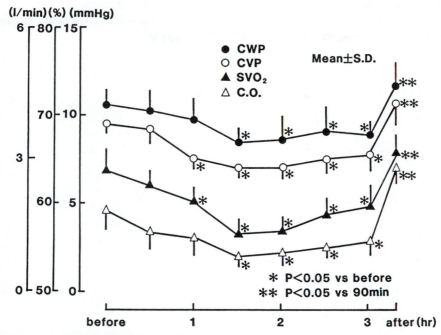

Figure 2. Hemodynamic changes during LDL apheresis.

angina, these devices should be attempted in the first place. Otherwise, if symptoms do not change, nitrates should be given quickly.

CONCLUSION

There were two patterns of anginal chest discomfort or pain during the LDL apheresis: one occurred at about 90 min after starting the procedure and the other at the end. The former is considered due to hypovolemia and the latter due to increases in preload. We suggest that the anginal chest discomfort or pain is avoidable by the following methods:

(i) Setting the blood recovery rate at 20 ml/min.

(ii) Using a small size plasma separator (FS-03).

(iii) Reducing the recovery volume to half by returning blood without the plasma component.

REFERENCES

1. H. Mabuchi. Use of LDL-apheresis in the management of familial hypercholesterolemia. *Curr. Opinion Lipid.*, 1, 43–47 (1990).
2. G. R. Thompson, M. Barbir and K. Okabayashi. Plasmapheresis in familial hypercholesterolemia. *Atherosclerosis*, 9, 152–157 (1989).
3. V. Hombach, H. Borberg and A. Gadzkowski. Regression of coronary arteriosclerosis in familial hypercholesteremia 2a by specific LDL plasma immunoadsorption. *Dtsch. Med. Wschr.*, 111, 1709–1715 (1986).

4. S. Yokoyama, A. Yamamoto and R. Hayashi. LDL apheresis; potential procedure for prevention and regression of atheromatous vascular lesion. *Jpn. Circ. J.*, **51**, 1116–1122 (1985).

5. T. Agishi, Y. Kitano and T. Suzuki. Improvement of peripheral circulation by low density lipoprotein adsorption. *Trans. Am. Soc. Artif. Intern. Organs*, **35**, 349–351 (1989).

Therapeutic Plasmapheresis (XII), pp. 757-759
T. Agishi *et al.* (Eds)
© VSP 1993

A New Hemofiltration Device with Reversible Roller Pump for Correcting Volume Controlled by a Precise Weight Balancer

Y. INAGAKI, K. KUMON, H. SUGIMOTO and N. YAHAGI

Surgical Intensive Care Unit, National Cardiovascular Center, Suita, Osaka 556, Japan

Key words: continuous venovenous hemofiltration; reversible roller pump; weight balance.

INTRODUCTION

Recently, continuous hemofiltration (CHF) has provided a great clinical advantage for patient with acute renal failure. The CHF has the following advantages: (i) it makes infusion management easy for patients with oliguria or anuria, (ii) it prevents the development of irreversible electrolyte abnormalities, and (iii) it removes unknown low molecular solutes to aid patients with multiple organ failure. CHF, however, also has the following disadvantages: (i) it is difficult to balance the accounts of removal of body water because of a large amount of ultrafiltration volume necessary for adequate control of uremia, (ii) it increases the opportunity for bacterial infection, and (iii) it decreases the filtration efficiency of solute removal. The removal of body water appears to be most important factor for the clinical application of CHF to patients requiring strict water management following cardiovascular surgery. Therefore, we evaluated a new continuous hemofiltration device (CHFD) with a reversible roller pump for correcting the volume controlled by a precise weight balancer (KM8001, Kuraray, Japan) in terms of the accuracy of the removal of body water, compared with a conventional CHFD (CHF-1, Ube, Japan). In addition, we examined the original polysulfone (PS) filter in terms of the clearance of solute during continuous venovenous hemofiltration (CVVH).

MATERIALS AND METHODS

Evaluation of the accuracy of removal of body water
The subjects of this study were nine patients, four male and five female, aged 45–70 years and weighing 56–72 kg, who suffered from acute renal failure following cardiovascular surgery in our intensive care unit.

In the 24 h period, we adopted the KM8001 with the original circuit and PS filter (membrane area: 0.4 m^2) for CVVH and CHF-1 with the original circuit and polyacylonitrile (PAN) filter (membrane area: 0.5 m^2) for the next 24 h period.

We evaluated the accuracy of removal of body water under the following six conditions, three times in each CHFD: (i) continuous infusion of supplemental fluid at the rate of 500 ml/h, (ii) blood flow at the rate of 60, 90 and 120 ml/min, and (iii) removal volume of body water at the rate of 100 and 200 ml/h. The prescribed conditions of CVVH were not altered for 24 h. The removal volume of body water was determined by a measuring cylinder every hour. We adopted Δremoval volume of body water (ΔRVBW), i.e. removal volume determined by a measuring cylinder minus prescribed removal volume, as an index of the accuracy, and evaluated the accuracy from the extent of variance of ΔRVBW.

Examination of the clearance efficiency of PS filter
We collected both samples of blood before PS filter and ultrafiltration fluid 3, 6, 12 and 24 h after the beginning of CVVH under the conditions of 60 ml/min of blood flow, 500 ml/h of infusion of supplemental fluid and 100 ml/h of removal of body water, and calculated the clearance ratio of sodium, potassium, creatinine or urea nitrogen from the following equation:

$$C_L/UFR = C_F/C_B$$

where C_L represents the clearance, C_F and C_B represent the concentrations of ultrafiltration fluid and blood before the filter, and UFR represents an ultrafiltration rate equal to an infusion rate of supplemental fluid in the present study, because supplemental fluid volume and ultrafiltration volume are controlled by the same roller pump via the twin lumen circuit.

The variance of ΔRVBW was analyzed by the F test and a P value less than 0.05 was considered significant.

RESULTS

Table 1 shows ΔRVBW in each CHFD under six conditions. The variance of ΔRVBW in KM8001 was significantly less than that in CHF-1 under every condition.
As shown in Table 2, the clearance ratios of the Ps filter were plotted on nearly 1.0 or 1.1.

Table 1.
ΔRVBW in KM8001 and CHF-1 [mean (SD)]

	KM8001 (ml)		CHF-1 (ml)	
Blood flow	100 ml/h	200 ml/h	100 ml/h	200 ml/h
60 ml/min	4.3 (11.6)[a]	1.6 (16.6)[b]	1.9 (45.0)	−47.2 (43.8)
90 ml/min	4.5 (8.8)[a]	3.1 (16.1)[b]	3.4 (66.3)	−50.3 (46.1)
120 ml/min	2.4 (9.8)[a]	3.2 (15.6)[b]	8.8 (56.2)	−54.2 (57.3)

[a] $P < 0.01$ vs CHF-1 at 100 ml/h
[b] $P < 0.01$ vs CHF-1 at 200 ml/h.

Table 2.
Time courses of the clearance ratio [mean (SD)]

Solute	Time after the beginning of CVVH (h)			
	3	6	12	24
Sodium	0.98 (.02)	0.97 (.01)	0.97 (.02)	0.98 (.01)
Potassium	1.03 (.01)	1.07 (.03)	1.05 (.03)	1.06 (.02)
Creatinine	1.05 (.08)	1.05 (.07)	1.05 (.04)	1.08 (.06)
Urea nitrogen	1.12 (.09)	1.11 (.10)	1.10 (.06)	1.12 (.05)

DISCUSSION

During CVVH, the variance of ΔRVBW in KM8001 had been significantly ($P < 0.01$) smaller than that in CHF-1. Similarly, KM8001 had removed body water which was nearly equal to the prescribed removal volume during CVVH regardless of the alterations of blood flow and removal volume. On the other hand, CHF-1 also removed body water nearly equal to the prescribed removal volume of 100 ml/h although its variance was large. However, the removal volume in CHF-1 at 200 ml/h decreased by 25% of the prescribed removal volume. There are a few factors which help to explain this difference between KM8001 and CHF-1. First, a reversible roller pump for correcting volume controlled by a precise weight balancer in KM8001 operates to maintain the account of weight balance within ±10 g, i.e. if the weight balance was beyond −10 g, the roller pump transfers the removal volume to ultrafiltration fluid and to maintain the weight balance zero; if the weight balance is beyond +10 g, the roller pump operates in the reverse direction. This mechanism was much precise and useful for providing stable body water removal and made water management easy. Second, the difference could arise from coordination of each original circuit or filter to each CHFD. The result obtained in this study suggests better coordination in KM8001 than in CHF-1. The PS filter, i.e. the original filter of KM8001, had kept an excellent clearance efficiency during CVVH for 24 h; the ratio (C_F/C_B) had been more than 1.0 except for sodium. In CVVH, the ultrafiltration volume is the most important factor to affect the clearance of solute [1], and the stable ultrafiltration volume is necessary for the ability to keep the clearance of solute stable. KM8001 has a clinical advantage over CHF-1 in terms of the stable clearance of solute.

In conclusion, the KM8001 with a PS filter has a high clinical advantage over conventional CHFD. Accurate body water removal could make water management easy for such patients with acute renal failure who require strict water management following cardiovascular surgery.

REFERENCE

1. A. Lauer, A. Saccaggi, C. Ronco *et al.* Continuous arteriovenous hemofiltration in the critically ill patients: clinical use and operational characteristics. *Ann. Intern. Med.*, **99**, 455 (1983).

Therapeutic Plasmapheresis (XII), pp. 761-765
T. Agishi *et al.* (Eds)
© VSP 1993

Hemolysis and Platelet Loss in Plasma Separation with Membrane-separator and Centrifugation Methods

T. SHIBAMOTO, T. AKIBA, H. OSHIMA, F. MARUMO, M. NARUSE, K. NAKAJIMA, H. OHBA and O. MATSUDA

Tokyo Medical and Dental University, Kidney Division and 2nd Department of Internal Medicine, Musashino Red Cross Hospital, Dialysis Division, Tokyo, Japan

Key words: therapeutic plasmapheresis; membrane; centrifugation; hemolysis; platelet loss.

INTRODUCTION

Therapeutic plasmapheresis has been applied widely to the treatment of immune diseases [1, 2], neurological diseases [3–5] and others [6]. Recently, the selective removal of target substances from separated plasma of patients has been tried. Plasma is separated from whole blood by use of either a membrane separator or centrifugation without destruction or loss of blood corpuscles.

We developed a hemolysis monitor during separation of plasma by a membrane-type separator. We validated whether the new device was applicable for monitoring hemolysis with a membrane separator.

The blood flow and centrifugation gravity were also investigated to minimize the loss of platelets during plasmapheresis using the centrifugation method.

MATERIALS AND METHODS

A plasma marker for hemolysis and the developed monitor
Hemoglobin had been measured by a cyanmethemoglobin method using 540 nm absorption *in vitro*. The monitoring system does not require so high a sensitivity as a cyanmethemoglobin method, but it should need less blood loss. Therefore, we developed a new monitoring device equipped with photoelectronics. We prepared hemoglobin solution using Sigma H-7876 at a concentration of 100 mg/dl in saline, and 0–20 mg/dl in plasma and in saline.

In vivo *study of hemolysis with a membrane separator*
Parameters of the membranes separator used for hemolysis tests were a polyethylene hollow fiber with 0.5 m^2 surface area and a 100 ml/min blood flow rate. Heparin was added as an anticoagulant. Transmembrane pressures were varied from 40, 60, 80, 100 and 120 mmHg to adjust the removal volume of plasma.

Platelet loss of centrifugation plasmapheresis
ACOBE 2997 (Cobe Lab., Denver, CO) and a plasma exchange set with a single-stage channel were used. Blood flow rates were changed from 40 to 60 ml/min. The centrifugation gravities were 1600 to 2200 r.p.m. Heparin (1000 u/h) was added as an anticoagulant.

We measured platelet counts in the whole blood and the separated plasma.

RESULTS

In hemoglobin solutions with concentrations from 0 to 20 mg/dl dissolved in the saline and the plasma it was difficult to discriminate the presence of hemolysis by visual inspection.

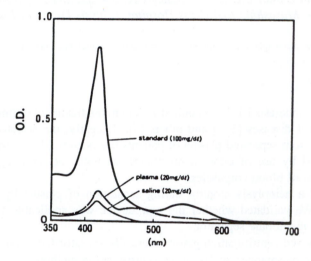

Figure 1. Absorption of hemoglobin from 350 to 700 nm.

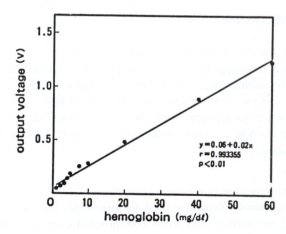

Figure 2. Hemoglobin concentration and output voltage of the new hemolysis monitor with plasma test solution.

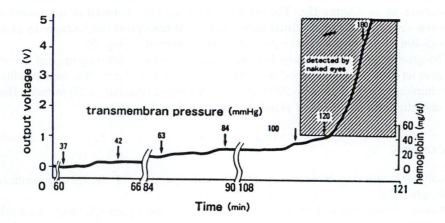

Figure 3. Transmembrane pressure and output voltage (*in vivo*).

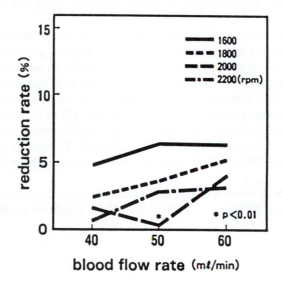

Figure 4. Percentages changes of platelet loss.

Figure 1 demonstrates optical absorption curves of hemoglobin between 350 and 700 nm. These absorption patterns had peaks at 420 nm, indicating the highest sensitivity at 420 nm in optical detection. Our hemolysis monitor measures the differences of optical density at 420 and 650 nm in separated plasma at the plastic tubing. The relationship between the hemoglobin levels and the output voltage of the developed device is shown in Fig. 2.

The relationship between the transmembrane pressure and the output voltage of the developed device was evaluated *in vitro*. The output voltage showed a slight increase of pressure up to 420 mmHg. The output voltage steeply increased at transmembrane pressures over 120 mmHg. Visual inspection could not detect the increase in plasma hemoglobin even transmembrane pressures over 160 mmHg (Fig. 3).

The greatest amount of platelet loss was seen at rotation at 1600 r.p.m. and the average platelet loss was 6% at blood flow rates from 40 to 60 ml/min. The best conditions for minimum platelet loss were 2000 r.p.m. with a blood flow rate of 50 ml/min. Under this condition, less than 1% of platelets were lost (Fig. 4).

DISCUSSION

Hemolysis monitoring is necessary for the safe operation of therapeutic membrane plasmapheresis.

Plasma hemoglobin had been measured *in vitro* by the cyanmethemoglobin method using 540 nm adsorption. A hemolysis monitoring system should be as sensitive as the cyanmethemoglobin method, and it is required to monitor hemolysis continuously. The spectrogram of hemoglobin from 350 to 700 nm showed maximum hemoglobin absorption at 420 nm. We developed a hemolysis device using red and blue optical photosensors.

The method of the newly developed hemolysis device was to detect the changes of discrepancies between red and blue optical densities. A green photosensor is effective to measure 420 nm optical absorption of hemoglobin liquid. A red photosensor detects the optical density around 560 nm to compensate for the draft and turbidity of tubing.

We conclude that this hemolysis monitor is applicable and necessary to therapeutic membrane plasmapheresis and membrane donor pheresis [7] to increase safety.

Next, we evaluated the best conditions of blood flow rate and centrifuge gravity to decrease platelet loss in the centrifugation plasmapheresis. Platelet loss increased when the blood flow rate was increased. Platelet loss decreased when the rotation r.p.m. was increased.

The best conditions of blood flow rate and rotation in the centrifugation plasmapheresis were 50 ml/min and 2000 r.p.m., respectively. These condition resulted in a platelet loss of 1%.

CONCLUSION

Our continuous hemolysis monitor is suitable for safe operation in therapeutic membrane plasmapheresis and membrane donor pheresis.

The best conditions of centrifugation plasmapheresis (COBE-2997) are a blood flow rate of 50 ml/min and a centrifugation gravity of 2000 r.p.m., in order to decrease platelet loss.

REFERENCES

1. W. A. P. Hamilton *et al.* Plasma exchange in SLE. *Lancet,* 1, 1249 (1980).
2. J. V. Jones *et al.* The role of therapeutic plasmapheresis in the rheumatic disease. *J. Lab. Clin. Med.,* 97, 589–598 (1981).

3. P. C. Daw *et al.* Plasmapheresis in multiple sclerosis: preliminary findings. *Neurology*, **30**, 1023–1028 (1980).

4. H. J. G. H. Oosterhuis *et al.* Antiacetylcholine receptor-antibodies in myasthenia gravis, Part 2. Clinical and serological follow up of individual patients. *J. Neurol. Sci.*, **58**, 371–385 (1983).

5. H. L. Weiner *et al.* Immunoregulation in neurological disease. *Ann. Neurol.*, **11**, 437–449 (1982).

6. G. R. Thompson *et al.* Assesment of longterm plasma exchange for familial hypercholesterolemia. *Br. Heart J.*, **43**, 680–688 (1980).

7. G. Rock *et al.* Plasma collection using an automated membrane device. *Transfusion*, **26**, 269–271 (1986).

Therapeutic Plasmapheresis (XII), pp. 767-770
T. Agishi *et al.* (Eds)
© VSP 1993

New Leukocyte Removal Filters: CF-1 and CF-2

Y. ENDO, T. TANI, H. ARAKI, Y. EBIRA, T. YOKOTA, Y. TSUTAMOTO,
H. ABE, K. NUMA, K. MATSUDA, H. AOKI, T. YOSHIOKA, K. HANASAWA,
M. KODAMA, S. OHNO[1] and H. HATTORI[1]

First Department of Surgery, Shiga University of Medical Science, Otsu, Japan
[1]*Nipro Medical Industries Ltd, Osaka, Japan*

Key words: leukocyte-removal filter; leukocyte depletion; flow cytometric technique; viral transmission; alloimmunization.

INTRODUCTION

The benefit of WBC-depleted blood products has been discussed because transfused leukocytes may increase the risk of adverse effects, such as febrile transfusion reaction, transfusion-associated HLA alloimmunization and the transmission of WBC-associated viral diseases such as cytomegalovirus. To reduce the severity and frequency of these transfusion-related complications, the number of WBCs are commonly reduced by filtration. We evaluated two new leukocyte removal filters, Nipro CF-1 and CF-2.

MATERIALS AND METHODS

Nipro CF-1 and CF-2 (Nipro Medical Industries, Osaka, Japan), non-woven polyester filters, gravity flow devices requiring no priming and no rinse after use, were developed to prepare 400 ml of whole blood or red cell concentrates (RBCCs) from 400 ml of whole blood. The filter column of CF-1 is small. Its priming volume was reported at 20 ml. CF-2 was developed to prepare 400 ml of whole blood or RBCCs from 400 ml of whole blood with a reduction in WBC counts greater than 3 log.

RBCCs prepared from 400 ml of whole blood purchased from Japanese Red Cross Blood Services, Shiga Region, and stored at 4 °C, and filtered within 3 days after collection.

Leukocyte counts were measured electronically using a Sysmex K-1000 (Toa Medical Electronics Corp., Kobe, Japan). Hemocytometric counts were performed in the standard manner. Flow cytometry was performed with a Coulter EPICS-C cytometer (Coulter Corp., Hialeah, FL). Samples were prepared in the following two ways.

Samples obtained using CF-1 were prepared by modified Takahashi's method [1]: 1 ml of each sample were placed in a tube; 7.5 ml of propidium iodide (PI) solution (5 μg/ml), 0.1% Triton X-100, 0.1% ribonuclease and 0.1 mg/ml sodium citrate was added to each tube. After a 10 min incubation, 50 ml of 0.87% ammonium chloride solution was added to lyse RBCs. The tubes were centrifuged for 5 min at 1580 *g*

(3000 r.p.m.) and the supernatant was discarded. The pellet was resuspended with 400 μl of PI solution and the samples were ready for flow cytometry.

For measuring leukocyte-depleted blood products filtered by CF-2, samples were prepared by the Wenz *et al.* method [2]. The following reagents from a WBC preparation system (Immunoprep EPICS) were added to 100 μl of RBCC: 600 μl of formic acid at 1.2 ml/l; 265 μl of carbonate buffer, pH 7.4, and 100 μl of paraformaldehyde at 10 g/l and 7 μl of Triton X-100; 100 μl of PI was added to the total volume and the suspension was placed in the dark for 30 min prior to flow cytometric analysis. Thereafter, 100 μl of WBC-reduced blood was diluted with Immunoprep, Triton X-100 and PI solution to 1172 μl. Then we counted 0.5 ml aliquots containing 42.7 μl of WBC-reduced blood. The lower limit of sensitivity for this WBC assay was reported 1×10^{-3} WBCs/μl.

The percentage depletion of WBC was calculated by dividing the postfiltration count measured by flow cytometry by the prefiltration count measured electronically.

RESULTS

To evaluate CF-1, a total of 21 units of RBCCs were studied using the flow cytometric technique, the visual hemocytometric technique and the automated cell analyzer. The residual WBCs were 2.57 ± 1.13 WBCs/μl (mean ± SD, $n = 14$) measured by flow cytometry. No residual leukocytes could be seen postfiltration with the hemocytometer in 20 units. The percentage depletion of WBC using CF-1 was $99.97 \pm 0.01\%$.

To evaluate CF-2, a total of 9 units of RBCCs were studied. Table 1 shows the postfiltration WBCs and the percentage depletion of WBCs using CF-2. Extremely low counts below the limit of sensitivity for this assay, less than 1×10^{-3} WBCs/μl, were detected in six of the 17 samples. More than a 6 log (> 99.9999%) depletion of WBCs was detected in six samples, a 6 log (99.9999%) despletion of WBC, was detected in two samples, a 5 log (99.999%) depletion was detected in seven samples and a 4 log (99.99%) depletion was detected in two samples.

DISCUSSION

To reduce the severity and frequency of transfusion-related complications, the number of WBCs is commonly reduced by filtration. The prevention of alloimmunization was reported to require less than 10^7 leukocyte contamination. However, when the efficacy of filters is evaluated, it is difficult to measure extremely low WBC counts correctly. The flow cytometric technique was developed to measure extremely low WBC counts. Wenz *et al.* reported flow cytometric counting procedures used to monitor the 6 log reduction in WBC count [2].

A small-sized leukocyte removal filter (Nipro CF-1) removed $99.97 \pm 0.01\%$ of leukocytes measured by flow cytometry. CF-1 recovered $90.7 \pm 4.47\%$ of RBC measured with the hemocytometer. With CF-1, which has a size and priming volume smaller than other commercial leukocyte removal filters, a 3 log reduction in WBC counts and more than 90% recovery in RBC counts are possible as with other commercial filters.

The transmission of viruses through transfusion has been a major problem. Screening for viruses still does not guarantee 100% safety. Although the transmission of viral agents occurs at low levels, the accumulated exposure that chronically transfused patients experience can potentially represent a significant increased risk of viral infection. It has been found that some viruses are transmitted by leukocytes and are highly cell-associated. Thus, the removal of leukocytes can decrease the transmission of these leukocyte-mediated viruses. A 3 log depletion may be adequate to reduce the incidence of cytomegalovirus in blood recipients. However, this level of depletion may not be satisfactory to protect the recipient against other WBC-associated viral infections. Recent reports suggest that a minimum of a 6 log WBC depletion may be necessary to reduce the transmission of human immunodeficiency virus [3]. This prompted the development of a leukocyte removal filter capable of a greater WBC depletion. Nipro CF-2 achieved a 4–6 log reduction of WBC counts. No commercial filters have been reported to achieve more than a 4 log reduction of WBC counts.

Table 1.
The postfiltration residual WBC count and the percentage depletion of WBCs through CF-2

No.	Initial WBCs $(\times 10^3/\mu l)$	Fluorescence events [a]	Residual WBCs $(/\mu l)$	Depletion of WBCs (%)	(log)
1	7.45	792	0.002	99.9999	6.56
2	7.45	525	< 0.001[b]	99.9999<	6.87<
3	7.6	388	< 0.001[b]	99.9999<	6.88<
3	7.6	461	< 0.001[b]	99.9999<	6.88<
3	7.6	467	< 0.001[b]	99.9999<	6.88<
3	7.6	550	< 0.001[b]	99.9999<	6.88<
3	7.6	587	< 0.001[b]	99.9999<	6.88<
3	7.6	818	0.002	99.9999	6.48
5	7.4	1131	0.023	99.9996	5.52
5	7.4	1188	0.032	99.9995	5.37
5	7.4	1631	0.271	99.9963	4.44
6	10	1157	0.026	99.9997	5.58
7	8.65	1196	0.033	99.9996	5.42
8	14	1289	0.055	99.9996	5.41
9	6.85	1159	0.027	99.9996	5.41
9	6.85	1300	0.058	99.9991	5.07
9	6.85	1625	0.264	99.9961	4.41

[a] These values were below the limit of sensitivity for this assay, less than 1×10^{-3} WBCs/μl.
[b] Fluorescence measured in total events per 42.7 μl of postfiltration blood.

Two new leukocyte removal filter were evaluated. CF-1, which has a size and priming volume smaller than other commercial leukocyte removal filters, accomplished as 3 log reduction in WBC counts as other commercial filters did. CF-2 achieved a 4–6 log depletion of WBCs assayed by flow cytometry.

REFERENCES

1. T. Takahashi, M. Hosoda and S. Sekiguti. A flow cytometric method to detect residual leukocytes in platelet and red cell concentrates. *Jpn. J. Transfus. Med.*, **36**, 429–437 (1990).

2. B. Wenz, E. R. Burns, V. Lee and W. K. Miller. A rare-event analysis model for quantifying white cells in white cell-depleted blood. *Transfusion*, **31**, 156–159 (1991).

3. S. M. Schnittman, M. C. Psallidopoulos, H. C. Lane *et al.* The reservoir for HIV-1 in human peripheral blood is a T cell that maintains expression of CD4. *Science*, **245**, 305–308 (1989).

Therapeutic Plasmapheresis (XII), pp. 771-774
T. Agishi *et al.* (Eds)

Clinical Evaluation of Newly Improved EVAL Second Filters

T. SUEHIRO, A. SUEOKA, J. HORIGUCHI, K. TAKAKURA and H. TSUDA[1]

Kuraray Co., Ltd, Kurashiki, Japan
[1]*Juntendo University, Tokyo, Japan*

Key words: plama fractionator; EVAL second filter; dextran rejection rate; pore distribution; EVAL-5A.

INTRODUCTION

The EVAL secondary membrane filters (Evaflux) provide excellent characteristics as a plasma fractionator in double filtration plasmapheresis (DFPP) [1]. Three types of EVAL secondary filters with different pore sizes are currently available, i.e. $2A_3$, $3A_3$ and $4A_3$, and they have been used widely for the treatment of various diseases according to the size of target substances to be removed. In order to increase furthermore their filtration performances, we have improved these conventional membranes and now three new versions ($2A_5$, $3A_5$ and $4A_5$) are becoming available. In addition, we have developed an entirely new type of membrane with much larger pore size ($5A_5$). This paper presents the results of our study on membrane structure and clinical performance test of those new membranes.

MATERIALS AND METHODS

We investigated the structure and property of membranes in the following manners: (i) observation by scanning electron microscope (SEM); (ii) measurement of water content as a rough measure of membrane pore volume; (iii) measurement of ultrafiltration rate (UFR); (iv) measurement of dextran rejection rate as measure of pore size. The clinical evaluation of these membranes was carried out by conducting a totally 54 sessions of DFPP on 31 patients, using Plasmacure as the plasma separator and the KM-8500 or KM-8800 (Kuraray, Japan) as a monitor (Table 1).

RESULTS AND DISCUSSION

Compared with the conventional types, the new versions have an inner diameter as small as $175\,\mu$m and a wall thickness of as thin as $40\,\mu$m (Table 2). Figure 1 shows SEM pictures of the inner surfaces of the $4A_3$ and $4A_5$ membranes. The $4A_5$ membrane clearly had a larger number of pores than $4A_3$. This closely corresponded with the fact that both $2A_5$ and $4A_5$ showed a water content 10% higher than their previous versions (Table 2). Figure 2 shows the dextran rejection curves of the membranes. The $2A_5$

Table 1.
Summary of clinical evaluation

EVAL filter	No. of patients	Disease	No. of treatments	
2A$_5$	7	RA(2), MCTD(2), SLE(2), PP(1)	14	⎫ partial discard
3A$_5$	8	RA(5), MCTD(1), DM(1), SS(1)	15	⎬ ($Q_D = 3.8 \pm 0.8$ ml/min)
4A$_5$	8	RA(5), SLE(2), PBC(1)	13	⎭
5A$_5$	8	FHC(6), SLE(1), PBC(1)	12	dead-end ($Q_D = 0$ l/min)

RA: rheumatoid arthritis, MCTD: mixed connective tissue disease, SLE: systemic lupus erythematosus, PP: pemphigus, DM: dermatomyositis, SS: Sjögren syndrome, PBC: primary biliary cirrhosis, FHC: familial hypercholesterolemia.
Plasma separator: Plasmacure-L (0.5 m^2, PVA, Kuraray).
DFPP monitor: KM-8500 or KM-8800 (Kuraray).
Q_B: 63.7 ± 14.2 ml/min, Q_F: 19.3 ± 4.2 ml/min, treated volume: 2.0 ± 0.21.

Table 2.
Characterizations of EVAL Second Filters

	Filter				
	2A$_3$	4A$_3$	2A$_5$	4A$_5$	5A$_5$
Inner diameter (μm)	200			175	
Wall thickness (μm)	50			40	
Surface area (m^2)	2.0			2.0	
Water content (vol%)	54.5	59.3	65.9	71.1	69.8
UFR (ml/min mmHg m^2)	0.51	1.86	0.53	1.92	3.90
MW of 90% rej. $\times 10^3$ (dalton)	135	614	144	340	570

displayed the same curves as the 2A$_3$ did. The 4A$_5$ revealed a sharp dextran rejection curve, or a high level of rejection on the whole, as compared with the 4A$_3$. The 5A$_5$ showed a sharp fractionation curve almost parallel with that of the 4A$_5$, displaying a low level of rejection in the low molecular weight range despite almost the same rejection curve as the 4A$_3$ in the region above a molecular weight of 500 000 dalton. Figure 3 shows the SCs of the new membranes for various plasma components, obtained in their clinical applications. The 2A$_5$ membrane showed a good ability to fractionate albumin (0.62) and IgG (0.19). The 5A$_5$ almost completely rejected LDL (0.02) while showing high SCs for albumin (0.92) and HDL (0.83). With the 5A$_5$ membrane in the dead-end method, DFPP could be successfully performed without having to use any infusion fluid. Comparing 4A$_5$ and 4A$_3$ as to their SCs for albumin (0.84/0.81), IgG (0.57/0.65) and IgM (0.00/0.10), the 4A$_5$ exhibited a sharper fractionation than the 4A$_3$ did. In addition, the 4A$_5$ showed a filtration pressure of 16 mmHg at the end of a DFPP session which the 4A$_3$ recorded 67 mmHg under the same operating condition, suggesting that the improved membrane could process more plasma than the conventional one.

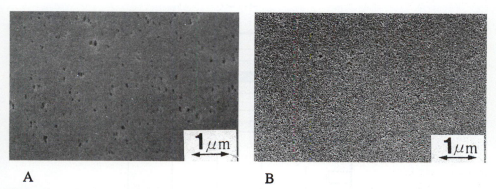

A   B

Figure 1. SEM micrographs of inner surface: (A) 4A₃ and (B) 4A₅.

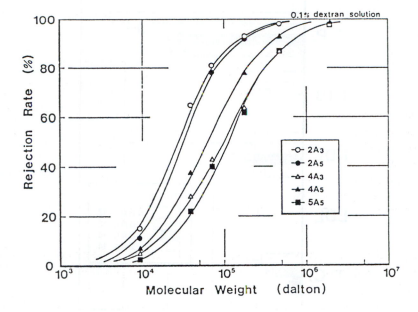

Figure 2. Dextran rejection curves.

CONCLUSION

The improved new membranes had a sharper pore distribution and a large number of pores per unit area compared with the conventional ones. Our clinical evaluation results also revealed that the new membranes could fractionate solutes more selectively than the previous ones. They also had an increased plasma processing capability. These results corresponded well with the modified membrane structure. The newly developed 5A₅ membrane almost completely rejected the passage of LDL while showing high SCs for albumin and HDL. With use of this membrane, it was possible to perform DFPP

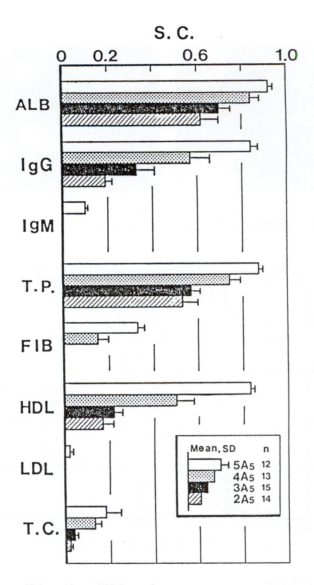

Figure 3. Sieving coefficients of new EVAL membranes.

without using infusion fluid such as albumin, and thus it seems that the 5A$_5$ membrane is particularly effective in the treatment of hyperlipidemia.

REFERENCE

1. A. Sueoka, T. Miyahara, K. Takakura *et al.* Study of filtration characteristics of EVAL secondary filters with diseased plasma. *Jpn. Artif. Organs*, **14**, 413–416 (1985).

Therapeutic Plasmapheresis (XII), pp. 775-777
T. Agishi *et al.* (Eds)
© VSP 1993

Machineless Double Filtration Plasmapheresis: A Novel and Cheap Method of DFPP in Developing Countries

R. SRIVASTAVA, R. HOTCHANDANI and A. DAR

Nephrology Department, Safdarjang Hospital, New Delhi, India

Key words: plasmapheresis; machineless.

INTRODUCTION

Plasmapheresis has today become an accepted method of treatment of many diseases of immunological nature. Many of these diseases were considered untreatable or used to require large doses of potentially toxic drugs. Double filtration Plasmapheresis (DFPP) results in prolonged remission and some cases even a cure of the disease process. However, due to the exorbitant cost of the filters and non-availability of the machine, this treatment has been denied to many, especially in the third world countries.

India is a poor country and the treatment of PP is normally not within the reach of everybody. The financial implication has two facts, one is the cost of the machine and second the price of filters. The cost of a PP machine, which is much higher than that of a HD machine, is the main limiting factor. It was to circumvent the need of a sophisticated PP machine and to reduce the cost that a simple, although novel, method was introduced by the author known as Srivastava's MLPP (machineless plasmapheresis).

PROCEDURE

To circumvent the non-availability of the PP machine, a method was devised using two or three roller pumps, two for SFPP and three for DFPP. These of pumps were made indigenously and give a blood flow of 50–500 ml/min.

In SFPP, blood was drawn from a large vein (left femoral vein), passed through the first roller pump and then into the plasma filter. It was returned to the patient after passing through the second pump.

In DFPP, plasma was sent to second filter by a second pump and the third pump returned the albumin and packed cells to the patient, while the globulin was discarded.

All the pumps were used at the same speed, so that there was no back pressure nor entry of air bubbles via the junction in the tubings.

RESULTS

Twelve cases of Srivastava's MLPP were performed and were compared with equally matched cases on a sophisticated PP machine, i.e. BT-796 (Dideco).

When compared, subjective, objective and immunological responses were unaltered and no-side effects were observed. This was suggestive of the utility, efficacy and cost effectiveness of this cheap method. See Table 1.

Table 1.
Comparison

	Treated with machine	Treated without machine
No. of patients	12	12
Response	good	good
Side effects	nil	nil

DISCUSSION

The machineless method gave the same results as with using the sophisticated machine.

The only drawback noticed during the procedure was the absence of monitoring facilities that are provided by the machine. Hence, the patients have to be very carefully monitored by the expert personnel conducting the procedure. Another defect was that the roller pumps have a lower limit of blood flow of 50 ml/min and, therefore, are not advisable in patients with hypotension.

Recently, apheresis has aquired a major role in the treatment of immune complex disorders. It has been used for the treatment of rheumatoid arthritis [1], myasthenia gravis [2], lupus nephritis [3], etc.

Different techniques have been used for effecting PP. For example, SFPP [4], DFPP [4], cascade filtration [6], plasma exchange [6], cryofiltration [7], thermofiltration, photofiltration and immunoadsorption techniques [7]. However, all these techniques necessarily require a sophisticated machine which is quite costly and sometimes may be beyond the reach of an average patient in countries like ours.

CONCLUSION

One reason why there is so little material in PP available from third world countries is the lack of availability of the PP machine. Hence, the importance of this method. We hope that with the more frequent use of this machineless method, many more patients requiring PP can be given the benefit of this modality of treatment and more data leading to a better understanding of PP will be available from these countries.

REFERENCES

1. D. J. Wallace, D. Goldfinger, R. Gatti *et al.* Plasmapheresis and lympopharasis in the management of rheumatoid arthritis. *Arthritis Rheum*, **22**, 703–710 (1979).
2. S. E. Levin *et al.* Successful plasmapheresis for fulminant myasthenia gravis during pregnancy. *Arch. Neurol.*, **43**, 197–198 (1986).
3. M. Amato *et al.* Can plasmapheresis improve lupus nephritis without its immunological markers? (Letter). *Nephron.*, **48**, 252–253 (1988).

4. R. Srivastava, A. Dar and A. Pasricha. Renal rehabilitation with DFPP in India. *Indian J. Apheresis*, in press.

5. K. Ota, H. Amemiya, N. Sugino *et al.* Double filtration plasmapheresis. *Trans. Am. Soc. Artif. Intern. Organs*, **26**, 406 (1980).

6. A. J. Rees. Plasma exchange: principles and practice. In: *Replacement of Renal Function by Dialysis*, W. Drukker, F. M. Parsons and J. F. Maher (Eds), p. 872. Martinus Nijhoff, Dordrecht (1983).

7. J. W. Smith, K. Kayashima, Kutsumec *et al.* Cryopheresis: immuno-chemical modulation and clinical response in auto immune disease. *Trans. Am. Soc. Intern. Artif. Organs*, **28**, 291 (1982).

Therapeutic Plasmapheresis (XII), pp. 779-783
T. Agishi *et al.* (Eds)
© VSP 1993

Newly Developed Adsorbent for Direct Hemoperfusion to Remove β_2-Microglobulin

S. FURUYOSHI, M. TSUNOMORI, S. TAKATA and N. TANI

Central Research Laboratories, Kaneka Corp., Kobe, Japan

Key words: β_2-microglobulin; dialysis; amyloidosis; adsorbent; hemoperfusion; hydrophobicity.

INTRODUCTION

It is well known that long-term hemodialysis patient frequently suffer from carpal tunnel syndrome and dialysis arthropathy due to deposition of amyloid substances [1, 2]. Since Gejyo *et al.* identified β_2-microglobulin (BMG) as a cause protein of the amyloid fibril by biochemical analysis in 1985 [3], various efforts have been made to eliminate BMG from the blood of dialysis patients. Our previous studies have demonstrated that a close relationship exists between the hydrophobicity of organic compounds and its affinity for BMG [4]. In this article, we will report on the BMG adsorbent designed on the basis of previous studies.

MATERIALS AND METHODS

Blood samples and adsorbent

Serum and fresh blood were obtained from patients with chronic renal failure and healthy volunteers, respectively. Hydrophobic compounds with long alkyl chains were immobilized to cellulose beads produced by Kaneka corporation (530 μm in diameter).

Evaluation of adsorption characteristics

Batch perfusion. One ml of the adsorbent was incubated with 6 or 36 ml of serum at 37°C for 2 h. The amount of adsorbed BMG and adsorption rates (%) of serum components were calculated from the concentrations of corresponding protein before and after incubation.

Column perfusion. Half ml of the adsorbent was packed into a syringe column and serum was passed through the column at the flow rate of 0.1 ml/min for 2 h. BMG and albumin (Alb) concentrations in effluent were determined.

Estimation of hemocompatibility

In vitro. One ml of the adsorbent was packed into a syringe column and heparin added (7 IU/ml) fresh blood was passed through the column at a flow rate of 0.5 ml/min at 37°C. The passage rate (%) of each blood cell was calculated by the following equation.

$$\text{passage rate (\%)} = 100 \times \text{outlet counts/inlet counts}$$

Ex vivo. Hemoperfusion was performed on mongrel dogs weighing about 10 kg with the column filled with 50 ml of the adsorbent. After whole body heparinization with 2000 IU of heparin, the perfusion was started at a blood flow rate of 10 ml/min and the rate was increased gradually up to 50 ml/min. Heparin was infused continuously at a rate of 1000 U/h during perfusion. Blood samples were taken from the upper reach of the column and the number of blood cells was counted.

RESULTS AND DISCUSSION

We have reported that a critical Σf value of organic compounds exists between 2 and 3 on which its affinity for BMG increases drastically [4]. On the basis of previous studies, hydrophobic alkyl compounds whose Σf value is over 7 were immobilized to cellulose beads. Σf is the sum of hydrophobic fragmental constants [5]. The capacity for adsorbing BMG was evaluated over 1 mg/ml adsorbent (Fig. 1). According to Karlsson's report [6], the BMG production rate is estimated about 160 mg/day in a man

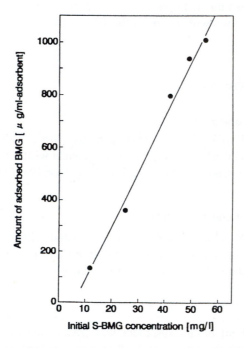

Figure 1. Relation between BMG concentration in serum and adsorption capacity for BMG in batch perfusion: serum/adsorbent = 36 (v/v), 37°C, 2 h.

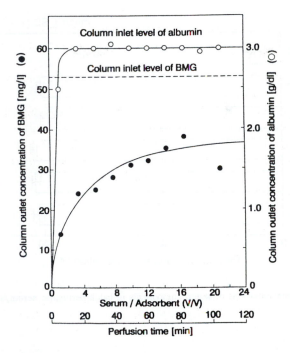

Figure 2. Adsorption characteristics of the adsorbent for BMG and Alb in column perfusion: column volume = 0.5 ml, Q_p = 0.1 ml/min, 37 °C.

weighing 50 kg, the device containing about 300 ml of the adsorbent is expected to adsorb BMG generated for 2 days.

In column perfusion, the Alb concentration in the effluent rose up the inlet level immediately, while the BMG concentration kept at 60% of the inlet level even after 120 min perfusion (Fig. 2). This material adsorbs BMG without affecting the concentrations of major serum proteins such as albumin and immunoglobulins (Fig. 3). This selectivity is attained by optimization of the surface pore size of adsorbent beads. The exclusion limit of the adsorbent is adjusted to about 20 000 daltons.

The adsorbent shows large passage rate on both WBC and platelets compared with commercially available charcoal coated by polyhydroxyethylmethacrylate (PHEMA) (Fig. 4). Furthermore, in the *ex vivo* perfusion with dog, the inlet counts of blood cells does not change (Fig. 5). These results indicate that the adsorbent has a good enough hemocompatibility for practical use.

CONCLUSIONS

An adsorbent based on the hydrophobic interaction for BMG has been developed. It has a capacity to adsorb over 1 mg of BMG/ml adsorbent, and shows good hemocompatibility in both *in vitro* and *ex vivo* studies. These results demonstrate that the adsorbent has good potential for direct elimination of BMG from circulating blood of dialysis patients.

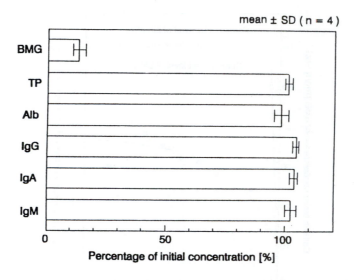

Figure 3. Changes in concentrations of serum components in batch perfusion: serum/adsorbent = 6 (v/v), 37 °C, 2 h.

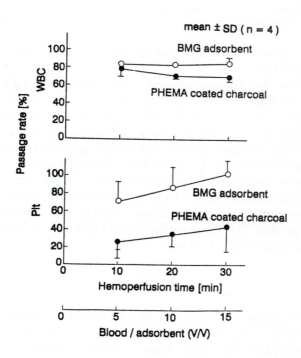

Figure 4. WBC and platelet passage through the adsorbent mini-column *in vitro*: column volume = 1.0 ml, Q_b = 0.5 ml/min, 37 °C.

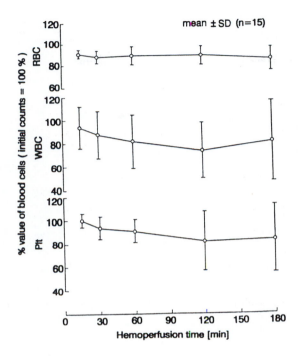

Figure 5. Changes of blood cell counts in the *ex vivo* hemoperfusion with dogs: column volume = 50 ml, Q_b = 10–50 ml/min, continuous heparin infusion = 1000 IU/h.

REFERENCES

1. B. Charra, E. Calemard, M. Uzan *et al.* Carpal tunnel syndrome, shoulder pain and amyloid deposits in long-term hemodialysis patients. *Proc. Eur. Dial. Transplant. Ass.*, **21**, 291–295 (1984).

2. T. Bardin, D. Kuntz, J. Zingraff *et al.* Synovial amyloidosis in patients undergoing long term hemodialysis. *Arthritis Rheum.*, **28**, 1052–1058 (1985).

3. F. Gejyo, T. Yamada, S. Odani *et al.* A new form of amyloid protein associated with chronic hemodialysis was identified as β₂-microglobulin. *Biochem. Biophys. Res. Commun.*, **129**, 701–706 (1985).

4. S. Furuyoshi, N. Tani and R. Nakazawa. New adsorbents for extracorporeal removal of β₂-microglobulin. In: *Amyloid and Amyloidosis*, T. Isobe (Ed.), pp. 629–634, Plenum, New York (1988).

5. W. T. Nauta and R. F. Rekker (Eds). *The Hydrophobic Fragmental Constant.* Elsevier, Amsterdam (1977).

6. F. A. Karlsson, T. Groth, K. Sage *et al.* Turnover in humans β₂-microglobulin: the constant chain of HLA antigens. *Eur. J. Clin. Invest.*, **10**, 293–300 (1980).

Therapeutic Plasmapheresis (XII), pp. 785-788
T. Agishi *et al.* (Eds)
© VSP 1993

Practice of Plasmapheresis using Centrifugal Devices

S. YOKOYAMA and T. HOSOI

Kyoto Red Cross Blood Center, Kyoto, Japan

Key words: donor plasmapheresis; centrifugal device; Haemonetics PCS; Ultralite-PCS.

INTRODUCTION

Recently, the Haemonetics plasma collection system (PCS) and Ultralite PCS (U-PCS) have become common, essential and routine machines in Japanese Red Cross Blood Centers. These centrifugal devices are fully automated systems which can be used to collect platelet-poor plasma (PPP) or platelet-rich plasma (PRP). PPP collection is a widely used method for fractionation of plasma components such as albumin and blood coagulation factor VIII. Platelets obtained by PRP collection are used as a random platelet concentrate (PC) and plasma is used for fractionation of plasma components. These devices are compact and easy to use and all operations are computer-guided and the different operating parameters can be modified during the procedure. However, some problems exist in the practice of plasmaphereses, particularly in terms of machine maintenance, quality of disposable kit and operation procedure. On the other hand, the operator must master the structure and features of the automated device in addition to collecting good quality platelets and plasma. For the past several years we have managed apheresis practices using PCS and U-PCS in our blood center.

MATERIALS AND METHODS

In 1985, PCS, and in 1987, U-PCS, which is a refined model for mobile plasmaphereses, were introduced in our blood center. Since 1990 over 20 000 donor plasmaphereses were carried out with these two devices every year, and about 45% in all cases with PCS and 55% with U-PCS. U-PCS is mainly used by mobile teams at various sites outside the blood center.

The donors all passed the selection criteria for apheresis donation set by the Ministry of Health and Welfare. For blood access, a 16G or 17G needle with a back-hole was used. From 450 to 700 g of plasma (PPP or PRP) including ACD-A solution according to donor's body weight was collected in each procedure. We have prepared a standard manual of which method (PPP or PRP) will be appropriate for the donor based on the accessibility of the vein, donor's body weight, pre-platelet count and Hematocrit value (Ht). Table 1 shows our standard selection criteria for the apheresis method based on the donor's condition.

When executing the PRP method, it is necessary to improve platelet collection efficacy (total collected platelet count: over 1×10^{11}/bag) by adjusting the blood collection

Table 1.
Standard selection criteria for apheresis method

Collection method	Pre-platelet count ($\times 10^4/\mu$l)	Pre Ht (%)	Body weight (kg)
PPP	15–18	$\leqslant$ 50	[a]40–50
PRP	18–60	$\leqslant$ 50	$\geqslant$ 50

[a] Female.

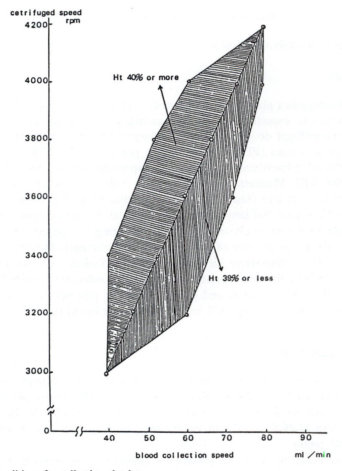

Figure 1. Conditions for collecting platelets.

pump speed and centrifuge speed of the bowl based on the donor's Ht (Fig. 1). In cases where the donor's body weight is 50 kg or less and pre-platelet count is $15 \times 10^4/\mu$l or less, the PPP method is executed. Our usual program parameters are shown in Table 2.

Our actual plasmarheresis technology with PCS or U-PCS is outlined below. The device draws donor's whole blood, mixes it with anticoagulant (ACD-A) in a prefixed ratio (1/16 for PPP, 1/12 for PRP) and fills a centrifuge bowl. When the bowl is filled with blood, PPP or PRP flows out and the draw cycle is completed, the bowl stops

Table 2.

Program parameters in Kyoto Red Cross Blood Center

Parameter	Pre-set value	Range	Steps
Cuff pressure	60 mmHg	0–200 mmHg	5 mmHg
Collection value	570 ml	0–1000 mmHg	10 ml
Blood pump speed			
draw PPP	80 ml/min	0–150 ml/min	5 ml/min
draw PRP	80 ml/min	0–150 ml/min	5 ml/min
return PPP	80 ml/min	0–150 ml/min	5 ml/min
return PRP	80 ml/min	0–150 ml/min	5 ml/min
Centrifuge speed			
PPP	5650 r.p.m.	2500–6000 r.p.m.	10 r.p.m.
PRP	4200 r.p.m.	2500–6000 r.p.m.	10 r.p.m.
Manual volume	200 ml	0–1500 ml	5 ml
Optics volume			
PPP	10 ml	0–1500 ml	5 ml
PRP	0 ml	0–1500 ml	5 ml

spinning and collected cellular components are pumped up through the feed tube and returned to the donor, then the next cycle starts. The procedure automatically ends when a pre-fixed plasma volume is obtained. An average of four to five cycles are needed to complete 500–600 g plasma collection within 40–50 min. It is important that an operator observes the donor's condition and the indicators on the device display panel.

This study examined device maintenance, disposable kit quality, problems which occurred during operation procedure (especially selection of the appropriate blood collection method and handling the machine), and quality of PPP or PRP obtained.

RESULTS

Device maintenance

In 1985, when PPP or PRP collection using PCS was begun, device trouble were frequently experienced with a few devices, including the inability to input the program, messages not appearing fully on the display panel, or the separator motor not functioning. After 1986 five new U-PCS and eight PCS devices were installed, none of these basic problems have occurred because of improvement of the devices and periodic dealer's inspection and maintenance services. However, with U-PCS, some incidents of malfunction of the bowl sensor, line sensor and optical sensor have occurred. These incidents all occurred when periodic inspection and maintenance services were not performed. Since 1987 the maintenance service's minimum requirement for the PCS and U-PCS has been designed. Our current maintenance services consist of cleaning the system lines, and assuring that the pump rollers are clean and free-rolling. It is necessary to write the date and type of service performed in the maintenance record book.

Quality of disposable kit

Since 1987 some quality problems with the kit were experienced. These problems were cases of defects of the bowl itself, so that the blood could not be returned to the donor during the return cycle. Another problem was leakage of blood from pinholes in the line tube and from the connecting part of the tube due to a defective kit. We believe the kit manufacturer has to make a greater effort to improve the quality of the products to avoid such problems.

Operation procedure

The average setting time required to install the kit to the device was 3 min. The average priming time with the kit was only 30 s, and even larger amounts of PPP or PRP (max 700 g) collection in each procedure can be performed within 50 min. However, operators sometimes make mistakes in setting the device or misunderstand the terms displayed on the panel. In some cases the procedure could not be completed due to dysfunction of the sensor, insufficient venous flow and blood leakage.

Quality of PPP or PRP

PPP collection using PCS or U-PCS exhibits perfect donor safety and a higher yield of plasma components. The yield of blood coagulation factor VIII and albumin were over 80%. When executing the PRP method, it is necessary to improve platelet collection efficiency by our indication showed in Fig 1. We have always obtained effective platelet counts (over 1×10^{11}/bag) from PRP collected.

DISCUSSION AND CONCLUSION

Plasmapheresis using PCS and U-PCS is widely used for PPP or PRP collection. These devices are more compact than other similar type devices and also are easy to operate. A number of reports [1–3] have described donor safety, operation procedure and quality of PPP or PRP collected. However, there are some problems resulting from device maintenance, defective kit and malfunction of the system (sensor, etc.). These problems also exist in other automated machines, and PCS and U-PCS are the superior devices which rarely experience these problems. When asked to select a device, the number of donors who chose the U-PCS was overwhelmingly high.

In order to improve platelet collection efficiency and reduce the time burden to the donors during PRP collection, operating conditions, such as the pump flow and centrifuge speed, must be adjusted based on the accessibility of the donor's vein, pre-platelet count value and Ht value. Thus the operator must master the operating technique.

It is concluded that any large-scale PPP or PRP collection program could be done safely and economically and could obtain sufficient source plasma and random PC.

REFERENCES

1. R. O. Gilcher. Plasmapheresis technology. *Vox Sang*, **51**, 33–39 (1986).
2. S. Yokoyama. Donor plasmapheresis with centrifuged method and its side effects. *Immunohaematology*, **10**, 184–188 (1988).
3. S. Yokoyama, T. Hosoi, Y. Maeda and K. Nanjo. The effect of frequent automated plasmapheresis on voluntary donors. *Jpn. J. Blood Transf. Med.*, **32**, 317–329 (1986).

Therapeutic Plasmapheresis (XII), pp. 789-792
T. Agishi *et al.* (Eds)
© VSP 1993

Cleaning of the Second Filter in Cryofiltration

M. MURAOKA, N. KAMII, K. ONODERA, M. TAKAHASHI,
H. WITMANOWSKI, J. MEGURO, K. KUKITA,
M. YONEKAWA and A. KAWAMURA

*Sapporo Hokuyu Hospital, Artificial Organ and Transplantation Hospital,
Sapporo, Japan*

Key words: cryofiltration; second filter; cleaning method.

INTRODUCTION

In cryofiltration, the loss of albumin and the supply of albumin are usually small. However, in washing out the cryogel trapped in the second filter when the inner pressure of the second filter reached 300 mmHg, not only the cryogel but also the plasma in the housing have to be washed away by saline solution by the following procedure. We tried to improve the procedure of washing out to save albumin.

METHODS

A (formal method): the second filter is washed out backward with 500 ml of saline solution. B (new method): the plasma in the housing of the second filter is forced out with 200 ml of saline solution prior to washing cryogel, then cryogel is washed out backward with 300 ml of saline solution. The two methods were applied to patients with rheumatoid arthritis, SLE and polymyositis. Serum protein, albumin and immunoglobulin were determined and compared in the two methods.

RESULTS

At first we tried *in vitro* cryofiltration with normal human plasma (Fig. 1). By method B, protein loss could be reduced in discharged solution and albumin supply could be decreased (Fig. 2). Furthermore, the reduction rate of immunoglobulin was significantly increased after changing the washing out procedure (Fig. 3).

CONCLUSIONS

  (i) By this method the protein loss could be reduced in the discharged solution and the albumin supply could be decreased.
 (ii) The reduction rate of immunoglobulin was significantly increased after changing the washing out procedure.

(iii) With this method the complications of hypotension could be decreased during cryofiltration.

(iv) This method might be useful not only in cryofiltration but also in double filtration plasmapheresis.

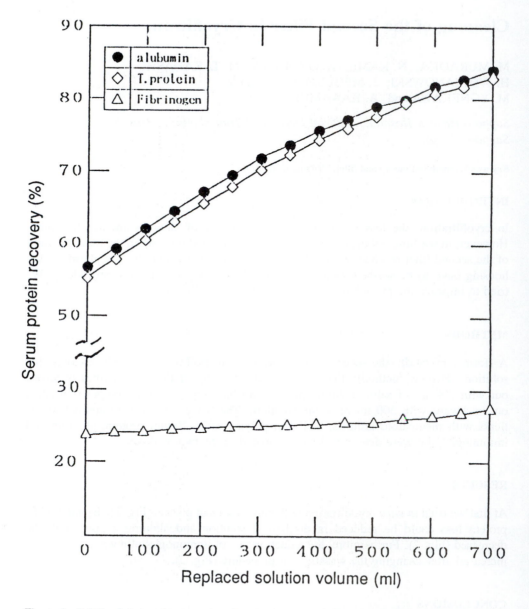

Figure 1. Relation between the serum protein recovery rate and the replaced solution volume. *In vitro* cryofiltration with normal human plasma (single pass).

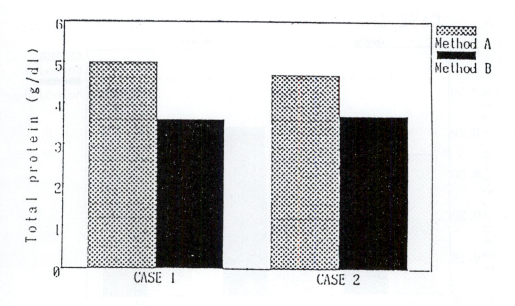

Amount of protein in discaharged solution

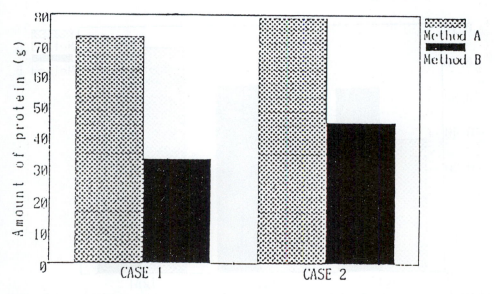

Figure 2. Top panel: total protein level in discharged solution. Bottom panel: amount of protein in discharged solution.

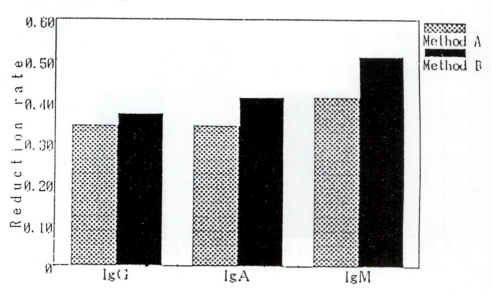

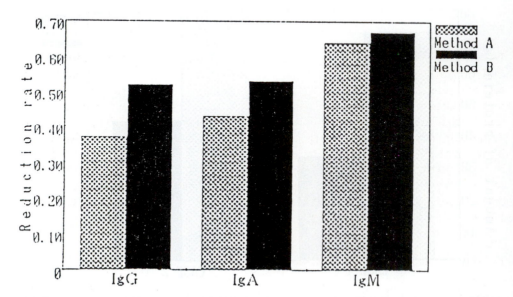

Figure 3. Reduction rate of immunoglobulin.

Therapeutic Plasmapheresis (XII), pp. 793-796
T. Agishi *et al*. (Eds)

Development of Selective Apheresis Devices: Application to Myasthenia Gravis Treatment

S. NAKAJI, K. OKA, M. TANIHARA, K. TAKAKURA and A. SUEOKA

Kuraray Co., Ltd, Kurashiki, Japan

Key words: myasthenia gravis; immunoadsorption; acetylcholine receptor; synthetic peptide; plasma fractionator.

INTRODUCTION

Myasthenia gravis (MG) is an autoimmune disorder in which neuromuscular transmission is impaired by anti-acetylcholine receptor (AChR) antibodies. It is of great importance to selectively remove these autoantibodies in the plasmapheresis treatment of MG.

This paper presents new types of apheresis devices for the treatment of MG. We have developed the plasma fractionator, EVAFLUX used in double filtration plasmapheresis (DFPP) and plasma immunoadsorption column, Medisorba MG.

PLASMA FRACTIONATOR (SECOND FILTER) IN DFPP: EVAFLUX

DFPP has been widely used in the treatment of various autoimmune diseases and hyperlipidemia, and its clinical usefulness has been demonstrated. In the DFPP treatment of MG with use of EVAL second filter, the reduction of anti-AChR antibodies as well as improvement of clinical symptoms has been reported [1]. As a second filter in DFPP, four types of EVAL filters with different pore sizes are presently available, i.e. 2A, 3A, 4A and 5A. The filter can be chosen according to the size of the target substance to be removed from the plasma. These filters have been improved with respect to their filtration performance. Of these filters EVAFLUX 2A has sieving coefficients of 0.62 for albumin and 0.19 for IgG, thus being the most suitable for selective removal of anti-AChR antibodies in MG treatment. The characteristic feature of new versions of EVAL second filters is presented in the Graphic Session (G-3) 200.

IMMUNOADSORPTION COLUMN: MEDISORBA MG

The anti-AChR antibodies involved in the pathogenesis of MG are classified into two subclasses; a blocking antibody and a binding antibody. The blocking antibody is known to block directly the ACh-binding with AChR, thus inducing MG (Fig. 1). Therefore, the removal of the blocking antibody is of importance in the treatment of MG. Takamori *et al.* [2] reported that the α183–200 segment of the *Torpedo californica* AChR is the

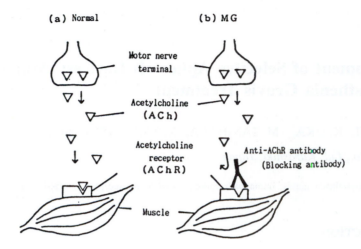

Figure 1. Mechanism of myasthenia gravis (schematic diagram).

ACh-binding site recognized by a blocking antibody, and this *Torpedo* peptide showed much more potent binding ability than the human peptide.

Based on these studies, we have designed a new immunoadsorbent for MG treatment by using the synthetic peptide (*Torpedo* α183–200, Fig. 2) as an affinity ligand to specifically remove the blocking antibody, as illustrated in Fig. 3. The immunoadsorbent column (Medisorba MG) we have recently developed is packed with 50 ml of porous cellulose beads (diameter 250 μm) immobilized covalently with this synthetic peptide and sterilized by autoclaving. The release of the peptide from the adsorbent was minimal. The safety of the immunoadsorbent has been confirmed by various toxicity tests. The size of Medisorba MG column is extremely small, with a plasma priming volume of only 17 ml (Fig. 4 and Table 1).

Table 1.
Specifications of immunoadsorption cartridge Medisorba MG

Adsorbent	
carrier	porous cellulose bead (diameter 250μm)
ligand	synthetic peptide
Filling liquid	physiological saline solution
Housing material	polypropylene
Shape of cartridge	cylindrical 34 mm Ø × 156 mm L
Volume	50 ml
Weight	145 g
Plasma priming volume	17 ml
Sterilization	steam autoclaving (121 °C, 20 min)

183
H-Lys-Lys-Gly-Trp-Lys-His-Trp-Val-Tyr-Tyr-Thr-Cys-Cys
200
-Pro-Asp-Thr-Pro-Tyr-Leu-Asp-Lys-Lys-Gly-OH

Figure 2. Amino acid sequence of the synthetic peptide corresponding to *Torpedo* α183–200.

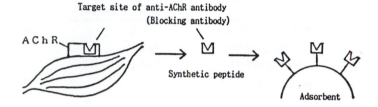

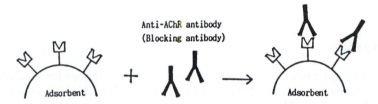

Figure 3. Adsorption mechanism of anti-AChR antibody by Medisorba MG, immunoadsorbent containing immobilized synthetic peptide of AChR (schematic diagram).

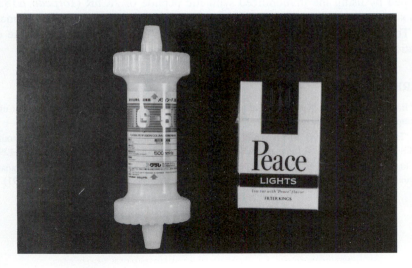

Figure 4. Immunoadsorption column Medisorba MG.

In the clinical evaluation [3], 77 treatments of plasma immunoadsorption were performed for 19 patients with MG at Kanazawa University and National Utano Hospital using a PVA plasma separator and KM-8800 monitor (Kuraray). The immunoadsorption treatment specifically removed the blocking antibody, without significantly reducing plasma protein levels, as shown in Table 2. Clinical improvement was found in 78% of the cases.

Table 2.
Removal rate of anti-AChR antibodies and plasma proteins in clinical tests

	Removal rate (%)
Anti-AChR antibody	
blocking antibody	40.2
binding antibody	12.4
Plasma protein	
total protein	5.7
albumin	2.4
IgG	10.2

CONCLUSIONS

We have developed two types of new selective apheresis devices for MG treatment, i.e. a plasma fractionator (EVAFLUX) used in DFPP and a plasma immunoadsorption column (Medisorba MG). Newly improved EVAFLUX 2A has sieving coefficients of 0.62 for albumin and 0.19 for IgG, and is most suitable for selective removal of anti-AChR antibodies in the DFPP treatment. To increase selectivity in anti-AChR antibody removal, a new immunoadsorbent against a blocking antibody (Medisorba MG) has been developed by using the immobilized synthetic peptide of AChR (*Torpedo* α183–200). It was shown that the blocking antibody was specifically removed in the plasma perfusion. The usefulness of these apheresis devices has been demonstrated in the clinical evaluation.

REFERENCES

1. T. Iida, K. Tanaka, M. Kitamura *et al.* Two cases of myasthenia gravis with improvement of clinical symptoms by plasmapheresis. *Jpn. J. Kidney Dialys.*, **22**, 735–739 (1987).
2. M. Takamori, S. Okumura, M. Nagata *et al.* Myasthenogenic significance of synthetic α-subunit peptide 183–200 of *Torpedo californica* and human acetylcholine receptor. *J. Neurol. Sci.*, **85**, 121–129 (1988).
3. Y. Ide, S. Okumura and M. Takamori. Treatment of myasthenia gravis with a specific immunoadsorbent bound to acetylcholine receptor peptide α183–200. *Ther. Plasmapheresis*, **9**, 147–152 (1991).

Therapeutic Plasmapheresis (XII), pp. 797-800
T. Agishi *et al.* (Eds)
© VSP 1993

Modified Polypropylene Membranes for Plasma Separation

M. ONISHI, K. SHIMURA, S. NAGAKI, T. FUJII, A. YAGISHITA, Y. SEITA, S. YAMASHITA, M. SADO and A. TAKAHASHI

Terumo Co. Ltd, R&D Center, Kanagawa, Japan

Key words: plasma separation; donor plasmapheresis; hemolysis; priming; modified polypropylene membrane.

INTRODUCTION

In order to collect large quantities of plasma from donors, it is important to develop a membrane-based donor plasmapheresis system that is designed to be utilized under various circumstances, such as mobile collection sites and at the bed side. We have developed microporous membranes that are made of polypropylene (PP) [1] and employed them in the disk-shape plasma separator of the constant pressure apheresis system II (CAPS-II) [2]. However, this plasma separator is of the wettype, which required priming by physiological saline prior to use. On the other hand, when blood first comes into contact with dry hydrophilic membranes, we observed hemolysis. In order to avoid this 'hemolysis', it was necessary to prime the membrane filters with saline or fill up microporous spaces inside the membranes with saline [3].

We produced a new composite membrane in order to abbreviate these problems. We describe the features of this innovative membrane in this paper. Since this new membrane does not cause hemolysis when blood first comes into contact with the membrane in a dry state, it does not require priming. We also comment on the possible mechanism by which this membrane does not cause hemolysis.

MATERIALS AND METHODS

We manufactured a microporous membrane with pore diameter of $0.45 \mu m$ and a wall thickness of $80 \mu m$ by our own method, namely a thermally-induced phase separation method from a mixture of PP, liquid paraffin and a nucleating agent [1]. The PP membrane was modified by surface graft copolymerization [4].

Wetting time, an indicator of hydrophylic property of microporous membranes, was determined according to ASTM D4199 (method B) procedures as follows. The membrane was placed on the surface of water. Wetting time is defined as the time required for water to travel through the pores and reach the opposite side of the membrane until it gets completely wetted.

Hemolysis caused by the hydrophilic membranes was assessed by the following procedure. Fresh bovine blood anticoagulated with ACD-A was run through a mini-module with a dry membrane without priming it by saline. Blood flow rate and wall shear rate were 20 ml/min and 400 s^{-1}, respectively. Transmembrane pressure was kept below 25 mmHg. Hemolysis ratio was defined by the following formula after measuring free hemoglobin concentrations (C_{Hb}) in plasma before and after the separation:

$$\text{Hemolysis ratio} = \frac{(C_{Hb} \text{ in the plasma filtered during the first 5 min})}{(C_{Hb} \text{ in the plasma from preblood by centrifugation})}.$$

In vitro plasma separation experiments using a PP-g-PMEA membrane was performed by the use of a disk-shape module with 0.16 m^2 effective area and a constant pressure plasma separation system without a priming step. The bag containing preblood was pressed with a pressure of 120 mmHg. The recovery rates of various protein components were calculated by the following equation:

$$\text{Recovery (\%)} = \frac{(\text{concentration in the plasma filtered})}{\substack{(\text{concentration in the plasma obtained} \\ \text{from preblood by centrifugation})}} \times 100.$$

RESULTS AND DISCUSSION

The PP membrane was successfully converted to a hydrophilic membrane by graft copolymerization of N,N-dimethylacrylamide (DMAA) or 2-methoxyethylacrylate (MEA) without using any wetting agent such as hydrophilic chemicals or surfactants [4]. This fact indicates that hydrophilic polymers are graft-polymerized on all surface areas of the membrane including pore walls and that water molecules can penetrate freely into the micropores and pass through the membrane without applying any pressure. Thus grafted polymers will not be washed away since they are chemically bound onto PP surface. PDMAA is a water-soluble polymer and more hydrophilic than PMEA. Consequently, the wetting time of PP-g-PDMAA is shorter than that of PP-g-PMEA.

Table 1.
Hemolysis ratios of modified PP membranes

Membrane	Wetting time (s)	Hemolysis ratio
PP-g-P(DMAA-EA)	30	1.0
PP-g-PMEA	10	1.0
PP-g-P(DMAA-MEA)	5	3.5
PP-g-PDMAA	< 1	7.8
PP coated with EVAL	< 1	7.8

PP, polypropylene; DMAA, N,N-dimethylacryamide; EA, ethylacrylate; MEA, 2-methoxyethylacrylate; EVAL, ethylene-vinylalcohol copolymer.

Table 1 shows a relationship between wetting time and hemolysis ratio. The membranes with a shorter wetting time caused hemolysis at the beginning of plasma separation. This type of hemolysis is seen when erythrocytes are trapped rapidly in the micropores of the membrane filter by capillary attraction and lysed. On the other hand, less hydrophilic membranes with a long wetting time, such as PP-g-PMEA, do not cause hemolysis. This can be explained by the fact that plasma penetrates into the pores slowly because of the less hydrophilic property of the membrane and consequently erythrocytes are not trapped in the micropores as badly. Our data may indicate that dry-type plasma separators with PP-g-PMEA membranes do not require priming with saline prior to use. Thus, separation procedures are simplified by eliminating a priming step. Another advantage is that the collected plasma will not be diluted by saline.

The PP-g-PMEA membrane has almost the same pore size, water filtration rate and plasma filtration velocity as the original PP membrane. An *in vitro* plasma separation experiment by a dry-type plasma separator with PP-g-PMEA was conducted without a priming step, using 460 ml fresh human blood with ACD-A. Hemolysis was not seen in this experiment as expected. The obtained plasma was not diluted by saline, so that the recovery rates of various plasma components were nearly 100% (Table 2). Another reason for the excellent recovery may be due to the PMEA grafted layer which could prevent proteins from adhering to the membrane. The PP membrane has lower recovery rates for coagulation factors such as fibrinogen when compared with those of total proteins and albumin [5]. This can be explained by the fact that hydrophobic polymers such as polyethylene and polypropylene adsorb these proteins through strong hydrophobic interactions [6].

Table 2.
Recovery rates of plasma components by PP-g-PMEA

Measurements	TP	Alb	T-cho	Fbg	F.VIII:C
Recovery (%)	100.0	102.1	99.6	99.7	99.1

($n = 3$, mean).

In order to test a hemo-compatibility of the membrane, C3a, C5a and β-TG levels were measured (Table 3). Although C3a concentration was higher after plasma separation, activation of these complement factors by PP-g-PMEA was found to be relatively mild compared with hydrophilic membranes that were already clinically used [7]. Since PP-g-PMEA does not contain reactive groups such as hydroxy groups, it does not activate C3 through the mechanism involving covalent attachment of C3 to the reactive groups [8, 9]. It is reported that anaphylatoxins are rapidly inactivated *in vivo* by carboxypeptidase and that more than 10^3ng/ml C3a and C4a can be found in the blood which was stored for a prolonged period of time to be utilized for transfusion [3]. Therefore, activation of complement factors by PP-g-PMEA may not present a serious problem.

Table 3.
Release of β-TG, f-Hb and complement activation by PP-g-PMEA

Measurements	Pre	Post	Plasma
f-Hb	0.6 ± 0.5	4.2 ± 1.1	0.5 ± 0.4
β-TG	78 ± 23	160 ± 14	87 ± 19
C3a	506 ± 61	581 ± 182	858 ± 393
C5a	9 ± 3	14 ± 7	9 ± 3

($n = 3$, mean $\pm$ SD).

CONCLUSIONS

A new type of hydrophilic membrane for plasma separation, PP-g-PMEA, was success-fully produced by conjugating PMEA onto PP membrane. The main advantage of this membrane is that it does not require priming by saline prior to use although it is in a dry state. A disk-shape plasma separator with this membrane had an excellent capacity for plasma separation, enabling good recovery of plasma components.

REFERENCES

1. Y. Seita and M. Onishi. A flat permeable membrane. *US Patent* 4,743,375 (1988).
2. T. A. Takahashi, T. Nakase *et al.* Clinical evaluation of the constant apheresis system type II. In: *Therapeutic Plasmapheresis (X)*, ICAOT Press, Cleveland (1992).
3. S. Sekiguchi, T. A. Takahashi *et al.* A New type of blood component collector: plasma separation using gravity without any electrical devices. *Vox Sang*, **58**, 182–187 (1990).
4. M. Onishi, K. Shimura, Y. Seita *et al.* Preparation and properties of plasma-initiated graft copolymerized membranes for blood plasma separation. *Radiat. Phys. Chem.*, **39**, 569–576 (1992).
5. T. A. Takahashi, M. Hosoda *et al.* A new donor plasmapheresis system with disk type membrane separator. *Jpn. J. Transfus. Med.*, **36**, 418–423 (1991).
6. J. D. Andrade (Ed). *Surface and Interfacial Aspects of Biomedical Polymers, Vol.2, Protein Adsorption.* Plenum, New York (1985).
7. T. Takaoka, J. B. Goldcamp, Y. Abe *et al.* Biocompatibility of membrane plasmaseparation. *Trans. Am. Soc. Artif. Intern. Organs*, **30**, 347–351 (1984).
8. S. A. Law. Non-enzymic activation of the covalent binding reaction of the complement protein C3. *Biochem. J.*, **211**, 381–389 (1983).
9. D. E. Chenoweth. Complement activation produced by biomaterials. *Artif. Organs*, **12**, 502–504 (1988).

Therapeutic Plasmapheresis (XII), pp. 801-805
T. Agishi *et al.* (Eds)
© VSP 1993

Immunoadsorption for ABO-Incompatible Kidney Transplantation

H. NAKASHIMA, A. IHARA,   T. KIHARA, M. ABE and T. MARUYAMA

Research and Development Center, Kawasumi Laboratories, Inc., Sagamihara, Japan

Key words: immunoadsorbents; ABO blood substance; anti-ABO antibodies; ABO-incompatibility; kidney transplantation.

INTRODUCTION

The ABO blood type is an important factor for transfusions and organ transplantations. ABO-incompatibility between donor and recipient has made transplantation impossible, especially kidney transplantation because of a high incidence of hyperacute rejection episodes after transplantation. However, it may be possible now to overcome ABO-incompatibility to have such transplantation if recipient's isoagglutinins are removed before transplantation by plasmapheresis and/or immunoadsorption (IA). In Japan, a multicenter trial of ABO-incompatible kidney transplantation, using an immunoadsorbent column called Biosynsorb™ (BS) to remove anti-A or anti-B antibody, has been performed since November 1989. In this report, we will describe basic and clinical data regarding specific-removal of anti-ABO antibodies by BSs.

MATERIALS AND METHODS

In vitro studies

We used Biosynsorb™-A (BS-A) and Biosynsorb™-B (BS-B), which were immunoadsorbent columns containing chemically synthesized human blood group A- and B-trisaccharides. The antigenic determinants are N-acetyl-D-galactosamine which expresses blood group A for BS-A and D-galactose which expresses blood group B for BS-B, respectively. The BSs were evaluated by batch and single pool assays. For batch assay, 1 g of BS-A or BS-B and 10 ml of human O plasma were incubated for 1 h at 37°C. After incubation, plasma was collected. The single pool assay simulated clinical perfusions was performed using small columns containing 1 g of BSs. The 30 ml of human O plasma as pool plasma was continuously stirred at 100 r.p.m., then recirculated through the column at 18 ml/h at 37°C. Samples were collected each 1 ml from inlet and outlet of a column at 2 and 5 h after recirculation. The collected samples were measured: total protein (TP), albumin (Alb), immunoglobulins (Igs) and electrolytes. The anti-A or -B titers of IgM and IgG types in plasma were also determined by standard saline agglutination test [1].

802   *H. Nakashima* et al.

CLINICAL STUDIES

All data were obtained from a multicenter trial of ABO-incompatible kidney transplantation by 'BS'. The BS, 45 × 120 mm column containing 80 g of immunoadsorbent described above was sterilized with ethyleneoxide gas, washed with 1 l of heparinized saline followed by washing with appropriate saline. During 7 days before transplantation, 51 of patients were treated by plasma-IA using BSs at 3–4 times and 31 of them were treated by double filtration plasmapheresis (DFPP) once before IA. Changes in plasma components and antibody titers were measured before or after IA by the protocols previously described [2].

RESULTS

Changes in plasma components and antibody titers in batch assays are shown in Fig. 1. BSs did not affect to plasma components, but could specifically remove anti-ABO titers. Indeed, BS-A could remove anti-A IgM from 1:128 to 1:8 and anti-A IgG from 1:128 to 1:16. BS-B could remove anti-B IgM from 1:32 to 1:1 and anti-B IgG from 1:32 to 1:4 in experiment 1. Similar results were obtained from experiment 2. In the single pool assay, BS-A could remove anti-A IgM from 1:128 to 1:8 for 5 h and BS-B could remove anti-B IgM from 1:32 to 1:1 for 5 h. Similar results were found in antibody titers in IgG (Fig. 2).

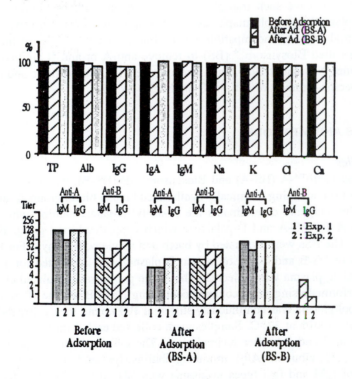

Figure 1. Changes of anti-ABO antibodies and plasma components by batch adsorption *in vitro* assays.

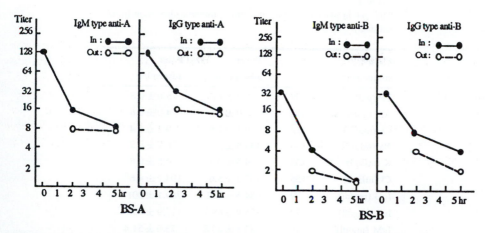

Figure 2. Changes of anti-blood antibodies in single pool assay (*in vitro*) using small BS columns.

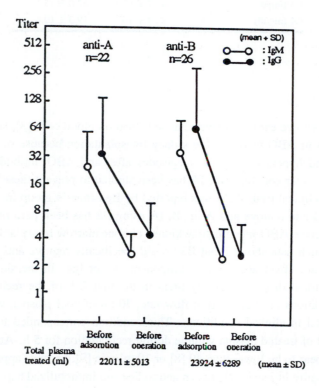

Figure 3. Reduction of anti-A and -B antibody titers before adsorption and before transplantation.

Clinical results concerning plasma components and antibody titers are summarized in Fig. 3 and Table 1. BSs showed specific-removal activities to antibody titers in plasma and did not affect plasma components during IA except Igs as well as *in vitro* data.

Table 1.
Changes in plasma components during immunoadsorption (clinical data)

Plasma components	n	Before adsorption	After adsorption
TP (g/dl)	139	5.9 ± 1.0	5.6 ± 0.8
Alb (g/dl)	110	4.0 ± 0.6	4.0 ± 0.6
Ca (mg/dl)	112	9.1 ± 1.5	9.2 ± 1.4
Na (mEq/l)	136	138.8 ± 3.3	138.7 ± 4.5
K (mEq/l)	135	4.5 ± 0.7	4.5 ± 0.8
Cl (mEq/l)	135	103.3 ± 5.6	104.1 ± 4.6
IgG (mg/dl)	79	884.5 ± 332.2	789.1 ± 301.1
IgA (mg/dl)	79	128.9 ± 68.7	113.9 ± 60.3
IgM (mg/dl)	79	83.8 ± 60.5	73.0 ± 51.4
CH50 (U/ml)	81	23.9 ± 12.1	16.8 ± 9.7
C3 (mg/dl)	93	41.7 ± 17.3	32.0 ± 13.1
C4 (mg/dl)	94	22.4 ± 9.7	19.3 ± 10.6

DISCUSSION

ABO antigens evolve earlier on epithelial cells than on blood cells [3], and may cause a major problem in ABO-incompatible kidney transplantation because of acute endothelium injury and hyperacute rejection episodes after anti-ABO antibodies react ABO antigens on vascular endothelium. IA has been studied to prevent these problems. The first result for clinical trial of BS was reported by Bensinger's group in 1981 [4]. Until recently, in order to remove anti-A or -B, IA using BS has been performed on patients who would achieve ABO-incompatible kidney or bone marrow transplantations [2, 5–7]. Our *in vitro* batch data showed that BSs could specifically remove anti-blood antibody titers and did not affect any plasma component except Igs. In the single pool assay, BS gave a marked drop of antibody titers in the first 2 h of the recirculation. This model, at conditions of at 18 ml/h of flow rate, 30 ml of pool plasma, was a simulated perfusion model in clinical conditions. This condition corresponded to 24 ml/min of flow rate, 7.2 l of treated plasma volume during recirculation for 5 h. An optimum flow rate would appear to be lower than 40 [8] or 10 ml/min [9], because appropriate contact time would require in reaction between antibodies and immobilized haptens. Therefore, the number of plasma volumes to be treated will depend directly on the flow rate and time. Although direct hemoperfusion has been reported [6], plasma perfusion may be useful because very fine particles in plasma can be removed by a post filter attached to the BS column. In clinical studies, 3 to 4 times of plasma-IA using BS could reduce isoagglutinins to acceptable transplant levels, below less than 1:16 titers, during 7 days before transplantation [7].

CONCLUSIONS

The Biosynsorb™ system could specifically remove anti-A or -B in plasma *in vitro* and clinically without any effect on another plasma components. Thus, it seems that Biosynsorb™ will be able to be used in ABO-incompatible kidney transplantation.

REFERENCES

1. F. K. Widmann (Ed.). *Technical Manual.* AABB (1985).
2. T. Agishi, K. Takahashi, T. Yagisawa *et al.* Immunoadsorption of anti-A or anti-B antibody for successful kidney transplantation between ABO incompatible pairs and its limitation. Japanese Biosynsorb Research Group. *ASAIO Trans.*, **37**, PM496–498 (1991).
3. R. Oriol, J. Le Pendu and R. Mollicone. Genetics of ABO, H, Lewis, X and related antigens. *Vox Sang,* **51**, 161–171 (1986).
4. W. I. Bensinger, D. A. Baker, C. D. Buckner *et al.* Immunoadsorption for removal of A and B blood-group antibodies. *N. Engl. J. Med.*, **304**, 160–162 (1981).
5. K. Watanabe, N. Kobayashi, K. Nakamura *et al.* An example of ABO-incompatible bone marrow transplant by use of immunoadsorbent. In: *Jpn. Clin. Haematol. Conf. Abs.*, p. 252 (1983).
6. R. Raja, R. McAlack, M. Mendex *et al.* Technical aspects of antibody immunoadsorption prior to ABO-incompatible renal transplant. *Transplant. Proc.*, **19**, 4525–4527 (1987).
7. K. Ota, K. Takahashi, T. Agishi *et al.* Multicenter trial of ABO-incompatible kidney transplantation. Japanese Biosynsorb ABO-incompatible kidney transplant study group. *Transplant. Int.*, **5** (Suppl. 1), S 40–43 (1992).
8. M. Kaplan and M. A. Mazid. Flow rate dependence of *in vitro* removal of anti-A and anti-B antibodies by immunoadsorbents with synthetic oligosaccharides representing blood group substances. *Int. J. Artif. Organs*, **12**, 799-804 (1989).
9. Y. Sasaki, H. Ogiwara, M. Mineshima *et al.* Immunoadsorption technique for removal of A and B blood-group antibodies. *Jpn. J. Artif. Organs*, **15**, 1659–1662 (1986).

Therapeutic Plasmapheresis (XII), pp. 807-810
T. Agishi *et al.* (Eds)
© VSP 1993

New Blood Processing Devices for Donor Plasmapheresis

Y. TAKENAKA, J. ISHIHARA, T. INOSHITA, H. NISHI,
T. TAKAHASHI[1] and S. SEKIGUCHI[1]

Asahi Medical Co., Ltd, Japan
[1]*Hokkaido Red Cross, Japan*

Key words: membrane; donor; plasmapheresis; leukocyte; depleted.

INTRODUCTION

In 1991 in Japan, about 500 000 l of plasma was collected by donor plasmapheresis for production of the coagulation factors used in domestic hemophilia therapy.

Asahi Medical has been involved for nearly two decades in development of blood treatment systems. In 1979, it introduced the world's first hollow fiber plasma separator for therapeutic use. Experience and development since then has brought continuing progress in plasma separation systems and has now led to new systems for donor plasmapheresis and a blood component collector based on a hollow fiber membrane.

APC-4000, Asahi Plasma Collector, is an automatic high-performance system for donor plasmapheresis. BCC-I-SP, Blood Component Collector, is one in a series of gravity-driven systems for separation and collection of red cell concentrate and plasma.

MATERIALS AND METHODS

APC-4000 system

This system consists of an APC-4000 machine and a disposable kit. This machine houses a blood pump, an anticoagulant pump, two air detectors, two pressure sensors and a touch panel display. Operation is controlled by a CPU. It weighs 14 kg and is smaller and lighter than any other donor plasmapheresis machine now on the market.

The disposable kit consists of a membrane plasma separator, blood tubing and two bags. These are connected beforehand. The plasma separation membrane is made of polyethylene by melt-spinning and heat-stretching. It is coated by hydrophilic polymer, ethylene-vinylalcohol or hydrophilic polyester. The average pore size is about 0.25 microns. The pores are charged with a small quantity of saline, for smooth blood flow without saline priming or rinsing.

On this system, blood is infused with anticoagulant and drawn from the donor, passing unaffected through the plasma separator, and collecting in the blood bag. When the blood bag is filled with blood, blood pump rotation is reversed and blood flows from the blood bag into the plasma separator, where plasma is separated, and then back to the donor.

BCC-I-SP

This disposable kit consists of a membrane plasma separator, a leukocyte removal filter, Sepacell RS-200 blood tubing and four bags. The first bag containing anticoagulant is for blood collection, the second bag containing additive solution is for red cell concentrate, the third is for separated plasma and the fourth is for additive solution for recovering residual blood in the leukocyte removal filter and plasma separator. These are connected beforehand as in the APC-4000 kit.

At first collected blood flows into Sepacell and then into the plasma separator, where plasma is separated, and then leukocyte depleted red cells flow into the RCC bag.

RESULTS

APC-4000 system

Table 1 shows the plasma collection time with various plasma collectors, as demonstrated at the Japan Society of Blood Transfusion. The APC-4000 system collected 450 ml of plasma in less than 30 min.

Table 1.
Plasma collection time with various collectors

	Donor number	Needle to needle time for 450 ml of plasma (min)
APC-4000	13	25.8 ± 1.6
NDP-200	8	42.0 ± 5.5
DONEX-100	5	40.9 ± 2.9
ULTRALITE-PCS	1	32.9

Table 2.
Recovery of plasma components ($n = 13$)

Plasma component	Recovery yield (%)
Total protein	95.0 ± 2.7
Albumin	95.0 ± 2.5
GPT	95.7 ± 17.2
BUN	98.1 ± 3.9
Total cholesterol	90.8 ± 2.5

Table 2 shows the permeability of plasma components using APC-4000 as observed in the same demonstration. The recovery rate was well over 95% for various plasma components, but total cholesterol was a little lower.

Table 3 shows the data on the safety of APC-4000 with hydrophilic polyester coated membranes. As shown, the level of complement activation was low. The activation of platelet and coagulation factor was also slight.

Table 3.
Safety features of APC-4000 ($n = 10$)

	C3a (ng/ml)	PF-4 (ng/ml)	FPA (ng/ml)
Pre	162.2 ± 62.6	5.0 ± 2.6	7.0 ± 8.0
100 g in	172.9 ± 36.3	7.0 ± 8.0	3.9 ± 1.6
100 g out	261.7 ± 84.1	24.4 ± 25.1	10.2 ± 9.5
Post	166.6 ± 75.8	8.2 ± 6.1	10.6 ± 10.0
Collected plasma	460.4 ± 269.9	48.2 ± 30.5	23.1 ± 24.9

BCC-I-SP

Separation performance of BCC-I-SP is shown in Table 4. About 200 ml of plasma and 350 ml of SAGM added red cell concentrate were obtained from 470 ml of whole blood, in an average time of 30 min.

Table 5 shows the removal of blood cell components and other performance parameters obtained with the BCC-I-SP. The average leukocyte removal rate of 5.49±0.53 $\log_{10}$ was quite high. The red cell recovery rate was 94.1% and the platelet removal rate was 99.6%.

Table 4.
Separation performance of BCC-I-SP

Whole blood (ml)	Separated plasma (ml)	RCC SAGM (ml)	Treatment time (min)
470.4 ± 11.5	197.4 ± 24.1	348.4 ± 21.6	30.7 ± 5.2

Table 5.
Blood cell change using BCC-I-SP

Hct of whole blood	Hct of RCC+SAGM	Red cell recovery (%)	WBC removal ($\log_{10}$)	Platelet removal (%)
38.2 ± 2.7	48.6 ± 4.2	94.1 ± 1.3	5.49 ± 0.53	99.6 ± 0.6

DISCUSSION

For donor plasmapheresis, it is important to develop a plasma collection system with high safety, easy handling, small-size and light-weight machine; and high performance such as fast collection time. Asahi Medical has been investigating a new plasma collection system with membrane to meet these demands, and has developed the APC-4000. The plasma separation membrane is made with polyethylene coated by hydrophilic polymer. This membrane has high plasma separation performance and it is not necessary to prime or rinse with saline.

In order to develop a small machine, it is important to simplify the extracorporeal system. The blood circuit of APC-4000 is simple, so the machine components of this are fewer than others. The weight of 14 kg of this machine is the lightest on the market.

As shown in Table 1, APC-4000 collected 450 ml of plasma in less than 30 min, well under the time required even by other membrane or centrifugal machines. Concerning the protein permeability, the recovery rate was over 95% for all of the protein, but it was somewhat lower for cholesterol, because of adherence to the membrane. So, it is suggested that by using this membrane, chylomicron in plasma can be removed. As shown in Table 3, by using hydrophilic polyester coated membrane, the activation of complement and coagulation system was slight, and the release of platelet factor was small.

On the other hand, the world's first gravity-driven membrane plasma collection system was announced by Dr Gurland in 1983. In Japan the system was not widely adopted, however, because it required a long plasma collection time and a complicated saline rinsing and priming process. Asahi Medical has long been studying gravity-driven membrane systems for separation of whole blood. This has led to the BCC-I systems [1], developed in collaboration with the Japan Red Cross Hokkaido Blood Center. This system can separate and collect plasma and red cell concentrate from whole blood using a plasma separation membrane. BCC-I-SP is the combination of BCC-I and a high performance leukocyte removal filter, Sepacell RS-200. As shown in Tables 4 and 5, whole blood is easily separated into leukocyte depleted RCC and plasma with only gravity. This leukocyte removal rate of 5.5 $\log_{10}$ is quite high. This is perhaps due to the 30 min processing time.

CONCLUSION

(i) APC-4000 system collected 450 ml of plasma in less than 30 minutes.
(ii) Recovery of plasma components was sufficiently high.
(iii) The activation of complement, coagulation system and platelets with APC-4000 was slight.
(iv) BCC-I-SP separated whole blood into leukocyte depleted RCC and plasma with only gravity.

REFERENCE

1. S. Sekiguchi, T. Takahashi *et al.* A new type of blood component collector. *Vox Sang*, **58**, 182–187 (1990).

Therapeutic Plasmapheresis (XII), pp. 811-814
T. Agishi *et al.* (Eds)
© VSP 1993

In vitro Serum (or Plasma)–Material Interaction

K. SAWADA, P. S. MALCHESKY,[1] J. M. GUIDUBALDI,[1] A. SUEOKA,[1]
S. NAKAYAMA,[1] M. KANO and T. SHIMOYAMA

Department of Internal Medicine IV, Hyogo College of Medicine, Hyogo, Japan
[1]*Department of Biomedical Engineering and Applied Therapeutics,*
The Cleveland Clinic Foundation, Ohio, USA

Key words: serum; plasma; material; interaction.

INTRODUCTION

It has been reported that hydroxyl group percent relates to complement activation [1];
however, our previous report suggested that bulk hydroxyl percent does not correlate
with membrane reactivity and surface property analyses may be more important in
quantitating their biocompatibility properties [2]. This study evaluates the relationship
between bulk hydroxyl and surface oxygen percent and serum/plasma–material interactions.

MATERIALS AND METHODS

Hydroxyl percent was calculated based on the bulk chemical structure of polymers.
Surface oxygen percents of native membranes were determined by electron spectroscopy
for chemical analysis (ESCA) [3].

Serum/plasma–material interactions were evaluated using six types of mini-membrane
modules including cellulose triacetate (CA), Cuprophan (CP), ethylene vinyl alcohol copolymers (EVAL), copolymer of acrylonitrile, methylene acrylate and acrylic
acid (PAN), polysulfone (PD-F) and a polymer alloy of polysulfone and polyvinyl pro-
lidone (PS-K).

The same five individuals' serums or plasmas were used to evaluate all materials
which have been constructed from the hemodialysis membranes by a single manufacturer, Kuraray Co., Japan. All membrane modules have 500 cm^2 of surface area and
are sterilized by 3% formadehyde solution.

Serums or plasmas were prepared from freshly drawn blood obtained by consent from
normal healthy donors. Twenty five ml of each serum or plasma/module was perfused
through only the inside of the mini-modules from top to bottom using a multi-channel
mini-pump. The pump flow rate used was 0.5 ml/min/module. As a sham control,
serum or plasma was perfused through the circuit without a module. Samples were
taken from pre- and each post-perfusion for measurements of biochemical solutes such
as total protein (TP), albumin (Alb), total cholesterol (TC), immunoglobulins (IgG, IgA,
IgM), complements (C3, C4, C5), and their des Arg components (C3a, C4a, C5a). The

individual serums from each perfusion were used to evaluate autologous mononuclear cell transformation function (MNCTF) to three mitogens: concanavalin A (Con A), phytohemaglutinin (PHA) and pokeweed mitogen (PWM). For the evaluation of the coagulation system, the concentration of fibrinogen, prothrombin time (PT), activated partial thromboplastin time (APTT) and thrombin time (TT) were measured using the plasmas. The differences between each true and sham perfusion and the percent changes from the sham among the six membranes were compared with paired *t*-tests. A *P* value of less than 0.05 is considered as a statistically significant difference.

RESULTS

CA, CP, EVAL, PAN, PS-F, and PS-K have 0, 31.5, 30.4, 1.5, 0 and 0% of hydroxyl, and the surface oxygen percents were 34.1, 37.5, 25.7, 9.7, 14.6 and 15.4%, respectively (Table 1). The differences of all biochemical solutes (TP, Alb, TC) for PAN and both PS membranes were significantly lower than sham and their percent changes were also lower than CA, CP and EVAL (Table 1). The differences of total protein and total cholesterol (TC) for CA were significantly lower than sham and their percent changes were also lower than CP and EVAL. The only significant decrease of TC was found in CP and EVAL versus sham. The decreases of immunoglobulins (IgG, M) for PAN and IgA for both PS membranes were significantly lower than sham, however, there were no significant percent changes among the membranes (Table 1). The differences of C3 for CA and of C3 and C4 for PAN and both PS membranes were significantly lower than sham and these percent changes were also significantly lower than CP and EVAL. The differences of C5 for PAN and both PS membranes were significantly lower than sham and these percent changes were also lower than CP. Though there was the tendency for all membranes to exhibit activation for all complements, there were no statistically significant differences in the activated complement components between true and sham perfusions. The percent change of C3a for PS-K was significantly lower versus CP and the percent change of C4a for PS-K was significantly lower than CA, EVAL and PS-F. The differences of MNCTF to all three mitogens for CA and CP were significantly suppressed versus sham and their percent changes were also greater than PAN and both PS membranes except PHA-induced MNCTF for CP. The only tendency of enhanced PHA-induced MNCTF was found for PS-K versus CA and CP (Table 1). There was a tendency of decreasing fibrinogen by perfusion over all membranes; however, statistically significant decreases of fibrinogen were found for only EVAL, PAN and PS-F versus sham. The only statistically significant prolongation of APTT was found for EVAL versus sham and its percent was also significantly greater than CA and CP (Table 1).

CONCLUSION

As no significant differences were noted in the C3a, C4a and C5a des Arg changes for CA and CP versus sham and differences were noted in MNCTF to the three mitogens for these versus sham and other membranes, this suggests that these individual components do not suppress MNCTF and multifactorial causes may be responsible or other yet unidentified humoral factors may be causative for suppression of MNCTF. Modification of cellulose by acetylation to reduce its hydroxyl content did not change the activation of

Table 1.
Percent changes vs sham control

	CA (n = 5)	CP (n = 5)	EVAL (n = 5)	PAN (n = 5)	PS-F (n = 5)	PS-K (n = 5)
−OH%	0	31.5	30.4	1.5	0	0
=O%	34.1	37.5	25.7	9.7	14.6	15.4
TP	−4.8±2*,c	−2.3±2.4	−1.1±2.5	−7.9±3*,d	−7.4±2.7*,d	−9.9±3*,d
Alb	−2.4±3	−0.4±1	0.0±0	−6.6±3*,d	−5.6±2.7*,d	−8.4±3*,d
TC	−4.9±1*,c	−2.3±1*	−1.7±1*	−6.9±3*,c	−6.7±2.8*,c	−8.7±4*,d
IgG	−8.4±5.5	−6.1±6.5	−4.5±6.5	−10.5±2*	−9.9±4	−9.5±4
IgA	−3.2±5.6	5.6±8.3	−1.8±3.2	−6.4±7	−4.9±3*	−9.2±7*
IgM	−7.6±6.6	−2.8±8.7	−5.1±9.3	−8.8±2*	−5.3±4	−1.7±9
C3	−5.7±2.7*,c	−1.3±2.7	0.5±2	−9.5±2*,c	−5.1±2.8*,c	−7.5±2*,c
C4	−4.2±4.1	−1.3±4.7	0.0±0	−7.7±2*,c	−4.8±3*,c	−7.6±5*,c
C5	−10.7±11	−12.7±13	−9±9	−21±14*,a	−24±8.6*,a	−17±10*
C3a	30±41	24±18	17±26	20±28	6.1±30	−12.9±18a
C4a	19±23	14±26	13±21	0.2±22	12±21	−29±12e
C5a	6.6±12	4.8±10	−4.8±11	2.8±17	−28±20	−22±17
MNC (Con A)	−71±25*,f	−60±36*,f	−37±54	−1.1±39	−10±22	−14±47
MNC (PHA)	−75±25*,f	−52±49*	−11±101	−14±67	−24±28	29±154
MNC (PWM)	−67±28*,f	−59±34*,f	−44±48	−15±12	−15±15	−27±39
Fibrinogen	−6.8±4.3	−3.8±3.9	−9.2±2.8*	−6.3±2.3*	−7.8±2.7*	−9.5±6.5
PT	70±6.0	0.8±4.5	5.8±6.9	4.8±3.6	3.0±4.1	2.8±3.6
APTT	0.7±1.5	2.7±2.2	8.8±2*,b	4.4±4.2	1.5±3.3	−0.4±3.2
TT	−0.1±3.8	−0.6±3.0	3.4±7.5	4.5±6.8	4.6±6.6	2.9±2.7

*$P < 0.05$ vs sham, [a]$P < 0.05$ vs CP, [b]$P < 0.05$ vs CA and CP, [c]$P < 0.05$ vs CP and EVAL, [d]$P < 0.05$ vs CA, CP and EVAL, [e]$P < 0.05$ vs CA, EVAL and PS-F, [f]$P < 0.05$ vs PAN, PS-F and PS-K.

complements and did not reduce suppression of MNCTF. EVAL membrane, which has middle level of oxygen percent content on the membrane surface among the membranes studied, showed a better biocompatibility with regards to changes noted for coagulation as less activation of APTT versus sham, CA, and CP. There was a tendency that the membranes with less oxygen percent on the surface adsorbed biochemical and complement components much more and the tendency that the serums from the membranes with more oxygen percent on the surface suppressed MNCTF much more. Though the only enhancement for PHA-induced MNCTF seemed to be associated with less activation for C3 and C4 for the PS-K membrane, there were no significant differences in the surface oxygen percent between PS-F and PS-K. This suggests that structural properties of the membranes must also be considered. This *in vitro* model provided comparative results among membranes and may be useful as a screening method for assessing biological reactivity of materials.

REFERENCES

1. D. Paul, G. Malsch, E. Bossin *et al.* Chemical modification of cellulosic membranes and their blood compatibility. *Artif. Organs*, **14**, 122–125 (1990).
2. K. Sawada, P. S. Malchesky, T. Ohshima, J. B. Goldcamp, J. M. Guildubaldi and S. Omokawa. Evaluation of materials for use in extracorporeal circulation. *In vitro* serum-material interaction. *Trans. Am. Soc. Artif. Intern. Organs*, **37**, 144–146 (1991).
3. A. Dilks. ESCA studies of natural weathering phenomena at selected polymer surfaces. *J. Polym. Sci., Polym. Chem. Ed.*, **19**, 2847–2860 (1981).

Therapeutic Plasmapheresis (XII), pp. 815-817
T. Agishi *et al.* (Eds)
© VSP 1993

Donor Plateletpheresis for Sufficient Supply of Single Donor Platelet Concentrates

N. UEDA, H. KIYOKAWA and Y. MAEDA

Fukuoka Red Cross Blood Center, Fukuoka, Japan

Key words: plateletpheresis; hospital demands; blood cell separator; computerization; cost effectiveness.

INTRODUCTION

The blood programme in Japan is completely monopolized by the Japanese Red Cross Society except for the production of plasma derivatives. Donor plateletpheresis and plasmapheresis were introduced to Japanese Red Cross Blood Centers under a new blood program in 1986. The number of apheresis donors has been increasing rapidly every year and has already expanded nearly 1 million donors last fiscal year. Fukuoka Red Cross Blood Center has been playing an important role as a pioneer of donor apheresis in Japan.

MATERIALS AND METHODS

The Fukuoka Red Cross Blood Center is one of the seven core blood centers of the Japanese Red Cross Blood Centers. It has one subcenter and two collection rooms. In the Fukuoka Red Cross Blood Center, 57 blood cell separators of seven different types are used for platelet and plasma procurement. Fifty registered nurses are working on both collection of whole blood and apheresis products. The number of apheresis platelets collected in the four fixed facilities is displayed by a computerized on-line system to coordinate supply and collection.

RESULTS

We compared yields and white cell contamination in donor plateletpheresis using several blood cell separators, retrospectively analyzing the samples during consecutive procedures throughout a 7 year time period. As a result, we conclude eligible criteria for machine selection for donors, such as blood flow rate, processing blood volume and centrifugal force of each machine for efficient platelet production with low white cell contamination, by referring to the gender, body weight, hematocrit and preprocedure blood platelet count.

Current status of plateletpheresis and plasmapheresis in our blood center is shown in Table 1. Forty five percent (11 543 donations) of plateletpheresis was performed in dual components. Side-effects and adverse reactions associated with apheresis donations

Table 1.
Current status of plateletpheresis and plasmapheresis in FRCBC (April 1991–March 1992)

Separators	No. of separator	HLA-PC	PC	PC+PPP	PRP	PPP
Cobe Spectra	3	186	56	910	—	—
CS-3000 Plus	11	214	72	6021	—	—
Haem. V-50	8	65	39	4612	121	184
Haem. PCS	8	—	—	—	6768	2233
Haem. U-PCS	12	—	—	—	6554	7565
Autopheresis	7	—	—	—	10	5812
Nipro NDP-200	8	—	—	—	—	3712
Total	57	465	167	11543	13453	19561

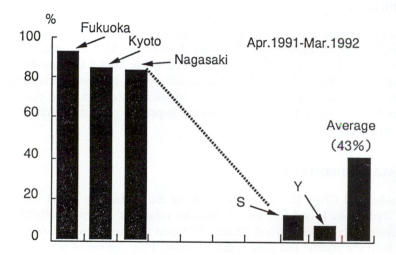

Figure 1. Rate of apheresis platelets in platelet concentrates issued. Total: 64 blood centers.

seem to be slightly higher (0.6%) than regular donation (0.4%/200 ml, 0.5%/400 ml). However, it shows no statistical significance. Regarding apheresis platelets in platelet concentrates (PC) issued, the Fukuoka Red Cross Blood Center has achieved more than 90% of PC from plateletpheresis (Fig. 1). The distribution of platelet yields is shown in Fig. 2. More than 50% of plateletpheresis procedures contained $> 2 \times 10^{11}$ platelets.

DISCUSSION

The Japanese government produced a 5-year specific plan to promote an apheresis program in 1986. The Ministry of Health and Welfare subsidized Japanese Red Cross Blood Centers to buy apheresis devices during the 5 years until the last fiscal year. The number of apheresis donors in the Japanese Red Cross Blood Centers is increasing year by year. Especially, after a change of hospital payments for blood components in 1990, donor apheresis is going forward rapidly.

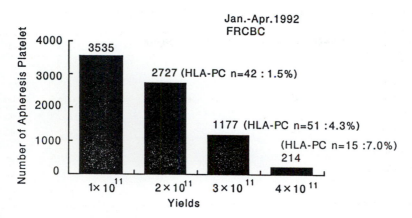

Figure 2. Distribution of platelet yields.

After achieving sufficient supply of apheresis platelets, we are going to pay much attention to leukocyte-poor or leukocyte-depleted platelets for prevention of alloimmunization to HLA antigen. Current devices for apheresis have sought to increase platelet collection yields while minimizing leukocyte contamination [1].

On cost effectiveness, it is very important to know the trend of hospital demands. Nurse training programs, donor selection and computerization will be most important factors to achieve cost performance.

CONCLUSIONS

Since 1986, donor plateletpheresis and plasmapheresis have been established to provide for hospital demands and plasma fractionation

The cost effectiveness of platelet production (platelet concentrates from 200 ml, 400 ml whole blood and plateletpheresis) is still controversial. However, it is likely that an increase of plateletpheresis would lead to a significant decrease of procedures of the blood processing laboratory and testing laboratory.

REFERENCE

1. M. F. Bertholf and P. D. Mintz. Comparison of plateletpheresis with two cell separators using identical donors (Abstract). *Transfusion*, **28**, 45 (1988).

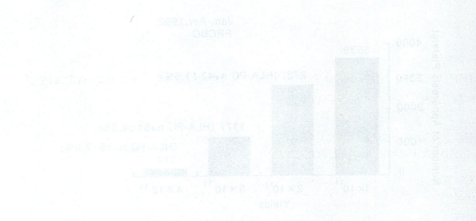

Therapeutic Plasmapheresis (XII), pp. 819-824
T. Agishi *et al.* (Eds)
© VSP 1993

Long-term Liquid Preservation of Platelet Concentratres in a Double-bag System

C. YAKUSHIJI, T. A. TAKAHASHI,[1]   K. ICHINOHE,
T. MARUYAMA and S. SEKIGUCHI[1]

Kawasumi Laboratories Inc., Tokyo, Japan
[1]Hokkaido Red Cross Blood Center, Sapporo, Japan

Key words: double-bag system; platelet preservation; colloidal osmotic pressure; platelet storage medium.

INTRODUCTION

Platelet concentrates (PC) derived from whole blood can be stored at room temperature in blood bags made of plastics such as polyolefin (PO) and polyvinyl chloride (PVC) with gentle agitation. In Japan, the storage period is limited to only 3 days after phebotomy, while other countries permit 5 days for storage. However, the PC prepared by platelet apheresis is highly concentrated and as the volume is large, it is difficult to store in one container. Because of the difficulty in finding donors for HLA-matched PC, extending the storage period of PC is highly desirable. We have succeeded in extending the liquid preservation period of PC by using a double-structured bag system (CC-201OE, Kawasumi) that was originally developed for continuous culture of cells, such as LAK cells.

MATERIALS AND METHODS

Storage container

The double-bag system has two compartments, an inner compartment with a semipermeable cellulose membrane (fractional molecular weight: 10 000, (Akzo, Wuppertal, Germany)) and an outer compartment made of PVC (Fig. 1A). As a control, a PO bag (capacity 600 ml, Nissyo, Tokyo) was used as a conventional storage container.

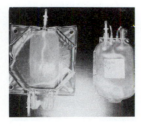

Figure 1A. Double-bag system (left) and PO bag (right).

Platelet preparation

PC was prepared from healthy volunteer donors by using a Fenwal CS-3000 Plus (Baxter Co., Deerfield, IL, USA). The ratio of PC to the anticoagulant citrate dextrose-A (ACD-A) solution was 10:1. Two hundred milliliters of PC and the same volume of platelet poor plasma (PPP) were collected. After mixing the PC and PPP, the diluted PC was divided into equal volumes, which were put into the double-bag system and PO bag, respectively.

Platelet storage medium

To the three kinds of platelet storage media shown Table 1, those developed by Holme, Murphy and Rock, 2.5% (w/v) dextran was added to adjust the colloidal osmotic pressure, and the pH was adjusted to 7.0 with 0.1 N NaOH or 0.1 N HCl. Five hundred milliliters of each medium was placed in the outer compartment of a double-bag for comparison, and 500 ml of sterilized air, filtered with a 0.22 μm pore-sized filter (Millipore Product Div., Bedford, MA, USA) was added to the medium for mixing.

Table 1.
Colloidal osmotic pressure

	Plasma	Albumin 3% (w/v)	Dextran			
			2% (w/v)	2.5% (w/v)	3% (w/v)	4% (w/v)
(mmHg)	20.8	7.8	13.5	17.5	21.3	30.1

Storage conditions

The double-bag was rotated at 5 r.p.m. with a the rotary agitator (KL-5001, Kawasumi) in the vertical position at an angle of 45° deg in a 22°C incubator (Fig. 1B). The PO bag was stored on a horizontal agitator (60 r.p.m., EKC-40, Ebara, Tokyo, Japan) at 22°C.

Platelet functions

Six milliliters of stored PC was analyzed for pH, CO_2 and O_2 by a pH/bloods gas analyzer (Model 170, Ciba Corning Diagnostics, Medfield, MA, USA). The platelet number and mean platelet volume were measured using a Coulter counter (Model S-PlusIV, Coulter Electronics, Hialeah, FL, USA). The platelet concentrate was adjusted to

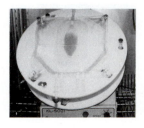

Figure 1B. Storage of double-bag system on rotary agitator.

$3.5 \times 10^5/\mu l$ with autologus PPP and the pH was adjusted to 7.4 ± 0.1. Platelet response to hypotonic stress (%HSR) was measured by the change of light transmittance at a wave length of 610 nm for 5 min by spectrophotometer (U-2000, Hitachi Ltd, Tokyo). Platelet aggregability was measured using an aggregometer (HEMA TRACER 801, Niko Bioscience, Tokyo) with the synergic aggregating reagent ADP (final concentration 5 μM, Boehringer, Mannheim, Germany) and collagen (final concentration 1 μg/ml, Hormon Chemie, München, Germany) in the presence of $CaCl_2$ (final concentration: 3 mM).

RESULTS AND DISCUSSION

Early in this study, the PC was stored in a double-bag system in which a cell culture medium with human serum albumin was used as the storage medium in the outer compartment. In that case, the platelet count, mean platelet volume and %HSR of PC stored in the double-bag system were worse than those stored in the standard PVC bag. In contrast, when the PC was stored in the double-bag system using PPP as the storage medium in the outer compartment, these platelet functions were dramatically improved. These observations brought to our attention two important points concerning the storage of PC in the double-bag system.

The first was that the regulation of colloidal osmotic pressure is necessary to maintain the volume balance between PC and the storage medium (Table 1). The colloidal osmotic pressure of the platelet storage medium was adjusted by the addition of dextran. If the concentration of dextran was not great enough, the medium in the outer compartment moved into the inner compartment through the semipermeable membrane, and the volume of PC increased. In contrast, if there was too much dextran, the volume of PC decreased and its concentration increased. Both conditions affect platelet functions adversely. We found that the colloidal osmotic pressure of the storage medium was the same as that of plasma when 2.5–3.0% (w/v) dextran was added to the medium. The addition of 2.5% (w/v) dextran resulted in minimal changes of PC volume and maximal maintenance of platelet functions.

Table 2.

Platelet storage media (components in mM)

	PAS (Holme)	PSM (Murphy)	Plasmalyte-A (Rock)
NaCl	110.0	98.0	90.0
KCl	5.1	5.0	5.0
$CaCl_2$ $2H_2O$	1.7	—	—
$MgSO_4$	0.8	—	—
Na_3 citrate	15.2	—	—
Citric acid	2.7	—	—
$NaHCO_3$	35.0	—	—
NaH_2PO_4 H_2O	2.7	25.0	—
Na acetate	—	—	27.0
Na gluconate	—	—	23.0
Glucose	35.5	—	—

The second point concerned the composition of the storage medium in the outer compartment (Table 2). Three kinds of platelet storage media developed by Holme, Murphy and Rock, respectively, were examined. As a result, we chose to use Holme's platelet storage medium, which had a better buffer effect than the others.

In the double-bag system, the maintenance of a suitable pH of 7.0–7.4 for PC depended on the pH of outer storage medium (Fig. 2). The pH of control PC stored in the PO container fell after the 5th day and on the 14th day was nearly pH 6.0.

Figure 3 shows changes in platelet count and mean platelet volume during the storage of PC. The platelet number was always higher in concentrate stored using the double-bag system than in that in the polyolefin container. The mean platelet volume of PC stored in the double-bag system was stable and was much better than that of PC stored in the polyolefin container.

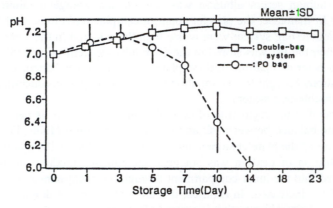

Double-bag system:N=10 PO bag:N=9

Changes in platelet count and mean platelet volume(MPV)
during storage of PC

Figure 2. Change in pH during storage of PC.

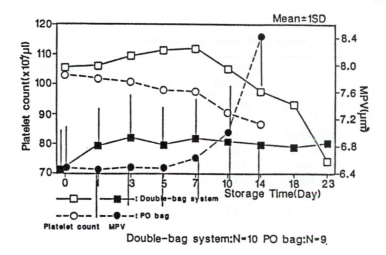

Double-bag system:N=10 PO bag:N=9

Figure 3. Changes in platelet count and mean platelet volume (MPV) during storage of PC.

The platelet response to hypotonic stress showed similar changes in the double-bag system and PO container before the 10th day (Fig. 4). After th 10th day, the PC stored in the double-bag system had a much higher %HSR than that stored in the PO container.

Platelet aggregability induced by a synergic aggregating reagent (ADP 5 μM + collagen 1 μg/ml) showed similar courses before the 10th day (Fig. 5). The response of the platelets stored in the PO container to the aggregating reagent almost vanished by the 14th day. However, in the double-bag system it was retained even after 23 days.

The liquid preservation of PC in a double-bag system has been successfully improved by the following modifications. First, the addition of proteins such as albumin is believed to protect platelets from shear stress when they are the stored and suspended in the storage medium. The %HSR, in particular, is affected by the concentration of plasma in PC. Therefore, the influx of storage medium, which causes a change of PC volume (an increase or decrease) and the following reduction of platelet functions should be prevented. We found that the appropriate concentration of dextran was 2.5% (w/v), which caused minimal changes in PC volume and sustained the maximal platelet functions (Table 2). Second, the composition of the medium in the outer bag was crucial. We compared three kinds of storage media for use in the outer compartment of the double-bag system (Table 1). Of the three, Holme's platelet storage medium best maintained the platelet functions.

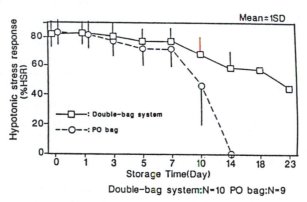

Figure 4. Change in hypotonic stress response during storage of PC.

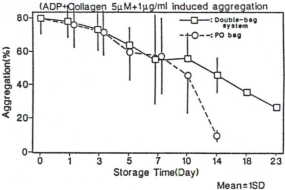

Figure 5. Change in platelet aggregability during storage of PC.

In conclusion, we found that storage of PC in the double-bag system could be improved as a result of adjusting the colloidal osmotic pressure by adding 2.5% (w/v) dextran to the storage medium, and by the use of Holme's medium in the outer bag. However, *in vivo* testing is required to more accurately evaluate this system.

Therapeutic Plasmapheresis (XII), pp. 825-828
T. Agishi *et al.* (Eds)
© VSP 1993

Clinical Study of a Disk-type Membrane Plasmapheresis System (CPAS-II) with a Hydrophilic Membrane

T. A. TAKAHASHI, T. NAKASE, M. YOKOYAMA, H. KODAMA, A. YAGISHITA,[1] M. SADO[1] and S. SEKIGUCHI

Hokkaido Red Cross Blood Center, Sapporo, Japan
[1]*Terumo Co., Ltd, Kanagawa, Japan*

Key words: donor plasmapheresis; Constant Pressure Apheresis System (CPAS); membrane plasma separator.

INTRODUCTION

We have been investigating a donor plasmapheresis system (Constant Pressure Apheresis System type-I, CPAS-I) which is capable of plasma collection by taking advantage of gravity alone without using any special devices [1, 2]. We improved the system by employing a special compact device which has a pressure-reducing and pressurizing chamber for whole blood collection and plasma separation, respectively (Constant Pressure Apheresis System type-II, CPAS-II). We conducted clinical evaluations of this system and confirmed that the system is applicable to operation in a blood mobile. Furthermore, we have evaluated the newly developed hydrophilized polypropylene plasma separation membrane which requires no saline rinsing or priming.

MATERIALS AND METHODS

The CPAS-II with hydrophobic membrane consists of three bags (a whole blood bag, a plasma bag and a drain bag), a disk-type membrane separator (0.6 μm pore sized polypropylene membrane, 0.16 m^2 effective surface area), tubing and a needle (Fig. 1). The hydrophobic separator is filled with doubly distilled water, and it is replaced with saline before the operation, but the hydrophilic membrane prepared by surface graft polymerization with hydrophilic monomer requires no saline rinsing or priming. The blood tubing set is simplified due to the development of a hydrophilic membrane. Figure 2 shows the outlook of the CPAS-II. The pressure-reduction in the bag chamber at blood collection mode is minus 180 mmHg, and the pressuring level in the blood return mode is 120 mmHg. The ratio of whole blood to anticoagulant ACD was 10 to 1. It is possible to collect 200, 300 and 400 ml of whole blood per cycle. Clinical evaluations were performed for healthy volunteer donors using either hydrophobic or hydrophilic separators. Written informed consent was obtained from each donor. Hematological values were measured pre- and postapheresis, as well as at the inlet and outlet of the plasma separator in the second infusion cycle.

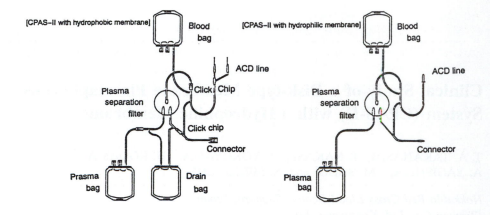

Figure 1. Disposable system for CPAS-II.

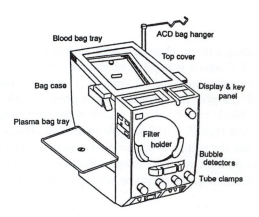

Figure 2. CPAS-II system.

RESULTS AND DISCUSSION

Each clinical evaluation was performed safety, and no donor developed side effects. Table 1 compares the properties of CPAS-I gravity-driven, CPAS-II with the hydrophobic membrane and CPAS-II with the hydrophilic membrane. The whole procedure time was shortened by using the hydrophilic membrane because no priming was required. There was no significant difference between the donation time in CPAS-I and CPAS-II with hydrophobic membrane and with the hydrophilic membrane. More plasma could be collected using CPAS-II with the hydrophilic membrane rather than CPAS-II with the hydrophobic membrane (Table 1).

Regarding the volume of collected plasma and needle to needle time, there was not significant difference between the hydrophobic and hydrophilic membranes. Figure 3 shows the comparison of plasma component sieving coefficient in plasma collected by the hydrophobic and hydrophilic membranes. Recovery rates using the hydrophobic

Table 1.
Properties of CPAS-I (gravity-driven) and CPAS-II (pressure-driven)

Machine	n	Priming time	Whole blood processed (ml)	Collected plasma volume (ml)	N–N time (min)
CPAS-I	54	6′20″ ± 1′14″	880	343.5 ± 33.2	34′43″ ± 7′19″
PAS-II (hydrophobic membrane)	8	6′28″ ± 1′15″	1141.1 ± 28.0	436.3 ± 1.0	33′24″ ± 3′42″
CPAS-II (hydrophilic membrane)	5	0	1262.0±92.7	457.2 ± 4.3	37′03″ ± 7′10″

Mean ± SD.

were as follows: total protein 90.9±3.5%, albumin 91.9±2.8%, coagulating factor VIII activity (F VIII:C) 78.4±11.8%, factor VIII related antigen (vWF:Ag) 90.6±6.7% (n = 15). In the case of the hydrophilic membrane, the recovery rates were as follows: total protein 98.8 ± 1.2%, albumin 99.7 ± 0.9%, F VIII:C 98.2 ± 10.4%, vWF:Ag 105.8 ± 16.5% (n = 10).The recovery rates of major plasma components were almost 100%. In all the plasma components compared, higher recovery was observed with the hydrophilized membrane.

Table 2 shows the results of complement activation and hemolysis prepared by the hydrophilic and hydrophobic membranes. Though the levels of C3a and C4a increased in the collected plasma, there was no significant difference in the levels of C3a and

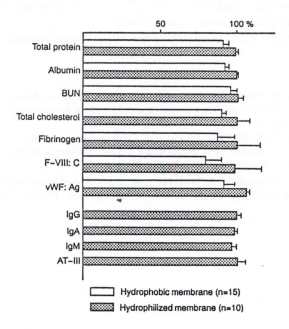

Figure 3. Sieving coefficient (PPP outlet/inlet) ×100%.

C5a between both membranes. However, C4a level increased with the hydrophilized membrane, significantly. The levels of C3a and C4a observed in the plasma separated by the CPAS-II may not be a very serious problem for the transfusion of these products [3]. Thus, the CPAS-II system seems to be a sample, compact and efficient donor plasmapheresis system suitable for blood mobiles.

Table 2.
Levels of complement activation and serum hemoglobin

		Blood collected in bag	Plasma collected
C3a	hydrophobic membrane	246 ± 69	958 ± 205
	hydrophilized membrane	176 ± 35	928 ± 1314
C4a	hydrophobic membrane	83 ± 12	413 ± 249
	hydrophilized membrane	100 ± 51*	8100 ± 5473
C5a	hydrophobic membrane	7.6 ± 5.0	7.7 ± 2.0
	hydrophilized membrane	2.1 ± 2.9	3.0 ± 4.5
S-Hb	hydrophilized membrane	8 ± 11	1 ± 0

Hydrophobic membrane, $n = 5$.
Hydrophilized membrane $n = 10$ (*$n = 7$).

CONCLUSION

We have developed a new donor plasmapheresis system, the CPAS-II. The system was improved by adopting a hydrophilized membrane. The improved system could obtain about 100% sieving coefficients of protein and coagulation factors. Plasma separation was successfully performed at constant pressure with easy operation.

REFERENCES

1. T. A. Takahashi, M. Hosoda, S. Yamamoto *et al.* A new donor plasmapheresis system with a disk-type membrane separator: plasma separation using gravity without any electrical devices. *Jpn. J. Transf. Med.*, **36**, 418–423 (1990).
2. T. Nakase, T. A. Takahashi, M. Yokoyama *et al.* Clinical evaluation of the constant pressure apheresis (CPAS-I): plasma separation using gravity with a disk-type membrane. In: *Therapeutic Plasmapheresis (IX)*, pp. 303–309, ICAOT Press, Cleveland (1991).
3. S. Sekiguchi, T. A. Takahashi, S. Yamamoto *et al.* A new type of blood component collector: plasma separation using gravity without any electrical devices. *Vox Sang*, **58**, 182–187 (1990).

Therapeutic Plasmapheresis (XII), pp. 829-832
T. Agishi *et al.* (Eds)
© VSP 1993

A Simple and Compact Hollow Fiber-type Membrane Donor Plasmapheresis System

T. A. TAKAHASHI, T. NAKASE, M. YOKOYAMA, H. KODAMA, Y. TAKENAKA,[1] T. INOSHITA[1] and S. SEKIGUCHI

Hokkaido Red Cross Blood Center, Sapporo, Japan
[1]*Asahi Medical Co., Ltd, Tokyo, Japan*

Key words: donor plasmapheresis; blood component collector system; blood plasma collector; membrane plasma separator.

INTRODUCTION

We have previously reported the development and evaluation of a gravity-driven blood component collector system (BCC-I) able to separate whole blood into plasma and red cell concentrate [1, 2]. We then tried to adapt this system to a donor plasmapheresis,

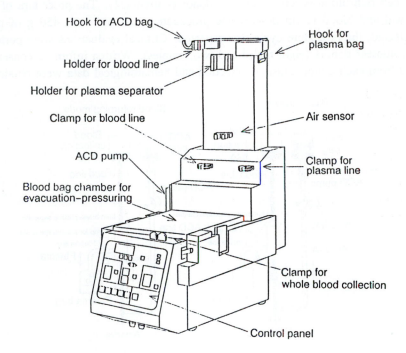

Figure 1. Schematic diagram of blood plasma collector (BPC).

and the donor plasma system is named BCC-II. Here we describe the clinical evaluation of a new donor plasmapheresis system, also based on a gravity membrane separator, for separation of plasma and return of red cell concentrate to the donor.

The new system, a pressure-driven BCC-II system named Blood Plasma Collector (BPC), employs an evacuator for blood collection routinely used at blood centers to reduce the blood collection time (Fig. 1).

MATERIALS AND METHODS

This membrane type plasma separator system employs porous hollow fibers which are hydrophylized polyethylene with a pore size of 0.24 μm and the effective surface area of the plasma separator is 0.22 m². The membrane of the plasma separator is wetted with about 10 ml of physiological saline to prevent hemolysis by capillary influx of red cells into the micropores of the hollow fiber. It was unnecessary to prime the separator with physiological saline prior to donor plasmapheresis. Figure 2 shows the system flow chart. During the procedure of blood withdrawal, 400 ml of blood is introduced into the blood collection bag going through the plasma separator without filtration. At the same time as the blood introduction, 1 volume of ACD-A per 12 volumes of blood is infused into the blood. The potential force of blood withdrawal into the collection bag is the evacuation within the apparatus. During blood return, the collected blood is pressurized to flow through the plasma separator. Within the plasma separator, plasma is separated and the cell rich blood is returned to the donor continuously. The procedure of blood withdrawal and blood return defines one procedure cycle and until 450 g of plasma was collected, the procedure cycle was repeated. Clinical evaluations were performed for 10 volunteer donors (eight males and two females). Written informed consent was obtained from each donor. Plasma collection and hematological data were obtained.

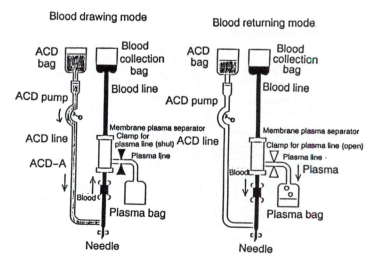

Figure 2. System flow chart.

RESULTS

Table 1 shows the data for the plasma collection. For the collection of 450 g of plasma, the blood collection time was 15.5 ± 4.0 min and the collection time was 16.8 ± 4.0 min. An average N–N time was 35.4 ± 4.0 min. No side effects were observed in any case. Table 2 shows the comparison of the plasma collection data between the BCC-II and new system BPC. The N–N time was drastically reduced in the BPC system compared with the BCC-II system for the collection of 452 g of plasma, i.e. from 50 min by BCC-II to 35 min by the BPC. Table 3 shows the comparison of plasma component concentrations in the blood collection bag and in the collected plasma bag. There was no significant change of concentrations between them in total protein (TP), albumin (ALB), cholesterol (CHOL), LDH, factor VIII and serum hemoglobin (S-Hb).

Table 1.

Results of plasma collection

Extra corporeal blood volume (g)	1238.1 ± 61.2
Collected plasma [a] volume (g)	450.0 ± 0
Whole blood[b] collection time (min)	15.5 ± 4.0
Plasma collection time (min)	16.8 ± 4.0
N–N time (min)	35.4 ± 4.0
Number of cycles	3.0 ± 0
Flow rate of plasma* collection (g/min)	28.0 ± 5.6

* $\frac{a)}{b)}$.

Mean $\pm$SD.

Table 2.

Performance of gravity- and pressure-driven BCC-II systems

Machine	(n)	Whole blood processed (ml)	Collected plasma volume (ml)	N–N time (min)
BCC-II (gravity-driven)	(20)	1181 ± 189	452 ± 75	50 ± 10
BCC-II (pressure-driven)	(10)	1320 ± 276	452 ± 37	35 ± 7

Mean $\pm$SD.

DISCUSSION AND CONCLUSION

The procedure of blood withdrawal and blood return was defined as one procedure cycle and until 450 g of plasma was collected, the procedure cycle was repeated. A shorter N–N time, 35.4 ± 4.0 min, was obtained by employing pressure-driven blood return.

Table 3.

Concentration of plasma components and coagulation factors ($n = 10$).

	Whole blood in bag	Collected plasma
TP (g/dl)	6.7±0.3	6.3±0.2
ALB (g/dl)	3.6±0.1	3.6±0.1
CHOL (mg/dl)	151±22	147± 23
LDH (IU/L)	267±32	247±33
FVIII:C (%)	134±27	130±30
FVIII:Ag (%)	95±28	92±27
S-Hb (mg/dl)	2.3±1.1	1.7±0.6

Mean ±SD.

The concentration of TP and ALB in collected plasma was 6.5 and 3.6 g/dl, respectively. More than 97% of TP and ALB was recovered. This shows the good permeability of the membrane.

Thus the donor plasma collection system BPC, incorporating a membrane plasma separator and an evacuator blood collection, appears to provide excellent safety and efficiency. N–N time for 450 g of plasma collection was 35 min. No adverse effects were observed among donors. In the collected plasma, most of the plasma component concentrations indicated good recoveries, which may largely be attributed to the freedom from a need for physiological saline priming and its diluting effect. The pressure-driven blood return system makes the system compact and no saline priming enables simple operation. The BPC system is considered to be a quite suitable donor plasmapheresis system for blood mobiles.

REFERENCES

1. T. A. Takahashi, S. Yamamoto, H. Hasegawa *et al*. A new type of blood component collector: plasma separation by gravity without any electrical devices. *Jpn. J. Transf. Med.*, **35**, 73–79 (1989).
2. S. Sekiguchi, T. A. Takahashi, S. Yamamoto *et al*. A new type of blood component collector: plasma separation using gravity without any electrical devices. *Vox Sang*, **58**, 182–187 (1990).

Therapeutic Plasmapheresis (XII), pp. 833-835
T. Agishi *et al.* (Eds)
© VSP 1993

Significance of Apheresis in Self-sufficiency of Blood Components and Source Plasma in Japan

T. NAKASE and S. SEKIGUCHI

Hokkaido Red Cross Blood Center, Sapporo, Japan

Key words: apheresis; source plasma; non-remunerated donor; plasma fractionation products; coagulation factor VIII.

Blood transfusion in Japan back to the period shortly after the World War II was supported mainly by paid donors. Non-remunerated donation increased since 1964 with the governmental declaration which requested the establishment of blood for transfusion by non-remunerated donation. Initially only 200 ml donation was accepted, and 400 ml donation and apheresis were accepted as of April 1986 by the change of donation criteria.

Numbers of donors reached a maximum of 8.76 million in 1985 but the donation volume increased thereafter and reached 2.2 million liters in 1991. The total volume consisted of 200 ml donation (47.6%), 400 ml donation (33.3%) and apheresis (18.7%).

Blood used for transfusion has been supported by non-remunerated donors only since 1974. Whole blood supply decreased since 1977 with the increase of concentrated red cell supply. Total red cell products reached a plateau in 1985 with about 6 million units (in terms of 200 ml products). Fresh frozen plasma (FFP) increased rapidly until 1985, when the new criteria for proper use of blood products was released and FFP supply decreased slightly to 5 million units per year. Platelet products increased rapidly and the ratio of apheresis-derived products increased recently (Fig. 1).

Plasma fractionation products had been dependent on imported materials mainly from USA (Fig. 2), but recently the government declared consecutively the self-sufficiency of plasma products in 1975, 1985 and 1989. The third declaration was forced by HIV infection of hemophiliacs by import coagulation factor products, and included self-sufficiency of coagulation factor products and step-wise increase of source plasma for albumin and globulins. The aim of collection of 500 000 l source plasma for coagulation factors was attained in 1991.

Promotion of plasmapheresis was the pivotal point of this accomplishment. The number of institutions for apheresis increased to 360, which includes 77 blood centers, 76 donation rooms and 207 blood mobiles for apheresis, with 1731 apheresis apparatuses as of March 1992.

The number of apheresis donors was 27 831 in the first year (1986) and doubled every year to reach 1.01 million in 1991. The ratio of apheresis at centers and rooms was dominant initially, but recently the ratio of apheresis at blood mobiles and at open sites increased with the development of portable and compact apparatuses (Fig. 3). An expandable mobile was introduced to Hokkaido Blood Center for the first time in the world, and has been used for blood collection at remote sites.

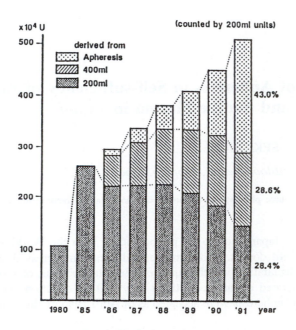

Figure 1. Yearly change of supply of platelet products in Japan.

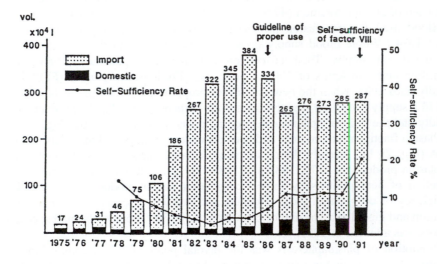

Figure 2. Self-sufficiency rate of plasma fractionation products in Japan.

Source plasma volume for coagulation factor increased progressively and attained the goal of 505 000 l in 1991, of which 320 000 l (63.3%) was obtained by plasmapheresis (Fig. 4).

Coagulation factor VIII products made from non-remunerated donation, 'Cross Eight M', were on the market as of March 1992. It will replace the imported products and will contribute to the prevention of HIV infection.

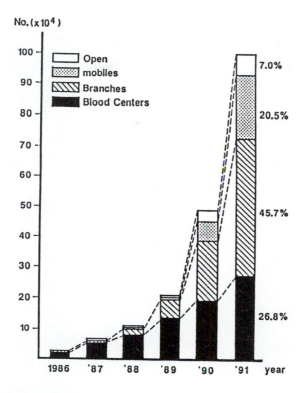

Figure 3. Yearly change of apheresis donor classified by type of institution.

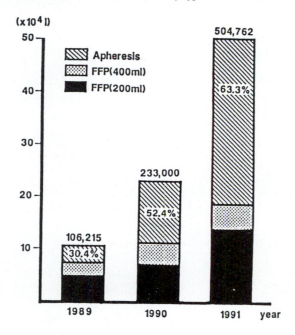

Figure 4. Volume of collected plasma for coagulation factor classified by origin.

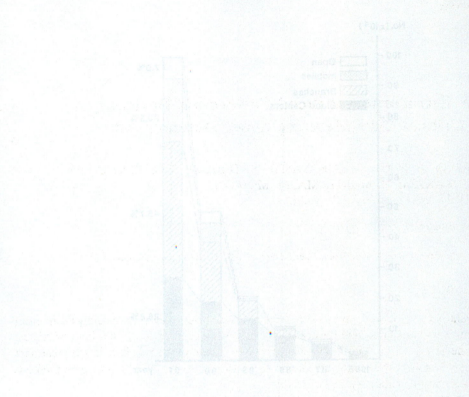

Figure 3. Yearly change of aphaeresis donor classified by type of institution.

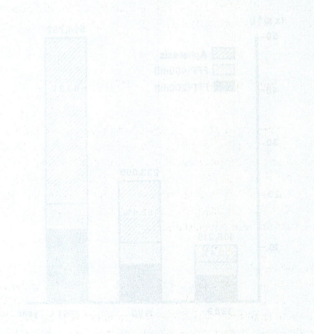

Figure 4. Number of collected plasma for anaphylatica frozen classified by origin.

Therapeutic Plasmapheresis (XII), pp. 837-842
T. Agishi *et al.* (Eds)
© VSP 1993

New Extracorporeal Blood Purification Devices for Critical Care Medicine under Development

Y. SAKAI, H. SHOJI, T. KOBAYASHI, R. TERADA, H. SUGAYA,
M. MURAKAMI, K. MORIYAMA, M. MINAGA,
T. KUNITOMO and T. TAKEYAMA

Toray Industries, Inc., Tokyo, Japan

Key words: critical care medicine; blood purification; sepsis; polymyxin; antithrombogenic.

INTRODUCTION

Conventional extracorporeal blood purification modalities, such as hemodialysis, hemofiltration, hemoadsorption and plasma exchange, have been applied in the field of critical care medicine. In this field, however, creative functions are required in the treatment of some morbid states, such as removal of endotoxins from the blood or new methods to ensure antithrombogenicity of devices.

We have developed two innovative devices incorporating such functions. One is polymyxin B immobilized fibers packed in a cartridge for direct hemoperfusion (DHP), called PMX. Another is an antithrombogenic continuous hemofilter, called ACUS or PANPEO.

POLYMYXIN B IMMOBILIZED FIBER CARTRIDGE

Intended use

The number of patients in septic shock or multiple organ failure has increased as a result of life saving of fatal patients. For those cases, detoxification of endotoxin is required even after the disappearance of living microorganisms as a result of antibiotic therapy. There are two candidate therapies in such states, one is anti-endotoxin antibody administration and another is removal of endotoxin from the blood by means of an adsorbent by DHP. We selected the latter because it can be used repeatedly, be more effective and exhibits less adverse effects.

Structure and materials

Figure 1 illustrates the chemical and physical structure of the polymyxin B immobilized fiber (PMX-F), 56 g of which is packed in the cartridge for DHP. Polymyxin B has been known as an antibiotic which neutralizes endotoxin by the affinity to the lipid A portion of endotoxin. A derivative of polystylene reinforced with polypropylene fiber is used as a carrier fiber binding polymyxin B covalently.

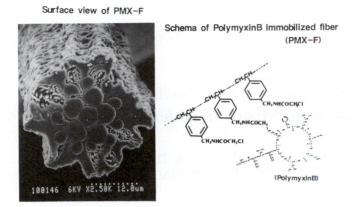

Figure 1. Chemical and physical structure of PMX-F.

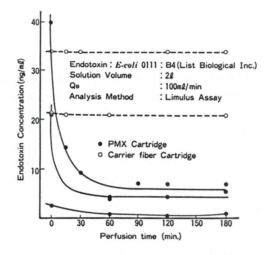

Figure 2. Endotoxin removal with PMX cartridge — *in vitro* perfusion test.

In vitro and ex vivo evaluations

The endotoxin removal by PMX was evaluated in perfusion tests with endotoxin being added to bovine blood. Typical data are shown in Fig. 2. Endotoxin removal lasts for about 1–2 h.

Evaluations with dogs to confirm the safety and effectiveness of PMX were conducted. Significant difference of the survival rate in the endotoxin challenged dogs were observed between the PMX and the control cartridge packed with the carrier fibers as shown in Fig. 3. In these tests thrombocytopenia was observed, the degree of which was similar to that of activated charcoal cartridges.

Results of clinical evaluations

The clinical evaluations were performed by Shiga University (Kodama, Tani) [1, 2], Chiba University (Hirasawa), Shohwa University [3], Nippon Medical School, Kitasato University, and Sapporo Medical College. As the clinical results are to be reported

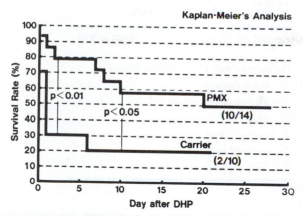

Figure 3. Survival rate in dog model treated with PMX and control cartridge.

elsewhere, only summaries are described here. The outline of the patients is shown in Table 1, where many patients that developed MOF were included. Nafamostat mesilate or heparin was used as an anticoagulant. The plasma endotoxin levels during DHP for 2 h decreased from 36 ± 7 to 20 ± 2 pg/ml ($n = 37$, $P < 0.01$). Other clinical findings are listed in Table 2. From these data, the DHP therapy with PMX has been shown to effectively ameliorate the critical manifestations in sepsis. It was also found that PMX was possibly effective for the patients in shock stage.

Table 1.
Outline of the patients treated with PMX (44 patients: male 33, female 11)

Underlying disease	Neoplasm	22
(main region or cause)	circulatory disease	11
	respiratory disease	4
	after surgery	19
	after trauma	9
Infectious region	abdomen	29
	breast	6
	others	9
Microorganisms	gram-negative	26
	gram-positive	8
	not detectable	10
Multiple organ failure	with	37
	without	7

Table 2.
Clinical findings of DHP with PMX

Survival rate ($\geqslant$ 14 days)	22/44 = 50%

Normalizing tendency in various indexes
    blood pressure
    amount of vasopressor
    heart rate
    cardiac index
    systemic vascular resistance
    body temperature

ANTITHROMBOGENIC HEMOFILTER FOR PROLONGED CONTINUOUS USE

Intended use

It is well known that in critical care medicine there are many patients who are origuric or anuric and resistant to diuretics, and who have some bleeding regions caused by surgery, trauma and underlying diseases. For these cases antithrombogenicity of the hemofilter is required because of the need for prolonged hemofiltration without anticoagulant. The PANPEO hemofilter was devised for such aim.

Structure and materials

The PANPEO hemofilter has been designed with the considerations on material and shape. Hollow fibers made of polyacrylonitrile–polyethyleneoxide copolymer (PAN-PEO) are used which are resistant to adhesion of blood components [4], and a material ionically binding heparin is used as a coating material on the surfaces of the tube sheet and header. The design of the shape of the headers and connectors facilitates the smooth blood flow pattern (Fig. 4).

Animal evaluations. PANPEO hemofilters were evaluated with the dog model without anticoagulant. The duration is shown in Fig. 5 comparing PANPEO hemofilters with conventional ones, where the superiority of PANPEO hemofilter is clearly demonstrated.

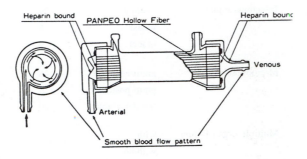

Figure 4. Design concept of PANPEO continuous hemofilter.

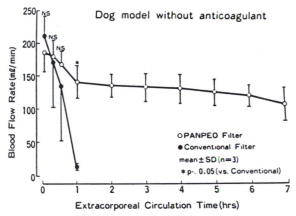

Figure 5. Duration with PANPEO and conventional hemofilters.

Results of clinical evaluations

The clinical evaluations were performed by Niigata University (Arakawa) [4, 5], Shin-rakuen Hospital (Hirasawa) and 12 other hospitals. The outline of the patients is shown in Table 3 and the histogram of the duration with the PANPEO hemofilter, without anticoagulant is shown in Fig. 6. The average duration was 34 h and much longer than that

Table 3.
Outline of the patients treated with
PANPEO hemofilter

32 patients:	
male	18
female	14
Age:	
average	65
range	17–85
Underlying disease	
neoplasm	8
cardiac disease	6
renal failure	5
liver cirrhosis	3
diabetes	3
collagen disease	2
accident	2
others	3
with bleeding region	9
postoperative	6

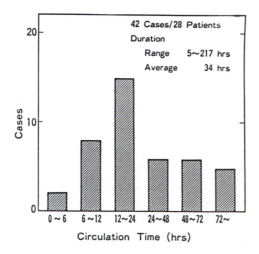

Figure 6. Clinical duration per one PANPEO hemofilter without anticoagulant.

of conventional filters whose duration is said to be a few hours from experience in general. The platelet counts were almost stable during hemofiltration, which demonstrates the antithrombogenicity of the filter, and bleeding episodes were not observed.

CONCLUSIVE REMARKS

The results obtained from the studies on both devices, PMX and PANPEO, are promising.

We will continue to work on improvements of devices in critical care medicine in cooperation with physicians.

REFERENCES

1. M. Kodama *et al.* Selective adsorbents of endotoxin in acute liver failure (Abstract). *Proc. Int. Soc. Artif. Organs,* Montreal (1991).
2. H. Aoki *et al.* Treatment of septic shock by extracorporeal elimination of endotoxin using fiber-immobilized polymyxin B (Abstract). *World Apheresis Ass.,* Sapporo (1992).
3. S. Kanesaka *et al.* Extracorporeal elimination of endotoxin by polymyxin B immobilized fiber in sepsis (Abstract). *Soc. Crit. Care Med.,* San Antonio (1992).
4. M. Arakawa *et al.* Development of a new antithrombogenic continuous ultrafiltration system. *Artif. Organs,* **15,** 171 (1991).
5. M. Arakawa *et al.* Antithrombogenicity of polyacrylonitrile–polyethyleneoxide hollow fiber membrane developed for designing an antithrombogenic continuous ultrafiltration system. *Artif. Organs,* **16,** 146 (1992).

Therapeutic Plasmapheresis (XII), pp. 843-845
T. Agishi *et al.* (Eds)
© VSP 1993

Extracorporeal Immunoadsorption with Immunosorba® Protein A

G. SAMUELSSON

Excorim AB, Box 10101, S-22010 Lund, Sweden

Key words: immunoadsorption; Immunosorba®; protein A.

Immunosorba® contains 62.5 ml of protein A Sepharose with a binding capacity of 20 mg of IgG/ml of gel. The column is tested for sterility and pyrogenicity and is reusable in the same patient. It works with a plasma flow of 35 ml/min. The leakage of protein A and Sepharose is below detection limits (1 ng/ml resp. 2 ug/ml). Side-reactions are very rare due to the low leakage and, if observed, mild.

Protein A binds 100% of available IgG1, 2 and 4, less (30–80%) of IgG3. Mean for total IgG 92%. IgA is adsorbed at a mean of 69% and IgM 56%. The variation correlates to the utilization of the human Ig heavy chain variable region of the V(H)-III subgroup.

This group-selectivity makes it possible to treat large volumes of plasma in a two-parallel-column setting working alternately without any clinically significant lowering of albumin, fibrinogen or anti-thrombin III. No replacement fluid is required. Using the microprocessor driven monitor Citem 10® three plasma volumes could easily be treated in 4–5 h and repeated as necessary. Theoretically this gives the possibility of decreasing the IgG level to 5% of the starting value. Practically, re-equilibration and synthesis of Ig has to be accounted for. This gives a reduction of IgG after two procedures of 90%, which should be compared with 68% for plasma exchange. After three procedures 120% of the starting IgG value is removed by immunoadsorption (IA) compared with 100% by plasma exchange.

To date more than 500 patients have been treated with Excorim's IA system. Some of the indications treated so far are: hyperimmunization, focal glomerulosclerosis (FGS), Goodpasture's syndrome, Guillain–Barré syndrome, hemophilia with antibodies, myastenia gravis, rapidly progressive glomerulonephritis (RPGN), SLE and Wegener's granulomatosis.

Three indications will be highlighted: (i) hypersensitized patients awaiting kidney transplantation, (ii) RPGN and (iii) hemophilia with antibodies.

Hypersensitized patients awaiting kidney transplantation
A multicenter study with participating clinics from Spain, France, Great Britain, Norway and Sweden was performed with the purpose to investigate if IA could sufficiently remove anti-HLA to increase the possibility of grafting highly sensitized patients and achieve acceptable graft survival.

The treatment protocol includes 4–6 IA procedures combined with cyclophosphamide and prednisolone. Post-transplantation immunosuppression was done according to the standard triple drug regime.

Forty-five patients were included in the study: 32 were transplanted, 13 untransplanted (one blood access problems, six awaiting Tx or repeated IA, six drop outs). Of the 22 patients with historic positive crossmatch, the 2 year graft survival was 59% (40% for 10 patients with historic negative crossmatch).

The conclusions from the study are:

(i) Immunoadsorption with Immunosorba® can safely and effectively remove anti-HLA in ESRF patients.

(ii) Anti-HLA removal increases the possibility for transplanting highly sensitized ESRF patients.

(iii) Graft survival rate in immunoadsorbed patients is 60% at a mean follow-up of 2 years.

(iv) Graft function is stable at a creatinine level of 150 μmol/l.

Rapidly progressive glomerular nephritis (RPGN)

The treated indications are: Wegener's granulomatosis, Goodpasture's syndrome, polyarteritis nodosa, SLE and idiopathic RPGN.

Palmer *et al.* treated 10 patients with RPGN and acute renal failure with IA, prednisolone and cyclophosphamide. Three patients had SLE, five had microscopic polyarteritis and two had Wegener's granulomatosis. All 10 patients were dialysis-dependent prior to IA. Nine of 10 rapidly regained renal function and seven continue to have independent renal function between 9 and 30 months after IA. Three patients were not dialysis dependent at presentation. Despite treatment with methylprednisolone, cyclophosphamide and oral prednisolone, renal function continued to deteriorate and they required dialysis. IA was started without altering baseline immunosuppression. Within a mean of 4.6 days (range 3–7), renal function improved and dialysis was not longer required.

Treated plasma volumes were in the range of 33.6–80.6 l.

Hemophilia with antibodies

The presence of high levels of antibodies against factor VIII or IX constitutes a major complication in the treatment of hemophiliacs. Inhibitor patients present a clinical problem because a titer greater than 10 Bethesda Units/ml (BU/ml) is difficult to overcome by infusion of large doses of factor concentrates.

The use of IA with Immunosorba® provides a very efficient solution to the clinical problem. The response is very fast and in 2–4 days the inhibitor level is usually brought down below 10 BU/ml. Hemostasis could thus be achieved by the infusion of coagulation factor.

In some patients immunological tolerance has been achieved by a combination of IA, cyclophosphamide, IVIG and coagulation factor.

Patients with aquired hemophilia are sometimes more difficult to treat since the inhibitor may be continuously produced. Still the data appears satisfactory with successful removal in six of 10 patients. An even higher rate could most likely be achieved with a more extensive IA.

If side reactions occur they are usually mild and of the same character as with other extracorporeal techniques. A cost comparison between IA with Immunosorba®/Citem 10® and plasma exchange has to take into consideration the market price for the columns as well as that of substitution fluids, i.e. albumin or FFP. The comparison we have made shows that the cost per litre of treated plasma on the average is lower for IA than PE after 3–7 procedures. This varies from country to country. The actual status is shown in Table 1. Extracorporeal immunoadsorption with Immunosorba® is thus a safe and cost-effective method for the removal of antibodies.

Table 1.

Sweden	3
Denmark	3
Norway	3
United Kingdom	6
Spain	4
Italy	7

REFERENCES

1. P. Gjörstrup. Anti-HLA antibody removal in hyperimmunized ESRF patients to allow transplantation. *Transplant. Proc.*, **23**, 392–395 (1991).

2. A. Palmer, T. Cairns, F. Dische, G. Gluck, P. Gjörstrup, V. Parson, K. Welsh and D. Taube. Treatment of rapidly progressive glomerulonephritis by extracorporeal immunoadsorption, prednisolone and cyclophosphamide. *Nephrol. Dial. Transplant.*, **6**, 536–542 (1991).

3. J. Uehlinger, G. R. Button, J. McCarthy, A. Forster, R. Watt and L. M. Aledort. Immunoadsorption for coagulation factor inhibitors. *Transfusion*, **31**, 265–269 (1991).

4. P. Gjörstrup and R. Watt. Therapeutic protein A immunoadsorption. A review. *Transfus. Sci*, **11**, 281–302 (1990).

Therapeutic Plasmapheresis (XII), pp. 847-849
T. Agishi *et al.* (Eds)

Single Donor Platelet or Platelet/Plasma Protocols using the Mobile Collection System

J. W. SMITH, L. PECK, M. MOORE and R. O. GILCHER

Oklahoma Blood Instiute Oklahoma City,
Oklahoma, USA

Key words: apheresis; platelets; plasma.

INTRODUCTION

Single donor apheresis platelets and plasma provide the safest, most efficacious transfusion therapy. An easily transportable apheresis instrument has been developed by Haemonetics Corporation which permits the collection of single donor platelets, platelet poor plasma, and/or platelets and plasma in a miniaturized apheresis system. This instrument incorporates and improves on the functions of the Haemonetics V-50 in a single line venous access device.

METHODS AND MATERIALS

The Mobile Collection System (MCS) is an easily transportable apheresis system incorporating a Latham style centrifugal bowl, a vacuum loading centrifugal chuck, an enhanced optics system, microprocessor-controlled surge elutriation platelet separation, and sophisticated donor and system pressure monitors permitting the collection of products in a functionally closed system [1] using disposable that permit 5 day platelet storage [2].

The evaluation of the MCS has been carried out in several phases. Phase I consisted of 20 procedures in which plasma was collected initially on each pass followed by surge elutriation of platelets at the end of each pass. Phase II consisted of 18 procedures in which there were three passes collecting plasma and then platelets plus one additional pass to collect additional plasma. This protocol was tested in order to collect a 500 ml apheresis fresh frozen product, one of our standard products and the only transfusible plasma which is used in the Oklahoma Blood Institute system. Phase III consisted of 57 procedures in which single donor platelets were collected using an average of seven passes. In addition, data has been made available from several European centers which evaluated either the platelet/plasma protocol or the single donor platelet protocol.

RESULTS

The initial evaluations of the platelet/plasma protocols at OBI yielded the information summarized in Tables 1 and 2. Donor precounts were in normal ranges with hematocrits of 41.9% ($\pm6.2\%$) platelet counts of $279 \times 10^3/\mu l$ ($\pm58 \times 10^3/\mu l$) and white blood cell counts of $6.89 \times 10^3/\mu l$ ($\pm1.76 \times 10^3/\mu l$). The volumes collected for the apheresis plasma, as noted in Table 1, indicates the collection of 500 ml in Phase II with acceptable Hematocrit and pH. Apheresis plasma showed acceptable QC parameters of factor VIII of $122\pm34\%$, fibrinogen of 210 ± 20 mg/dl and total protein of 6.4 ± 0.57 g/dl. Apheresis platelet products from platelet/plasma protocols are summarized in Table 2 and indicate the collection of approximately one-half of a typical apheresis platelet product with all other parameters being acceptable. In summary for Phase I, three passes were required and took 41.9 ± 6.2 min. For Phase II there were three passes in which platelets were collected and 3.89 ± 0.68 passes in which plasma was collected with a total procedure

Table 1.

MCS apheresis plasma

	Volume (ml)	Hematocrit (%)	pH
Phase I ($n = 20$)	266±64	0.06±0.07	7.18±0.10
Phase II ($n = 18$)	487±27	0.06±0.07	7.15±0.05

Table 2.

MCS apheresis platelets

	Platelet yield ($\times10^{11}$)	Hematocrit (%)	WBC ($\times10^8$)	Volume (ml)	pH
Phase I ($n = 20$)	1.90±0.51	0.085±0.093	1.59±0.84	229±44	7.17±0.15
Phase II ($n = 18$)	1.79±0.39	0.16±0.23	4.04±4.43	185±39	7.15±0.05

Table 3.

MCS clinical results — Europe

	Platelet/plasma protocol[a] (mean ± SD)	Single donor platelet protocol[b] (mean ± SD)
Number of procedures	54±21 ($n = 217$)	25±14 ($n = 75$)
Volume processed (ml)	2395±267	3392±1314
Length of procedure (min)	66±9	105±44
Efficiency (%)	63.7±4.7	55±9.6
Number of cycles	5.25±0.5	7±2.6
Platelet precount ($\times10^3/\mu l$)	265±13	274±11
Total platelets ($\times10^{11}$)	3.3±0.7	3.8±0.8
Total WBC ($\times10^8$)	2.0±2.15	2.1±1.5
Concentrate volume (ml)	256±27	335±126
Plasma collected (ml)	364±50	

[a] Lausanne, Oxford, Dordrecht, Besancon (4/03/92).
[b] Dordrecht, Berlin, Besancon (4/03/92).

collected and 3.89 ± 0.68 passes in which plasma was collected with a total procedure time of 52.8 ± 7.8 min. The next phase evaluated single donor platelet protocols. During a 3 month period in which 57 procedures were performed, platelet yield was $4.39 \pm 1.15 \times 10^{11}$ platelets with $0.42 \pm 0.54 \times 10^9$ white cells in a total product volume of 399 ± 80 ml. The data from Europe is summarized in Table 3 and includes both the platelet plasma protocol and single donor platelet protocol. The platelet yields are quite acceptable in either product, meeting FDA criteria of 3.0×10^{11} platelets. The plasma volume collected is larger than would be typically taken from a whole blood unit, though not a double product.

DISCUSSION

The studies summarized in this report indicate the capability of the MCS to collect single donor platelets, apheresis plasma and one-half of a single donor platelet product, or single donor platelets plus apheresis plasma. These various products can be collected in single procedures using an instrument which can be transported to multiple collection sites. Depending upon the collection parameters specified, this instrument allows the option of several products to be drawn which are able to meet customer needs in a more effective manner. The easy transportability also facilitates collection of various products from donors in remote mobile locations.

CONCLUSIONS

The MCS provides flexibility of product collection by virtue of the Latham apheresis bowl. This facilitates the collection of plasma and the surge elutriation of platelets in one of several protocols. The system is set up in a functionally closed manner so that platelets have a 5 day outdate. The system is easily transportable and permits the collection of apheresis products in the mobile collection environment.

REFERENCES

1. M. S. Jacobson, S. V. Kevy, G. M. Thorne *et al.* Microbial challenge of a blood cell separator outside seal bowl system. *Transfusion*, **30**, 146–149 (1990).
2. D. M. Kenney, J. J. Peterson and J. W. Smith. Extended storage of single-donor apheresis platelets in CLX blood bags, effect of storage an platelet morphology, viability and *in vitro* function. *Vox Sang.*, **54**, 24–33 (1988).

Therapeutic Plasmapheresis (XII), pp. 851-855
T. Agishi *et al*. (Eds)
© VSP 1993

New Features of the Fresenius Blood Cell Separator AS 104

V. KRETSCHMER,[1] M. BIEHL,[2] C. COFFE,[3] R. ECKSTEIN,[4] D. KIPROV,[5]
G. MENICHELLA,[6] H. MITSCHULAT,[2] R. MOOG,[7] H. J. NEUMANN,[2]
T. PUSINELLI,[2] M. VALBONESI,[8] T. WEISSWANGE,[2]
D. WIEBECKE[9] and J. ZINGSEM[4]

[1]*Dept. Transf. Med. Coagulat. Physiolog., Univ. Marburg, Germany*
[2]*R&D, FRESENIUS St. Wendel, Germany*
[3]*Inserm-CRTS, Besancon, France*
[4]*Dept. Hematol. Oncolog., Univ. Rudolf Virchow, Berlin, Germany*
[5]*Dept. Medic. Immunotherapy, Children's Hosp., San Francisco, USA*
[6]*Dept. Hematol. Transfus., Univ. Cat. Sacre Cuore, Rome, Italy*
[7]*Dept. Transf. Med., Univ. Hosp., Essen, Germany*
[8]*Immunhematol. Services, San Martino Univ. Hosp., Genova, Italy*
[9]*Dept. Transf. Med. Immunohem., Univ. Clin., Würzburg, Germany*

INTRODUCTION

The Fresenius blood cell separator AS 104 belongs to the third generation of blood cell separators. It works as a continuous flow centrifuge with a sealless disposable system that collects blood products outside the centrifuge. All separation procedures work under full automatic control by an interface control system (IFC) and several sensitive detectors and monitors. The safety system consists of a redundant back up circuit that is independent of the microprocessor, and a software control. Up to now 12 application protocols are implemented in the ROM, which can be easily altered for individual applications and stored by the user in the RAM storage. The machine has a good and complete user guidance that is shown on the display.

MATERIALS AND METHODS

The AS 104 possesses a hardware safety system which includes detection of the alarm free condition of the sensors and monitors, detectors for power failure, ACD ratio (lower limit), pressure (in inlet and return line) and a blood leak detector in the centrifuge housing. The speed of the pumps is monitored and the correct closing of the centrifuge cover is detected. This hardware system works independently of the microprocessor. In addition, there is a software safety system which observes the microprocessor and includes detectors for ACD ratio (upper limit), hemolysis and hematocrit in the plasma (PLS) line, and centrifuge imbalance. Temperature in the centrifuge compartment is controlled by air ventilation. Further, a halt alarm is implemented and a leak will cause a pressure check failure in the disposable system. The following standard protocols are implemented: platelet (PLT) collection and depletion, peripheral blood stem cell (PBSC) collection, lymphocyte depletion, granulocyte collection, monocyte collection, bone marrow stem cell (BMSC) separation, plasma exchange and red cell exchange. The PLT collection can be done by a single needle (SN) or a dual needle (DN) procedure with special disposables for 1 day (C4) or 5 day (C4L) storage. It is possible to change from DN to SN during a running procedure. PLT collection can be done automatically after input of precount of the donor. Then the machine will produce a standard concentrate of 250 ml with 3.3×10^{11} PLT (values for Germany). Individual preparations are although possible. Standard protocols are listed in Table 1.

Table 1.

Standard protocols, version 4.4

Program	PLT		PBSC	BMSC	Gran	PLS
	DN	SN				
Blood volume (l)	3.5	3.5	10	***	5.2	4000
Blood flow (ml/min)	50	50	50	50	50	50
Interface position	7:1	7:1	6:2	6:2	6:2	4:4
ACD:WB ratio	1:10	1:10	1:10	1:10	1:10*	1:10
Concentrate volume (ml)	250	250	360	***	260	—
Centrifuge speed (r.p.m.)	1900	1900	1700	1200	750	2000
Duration (min)	70	86	215	***	120	80
Cycles	—	10	36	3	13	—
Phases per cycle	—	2**	4	3	3	—

*Citrate (500 ml HES 6% (450 kD) + 50 ml Na Citrate 33.3%)
**Blood donation with intermitted reinfusion by bag press (150 mmHg) with partial recirculation to centrifuge and automatic cuff control.
***Depending on the volume of the BM.

RESULTS

For PLT separation there is significant improvement when changing the protocols: whereas with protocol 4.1, 73% of the platelet concentrates have a contamination of less than 10^7 WBC, with protocol 4.4 more than 90% are within this range (Table 2). The medium WBC and RBC counts seem to be higher with a higher deviation due to a few extremely high values.

Table 2.

AS 104 PLT dual needle (1)

Protocol	4.1	4.4
Runs	610	340
PLT ($\times 10^{11}$)	3.5±1.0	3.6±1.0
Efficiency (%)	53±13.5	59±12.4
WBC ($\times 10^6$)	9±23	15±74
RBC ($\times 10^6$)	17±70	20±44

In comparison to the DN procedures the PLT-SN results (Tables 2 and 3) show the same efficiency of PLT collection due to the recirculation phase but a slightly increased WBC contamination and donation time.

PBSC collection yields (Table 4) and efficiencies are good, contamination with RBC and PLT is rather low.

BM harvest (Table 5) shows that the GFU-GM recovery (62%) was better than MNC recovery (43%). In no case was the cell viability (tested by trypan blue exclusion) affected by the procedure.

With the 'grancollect' protocol mean yields of $4.6 \times 1.7 \times 10^9$ can be obtained; contamination with RBC is $2.7 \pm 1.0 \times 10^6/\mu l$ and with PLT $243 \pm 59 \times 10^3/\mu l$, respectively (Table 6).

Plasma exchange has a very high efficiency (more than 90% of total plasma is separated). The PLT decrease in the patient and the PLT count in the plasma is low (Table 7 and 8).

Table 3.
AS 104 PLT single needle

Runs	I	II
n	20	52
Blood volume (ml)	3000	3200 (− ACD)
PLT ($\times 10^{11}$)	5.8	3.0
Efficiency (%)	76	59.3
Concentrate volume (ml)	340	250
WBC ($\times 10^6$)	28	30.5
Duration (min)	82	88

Table 4.
AS 104 PBSC collection ($n = 83$)

	Yield	Efficiency (%)
WBC ($\times 10^9$)	10.3±3.6	33±20
MNC ($\times 10^9$)	5.7 ± 2.1	56 ± 17
CFU-GM ($\times 10^4$)	153 ± 91	123±179

Table 5.
AS 104 BMSC collection (adults, $n = 17$)

BM volume (ml)	1450± 0.42	
Concentrate volume (ml)	138±34	
	Yield	Efficiency (%)
WBC ($\times 10^9$)	65 ± 22	32 ± 16
MNC ($\times 10^9$)	57 ± 10	43 ± 20
CFU-GM ($\times 10^4$)	401 ± 189	62±46
RBC ($\times 10^{11}$)	2.1	

Table 6.

AS 104 granulocyte collection* $(n = 9)$ [2]

Blood volume (ml)	5200 (−ACD)	
Concentrate volume (ml)	260	
	Yield	Efficiency (%)
WBC ($\times 10^9$)	9.2 ± 2.8	29.0 ± 22.5
Granulocytes ($\times 10^9$)	4.6 ± 1.7	22.5 ± 5.6

*Without donor stimulation.

Table 7.

AS 104 plasma exchange $(n = 1050)$

Blood volume (ml)	4000
Plasma volume (ml)	2800
PLT decrease ($\times 10^3/\mu$l)	90

Table 8.

AS 104 plasma exchange $(n = 13)$

Blood volume (ml)	4100	
Plasma volume (ml)	2800	
PLT ($\times 10^3/\mu$l)	Patient	pre 222.1
		post 158.9
	PLS waste	bag 27.4±12.1*

*One case $> 40 \times 10^3/\mu$l.

DISCUSSION AND CONCLUSIONS

Regarding PLT yield and donation time, the plateletpheresis results are good. The efficiency of the SN procedure is very high due to the recirculation phases during reinfusion cycles. Predicted and measured yields correlate rather good.

The BMSC collection — the only one available running automatically — is very efficient and the obtained reduction of RBC (92.6%) and granulocytes (84.8%) is sufficient for purging as well as for successful freezing, thawing and transplanting.

The PBSC protocol is a reliable and safe automatic procedure, with a high MNC and CFU-GM efficiency. Contamination of PLT and RBC is very low. The CFU-GM efficiency is much more important than MNC efficiency. This can be due either to the loss of potentially inhibitory cells or to high selectivity of the protocol.

The 'grancollect' procedure is still in its optimization phase.

Plasma exchange procedures with high separation efficiency can be performed very easily and quickly. Compared with the Cobe Spectra, both the PLT decrease in the blood of the patient ($90 \times 10^3/\mu$l AS 104; $180 \times 10^3/\mu$l Cobe Spectra) and the ACD volume necessary are rather small.

Priming of the disposables only takes between 3 and 5 min (C4L).

The Fresenius blood cell separator AS 104 has a high donor safety, a broad applicability and good separation efficiencies resulting in rather pure products. The protocols are individually adaptable for special clinical demands and there is still a great development potential. The machine is very easy to handle and there is full time help function available that will provide the user with answers in case of error, alarm or handling problems.

REFERENCES

1. N. Müller *et al.* Improvement of the separation efficiency and concentrate purity of Fresenius cell Separator AS 104: results of a multicentre study. *Tranf. Sci.*, **14**, 105–114 (1992).
2. N. Müller *et al.* Leukocytapheresis: evaluation of a new procedure for the blood cell separator Fresenius AS104. *Infusionsther*, **19**, 70–72 (1992).

Therapeutic Plasmapheresis (XII), pp. 857-859
T. Agishi *et al.* (Eds)
© VSP 1993

Heparin-Induced Extracorporeal Low Density Lipoprotein and Fibrinogen Precipitation (HELP): State of the Art June 1992

N. L. STROUT and B. BAYER

B. Braun Melsungen AG, Medical Technology Division, Melsungen, Germany

Key words: HELP.

The precipitation of low density lipoproteins (LDL) and fibrinogen at low pH levels in the presence of heparin as a therapeutic measure was developed by Seidel and co-workers at the University of Göttingen and was first described by them in the early 1980s [1]. In cooperation with the B. Braun Melsungen AG, a system for performing HELP treatments as a regular clinical procedure was developed. The basic concept of the system and the clinical results of HELP treatment have been reported extensively [2–4]. Since the introduction of the device in 1986 it has been used to perform over 25 000 treatments worldwide. This extensive clinical experience has helped to identify aspects of the system which play a key role in optimizing specific performance characteristics and minimizing operator problems.

Technologically the HELP procedure consists of five steps: separation of plasma from cellular components, acidification of the plasma and addition of heparin to cause precipitation of LDL and fibrinogen, filtration of the heparin/LDL and heparin/fibrinogen complexes, adsorption of excess heparin, and readjustment of plasma to physiological pH and correct volume by bicarbonate dialysis and ultrafiltration. All of these steps are performed on a single machine (Plasmat secura) using specific filters, fluid components and connection lines.

In optimizing the HELP system, a great deal of attention was paid to the plasma separation process, which is the heart of any plasmapheresis procedure. The separation of plasma and blood cells in the HELP system is achieved using a standard polypropylene plasma filter. To prevent the arterial needle from adhering to the wall of the patient's blood vessel, the pressure in the connection line between the needle and the blood pump (AP 1) is monitored continuously, and a user-adjustable lower pressure limit alarm warns of excessively high negative pressure (relative to the patient's blood pressure) in the line.

To avoid unnecessary alarms caused by temporary blockage of the needle, the Plasmat secura now reduces the blood pump speed by 50% the first time the lower pressure limit set by the user is exceeded. This will usually suffice to release the needle from the vessel wall and restore normal pressure levels. In this case the blood pump gradually returns to the previous speed, without manual adjustment or nurse intervention. If the pressure does not return to normal and remains outside the lower limit value for a period of 20 s, then the blood pump stops and an alarm notifies the nursing staff of the problem. This change should greatly reduce the number of blood pump alarms during treatment.

In previous versions of the Plasmat secura the transmembrane pressure (TMP) was calculated as ((blood in + blood out)/2) − plasma out. This has been changed so that plasma separation is governed solely by the inlet pressure (AP 2) and plasma outlet pressure (PLP 1). A plasma pump runs at whatever speed is necessary (up to 50 ml/min) to maintain a constant pressure difference between AP 2 and PLP 1, thus accounting for changes in blood pump speed or plasma separability. The desired pressure difference is defined by the operator; the maximum pressure difference is limited to 100 mmHg, in order to prevent possible hemolysis. The PLP 1 pressure is no longer set automatically to 50 mmHg below AP 2 after an alarm, as was previously the case. Instead, an alarm limit is set 10 mmHg below the pressure difference chosen by the operator. This saves the operator time and trouble. There is thus no not volume change for the patient.

The acidification of the plasma is achieved by adding a sodium acetate buffer with 100 000 IU heparin per liter. The buffer pump speed is keyed to the speed of the plasma pump at a ratio of 1:1 for adults and up to 3:1 for small children (to reduce the extracorporeal volume of plasma in the system). Thus with one 3 l bag of buffer up to 3 l of plasma can be treated with the HELP system. The plasma pump and the buffer pump feed into a precipitation chamber, where the precipitation of LDL and fibrinogen takes place. The heparin/LDL and heparin/fibrinogen complexes are removed from the plasma by a polycarbonate precipitate filter.

For a small percentage of patients the precipitate filter has in the past had to be replaced during treatment in order to treat the desired amount of plasma, usually 2.5–3 l [4]. A change in the filter membrane support material has been made to increase the effective usage of the available surface area. A change in the preparation of the filter prior to treatment may further increase the effective usage.

Plasma is drawn from the recirculation circuit through the precipitate filter by a filtrate pump. Since the speed of the filtrate pump is equal to the sum of the plasma pump and buffer pump speeds, the volume in the recirculation circuit is essentially constant. Two sensors at the upper and lower ends of the precipitation chamber ensure that the fluid volume does not increase or decrease significantly. Pressure between the precipitate filter and the filtrate pump (FP 1) is also monitored, and an operator-adjustable lower alarm limit serves to prevent excessive negative pressure due to a clogged filter.

The filtrate pump draws the LDL and fibrinogen-free plasma to the heparin adsorber, where excess heparin not required for precipitation is adsorbed to a DEAE cellulose membrane. The pressure between the filtrate pump and the heparin adsorber (FP 2) is also monitored continuously. An upper alarm limit prevents excess pressure due to a clogged heparin adsorber or kinked line. To prevent operator error in connecting the lines to the FP 1 and FP 2 transducers a fixed alarm has been added at 20 mmHg for FP 1 and −50 mmHg for FP 2.

To date HELP treatments have been performed using two small heparin adsorbers (model 250) in series. Since each heparin adsorber can bind up to 150 000 IU of heparin, the two adsorbers together would be capable of binding the total amount of heparin used in the HELP system if no precipitation were to occur. These are being replaced by a single heparin adsorber (model 500) with the same total binding capacity. This single heparin adsorber has the advantage of a significantly reduced resistance to flow and eliminates the need for a connecting line between the two previous heparin adsorbers, improving handling and hygiene. The new heparin adsorber can also be prepared for use in a shorter period of time, reducing operator time for preparation. An additional air detector will help maintain the efficiency of the heparin adsorber by preventing the influx of air, which would reduce the effective membrane surface area available for heparin adsorption.

Following the heparin adsorber the plasma flows directly through an ultrafilter, where excess fluid volume is removed and physiological pH is restored by bicarbonate dialysis. Fluid removal is induced by the difference in speed between the filtrate pump and the substitution pump. Since the substitution pump and plasma pump run at the same speed, and the filtrate pump speed is equal to the plasma pump speed plus the buffer pump speed, the volume that is provided by the buffer pump is removed in the ultrafilter, and the plasma volume removed from whole blood by the plasma pump is returned to the patient by the substitution pump.

The plasma outlet pressure of the ultrafilter (PLP 2) can be set by the operator according to the patient's needs. The dialysate inlet pump and negative pressure pump are then adjusted automatically to create the TMP needed to remove the correct amount of fluid. This allows the system to respond to changing conditions within the ultrafilter during HELP treatment. Excessive fluid removal is prevented by an alarm set at 20 mmHg below the PLP 2 value set by the operator.

The HELP system has proven itself to be a highly safe and effective system for the selective removal of atherogenic compounds such as LDL and fibrinogen. The changes made to the system based on broad clinical experience have optimized the performance characteristics and have helped minimize operator problems. A further development of the original HELP system is the adaptation of the system for dialysis patients, which allows a HELP treatment and a normal hemodialysis treatment to be performed simultaneously on one machine. This system is currently in trials, and first reports of the clinical results are very promising [5].

REFERENCES

1. H. Wieland and D. Seidel. A simple specific method for precipitation of low density lipoproteins. *J. Lipid Res.*, **24**, 904–909 (1983).

2. T. Eisenhauer, V. W. Armstrong, H. Wieland *et al.* Selective continuous elimination of low density lipoproteins (LDL) by heparin precipitation: first clinical application. *Trans. Am. Soc. Artif. Intern. Organs*, **32**, 104–107 (1986).

3. P. Schuff-Werner, E. Schütz, W. C. Seyde *et al.* Improved haemorheology associated with a reduction in plasma fibrinogen and LDL in patients being treated by heparin-induced extracorporeal LDL precipitation (HELP). *Eur. J. Clin. Invest.*, **19**, 30–37 (1989).

4. D. Seidel, V. W. Armstrong, P. Schuff-Werner *et al.* The HELP-LDL-apheresis multicentre study, an angiographically assessed trial on the role of LDL-apheresis in the secondary prevention of coronary heart disease. *Eur. J. Clin. Invest.*, **21**, 375–383 (1991).

5. T. Eisenhauer, U. Müller, P. Schuff-Werner *et al.* Simultaneous heparin extracorporeal LDL precipitation and hemodialysis: first clinical experience. *Trans. Am. Soc. Artif. Intern. Organs*, **37**, M494–M496 (1991).

21
Autologous Transfusion

Therapeutic Plasmapheresis (XII), pp. 863-869
T. Agishi *et al*. (Eds)
© VSP 1993

The Stat Compact as a Simplified Cell Separator

G. FLORIO, R. FRISONI, M. VALBONESI, C. CAPRA,
P. CARLIER and G. GIANNINI

Immunohematology Services, San Martino University Hospital, Genova, Italy

Key words: therapeutic apheresis; thrombocytapheresis; platelet apheresis; therapeutic thrombocytapheresis; therapeutic leukapheresis; erythro exchange; intraoperative blood salvage.

INTRODUCTION

Dictated by considerations of cost efficiency, volumes of blood salvaged and surgical volumes, as well as of risks of homologous blood transfusion, intraoperative blood salvage machines (IOBSM) are presently becoming an integral part of the apparatus used in transfusion medicine. Such apparatus, initially used to salvage red blood cells (RBC) from the operatory field, has been progressively modified and presently can be used to make preoperative hemodiluition and platelet rich plasma (PRP) sequestration [1] using the same kit that will be used later on, during operation. This technique, described in 1987 by our group, has been applied in more than 700 procedures. A similar technique rediscovered in 1991 by Silva *et al*. [2], proved effective in the preoperative collection of 800–1000 ml of autologous plasma containing approximately 1.9×10^{11} platelets, along with 2–3 units of packed RBC. In their hands, PRP transfusion after by-pass surgery and heparin neutralization contributed to reduced blood losses, with the chance for receiving no or only one homologous blood product exposure increased from 20 to 50%. In Silva's *et al*. experience an Electromedics AT 1000 system was used, whereas in our original experience a Dideco Autotrans BT 795-A was employed. Both experiences confirmed that not only are IOBSM derived from discontinuous flow cell separators, but also that they can be used as cell separators. Taking advantage of our long lasting experience with this type of machine, as well as of their inherent capabilities [3], we have initiated the use of the Autotrans apparatuses to carry out therapeutic procedures to be performed in the intensive care units. We recently have adapted the Dideco Stat-Compact apparatus both to preoperative PRP collection and emergency therapeutic procedures. Here we report very preliminary results of both techniques.

THE STAT-COMPACT APPARATUS

The machine is an evolution of the Stat Apparatus, produced by Dideco Srl, Mirandola, Modena, Italy. It weighs only 34.5 kg and its transportation is facilitated by the transport-cart. Its heart is the 175 cm^3 bowl that is spun by a centrifuge whose speed can be regulated by the operator. There are three lines which arrive to the bowl. The first is for the blood arriving from the reservoir, the second for the washing solutions and the last brings the effluent out of the bowl to an air/waste bag. The lines are under the control of three clamps which close and open automatically depending on the operational phases of the procedure. Immediately after the clamps, the three lines converge into a single line with a segment dedicated to a high flow peristaltic pump. During the filling phase, blood is aspirated from the reservoir into the bowl at 300–350 ml/min. Subsequent washing is done with saline pumped into the bowl at the same velocity for 3 min. After washing, RBC are sent into a reinfusion bag by the action of the same peristaltic pump that reverses its rotation in this phase. There are only four essential commands for the semi-automatic operation of the system: prime, wash, empty and stand-by. Two adjunctive arrow systems are used for the regulation of blood flow rate and revolutions per minute. A 'help' display is also provided to solve the most frequent technical problems.

The transformation of the Stat-Compact into a discontinuous flow cell separator requires only minor modifications:

(i) The line that normally comes from the reservoir is connected with a 16 gauge needle and works as an arterial line during the priming phase. Blood is anticoagulated with ACD-A by gravity as shown in Fig. 1. The ACD to blood ratio is regulated with a dropper or a roller clamp.

(ii) Before the waste bag a Y connection is inserted and the two branches connected with the waste bag and second transfer bag which, depending on the procedure to carry out, is destined to collect PRP or to contain the replacement solutions.

(iii) Only a couple of hemostats are required to close or to open the effluent lines depending on the desired procedure.

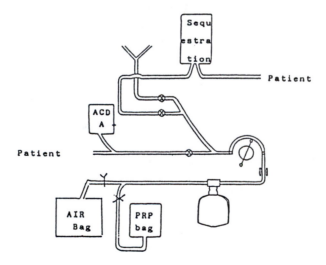

Figure 1. Configuration A — autologous PRP and PRBC sequestration. Patient's blood is anticoagulated by gravity with ACD-A. The blood flow is from 50 to 120 ml/min at 2880 r.p.m. When the bowl is full PRP is collected by moving the hemostat from X to Y. With the 'empty' command air comes back into the bowl and WRBC are sent to the sequestration bag. At each pass 0.68×10^{11} platelets can be collected along with 200 ml of plasma and 175 ml of packed red blood cells.

THE ADAPTED PROCEDURES

The main task of our job was to adapt the apparatus to perform preoperative hemodiluition and preoperative autologous PRP sequestration. This goal was met by aspirating ACD-A anticoagulated blood directly from the vein through the priming line, sending it into the bowl rotating at 2800 r.p.m. at blood flow rates ranging from 50 to 90 ml/min and collecting the autologous PRP in a dedicated collection bag. A working diagram of this procedure is presented in Fig. 1. In this empty phase the packed RBC were either reinfused or sequestered in the reinfusion bag (Fig. 1).

Taking advantage of the great simplicity of the system, the Stat-Compact was adapted in order to carry out therapeutic procedures. RF or thrombocytapheresis and leukapheresis, the main variation of the thrombocytapheresis procedure, was the collection of plasma and air in a dedicated bag, whereas the cell product was sent into the waste bag. The working diagram is depicted in Fig. 1. For therapeutic plasma exchange, plasma to be removed was sent into the waste bag whereas the replacement solutions were given back through the air bag, as shown in Fig. 2.

For erythroapheresis with RBC exchange, air and plasma were collected in a dedicated bag with air left on top of plasma. During the empty 'phase' RBC were sent in the reinfusion bag for subsequent elimination. Autologous plasma and substitution RBC were given back without passing through the bowl, by gravity, as shown in Fig. 3.

THE CLINICAL EXPERIENCE

The hemodiluition-autologous PRP application of the system was carried out in 45 cases in patients undergoing coronary by-pass surgery or major plastic or orthopedic and

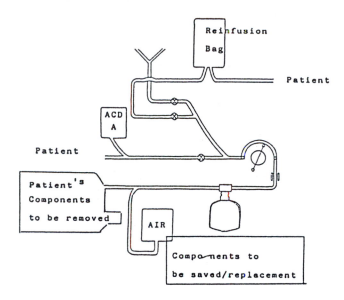

Figure 2. Configuration B — therapeutic apheresis. ACD-A anticoagulated blood is aspirated into the bowl rotating at 5800 r.p.m. Leaving the bowl after separation, the component to be eliminated is deviated into the waste bag. During the 'empty' phase air and replacement fluid are aspirated into the bowl where they are mixed with the PRBC prior to collection into the reinfusion bag.

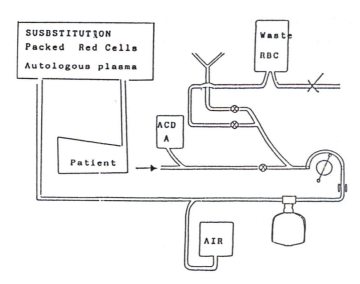

Figure 3. Configuration C — therapeutic erythroapheresis and exchange. After blood separation the patient's plasma is directly sent into the donor's RBC bag for direct transfusion. The air that is contained in the air bag is used to substitute for the patient's erythrocytes which are sent from the bowl in the waste RBC bag.

vascular surgery. In these operations the anticipated need for homologous blood products is of 2.5 units of PRBC and 1.7 units of PRP with only 10% chance of none or one homologous blood product exposure. Prior to operation these patients had no acute myocardial injury and no significant pulmonary, renal or liver disease. Their average hematocrit was 38.3%, ranging from 33 to 41.7% at the beginning of operation. The platelet precount averaged $238 \times 10^3/\mu l$. In 23 cases, 3 units of autologous RBC (175 ml) were sequestered. In the other 22 case, only 2 units could be collected. Isovolemia was maintained with cristalloids. The average procedure time was 10.8 min per pass. Autologous PRP was collected at each pass. Between 480 and 820 ml of PRP was collected and the platelet yield was of 0.68×10^{11} per pass. No attempt was made to prevent leukocyte or erythrocyte contamination, working in an autologous system. In five cases, transient hypotension was recorded after finishing blood collection. These episodes were easily managed by faster infusion of Hespan and phenylephrine. In these patients the chance of receiving none or only one homologous blood product exposure increased from the expected 10% to an observed 65%. No untoward effect was observed during the IOBS procedures, either during RBC retransfusion or at the end of the operation when autologous PRP was transfused. Some technical aspects of these procedures are given in Table 1.

As to therapeutic procedures, 24 patients had Stat-Compact treatment; these patients and the characteristics of their treatments are summarized in Tables 2 and 3. During plasma exchange 3.8–4% albumin was used as replacement, whereas fresh packed RBC were used as replacement in the case of therapeutic cytapheresis. Most of these procedures have been carried out as emergency therapies in intensive care units. From

Table 1.
Autologous RBC and PRB plasma sequestration with the Stat-Compact

Procedures	45 (cardiovascular surgery, plastic, orthopedic surgery)
Preoperative HCT	38.5%
Preoperative platelets	$238 \times 10^3/\mu l$
PRBC sequestration	2.54 units (175 ml)
Platelet yield/pass	0.68×10^{11}
PRP collection/pass	258 ml
Average plasma collection	530 ml
Average time/pass	10.8 min
Chance for receiving more than 1 unit of hoimologous blood	37%

Table 2.
Therapeutic plasma exchange with the Stat-Compact

Diagnosis	Cases	Procedures	Volume (l)	Procedure time (min)
Myasthenia Gravis	3	8	3.1	78
Acute GBS	3	10	2.7	73
TTP	2	7	2.9	84
Cryoglobulinemia	3	4	2.6	71
RPGN, ANCA+	1	2	3.1	67
Waldenstrom M.	2	4	2.8	71
Secondary hyperbilir.	2	4	3.2	84
	16	39	∼ 2.8	∼ 75

Table 3.
Therapeutic cytaphereses with the Stat-Compact

Diagnosis	Cases	Sessions	Volume of blood (l)	Procedure time (min)
CML thrombocytemia	5	8	6	95
CML leukostatic synd	2	3	4.9	100
Erythro exchange (cerebral malaria)	1	1	5.8	137
	8	12	∼ 5.5	∼ 120

a clinical point of view the results of these treatments were the ones expected when carying out the same procedures with the usual discontinuous or continuous flow cell separators. The same holds for the observed untoward effects.

COMMENTS

Our study has demonstrated that the Stat-Compact, like other machines for IOBS, can be safely employed as a limited performance DFC cell separator. The advantages of the systems are that:

  (i) Intentional preoperative hemodiluition and autologous PRP sequestration can be carried out using the same kit that immediately after is employed for intraoperative blood salvage.

  (ii) Simple therapeutic procedures, such as plasma exchange, thrombocytapheresis, leukapheresis and erythroapheresis with erythro exchange, can be done without any technical problems.

  (iii) The high speed of the centrifuge helps fast separation of the blood components for fast operations.

  (iv) The system cannot complete with full-option cell separators but can be of absolute utility when emergency treatments are required.

  (v) This depends on the excellent transportability of the machine even in hospitals such as ours with many blocks spread in the hospital complex, where surgery resuscitation units operate.

  (vi) The personnel normally dedicated to IOBS can operate the machine, avoiding the personnel operating in the blood bank to be compelled to move with cell separators to the operatory blocks.

  (vii) This holds mostly for patients who need apheresis as preparation for surgery, such as in the case of hyperbilirubinemia in preparation for liver transplantation, myasthenic crisis prior to or after thymectomy.

  (viii) The cost of the procedure is reduced compared with the procedures carried out with normal separators. In our conditions the cost of the harness is US$ 95 for the IOBSM and US$ 140 for the cell separators.

  (ix) These advantages, along with the possibility of preoperative sequestration of RBC and PRP, contribute to make the Stat-Compact machine even more cost effective. The machine presently needs only the automation of these manual procedures.

CONCLUSION

The Stat-Compact is a safe and fast apparatus for IOBS. It can be used for RBC and PRP preoperative sequestration. As the Dideco Autotrans BT 795-A it can be used to carry out therapeutic procedures such as PEX, thrombocytapheresis, leukapheresis and erythro exchange. These procedures are fast as the blood flow rate is 50–300 ml/min. The machine cannot compete with full cell separators. The cost of the machine and of the kits is 60% of the costs to be sustained with cell separators. An automatic delivery of anticoagulant is necessary. Total automation of the procedures is the next step.

REFERENCES

1. M. Ferrari, S. Zia, M. Valbonesi *et al.* A new technique for hemodiluition, preparation of autologous platelet-rich plasma and intraoperative blood salvage in cardiac surgery. *Int. J. Artif. Organs*, **10**, 47 (1987).

2. V. A. Silva, G. J. Despotis and G. C. Pond. Effectiveness of intraoperative platelet-rich plasma collection and blood salvage in reducing homologous blood exposure in cardiac surgery (Abstract). *American Society for Apheresis: 12th Annual Meeting.* New Orleans (1991).

3. M. Valbonesi, M. Ferrari, S. Zia *et al.* New application of the Autotrans: Autologous support of the organ donor and salvage of the donor's red blood cells for the transfusion support of organ recipients. *J. Clin. Apheresis*, **4**, 166 (1988).

Therapeutic Plasmapheresis (XII), pp. 871-874
T. Agishi *et al.* (Eds)
© VSP 1993

Rheological Changes of Rat Blood upon Administration of Recombinant Human Erythropoietin

N. MAEDA,[1] K. KON,[2] N. TATEISHI,[1] Y. SUZUKI,[1]
T. TANIGUCHI[2] and T. SHIGA[3]

[1]*Department of Physiology, School of Medicine, Ehime University, Shigenobu, Onsen-gun, Ehime, Japan*
[2]*Department of Physiology, Ehime College of Health Science, Tobe, Iyo-gun, Ehime, Japan*
[3]*Department of Physiology, School of Medicine, Osaka University, Suita, Osaka, Japan*

Key words: recombinant erythropoietin; blood viscosity; red cell deformability; red cell aggregation; hemorheology.

INTRODUCTION

Recombinant human erythropoietin (rhEPO) is effective in ameliorating anemia in chronic renal failure through a rapid rise in hematocrit [1, 2] and it may dramatically alter the function of the blood bank [3]. However, the inevitable increase of blood viscosity accelerates the risk of cardiovascular diseases [4].

This paper describes the rheological changes of blood upon intravenous administration of rhEPO to normal rats daily for 1 week, with the hematological properties and the red cell metabolism.

MATERIALS AND METHODS

rhEPO administration
Either 180 or 1800 IU/kg rhEPO (a gift from Chugai Pharmaceutical Co., Japan) [5] was administered to 6 week old Sprague–Dawley rats daily for 1 week through the tail vein (only vehicle was administered to control rats). The growth of rats as measured by body weight was not affected by rhEPO administration.

All measurements were performed within 20 min after collection of blood from the abdominal aorta, in order to avoid the effect of echinocytic transformation of red cells, which inevitably occurs [5].

Rheological measurements
Viscosity of whole blood and plasma was measured at various shear rates at 25 °C with a cone-plate viscometer.

Using a high shear rheoscope [6, 7], red cells were deformed in isotonic HEPES-buffered saline containing 14 or 20 g/dl Dextran T-40 at 25 °C by shear force. By measuring the long radius (L) and short radius (S) of 50–100 ellipsoidally deformed cells on flash photographs, the 'deformability' was expressed by the deformation index, $(L - S)/(L + S)$.

The red cell aggregation at a shear rate of 7.5 s^{-1} in autologous plasma was measured at a hematocrit of 0.4% at 25 °C, using a low-shear rheoscope [6, 8]. The 'velocity of red cell aggregation' (v, μm^2/min) was expressed by the growing rate of averaged projected area of individual rouleaux.

Hematological examinations
The standard method was used for the determination of hematological parameters. Reticulocytes were counted on blood smears with supravital staining. The density distribution of red cells was determined using phthalate esters. Electrophoresis on cellulose acetate membrane was adopted to determine the relative amount of plasma proteins.

Organic phosphates in red cells
2,3-DPG was determined by an enzymatic method. The content of purine nucleotides was determined for acid extract by high performance liquid chromatography [9]. The energy charge of adenylates was calculated by (2 [ATP] + [ADP])/2 ([ATP] + [ADP] + [AMP]).

RESULTS AND DISCUSSION

Blood viscosity
Blood viscosity–hematocrit relations of control and rhEPO-administered rats at shear rate of 40–380 s^{-1} corresponded well with a standard relation obtained for normal blood from 6 week old rats, in spite of the considerable increase of reticulocytes and young red cells (see below). The cell–cell interaction may be considered to interpret the blood viscosity [7]. Upon rhEPO administration, the plasma viscosity and the composition of plasma proteins were not altered.

Red cell deformability
No significant alteration of the deformation index was observed at shear stresses of 9–160 dyn/cm^2, in spite of the large MCV and low MCHC (Table 1). However, the deformed red cells in rhEPO-administered rats were longer than those in control rats, and the statistical distribution was unsymmetrical (i.e. the red cells were heterogeneous).

Red cell aggregation
The rouleaux were clearly shorter in rhEPO-administered rats than in control rats. The velocity of red cell aggregation was lower in rhEPO-administered rats than in control rats (Table 1). The suppressed aggregation in rhEPO-administered rats is probably due to the high density of negative charges (mainly of sialic acid) on the surface of young cells [5, 10], which increases the electrostatic repulsion between red cells [6].

Table 1.
Hematological, biochemical and rheological changes of rat blood upon rhEPO administration

	Control	rhEPO-administered	
		180 IU/kg	1800 IU/kg
RBC (/pl)	7.28 ± 0.17	8.03 ± 0.11**	8.50 ± 0.26**
Hb (g/dl)	15.2 ± 0.3	17.9 ± 0.5**	18.2 ± 0.7**
Ht (%)	43.4 ± 0.9	53.8 ± 1.7**	56.7 ± 2.4**
MCV (fl)	59.6 ± 1.5	67.0 ± 2.2**	66.7 ± 1.3**
MCH (pg)	20.9 ± 0.4	22.3 ± 0.7	21.4 ± 0.4
MCHC (g/dl RBC)	35.0 ± 0.3	33.3 ± 0.3**	32.0 ± 0.4**
Reticulocyte (%)	3.1 ± 1.2	7.9 ± 1.9**	15.7 ± 1.7**
2,3-DPG (mM/1 RBC)	8.45 ± 0.51	8.47 ± 0.39	7.92 ± 0.47
AMP (mM/1 RBC)	0.030 ± 0.004	0.030 ± 0.015	0.026 ± 0.003
ADP (mM/1 RBC)	0.223 ± 0.032	0.208 ± 0.051	0.203 ± 0.008
ATP (mM/1 RBC)	1.019 ± 0.123	1.216 ± 0.137*	1.201 ± 0.070*
EC	0.889 ± 0.006	0.908 ± 0.025	0.910 ± 0.007**
GTP (mM/1 RBC)	0.183 ± 0.036	0.221 ± 0.029	0.254 ± 0.034**
DI	0.333 ± 0.019	0.346 ± 0.016	0.324 ± 0.008
v (μm^2/min)	8.3 ± 1.8		6.4 ± 1.5

Values are presented by mean ± SD ($n = 6$). Statistical significance to control rats (**$P < 0.01$, *$P < 0.05$). EC, energy charge of adenylates; DI, deformation index, measured at 22 dyn/cm^2; v, velocity of red cell aggregation (control, $n = 9$, for 6 week old rats; rhEPO-administered, $n = 4$ for 7 week old rats).

Hematological and biochemical properties

During growth of rats, red cell count, hematocrit and hemoglobin concentration increased. These values and reticulocytes further increased upon rhEPO administration in a dose-dependent manner (Table 1).

MCV was larger in rhEPO-administered rats than in control rats (not significant between 180 and 1800 IU/kg). MCHC decreased upon rhEPO administration (MCH, not altered significantly). Probably, red cells produced acutely by rhEPO are characteristic in young cells (with large MCV and low MCHC) [6, 9]. Analysis of the density distribution of red cells showed that red cells in rhEPO-administered rats were light and inhomogeneous, probably due to the appearance of reticulocytes and low MCHC cells.

2,3-DPG content and the molar ratio to hemoglobin were not altered upon rhEPO administration. Probably, the oxygen-binding properties of hemoglobin in red cells is not altered in the polycythemic state. The ATP level and the energy charge of adenylates were slightly higher in rhEPO-administered rats than in control rats (no differences in ADP and AMP levels between both rats). The increase of ATP is characteristic of young cells [9]. GTP increased in rhEPO-administered rats, in a dose-dependent manner.

In conclusion, clinical attention should be given to the control of hematocrit upon rhEPO administration to avoid adverse effects due to polycythemic hyperviscosity; special attention to the alterations of red cell deformability and red cell aggregation is not needed.

Acknowledgments

The authors are indebted to Chugai Pharmaceutical Co. for cooperation. This work was supported in part by grants from the Ministry of Education, Science and Culture of Japan and from the Ehime Health Foundation.

REFERENCES

1. E. D. Zanjani and J. L. Ascensao. Erythropoietin. *Transfusion*, **29**, 46–57 (1989).

2. K.-U. Eckardt and C. Bauer. Erythropoietin in health and disease. *Eur. J. Clin. Invest.*, **19**, 117–127 (1989).

3. D. W. Golde and J. C. Gasson. Hormones that stimulate the growth of blood cells. *Sci. Am.*, **259**, 34–42 (1988).

4. A. E. G. Raine. Hypertension, blood viscosity, and cardio-vascular morbidity in renal failure: implications of erythropoietin therapy. *Lancet*, **i**, 7–100 (1988).

5. N. Maeda, K. Kon, N. Tateishi *et al.* Rheological properties of erythrocytes in recombinant human erythropoietin-administered normal rat. *Br. J. Haematol.*, **73**, 105–111 (1989).

6. T. Shiga, N. Maeda and K. Kon. Erythrocyte rheology. *Crit. Rev. Oncol. Hematol.*, **10**, 9–48 (1990).

7. K. Kon, N. Maeda and T. Shiga. Erythrocyte deformation in shear flow: influences of internal viscosity, membrane stiffness, and hematocrit. *Blood*, **69**, 727–734 (1987).

8. T. Shiga, K. Imaizumi, N. Harada *et al.* Kinetics of rouleaux formation using TV image analyzer. I. Human erythrocytes. *Am. J. Physiol.*, **245**, H252–H258 (1983).

9. T. Shiga, M. Sekiya, N. Maeda *et al.* Cell age-dependent changes in deformability and calcium accumulation of human erythrocytes. *Biochim. Biophys. Acta*, **814**, 289–299 (1985).

10. H. Walter, E. J. Krob, C. H. Tamblyn *et al.* Surface alterations of erythrocytes with cell age: rat red cell is not a model for human red cell. *Biochim. Biophys. Res. Commun.*, **97**, 107–113 (1980).

Therapeutic Plasmapheresis (XII), pp. 875-878
T. Agishi *et al.* (Eds)
© VSP 1993

Application of Recombinant Human Erythropoietin for Preoperative Autologous Blood Banking on Patients Undergoing Cardiac Surgery

K. KUMON, H. SUGIMOTO, H. KITAHARA, Y. INAGAKI, N. YAHAGI,
Y. KITOH,[1] N. NAKAJIMA[1] and Y. KAWASHIMA[1]

Surgical Intensive Care Unit and [1]Cardiovascular Surgery, National Cardiovascular Center, Suita, Japan

Key words: erythropoietin; subcutaneus administration; autologous transfusion; cardiac surgery.

INTRODUCTION

Cardiac surgery has hitherto required a large volume of homologous transfusion (HT). The complications inherent in the HT have worsened the morbidity and mortality of patients who successfully received cardiac surgery, and have made increased efforts to avoid HT. Recently, the use of autologous transfusion (AT) has become a standard of care for avoiding HT [1]. Recombinant human erythropoietin (rh-EPO), which enhances endogenous erythropoiesis [2], may shorten the periods for preoperative autologous deposit (PAD). However, little is known about the administration of it for PAD.

We applied rh-EPO on patients who were scheduled to undergoing cardiac surgery with AT, and studied the application of it for PAD, including the administration methods, its efficacies, etc.

PATIENTS AND METHODS

This study was performed on 71 patients who were scheduled to undergo cardiac surgery with AT. We employed five protocols for the administration of rh-EPO and the PAD (Table 1). The intravenous (i.v.) administration of rh-EPO was for Protocol A, B, C and D, and the subcutaneous (s.c.) administration of it was for Protocol E. rh-EPO was initiated 1–3 weeks before operation and one unit (400 g)/week of PAD was donated 1 or 2 weeks before operation. Doses and times of the rh-EPO are listed in Table 1. Daily, 200 mg of Fe was given orally in all patients during the study periods.

We detected plasma levels of erythropoietin (EPO), reticulocyte and hemoglobin (Hb) before and after the administration of rh-EPO. Moreover, we calculated increased volumes of Hb per week from the changes in blood levels of Hb, donated volume of hemoglobin and circulating blood volume.

Table 1.
Protocols and patients summary for the administration of rh-EPO and PAD

	rh-EPO				PAD				
	dose (unit)	site	initiation (w.b.o.)	times (/w)	unit	volume (g)	patients no.	age (yr)	body weight (kg)
A	6000	i.v	3	2–3	2	800	10	49 ± 7	65 ± 11
B	6000	i.v.	2	daily	2	800	12	49 ± 15	61 ± 8
C	9000	i.v.	2	2–3	2	800	10	56 ± 6	63 ± 9
D	9000	i.v.	1	daily	1	400	6	43 ± 8	60 ± 11
E	24000	s.c.	1	1	1	400	33	51 ± 15	56 ± 11

w.b.o.: week(s) before operation. w: week.

RESULTS

The 1 unit/week of PAD treatments were safely carried out in all patients during the study periods.

Plasma levels of EPO just before operation increased significantly in all groups except group A. The plasma EPO levels of group E increased dramatically from 37 ± 42 to 489 ± 234 mU/ml 1 day after the administration, and then decreased gradually but kept a significantly high level of 58 ± 41 mU/ml even 1 week after administration (Fig. 1). Reticulocyte levels increased significantly just before operation in all groups, as shown in Fig. 2. Average increased volumes of Hb/week were 24.1 g in group A, 44.8 g in group B, 44.9 g in group C, 50 g in group D and 18.2 g in groups E. Figure 3 shows the weekly increased volume of Hb of group A and E. There was little increase in the Hb volume for the initial week in group A, but thereafter it escalated and subsequently reached 68.1 g at the third week. The increased Hb volume of the initial first week in group E was significantly higher than that of group A.

Antibody for erythropoietin was not detected in any patients through the study periods.

HT was evaded completely in 92% of the study patients during and after operation (400 g of PAD for 85.7% and 800 g of PAD for 94.4%).

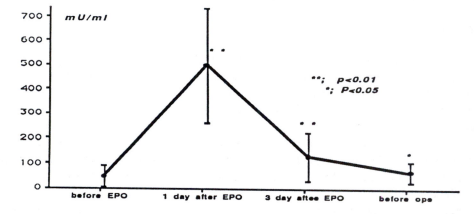

Figure 1. Plasma EPO levels (mean ± SD) after s.c. administration of 24 000 units of rh-EPO in group E.

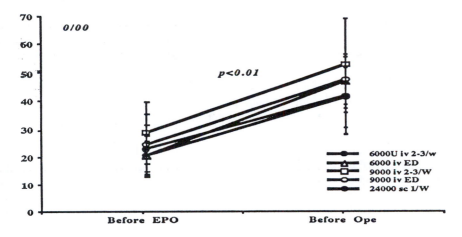

Figure 2. Reticulocytes before rh-EPO and just before operation.

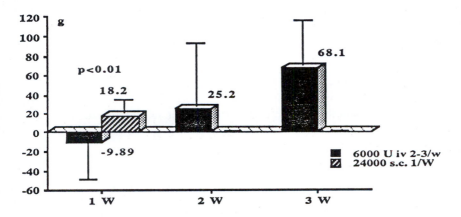

Figure 3. Weekly increased volume of Hb in groups A and E.

DISCUSSION

The HT free ratio of the study patients was significantly high compared with that of 29 patients who received cardiac surgery without PAD, which accounted for 62.1%. PAD, therefore, should reduce hologous blood use, which should diminish the complications of HT and subsequently result in improving the morbidity and mortality of cardiac surgical patients.

The use of rh-EPO enabled us to do the PAD safely in the short preoperative periods, as verified in this study. There has been little information about the method of administration of rh-EPO for PAD, but all methods applied in this study were shown to be effective.

Increased EPO levels associated with increased reticulocytes just before operation, as observed in this study, elucidated accelerating erythropoiesis by the administration of exogenous EPO in the PAD, which, moreover, should accelerate postoperative erythropoiesis and also result in reducing the requirements of homologous transfusion.

The changes in EPO levels of group E suggest that subcutaneus administration of rh-EPO may keep accelerating erythropoiesis for a long period (1 week) after s.c. administration.

Around 50 g of Hb is identical with hemoglobin volumes in 400 g of whole blood. Average weekly increased volume of hemoglobin in group B, C and D reached levels equal to the lost hemoglobin volume by blood donation, but were not sufficient in either group A and E.

As shown in Fig. 3, however, the increased volume of Hb at the third week of group A exceeded 50 g. There are some lag periods for the accelerating erythropoiesis after the administration of rh-EPO. We, therefore, recommend initiating the administration of rh-EPO 2–3 weeks before operation for PAD.

Increased volume of Hb at the initial week of group E was significantly higher than that of group A, which indicates that subcutaneous administration of rh-EPO has more potent enhancing effects on erythropoiesis than the i.v. administration because of its continuous stimulation to the erythropoietic systems. Moreover, s.c. rh-EPO administration is required only once per week for the PAD, which is very convenient for both patients and physicians.

CONCLUSION

From these results, we conclude that PAD with rh-EPO is effective for avoiding HT, and that all methods for the administration of rh-EPO applied in this study were effective for PAD, but we recommend 400 g of PAD per week under s.c. administration of rh-EPO once per week.

REFERENCES

1. M. A. Popovsky. Autologous blood transfusion in the 1990s. Where is it heading? *Am. J. Clin. Pathol.*, **97**, 297–300 (1992)
2. A. Edward, M. D. Levine, A. Steven *et al.* Perioperative recombinant human erythropoietin. *Surgery*, **106**, 432–438 (1989).

Therapeutic Plasmapheresis (XII), pp. 879-882
T. Agishi *et al.* (Eds)
© VSP 1993

The Efficacy of Recombinant Human Erythropoietin (rHuEPO) in Predeposited Autologous Blood Transfusion for Orthopedic Surgery

H. MAEDA, Y. HITOMI, R. HIRATA, H. TOHYAMA,
J. ODA and N. TSUZUKI

Blood Transfusion Service and Department of Orthopedic Surgery, Saitama Medical Center, Saitama Medical School, Kawagoe, Saitama 350, Japan

Key words: predeposited autologous blood transfusion; erythropoietin.

INTRODUCTION

Recent transfusion medicine has entered a new era marked by the risks of diseases transmitted by homologous transfusion. In particular, transmission of human immuno-deficiency virus (HIV) or non-A non-B hepatitis virus and transfusion-associated graft-versus-host disease cause lethal adverse effects to patients, and the safety of the blood transfused is the public and physicians' concern. Autologous blood is an alternative and the safest blood for transfusion. We have practiced predeposited autologous blood transfusion in patients undergoing orthopedic surgery. The advantage of predeposits of whole blood and storage in the liquid phase is simple and convenient. However, the blood in liquid is effective in 21 days in Japan and collection of a certain amount of blood in the limited time leads the patient/donor to the anemic state and hence makes it difficult to collect further blood. One strategy to overcome this disadvantage is to utilize recently developed recombinant human erythropoietin (rHuEPO) during donations [1, 2]. rHuEPO has been demonstrated to be effective in improving the anemia of uremic patients on dialysis [3]. In this study, we designed the use of rHuEPO in an autologous blood donation program and evaluated the efficacy of rHuEPO in such a program.

PATIENTS AND METHODS

The subjects were 31 patients who underwent hip joint surgery and consented to prede-posited autologous blood donation and administration of rHuEPO (EPOCH) provided by Chugai Pharmaceutical Co., Tokyo, Japan. All patients donated 400 ml of autolo-gous blood at 17, 10 and 3 days before operation, if their hemoglobin (Hb) levels were greater than 11.0 g/dl. Twelve patients donated blood without dosing rHuEPO and were given two tablets of ferrous sulphate (210 mg iron) orally every day from 2 weeks be-fore the first donation (the control group). Nine and 10 patients donated the same three units of autologous blood but received 6000 IU rHuEPO twice or thrice a week from

1 week before the first donation until operation, a total of 8 or 11 injections, together with 40 mg saccharated ferric oxide intravenously at each donation (the EPO 2/W and EPO 3/W group, respectively). The sex, age, body weight, the initial Hb level, serum iron and ferritin levels, the type of operation, and perioperative blood loss among three groups is shown in Table 1.

Table 1.
The background of the patients studied

		Control	6000 U 2/W	6000 U 3/W
Number of patients		12	9	10
sex (M; F)		1; 11	1; 8	1; 9
age		33.6 (9.5)	40.1 (21.3)	48.6 (15.1)
body weight		50.9 (5.9)	52.0 (3.5)	51.9 (5.2)
Type of surgery	RAO	10	5	4
	THR	1	4	5
	others	1	0	1
Initial Hb (g/dl)		13.8 (1.0)	12.9 (1.0)	12.7 (0.8)
Fe (μ g/dl)		96.2 (27.4)	83.5 (31.5)	124.3 (51.7)
Ferritin (ng/ml)		42.8 (30.7)	53.1 (35.9)	48.4 (25.9)
Blood loss (ml)		1001 (270)	1014 (522)	835 (287)

Mean (SD).

RESULTS AND DISCUSSION

The change of Hb values during donations
The Hb values of the control group before donation were 13.8 (1.0) g/dl on preoperative day −24 and 13.8 (1.2) g/dl on day −17, respectively. After each 400 ml weekly donation, these Hb values decreased to 12.5 (0.9) on day −10, 11.9 (1.2) on day −3 and 10.9 (0.7) g/dl on day −1, respectively. Ten of 12 patients completed 1200 ml donations. The mean initial Hb levels of the EPO 2/W ($n = 9$) and EPO 3/W ($n = 10$) groups were 13.0 (1.1) and 12.7 (0.8) g/dl, respectively, and were slightly lower than that of the control group. The Hb values of the EPO 3/W group slightly but significantly increased to 13.2 (0.7) g/dl on day −17 after a weekly administration of rHuEPO, while that in the EPO 2/W group remained unchanged. After each donation, the Hb values in the 2/W and EPO 3/W groups decreased to 12.5 (1.2) and 13.1 (1.1) g/dl on day −10, 12.4 (0.8) and 12.5 (0.9) on day −3, and 12.0 (1.4) and 12.0 (1.4) on day −1, respectively. All 19 patients succeeded in 1200 ml donations. The Hb levels of the EPO-treated groups after the third donation (i.e. just before operation) were significantly higher than that of the control group not given rHuEPO.

The decreased Hb values during donations
To evaluate the efficacy of rHuEPO, the decreased Hb values were calculated by subtracting Hb values at each donation time and just before operation from that of pretreatment. The decreased Hb values after the first, second and third donation in the

control group were 1.35 (0.16), 1.88 (0.19) and 3.07 (0.18) g/dl, respectively, while those Hb values were 0.46 (0.23), 0.52 (0.24) and 1.09 (0.33) in the EPO 2/W group and 0.38 (0.26) increase, 0.20 (0.34) and 0.66 (0.31) g/dl in the EPO 3/W group (Fig. 1). The decreased Hb values after the second and third donations in the control group were significantly greater than those of the EPO 2/W and EPO 3/W groups ($P < 0.0001$). Thus, administration of rHuEPO (6000 IU) twice or thrice a week for 4 weeks before operation was efficacious in preventing anemia induced by autologous blood donation.

The Hb values after operation

The Hb values on postoperative day 3 in the EPO 2/W and EPO 3/W groups were 9.8 (1.9) and 10.4 (1.3) g/dl, respectively, and significantly higher than 8.7 (1.9) g/dl in the control group. Three patients with Hb values of 6.2, 7.3 and 7.5 g/dl in the control group received 2 or 3 units of homologous blood. None in the EPO-treated groups received homologous blood. The Hb values in the control group, however, reached 10.9 g/dl on postoperative day 14 and were not significantly different from 10.3 g/dl in the EPO 2/W group and 11.2 g/dl in the EPO 3/W group.

Conclusion

To avoid the adverse effects of homologous transfusion, we have performed predeposited autologous blood transfusion in patients undergoing orthopedic surgery with or without dosing of rHuEPO. All the patients donated three 400 ml autologous blood, a total of 1200 ml, on preoperative days −17, −10 and −3, if their Hb values were greater than 11.0 g/dl. The Hb values in the control group ($n = 12$) who were not given rHuEPO decreased to 3.07 (0.18) g/dl after three 400 ml donations, while those in the

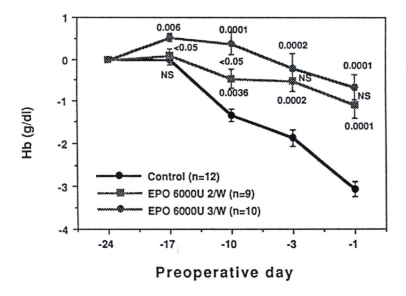

Figure 1. Decreased Hb values during autologous blood donations.

EPO 2/W ($n = 9$) and EPO 3/W ($n = 10$) groups who received rHuEPO (6000 IU) twice or thrice a week for 4 weeks before operation slightly decreased to 1.09 (0.33) and 0.66 (0.31) g/dl, respectively, which were significantly less than that of the control ($P < 0.0001$). Three of 12 patients in the control group received 2 or 3 units of homologous blood transfusion postoperatively, while none in the EPO-treated groups received homologous blood. Thus administration of rHuEPO in predeposited autologous blood donation setting was not only efficacious in preventing the anemia induced by donations but also promising for avoiding homologous blood transfusion.

REFERENCES

1. H. Maeda, Y. Hitomi, R. Hirata *et al.* Erythropoietin and autologous blood donation. *Lancet*, **2**, 284 (1989).
2. L. M. Goodnough, S. Rudnick, T. H. Price *et al.* Increased preoperative collection of autologous blood with recombinant human erythropoietin therapy. *N. Engl. J. Med.*, **321**, 1163 (1989).
3. J. W. Eschbach, J. G. Egrie, M. R. Downing *et al.* Correction of the anemia of end-stage renal disease with recombinant human erythropoietin. *N. Engl. J. Med.*, **316**, 73 (1987).

Therapeutic Plasmapheresis (XII), pp. 883-886
T. Agishi *et al.* (Eds)
© VSP 1993

Effect of Recombinant Human Erythropoietin (rHuEPO) and Autologous Blood Transfusion in Open Heart Surgery

M. TAKINAMI, M. OSAWA, K. HORIBA, N. ISHIGAMI,
T. KIMURA and Y. HARADA

First Department of Surgery, Hamamatsu University School of Medicine, Hamamatsu, Japan

Key words: autologous blood transfusion; recombinant human erythropoietin.

INTRODUCTION

Currently, for the prevention of complications caused by allotransfusion, there is a trend to perform surgery without transfusion, or with autotransfusion using recombinant human erythropoietin (rHuEPO).

Although the latter method has been performed not only in adults but also in children, there are many important issues such as the side effects of rHuEPO and the complications caused by the method.

In the present study, we investigated the timing of the autotransfusion of the stored blood and the safety of the method.

MATERIALS AND METHODS

A total of 27 children received open heart surgery in our department in July 1990 and thereafter. They were divided into three groups, those where autotransfusion with administration of EPO was performed during extracorporeal circulation (ECC) (Group A: nine cases: ASD, five; VSD, four; age 5–11 years; mean 7.8 years; body weight 25.5 ± 10.5 kg); those where autotransfusion with administration of EPO was performed after ECC (Group B: nine cases: ASD, four; VSD, two; PAPVR, one; TR, one; age 4–15 years; mean 9.8 years, body weight 31.9 ± 13.7 kg); and those where allotransfusion was performed (Group C: nine cases: VSD, seven; ASD, one; T/F, one; age 9 months–6 years; mean 2.9 years, body weight 12.1 ± 4.2 kg). In Groups A and B, 150–400 ml/time of blood was withdrawn from the patient at approximately 2 weeks and 1 week before surgery, and EPO at 100 U/kg was administrated to the patient twice a week for 2 weeks. RBC, Hb, Ht, reticulocyte, serum iron, UIBC, WBC and platelet were measured before blood collecting and immediately before surgery, the minimum values of BE and SvO_2 were measured. During ECC serum total hemoglobin and serum free hemoglobin were measured as parameters of hemolysis before ECC, at 1 h after its start, at its completion, at 2 h after its completion, and on day 1 after surgery.

Also, endotoxin [Toxicolor (TC) test, Endotoxin specific (ES) test], BUN, Crt, LDH, GOT, GPT, T.Bil, D.Bil, RBC, Hb and platelets were measured before and after surgery, and at 1 week after surgery, and compared among the groups.

RESULTS

The effect of rHuEPO and blood collecting

RBC was significantly reduced but the value immediately before surgery, $4.16 \pm 0.44 \times 10^6/mm^2$, was still within the normal range. Hb and Ht tended to be reduced but no significant difference was observed. Reticulocyte was significantly increased from 12.2 ± 4.9 to $35.8 \pm 16.7‰$ suggesting accelerated hemopoiesis. Serum iron was reduced from 73 ± 29 to 64 ± 43 $\mu g/dl$ within the normal range. UIBC was slightly lowered from 300 ± 46 to 274 ± 58 $\mu g/dl$, but no significant difference was observed. WBC tended to be reduced and platelet tended to be increased but no significant difference was observed.

The minimum value of BE and SvO$_2$

The ECC was performed at a rate of 80 ml/kg/min using a membranous oxgenator. The minimum values of Ht were 16.1 ± 1.9, 17.6 ± 3.3 and $21.7 \pm 5.7\%$ in Groups A, B and C. The minimum values of BE were -5.43 ± 1.2, -4.8 ± 1.9 and -3.7 ± 2.5 mEq in Groups A, B and C. It was significantly lower in Group A. The minimum value of SvO$_2$ was 51 ± 11, 63 ± 12 and 58 ± 10 in Groups A, B and C. It was significantly lower in Group A.

Changes of serum total Hb and free Hb (Fig. 1)

Total Hb reached a peak (A: 58.5 ± 32.4 mg/dl; C: 127 ± 83 mg/dl) after the start of ECC in Groups A and C, where transfusion was performed during ECC, and thereafter it was gradually reduced. In group B, where transfusion was not performed during ECC, it reached a peak (21.7 ± 24 mg/dl) immediately after its completion, and at 2 h after it was almost not detected. Serum free Hb reached a peak (A: 38.2 ± 31.5 mg/dl; B: 14.3 ± 14 mg/dl) immediately after ECC in Groups A and B, and it was almost not detected on day 1 after surgery in Group A and at 2 h after in Group B. In Group C it reached a peak (24.1 ± 20.8 mg/dl) at 1 h after start of ECC, and it was still high on day 1 after surgery (32.4 ± 32.7 mg/dl).

Endotoxin (TC method, ES method)

It has been reported that an increase of endotoxin during open heart surgery is frequently observed during transfusion. Endotoxin measured by the TC method was increased immediately after surgery in all of the three groups (A: 21 ± 15; B: 28 ± 22; C: 46 ± 24 $\mu g/ml$). Endotoxin measured by the ES method was slightly increased during surgery in all of the three groups. Although blood was stored for 2 or 3 weeks in Groups A and B, it seems no problem from the viewpoint of endotoxin.

Other parameters

BUN tended to be slightly higher on day 1 after surgery in Group C where allotransfusion was performed. Creatinin was within the normal range in all of the groups. T.Bil, LDH and GOT reached a peak on day 1 after surgery, but there was no significant difference in the three groups. After surgery no significant difference was observed in either RBC or Hb among the groups. Hb was more than 10 g/dl in all of the groups, suggesting success without transfusion. No significant difference was observed in either WBC or platelets among the groups, and they returned to the preoperative level on day 7 after surgery.

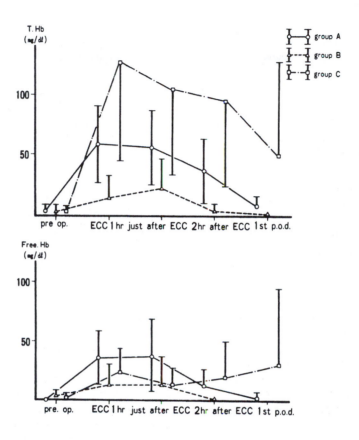

Figure 1. Change of total and free hemoglobin.

DISCUSSION

Recently, experiences of autotransfusion in children have been reported; however, criteria for blood withdrawal, its method, and dose and dosing method of EPO are varied depending on the institution [1–4]. Our subjects were children with a simple congenital heart malformation and who were in stable systemic conditions. However, considering that the age where blood withdrawal is able to be performed safely, children aged 4–5 years or above and of body weight of approximately 15 kg or more seems to be possible. As a complication caused by blood withdrawal, vomiting was observed only in one subject, but specific corrective treatment was not required. In the present study, we administered EPO twice a week by the intravenous route, and preoperative progress of anemia was mild and effective erythropoietiesis was obtained. Although there has not been an established theory on where the lowest limit of Hb at which open heart surgery can be performed safely without transfusion is, it is presumed that approximately 15% is the lowest limit for safety as far as we can judge from the data on BE and SvO$_2$. We usually adopt a simple and easy method for storage of blood in liquid from using a common transfusion pack. Concerning so-called stored blood, the influence of hemolysis sometimes causes a problem [5]; however, in the present study there was almost no problem if the blood was used after extracorporeal circulation and the influence of hemolysis was milder than the case of allotransfusion of fresh blood. Also, it has been confirmed that stored blood is safe from the viewpoint of endotoxin.

As aforementioned, we have shown the results of the study on the safety of stored blood using EPO and the timing of its use.

CONCLUSION

(i) Preoperative autotransfusion of stored blood of the patient using EPO was performed in 18 children. In all cases, surgery without transfusion was able to be performed without complications.

(ii) Free hemoglobin and LDH tended to be lowered in the group with autotransfusion following ECC. Considering the influence of hemolysis, it seems that transfusion during ECC should be avoided if possible.

REFERENCES

1. R. W. Novak. Autologous blood transfusion in a pediatric population: safety and efficacy. *Clin. Pediatr.*, **27**, 184 (1988).

2. A. J. Silvergleid. Safety and effectiveness of predeposite autologous transfusion in preteen and adolescent children. *J. Am. Med. Ass.*, **257**, 3403 (1987).

3. L. T. Goodnough *et al.* Increased preoperative collection of autologous blood with recombinant human erythropoietin therapy. *N. Engl. J. Med.*, **321**, 1163 (1989).

4. K. M. Shannon. Recombinant erythropoietin in pediatrics: a clinical perspective. *Pediatr. Ann.*, **19**, 197 (1990).

5. J. J. Osborn, K. Cohn, M. Hait, M. Russi, A. Sale, G. Harkins and F. Gerbode. Hemolysis during perfusion source and means of reduction. *J. Thorac. Cardiovas. Surg.*, **43**, 459–464 (1963).

Therapeutic Plasmapheresis (XII), pp. 887-890
T. Agishi *et al.* (Eds)
© VSP 1993

Autologous Blood Donation Programs in the Patients Undergoing Gastroenterological Surgery

S. OMOKAWA, T. NOTOYA, Y. WATANABE, A. B. MIURA, H. ANDOH,[1]
Y. ASANUMA[1] and K. KOYAMA[1]

Division of Blood Transfusion and [1]Department of Surgery,
Akita University School of Medicine, Akita, Japan

Key words: autologous blood donation; gastroenterological surgery; erythropoietin.

INTRODUCTION

The risks of homologous blood transfusion such as transmission of infectious disease can be minimized with autologous blood donation programs. In addition autologous blood may conserve the limited blood resource. Therefore, autologous blood donation programs have been widely carried out as a good transfusion practice in elective cardiovascular and orthopedic surgery [1, 2]. However, in gastroenterological surgery, autologous blood donation has not been well accepted because the preoperative period for most of them is limited due to their disease status with cancer. The objectives of this study are to investigate the safety and efficacy of autologous blood donation programs in patients undergoing gastroenterological surgery and to evaluate the effects of erythropoietin on blood donation for the patients with a short preoperative period.

SUBJECTS AND METHODS

Thirteen cases, three of total or proximal gastrectomy, four of rectal resection, four of hepatectomy, one of pancreatic resection and one of ileoproctostomy, were entered in the program as listed in Table 1. In four cases, recombinant human erythropoietin (r-HuEPO, 6000 U ×3/week, i.v.) was used [3]. Two hundred or 400 ml (when donor's Hb > 13 g/dl) of blood was donated with transfusion of saccharated ferric oxide each time. The time of phlebotomy, predeposit blood volume, preoperative donation period and hematological changes during blood donation were studied.

RESULTS

Table 1 summarizes the cases studied. Average predeposit blood volume was 638 (250–1200) ml and the average time of phlebotomy was 2.3 (1–5) times. The preoperative blood donation period ranged 4 to 31 days, but in nine cases (75%), blood donation was completed within 15 days. Blood loss during operation was 90–1243 ml, especially in the cases of hepatectomy (more than segmentectomy), 749–1243 ml of blood was lost.

Table 1.
Cases of autologous blood transfusion

Case	Age	Sex	Disease	Operative procedure	Predeposit blood volume (ml)	No. of phlebotomy	Preoperative period (day)	Blood loss (ml)	Homologous blood transfusion
1	65	M	gastric cancer	proximal gastrectomy	250	1	5	392	—
2	60	M	gastric cancer	total gastrectomy	600	2	14	90	—
3	65	M	malignant lymphoma	total gastrectomy	800	3	17	156	—
4	60	M	rectal cancer	low anterior resection	600	2	14	550	—
5[a]	55	M	rectal cancer	low anterior resection	800 (400)	1	6	684	—
6	49	M	rectal cancer	low anterior resection	800 (400)	1	4	689	—
7[a]	60	M	rectal cancer	low anterior resection	600	2	9	507	—
8	34	M	ulcerative colitis	ileoproctostomy	400	2	15	137	—
9[a]	55	M	gallbladder cancer	hepatic segmentectomy	1000	3	14	749	—
10	56	M	gallbladder cancer	partial hepatectomy	(400)			280	—
11	15	F	pancreatic tumor	enucleation of tumor	600	3	19	158	—
12	52	M	liver tumor	left hepatic lobectomy	800	3	12	1243	—
13[a]	39	M	liver cell cancer	hepatic segmentectomy	1200	5	31	1100	—

[a] Erythropoietin administered.
( ) : Autologous blood by hemodilution.

However, no homologous blood was given in any of the cases studied. Although Hb, Ht and RBC counts significantly decreased immediately after each phlebotomy, no differences were observed between 200 and 400 ml of donation. All patients developed slight anemia before surgery (Hb: 12.8 g/dl) compared with prephlebotomy value (Hb: 13.5 g/dl); however, plasma coagulation factors did not show much differences (data not shown).

Figure 1 shows the clinical course of the case who underwent hepatic segmentectomy. The autologous blood donation was initiated only 14 days before operation. Although a total of 1000 ml of autologous blood was obtained before operation with the use of r-HuEPO (6000 U × 6 times, i.v.), no significant anemia was seen before and after operation. The blood loss of this case was 749 ml and was treated only with predeposit autologous blood.

In the four cases with the use of r-HuEPO, the decrease of Hb before operation was minimized compared with the cases without r-HuEPO (data not shown).

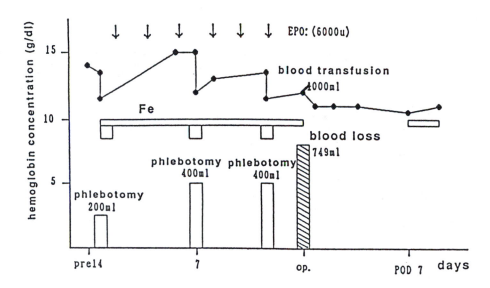

Figure 1. A case who underwent hepatic segmentectomy. r-HuEPO (6000 U) was intravenously administered 3 times per week.

DISCUSSION

Autologous blood donation is a desirable clinical transfusion practice. Benefits of autologous blood transfusion include: autologous blood is the safest transfusion material and that less use of homologous blood may contribute to the limited blood source. The surgeries in which autologous blood donation is widely applied are mainly cardiovascular and orthopedic operations [1, 2]. Erythropoietin has been used in an aggressive blood donation [3]. However, 3–5 weeks of preoperative period should be allocated to obtain sufficient blood volume. In gastroenterological surgeries, autologous blood donation may be carried out depending on the volume of preoperative blood loss, but clinical status includes malignant disease such as cancer. Therefore, the preoperative period is quite limited and usually less than 2–3 weeks in the surgical department. The objectives of this study were to evaluated the safety and efficacy of autologous blood donation in a short period.

The results obtained clearly demonstrated that 600–800 ml of autologous blood could be obtained within 2 weeks without preoperative severe anemia. The blood donation program did not disturb the preoperative examination or operation schedule. In the cases with hepatectomy, more than 1000 ml of autologous blood was needed and could be collected with the use of erythropoietin. This result indicates the effectiveness of erythropoietin in collecting a relatively large volume of blood in a short period.

In this study, the safety and efficacy of autologous blood donation in gastroenterological surgery, for which the preoperative donation period is limited, was evaluated and demonstrated. In addition, the effect of r-HuEPO on an aggressive donation program was shown in the patients undergoing hepatectomy.

Acknowledgments

The authors thank Ms Noriko Fujita for her expert secretarial assistance in preparing this manuscript.

REFERENCES

1. P. T. Toy, R. G. Strauss, C. C. Stehling *et al.* Predeposited autologous blood for elective surgery: a national multicenter study. *N. Engl. J. Med.*, **316**, 517–520 (1987).

2. M. S. Kruskall, E. E. Glazer, S. S. Leonard *et al.* Utilization and effectiveness of a hospital autologous preoperative blood donor program. *Transfusion*, **26**, 335–340 (1986).

3. L. T. Goodnough, S. Rudnick, T. H. Price *et al.* Increased preoperative collection of autologous blood with recombinant human erythropoietin therapy. *N. Engl. J. Med.*, **321**, 1163–1168 (1989).

Therapeutic Plasmapheresis (XII), pp. 891-895
T. Agishi *et al.* (Eds)
© VSP 1993

Autologous Transfusion of Erythrocyte-rich Blood Component Aided with Erythropoietin in Transurethral Resection of the Prostate

N. GOYA, N. KATO, H. ITO, O. RYOUJI, R. NAKAMURA, H. NAKAZAWA, H. TOMA, T. AGISHI, K. OTA, H. FUJII[1], M. SHIMIZU[1] and M. KAWAMATA[2]

Department of Urology and Third Department of Surgery, Kidney Center, [1]Department of Transfusion Medicine and [2]Department of Anesthesiology, Tokyo Women's Medical College, Tokyo, Japan

Key words: autologous blood transfusion; red cell concentrate; membrane plasma separater.

INTRODUCTION

Autologous blood transfusion has many advantages compared with allotransfusion. We designed a method for producing auto-CRC (concentrated red cells, erythrocyte-rich blood component) by using a membrane plasma separator.

This report describes our experience and its usefulness in autotransfusion of CRC along with the use of erythropoietin (EPO) in transurethral resection of the prostate (TUR-P).

SUBJECTS AND METHODS

The subjects were five benign prostatic hypertrophy (BPH) patients (mean age; 68 years) who needed TUR-P. EPO (12.000 units) was subcutaneously administered with a concomitant iron preparation. Administration was conducted three times beginning 3 weeks preoperatively (Fig. 1).

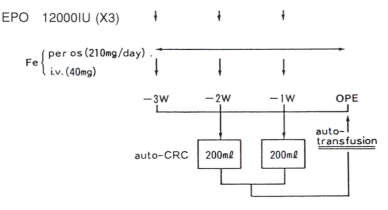

Figure 1.

Methods of producing CRC
A sterilized system was prepared in which the outlet line, plasma separator, returning line and collecting bag were connected. The membrane plasma separator used was a APC-F240 (Hydrophylized polyethylene, 0.2 m^2, Asahi Medical Co. Ltd). The instrument used was a continuous hemofilter apparatus ACH-07 (Asahi Medical Co. Ltd). Auto-CRC was collected from the patient (about 200 ml) each time at 2 and 1 week before operation and was used at TUR-P.

RESULTS

Ten bags of auto-CRC were produced.

Components of CRC
   Erythrocyte ($n = 9$): $(613 \pm 54) \times 10^4/mm^3$.
   Leucocyte ($n = 9$): $8200 \pm 2300/mm^3$.
   Platelet ($n = 9$): $(21.3 \pm 12.6) \times 10^4/mm^3$.
   Na ($N = 6$): $144 \pm 9.1\,mEq/l$.
   K ($N = 6$): $27.4 \pm 7.2\,mEq/l$.
   LDN ($N = 6$): $599 \pm 227\,IU/l$.
   Mean Ht value before blood taking ($N = 9$) was $46.6 \pm 3.5\%$ and that of the CRC was $58.2 \pm 5.1\%$ (Table 1).

Table 1.
Ht value of pre-concentrated blood and CRC

Case	No.	Pre-concentrated blood	CRC
(1) NW	1	44.7	52.6
	2	45.6	58.2
(2) ST	3	48.0	52.2
	4	44.6	57.8
(3) ST	5	52.4	60.7
	6	50.8	65.7
(4) KK	7	47.0	56.2
	8	45.5	65.9
(5) KA	9	40.7	54.4
	10	37.3	
Mean ($N = 9$)		$46.6 \pm 3.5\%$	$58.2 \pm 5.1\%$

Changes of leucocyte ($N = 8$) (Fig. 2)
The mean leucocyte count was $8000 \pm 1600/mm^3$ in the untreated blood. This diminished somewhat to $7200 \pm 1800/mm^3$ 15 min following commencement. The granulocyte percentage in both materials was nearly identical.

Changes of leucocyte

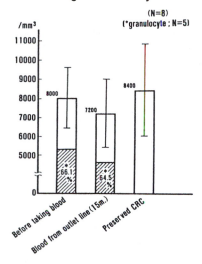

Figure 2. Changes of leucocyte.

Changes of complements (N = 6)
The mean CH50 value of the blood on the outlet side 15 min after commencement was 93% (44.8 ± 8.3 U/ml); and that of the plasma on the returning line was 79% (37.9±5.5 U/ml) compared with that of the untreated blood (48.0±7.5 U/ml). The mean CH50 value of the blood at completion recovered slightly to 91% (43.7±8.0 U/ml). The mean CH50 value of CRC after 1–2 weeks of preservation was 61% (29.1 ± 6.2 U/ml) of that of untreated blood (Fig. 3). The changes of C3c and C4 were almost similar to that of CH50 (Figs 4 and 5).

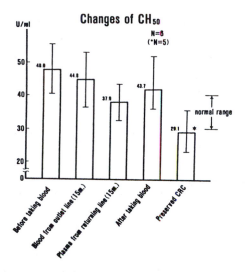

Figure 3.

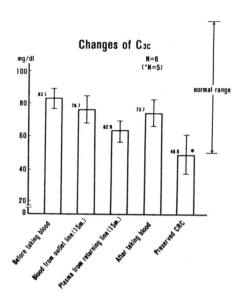

Figure 4.

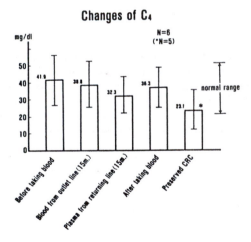

Figure 5.

Transfusion at TUR-P
Of five patients, four were given only auto-CRC. One patient, however, needed 400 ml of allotransfusion because one bag of auto-CRC was lost during the preservation (Table 2).

CONCLUSION

Component blood transfusion has been widely applied in allotransfusion of blood. The merit of auto-CRC is donor safety in the aspect of hemodynamics, even among elderly

Table 2.

No.	Case	Age (years)	Volume of taking CRC (ml)	Time of TUR-P (min)	Weight of resected prostate (g)	Blood transfusion at TUR-P	
						auto-CRC (ml)	allo-CRC (ml)
1	NW	70	400	100	40	400	(–)
2	ST	71	400	60	22	400	(–)
3	ST	64	400	80	27	400	(–)
4	KK	64	400	40	22	400	(–)
5	KA	71	400	100	39	200	400

patients. In as much as the irrigating solution is absorbed by the body via the prostatic bed during TUR-P, a tendency for overhydration may always exist.

The Ht value of the CRC we produced is somewhat low compared with conventionally used CRC (65–75%). Thus, in the future we must make more concentrated blood cells by changing the conditions of the instruments. The changes, however, in leucocyte and complements during the sampling operation are not serious.

Accordingly, transfusion of CRC produced by using a membrane plasma separator is clinically worth applying, especially among elderly patients, because it induces a minimal increase in the circulating volume.

REFERENCES

1. L. T. Goodnough, S. Rudnick, T. H. Price *et al.* Increased preoperative collection of autologous blood with recombinant human erythropoietin therapy. *N. Engl. J. Med.*, **321**, 1163–1168 (1989).

2. S. Yokoyama and H. Takemitsu. Donor plasmapheresis using an automated device with polyethylene membrane filtration. *Jpn. J. Transfusion Med.*, **35**, 611–615 (1989).

3. N. Goya, H. Yanagisawa, K. Osanai *et al.* Autologous blood transfusion aided with erythropoietin in transurethral resection of the prostate. *Jpn. J. Urol.*, **82**, 1978–1985 (1991).

Therapeutic Plasmapheresis (XII), pp. 897-899
T. Agishi *et al.* (Eds)
© VSP 1993

Autotransfusion is Safe and Effective on Patients Undergoing Hepatectomy for Hepatocellular Carcinoma

J. FUJIMOTO, E. OKAMOTO, N. YAMANAKA, T. ORIYAMA, K. FURUKAWA, E. KAWAMURA, T. TANAKA and F. TOMODA

The First Department of Surgery, Hyogo College of Medicine, Hyogo, Japan

Key words: autotransfusion; hepatectomy; hepatocellular carcinoma.

INTRODUCTION

Autologous transfusion is widely used in a variety of surgical procedures, including cardiovascular, orthopedic and gynecologic procedures, liver transplantation, and emergency medical situations [1–3]. It can decrease the demand for banked blood and eliminate the risk of infection and alloimmunization. Intraoperative blood salvage (IBS) in cancer patients has not been widely investigated in the past. Despite the concern about the dissemination of malignancy by IBS, these authors are not aware of any reports that dissemination or metastasis has occurred by IBS so far. In January 1988, we started a program of autotransfusion for patients with hepatocellular carcinoma (HCC) who underwent hepatectomy. We have now reviewed and analyzed the clinical and laboratory data for 54 patients who received autologous transfusions, and these were matched for comparison with 50 patients receiving homologous blood before December 1987.

MATERIALS AND METHODS

This autotransfusion study was done in 54 patients receiving hepatectomy for HCC during the period from January 1988 to April 1989 (group 1). To compare results with previous transfusion practice, we used a group of 50 patients with HCC undergoing hepatectomy from September 1986 to December 1987 who were operated on by the same surgeon without autotransfusion (group 2). Two methods, preoperative phlebotomy and intraoperative blood salvage, were combined for each patient of group 1. Preoperative blood donation was done according to the autologous blood donation programs [4]. The Haemonetics Cell Saver (HCS) was employed as an intraoperative scavenger of blood. The HCS was used with consent of the patient, anticipation of intraoperative loss of blood, availability of the autotransfusion device and cost of it. The following factors were recorded for comparison between group 1 and 2: intraoperative bleeding volume, intra- and postoperative blood product usage, hemoglobin, serial platelet counts, coagulation tests: prothrombin time (PT) and partial thromboplastin time (PTT), (preoperative, 24 h postoperative, 2 and 3 days postoperative, 1 and 2 weeks postoperative).

A cytological study was done from processed blood products for the first 20 patients of group 1. Follow-up was continued until death or December 1991. Life-table analyses were presented as Kaplan–Meyer plots. The generalized Wilcoxon's test was used to determine if significant differences existed between the curves.

RESULTS

In group 1, the mean intraoperative loss of blood was 1666 ml. Fifteen patients (27.7%) underwent the operation with their own autologous blood transfusion and no homologous RBCs, plasma or whole blood. Eleven out of these 15 patients avoided the use of any homologous blood components for the entire hospitalization (Table 1). The mean volume of autotransfused blood was 831 ml; 392 ml by preoperative donation and 439 ml by intraoperative salvage. The total volume of transfusion (autologous and homologous) was 1645 ml (mean), of which 831 ml (50.5%) was autologous component and 814 ml (49.5%) was homologous requirements (RBCs or whole blood: 706 ml, FFP: 108 ml). In contrast, 49 patients (98%) in group 2 required homologous blood ($P < 0.05$). There was a significant difference ($P < 0.05$) in volume of homologous blood used between the patients in group 1 (814 ± 397 ml [mean $\pm$ SD]) and group 2 (3466 ± 1811 ml). In group 1, the mean hemoglobin value decreased from 13.3 to 10.8 g/dl 3 days after the operation, then returned to about 90% of the value before the operation within 2 weeks (11.5 g/dl). Platelet counts decreased from a preoperative mean value of 13.1 ($10/\mu l$) of a third day's mean of 7.1. The mean level returned to normal within a week then increased to 16.5 at 2 weeks after the operation. There are no significant differences in the mean hemoglobin level or the platelet counts between the patients of group 1 and group 2. A cytological study of the processed RBCs revealed no malignancy in all specimens. All of the 100 specimens (five sample from each of 20 patients) were diagnosed as class 1 by the pathologists. The cumulative intrahepatic recurrence rates of the patients who underwent curative resection for HCC are group 1: 62.8% and group 2: 67.3%, no significance was recognized between the two groups. The cumulative survival rates were 61.9% in group 1 patients and 52.8% in group 2 pateints at 3 years.

DISCUSSION

Hart and coworkers performed pioneering studies in the use of IBS in patients with carcinoma of the bladder [5]. The mean volume of IBS was nearly 500 ml, which accounted for 40% of the total transfusion requirements. In 33 patients, radical cystectomy was done using HCS and follow-up was continued for a mean of 24 months. Their data failed to show any evidence for dissemination of tumor caused by autotransfusion. In this study, the cumulative recurrence rate of patients of group 1 (62.8%) was lower than that of group 2 (67.3%), and they were similar to a previous report [6]. The pattern and frequency of recurrence suggest that autotransfusion is not responsible for the recurrence or metastasis. However, the follow-up period is not long enough, we must continue to follow these patients carefully. Another criticism of autotransfusion for HCC with cirrhosis is coagulopathy. The centrifuge washing removes platelets and plasma which contains coagulation factors. In the patients of group 1, 51 out of 54 patients (94.4%) had liver disease. A decreased platelet count and prolonged PT and PTTs were notice in them. Fifty-three patients followed an uneventful postoperative course, the mean level of platelet count and PT, PTTs were similar to those of group 2. Platelet counts do decrease but to levels that generally do no need platelet transfusion. We succeeded to reduce the volume of bank blood transfusion by combining an autologous blood program, preoperative phebotomy and intraoperative blood salvage. About 20% of the patients underwent hepatectomy without any bank blood requirements, nearly 50% of the patients required less than 1000 ml of homologous transfusion. Our data suggest that autotransfusion can be used safety in liver surgery for HCC, it was effective and practical. Further studies are still required to investigate the long-term safety of autotransfusion, and of potential benefits of avoiding immunosuppressive effects.

REFERENCES

1. J. W. Hallet, M. Popovsky and D. Ilstrup. Minimizing blood transfusions during abdominal aortic surgery: Recent advances in rapid autotransfusion. *J. Vasc. Surg*, **5**, 601–606 (1987).
2. W. H. Dzik and R. Jenkins. Use of intraoperative blood salvage during orthotopic liver transplantation. *Arch. Surg.*, **120**, 946–948 (1985).
3. K. R. Williamson and H. F. Taswell. Intraoperative blood salvage: a review. *Transfusion*, **31**, 662–675 (1991).
4. R. O. Gilcher and L. Belcher. Preoperative autologous blood donation programs. In: *Autologous and Directed Blood Programs*, pp. 15–29, American Association of Blood Banks, Arlington (1987).
5. I. Klimberg, R. Sirois, Z. Wajsman and J. Baker. Intraoperative autotransfusion in urologic oncology. *Arch. Surg.*, **121**, 1326–1329 (1986).
6. J. Belghiti, Y. Panis, Farges *et al.* Intrahepatic recurrence after resection of hepatocellular carcinoma complicating cirrhosis. *Ann. Surg.*, **214**, 114–117 (1991).

Therapeutic Plasmapheresis (XII), pp. 901-904
T. Agishi *et al.* (Eds)
© VSP 1993

Several Attemps at Complete Autotransfusion in Surgical Patients

M. TAKAORI, A. FUKUI and K. KIMURA

Department of Anesthesiology, Kawasaki Medical School, Kurashiki, Japan

Key words: red cell salvaging; hemodilution; cancer; colloid solution; postoperative autotransfusion.

INTRODUCTION

Since 1982, several attempts have been made in our clinic to avoid the use of homologous blood transfusion in the performance of surgical operations. Blood loss of 3000–4000 ml has been treated with autologous blood transfusion alone by means of the intraoperative red cell salvaging technique (SAT) combined with preoperative blood preservation associated with hemodilution (HAT) [1]. In addition, a few studies are presently in progress to expand the indication for perioperative autotransfusion.

EFFECTIVE REGIMEN FOR THE USE OF HAT BLOOD

The amount of HAT blood preserved immediately before surgery for each patient is based upon the suspected blood loss during the operation. Nevertheless the total amount should not exceed 1200 ml in adults in order to prevent coagulopathy. As shown in Table 1, 2600 ml of blood loss usually can be treated well with 1200 ml of HAT

Table 1.

Blood volume replacement with colloid and HAT blood for intraoperative hemorrhage

blood loss (ml)	replacement	(ml)
0 —→ 400	crystalloid	alone
400 —→ 600	HAT blood	200
600 —→ 800	Plasmanate®	500
800 —→1000	HAT blood	200
1000 —→1200	Plasmanate®	500
1200 —→1400	HAT blood	200
1400 —→1600	dextran 70	200
1600 —→1800	HAT blood	200
1800 —→2000	dextran 70	200
2000 —→2200	Hat blood	200
2200 —→2400	dextran 70	200
2400 —→2600	HAT blood	200

blood and some colloids. In the meantime, red cell concentrate is being prepared from salvaged blood and is transfused into the patient.

BETTER RECYCLING OF RED CELLS

When SAT was introduced in our clinic, plain physiological saline solution with heparin was used as the irrigation fluid. The red cell recycle rate, which is calculated by the following formula, was $81.0 \pm 6.6\%$.

$$\frac{A}{A + B} \times 100\,(\%),$$

where A is the red cell mass collected for SAT and B is the red cell mass loss due to hemolysis.

We added poloxamer 188, namely Pluronic F68, to the saline, but the red cell recycle rate was not improved. Then two colloid solutions, Haemaccel® and Hespander®, were used as the irrigation fluid with the expectation that these would have a membrane protecting effect. Consequently, the red cell recycle rate increased to 87.3 ± 5.6 with Haemaccel® and $87.2 \pm 3.9\%$ with Hespander®.

POSTOPERATIVE SAT

The usefulness of blood drained postoperatively from the operated wound has been established in foreign countries [2] but not in our country, as yet. In 1991, we sent a questionnaire to 171 departments of cardiovascular surgery and orthopedics for a survey of the applicability of drained blood. Postoperative SAT is being performed or there are plans to do so in 57.3% of the institutes that responded. However, 42.7% opposed its use or had no plan to use it. The reason most often given for opposition to its use by 33.6% was the fear of bacterial contamination into the red cell concentrate. However, we have examined blood drained from the mediastinum after open heart surgery for bacterial contamination and no positive findings of bacteria culture were noted in 27 cases in whom specimens were obtained 24 h after the surgery.

Table 2.
Chemical characteristics of blood collected

	Ht	K	Hbf	Pi	2,3-DPG
Group A	11.6 ± 2.7	8.2 ± 2.1	286 ± 113	6.9 ± 1.9	102 ± 16
	(25.4 ± 2.9)	(3.3 ± 0.3)	(10.4 ± 2.9)	(3.3 ± 0.5)	(100 ± 19)
Group B	11.2 ± 2.5	6.3 ± 1.9	213 ± 71	3.8 ± 0.9	99 ± 22
	(25.2 ± 5.3)	(2.8 ± 0.5)	(12.2 ± 8.3)	(3.1 ± 0.8)	(88 ± 34)

Ht: hematocrit (%), K: serum potassium (mEq/l), Hbf: serum free hemoglonin (mg/dl), Pi: inorganic phosphate (mg/dl), 2,3-DPG (μmol/lHb), $n = 5$, mean $\pm$ SD.
Value in the circulating blood is given in parentheses.
Group A: blood collected into a plastic box at room temperature.
Group B: blood collected into a CPD bag at $4\,^\circ$C.

Some objections to the use of drained blood concerned with abnormalities of the blood salvaged has been also stated. Therefore, the blood was drained into a CPD bag and kept at 4 °C. In comparison with other blood which was collected in a regular plastic box at room temperature, the concentrations of serum potassium and inorganic phosphate were less in the blood drained into a CPD bag, as shown in Table 2. No significant difference was noted in the 2,3-DPG level per hemoglobin either between the two types of blood collected or between the drained blood and the circulating blood.

APPLICATION OF SAT IN SURGERY FOR MALIGNANCIES

SAT is usually contraindicated in surgery involving the removal of malignancies. The massive hemorrhage which so often accompanies those operations has led us to adopt a modified use of SAT. The idea that malignant cells, which might contaminate the red cell concentrate, should be made non-viable for metastasis by anticancer drugs was adopted by us for clinical application. Very little data, however, have been published on the cytocidal effect of anticancer drugs *in vitro*. Therefore, a number of experimental studies were conducted to determine the minimum concentration of anticancer drug required to cause a cytocidal effect *in vitro*.

First, 2×10^6 cells of Ehrlich ascites tumor were exposed to 0–400 μg/ml of mitomycin C (MMC) for either 5, 10, 15 or 20 min and washed with saline. Then these cells were implanted into the abdominal cavity of normal mice. When no positive implantation was observed in nine animals under certain exposure condition, the same procedure was carried out in 50 other animals. Against Ehrlich ascites tumor, the minimum cytocidal effect was obtained by exposure to 100 μg/ml of MMC for 15 min. Against Harding Passey B-16 melanoma the minimum cytocidal effect was obtained by exposure to 400 μg/ml for 15 min. Against either rat hepatoma AH66 or AH130 it was obtained by exposure to 100 μg/ml for 20 min.

Next, four other anticancer drugs were tested to determine their minimum cytocidal effect against Harding Passey B-16 melanoma. As a result, 20 min exposure to 10 mg/ml of doxorubicin, 15 min to 500 μg/ml of chromomycin and 20 min to 1 mg/ml to aclarubicin were determined to be the minimum cytocidal exposure. Twenty minutes exposure to 400 μg/ml of carboquone, however, prevented implantation only in 67% of the tested animals.

To date, SAT has been carried out in nine cases involving the removal of a malignant tumor. Forty-five milligrams of MMC was mixed with 225 ml of red cell concentrate in a centrifuging bowl of Cell Saver®, and the concentration of MMC was kept at approximately 400 μg/ml for 20 min. During 3 years of follow-up none of the patients has suffered metastasis. Therefore, our experience suggests that the effective use of anticancer drugs may lead to the use of SAT during operations for the removal of malignancies.

UNEXPECTED HOMOLOGOUS BLOOD TRANSFUSION

More than 200 cases with intraoperative blood loss exceeding 1500 ml have been treated with our autotransfusion technique in the past. None of these patients were transfused with homologous blood in our operating theater or recovery room. Twenty-nine patients (18.3%) out of 159, however, were transfused with homologous blood in their wards. Multivariant analysis used with the discriminant linear function indicated that the hematocrit value on the first postoperative day most likely promoted their attending surgeons to transfuse homologous blood. Namely, the hematocrit value was $17.6\pm2.5\%$ in patients who were transfused with homologous blood whereas it was $24.8 \pm 3.4\%$ in the patients without homologous blood transfusion. It could not be determined accurately whether or not postoperative morbidity would have increased in the former patients if the additional transfusion had not been done. Nevertheless the additional transfusion might have been unnecessary. We have had many experiences in treating severely hemorrhaging patients with colloid solution alone. Although their hematocrit value decreased below 15% and did not increase up to 20% within the subsequent 24 h, the patients passed their postoperative period uneventfully.

In conclusion, it is essential to remember that '20% of hematocrit is not the critical level' [3] for the complete performance of autotransfusion.

REFERENCES

1. M. Takaori. Perioperative autotransfusion: hemodilution and red cell salvaging. *Can. J. Anaesth.*, **38**, 604–607 (1991).
2. The National Blood Resource Education Program Expert Panel. The use of autologous blood. *J. Am. Med. Ass.*, **263**, 414–417 (1990).
3. M. Takaori and P. Safar. Critical point in progressive hemodilution with hydroxyethyl stach. *Kawasaki Med. J.*, **2**, 212–222 (1976).

22
Donor Apheresis

Therapeutic Plasmapheresis (XII), pp. 907-910
T. Agishi *et al.* (Eds)
© VSP 1993

Donor Plasmapheresis using New Membrane Devices

S. YOKOYAMA and T. HOSOI

Kyoto Red Cross Blood Center, Kyoto, Japan

Key words: membrane device; APC-4000; AC-300; donorplasmapheresis.

INTRODUCTION

Since 1986 several types of domestic membrane devices have been introduced in order to procure fresh plasma for national self-sufficiency of coagulation factors. Since
the results of plasma collection using several of the membrane devices, i.e. NDP-100,
NDP-200, Nipro; APC-2000, Asahi medical; Ube Donex-100, Ube Industry were unsatisfactory [1], there was an urgent need for augmentation of plasmapheresis donation.

In 1992 two new domestic membrane devices, APC-4000 and Hemoquic-II AC-300
(AC-300), were introduced in our blood center. The purpose of this study was to verify
donor safety, plasma quality, operational procedure and cost efficacy with regard to
these two devices.

METHOD

Since February 1991 we have carried out 351 plasmaphereses using these two devices:
306 cases with APC-4000 (Asahi Medical) and 45 cases with AC-300 (Terumo).

The donors all passed the selection criteria for apheresis donation set by the Ministry
of Health and Welfare [2]. For blood access a 17 G needle with a back-hole was used.
From 450 to 700 g of plasma, including ACD-A solution according to donor's body
weight, was collected during each procedure. With APC-4000, blood drawing flow
was an average of 90 ml/min and blood returning flow was an average of 110 ml/min.
With AC-300, average pressure in drawing phereses was −180 mm Hg and in returning
phereses was +100 mm Hg.

All donors underwent hematological and biological tests according to the Japanese
Red Cross Technical Manual. Immunoglobulin determination using the RIA method
was carried out on the collected plasma and also on samples taken at points pre-, post-
and at the membrane outlet.

RESULTS

Operation of plasmapheresis
Table 1 shows the average setting time, priming time and needle to needle time using
these two different devices. The average time required to install the kit to the devices
was almost 3 min in all cases.

With APC-4000 the average priming time was only 30 s because the membrane module was already coated with a hydrophilic substrate. The priming procedure to the membrane module was not needed. On the other hand, using AC-300, the average priming time was about 7 min because of the need to prime the membrane separator. Needle-to-needle (N–N) time using both APC-400 and AC-300 was almost 30 min for 450 g plasma collection. The differences between these two devices was not significant; however, the APC-40000 appeared slightly better than the AC-300.

Table 1.
Procedure time (smoothly operated cases)

	APC-4000	Hemoquic-II (AC-300)
Average setting time	3 min	3 min
Average priming time	30 s	6–7 min
N–N time at plasma volume		
450 g	28 ± 6 min	32 ± 10 min
500 g	33 ± 11 min	38 ± 3 min
600 g	37 ± 13 min	—

Effects of plasmapheresis on donor
Hematological and biochemical donor tests were within normal ranges in all cases. Donors experienced no physical or psychological adverse effects due to the plasmapheresis, except three cases of slight subcutaneous hemorrhage caused by venipuncture.

Cases of incomplete plasmapheresis
Using APC-4000, in three cases the procedure could not be completed. In one case, due to a membrane crack which occurred during operation, red cells mingled with the collected plasma. In the other two cases, the blood leaked from the connecting part of the tube due to a defective kit.

Using AC-300, in two cases the procedure could not be completed. In one case blood leakage due to the defective kit was observed. In another case, the device did not run normally due to trouble in the Hemoquic system.

Yield of plasma component
With APC-4000, the yield of coagulation factor VIII, factor IX, total protein, albumin and IgG (particularly factor VIII and albumin) were over 90%. With AC-300, the yield of each component was about 80% and appears lower than APC-4000 because of the effect of dilution by physiological saline used for priming.

Activation of β-TG
Activated complement and β-TG were determined on samples taken at the membrane outlet and on product plasma. The results are shown in Fig. 1. Using both devices, anaphylatoxines at the membrane outlet showed a slightly high value, but no effect on the donor was observed. C3a and C4a in the collected plasma showed a relatively higher value, but C5a was always within normal ranges in all samples.

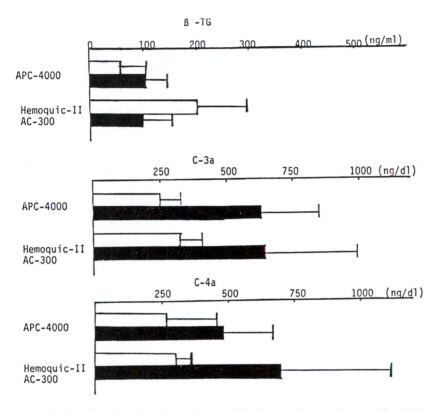

Figure 1. Activation of β-TG and anaphylatoxine: □, blood at membrane outlet; ■, collected plasma.

DISCUSSION

Our requirements for membrane devices were (i) donor safety, (ii) short operation time, (iii) ease of operation, (iv) higher yield of components such as albumin and coagulation factor VIII, (v) a device both small and light weight, and (vi) validity of device and disposable kit. Number (v) is especially indispensable because plasmapheresis is more and more often carried out by mobile teams at various sites outside the blood center.

The APC-4000 is a refined model of APC-2000 which has been used in our blood center during the past 3 years. This device is very small and light (a total weight of 14 kg). The AC-300 is also very light (a total weight of 16 kg) and consists of a Hemoquic system creating an air compressed force without electrical pumps, so that it is possible to use whole blood donation.

With regard to donor safety, the results obtained were as satisfactory as the results described in previous reports [3]. However, the disadvantage of AC-300 lies in both pumping time and coagulation factor yield; therefore improvement of the membrane is desirable.

The cost of the APC-4000 kit is 3090 yen. It is favorably priced compared with the AC-300, the price of which is unknown. However, it is expected that a lower kit price will be offered for an economical advantage.

CONCLUSION

From a standpoint of plasma procurement for fractionation, two kinds of domestic membrane devices were evaluated and compared. The APC-4000 can be used in the routine work of our blood center. The AC-300 should improve its membrane material by deleting the priming procedure.

REFERENCES

1. S. Yokoyma and T. Hosoi. Donorplasmapheresis using automated membrane device. *Jpn. J. Transf. Med.*, **36**, 5–9 (1990).
2. Ministry of Health of Welfare. Criteria for donor selection. *Yakumu koho No. 1328* (1986).
3. S. Yokoyama and T. Hosoi. Donor plasmapheresis using an automated device with polyethylene membrane filtration. *Jpn. J. Transf. Med.*, **35**, 611–615 (1989).

Therapeutic Plasmapheresis (XII), pp. 911
T. Agishi *et al.* (Eds)
© VSP 1993

Selection of Apheresis Donors:
Recruitment and Education

B. BERG and A. SHANWELL

Stockholm Blood Transfusion Service, Huddinge University Hospital,
S-141 86 Huddinge, Sweden

Key words: apheresis; donors; recruitment; education.

INTRODUCTION

In 1986 the Stockholm Blood Transfusion Service started preparing apheresis platelets (AP) at Huddinge University Hospital. Only CMV seronegative donors were recruited.

MATERIAL AND METHODS

After initial written information, groups of eight to ten donors were invited to receive additional information. At this meeting the donors were informed about the goals and the procedures by a doctor. The donors were instructed not to take any aspirin 7 days before donation and informed of the importance of keeping their scheduled appointments. Adverse side-effects such as citrate toxicity and how to deal with it was discussed and there was also an opportunity for questions. The donors arms were examined by an apheresis nurse and bloodsamples were drawn to count the donors peripheral platelets counts. Donors with platelets less than 200×10^9/l and bad peripheral vein access were excluded.

RESULTS

From September 1986 to May 1991, 1004 donors were invited for information. Of these 52% were accepted. A total of 5563 scheduled appointments resulted in 5383 AP (Baxters CS 3000). Of these, 1.4% did not appear for donation as agreed, 2.4% called the same day and cancelled the appointment because of sudden illness, and 1.3% of the donations failed while trying to puncture the donors veins.

CONCLUSION

By selecting motivated donors and educating them you can assure high attendance and co-operation. Together you can make better use of the resources available.

Therapeutic Plasmapheresis (XII), pp. 913-914
T. Agishi *et al.* (Eds)
© VSP 1993

Repeat Plateletpheresis — the Effect on the Donor and the Yield

G. ROCK,[1] P. TITTLEY,   M. STERNBACH,
N. BUSKARD and M. SCHROEDER

[1]*Department of Medicine, University of Ottawa, Ottawa, Ontario, Canada
Canadian Red Cross Society*

Key words: plateletpheresis; single donor; platelet count.

INTRODUCTION

Repeat plateletpheresis of a single donor is often required to provide continuous and appropriate support of platelets to an individual patient. This is especially relevant with the recent increases in bone marrow transplantation and the subsequent need for HLA-matched, single donor platelets. To determine the effects of concentrated, repeat procedures, we have prospectively evaluated the hematological values in 13 donors undergoing plateletpheresis procedures every other day over a 22 day interval and have also evaluated the yields obtained from such procedures.

METHODS

Thirteen individuals underwent repeat plateletpheresis procedures at 48 hour intervals (3 times per week) over a 22 day period. All individuals were regular donors of platelets and were required to sign a consent form. All were clinically observed throughout the procedure. Ten procedures were scheduled for each of the donors participating in this study at four different Canadian Red Cross Blood Transfusion Centers. All procedures utilized the Haemonetics V50 Surge machine (Haemonetics Corp., Braintree, MA) in the autosurge mode, with ACD-A as the anticoagulant in a 1 to 8 ratio. Blood was taken from the donor before each procedure to assess baseline values then following the procedure to determine changes, as well as 7 days after the last apheresis procedure. In addition, samples were taken from the plateletpheresis product.

The following investigations were performed on all samples: platelet count and size distribution with mean volume and peak volumes determined (model ZB with Chan-nelyzer, Coulter Electronics, Hialeah, FL); white blood count (WBC; Coulter Elec-tronics); and total platelet and WBC counts on the product. Additional studies were performed on the donor prior to the first, seventh and 10th procedure, and 7 days fol-lowing the last procedure as follows: IgG, IgM and IgA by laser nephelometry and immunodiffusion techniques, quantitation of T_3, T_4, and T_8 lymphocytes by flow cy-tometry and platelet aggregation response using both ADP and collagen as stimulating agents.

Results are expressed as a mean ± SD. Statistical comparisons were done using a Student *t*-test; *P* values of less than 0.05 were considered statistically significant.

G. Rock et al.

RESULTS

After eight passes (cycles) with the V50 machine a product was produced with a yield ranging from 3.2×10^{11} to 2.3×10^{11} platelets in volumes ranging from 293 ± 87 to 346 ± 77 ml of plasma. Depending on the blood volume of the donor, 2.6 to 4.4 l of blood was processed. No clinical complications were observed.

The donor's platelet count was significantly decreased by the third donation (procedure day 5) in all instances, falling to $79 \pm 13\%$ of the baseline count. This corrected to within 10% of the starting level by the sixth procedure but at no time did the platelet count exceed the value of the first day. Ten minutes following each procedure the platelet count was found to be 20% lower than at the start. Platelet size distribution increased from $7.3 \mu m^3$ (peak volume) on the first day to $7.8 \mu m^3$ by the fourth procedure ($P > 0.05$); this subsequently decreased prior to the seventh donation. Responses to ADP and collagen were normal and unchanged throughout the study. The hematocrit and WBC did not alter significantly. The total number of lymphocytes did change by the third procedure but levelled off by the fifth procedure; there was no significant difference in the ratio of T_4 and T_8 cells throughout.

IgG levels were significantly decreased by the seventh donation with a further decrease at the end of the study. This was partially corrected 7 days after the last procedure. The IgM levels also showed significant decreases, however IgA did not vary significantly.

RESULTS

The results demonstrate that ten plateletpheresis procedures repeated within a 22 day period on the same individual produced little change in the hematological values. While the platelet count of the donors did drop significantly, relatively little change was noticed in the yield of the platelet product. This is likely due to the overall scatter in results but is an interesting finding given the generally accepted good correlation between donor pre-count and yield. The study indicates the relative safety and efficacy of repeat plateletpheresis of a single donor who is committed to a maintenance regime for a designated patient.

Therapeutic Plasmapheresis (XII), pp. 915-918
T. Agishi *et al.* (Eds)
© VSP 1993

Permeation of Plasma Proteins through Polyolefin Membranes for Spontaneous Donor Plasmapheresis

T. TOMONO, T. SUZUKI, S. IGARASHI, N. MUROI,
T. OHORI and S. SEKIGUCHI

Department of Research and Development, Japanese Red Cross Plasma Fractionation Center, Tokyo, Japan

Key words: donor plasmapheresis; membrane; polyethylene; polypropylene; hydrophilization.

INTRODUCTION

In order to supply coagulation protein concentrates exclusively to Japanese hemophiliacs, we must collect about 500 000 l of plasma a year. In Japan, most blood is donated from healthy volunteers in special mobiles. We therefore need such a simple, convenient and efficient systems as the spontaneous donor plasmapheresis system using gravity in addition to the motorized systems. From this point of view, we characterized polyolefin membranes which were originally developed for spontaneous donor plasmapheresis using pooled fresh frozen plasma under normalized conditions.

METHODS

Non-grafted or hydrophilic polyacrylate grafted polypropylene (PP) disk-type membranes (CPAS Systems, Terumo Co.) and hydrophilic polyester coated polyethylene (PE) hollow-fiber membranes (BCC Systems, Asahi Medical Co.) were chosen for the tests. The specification of these membrane modules are summarized in Table 1.

Table 1.
Specification of polyolefin membrane modules

System	Supplier	Type	Material	Pore size (μm)	Area (m^2)	Flow rate (ml/min)
CPAS (old)	Terumo Co.	disk	PP	0.60	0.16	17.5
CPAS (new)	Terumo Co.	disk	hydrophilized PP[a]	0.60	0.16	17.5
BCC	Asahi Medical Co.	hollow-fiber	hydrophilized PE[b]	0.20	0.12	10.4

[a] Hydrophilic polyacrylate grafted polypropylene.
[b] Hydrophilic polyester coated polyethylene.

After priming the module with saline, 700 ml of thawed and pooled fresh frozen plasma (from 10 donors with same blood type) was allowed to pass through the modules at constant flow-rates of 17.5 ml/min [1] for PP and 10.4 ml/min [2] for PE modules at 25 °C. Aliquots (3 ml) of the sample were collected and subjected to protein and activity analysis.

Coagulation factor VIII (FVIII) and IX (FIX) activity were assayed by the one-stage method. Fibrinogen (Fib) was determined by the thrombin time method. Albumin, immunoglobulin G (IgG) and M (IgM) were measured by the single radial immunodiffusion method.

RESULTS AND DISCUSSION

Figure 1 shows protein concentration or activity changes using the CPAS (old) module. Albumin and IgG almost perfectly permeated thorough the module at the steady state. However, approaching the steady state of coagulation, proteins were delayed as compared with albumin or IgG and the sieving coefficients of higher molecular weight proteins (IgM and FVIII) were somewhat decreased. These phenomena could be due to the protein adsorption on the membrane and the pores of membrane becoming narrower with the adsorbed proteins.

To normalize conditions among the three modules concerning the dead volume of the experimental circuit, the recovery of albumin were fixed as 100%. Then the quantity or activity $R(v)$ of non-permeated protein could be estimated to be

$$R(v) = C_p(0) \cdot \sum_{P_v=0}^{v} (T_a - T_p)/100$$

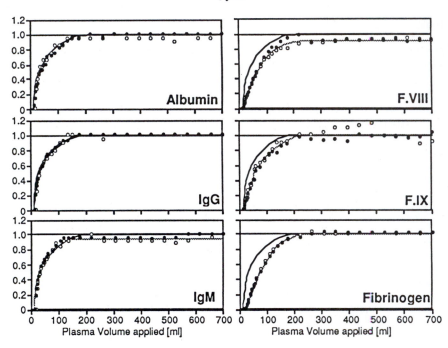

Figure 1. Change of protein concentration in CPAS (old) module.

where $C_p(0)$ is the protein content or activity in 1 ml of plasma pool (mg or unit), T_a and T_p are albumin and other protein contents in v ml of fed plasma (100%: initial protein content), respectively, and P_v is a total plasma volume applied.

Table 2.
Non-permeated proteins at 700 ml plasma applied

Protein	CPAS (old)	CPAS (new)	BCC
Alb (mg)	0	0	0
IgG (mg)	0	0	0
IgM (mg)	8	0	0
FVIII (units)	100	19	21
FIX (units)	27	17	24
Fib (mg)	87	49	24

Table 2 shows the quantities or activities of non-permeated proteins at 700 ml plasma applied. The amounts of non-permeated protein with hydrophilized membranes, i.e. CPAS (new) and BCC, were less than those of non-hydrophilized membranes, and choking was not observed. These significant improvements might be due to the reduction of protein adsorption on the membranes. The amounts of protein adsorption on CPAS (new) and BCC membranes were similar, but the profiles of protein permeation were slightly different. BCC membranes adsorbed coagulation proteins only at the initial stage, and all proteins almost perfectly permeated at steady state. On the other hand, CPAS (new) membranes adsorbed proteins very little at the initial stage, although the sieving coefficients of coagulation proteins were slightly lower albumin, which was comparable to BCC.

The recovery of FVIII and FIX are shown in Fig. 2. Because of the initial adsorption, the recoveries using BCC modules were rather low at the start as seen with the non-hydrophilized CPAS (old) modules. However, after 300–400 ml of plasma was applied,

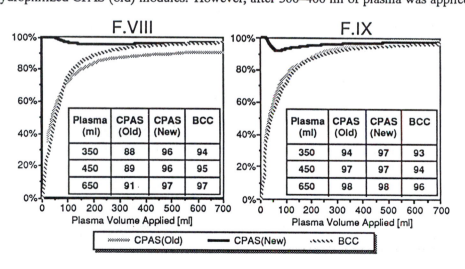

Figure 2. Recovery of FVIII and FIX.

no difference in the recoveries using the CPAS (new) and BCC modules was observed. When 450 ml of plasma was applied to the hydrophilized modules, FVIII and FIX recoveries were over 94%.

CONCLUSION

We tested three polyolefin membranes for spontaneous donor plasmapheresis. It was confirmed that hydrophilization of the membrane was very effective to increase the recoveries of coagulation proteins, although there still remained a little adsorptivity. We therefore conclude that in spontaneous donor plasmapheresis we should collect more than 300 ml plasma at each donation so that we could recover sufficient plasma proteins for fractionation. Moreover, since the hydrophilized membranes do not require priming in use, we could minimize protein dilution with saline or anti-coagulant.

REFERENCES

1. M. Yokoyama, T. Nakase, T. Takahashi *et al.* Development of plasmapheresis system to separate plasma using gravity. *Jap. J. Trans. Med.*, **37**, 114–115 (1991).
2. T. Takahashi, M. Hosoda, S. Yamamoto *et al.* A new donor plasmapheresis system with disk type membrane separator. *Jap. J. Trans. Med.*, **36**, 418–423 (1990).

Therapeutic Plasmapheresis (XII), pp. 919-922
T. Agishi *et al.* (Eds)
© VSP 1993

WBC-Depletion of Blood Components by a New Plant Vesicular Packing Material

G. MATTHES,[1] L. MAVRINA[1] and R. EHWALD[2]

[1]*Institute of Trasfusiology and Transplantology, School of Medicine (Charité)*
[2]*Institute of Plant Physiology, Biological Faculty, Humboldt University of Berlin, Germany*

Key words: leucocyte depletion; red cell concentrates; blood transfusion; plant vesicular material; preparative extraction; exclusion chromatography.

INTRODUCTION

Leucocyte depleted blood components are commonly used to prevent, decrease or delay alloimmunization, the risk of transfusion-transmitted diseases, the incidence of non-infectious transfusion reactions, transfusion complications in transplant recipients, etc. The efficacy of leucocyte removal varies with different filters from 80 to 99.9% and the extent of product loss varies from 5 to 30%.

We introduce a new type of biotechnologically produced chromatographic separation material consisting of purified plant cell wall ghosts (vesicular packing material) for filtration and separation of contaminating cells and substances.

MATERIALS AND METHODS

In all experiments ACD- or CPD-A1-anticoagulated whole blood resp. SAGM-resuspended packed red cells from normal blood donors were used.

The vesicular plant cell packing material is prepared by enzymatic digestion of mechanically undestroyed plant cells (*Wolffia arrhiza* L. or *Chenopodium album* L.) and subsequent extractive purification of the cell walls [1]. The vesicular particles are between 0.2 and 0.8 cm in size. They are hollow and consist of a cellulose network and semipermeable pectin matrix of primary plant cell wall, about 1 mm in thickness. The surface of the carrier is smooth and negatively charged. The material in packed condition is of reduced hydrodynamic resistance and suitable for filtration of blood and plasma in order to eliminate contaminating cells or to exclude low molecular substances. The exclusion limit for proteins is 35 kD.

The plant cell material, so far investigated, could be sterilized by gamma irradiation and is compatible with blood as was shown by *in vivo* and *in vitro* test [2].

RESULTS AND DISCUSSION

Leucocyte depletion of blood components

The *Chenopodium* plant material has a strong affinity to leucocytes [3, 4] and is especially suitable for elimination of white blood cells (Table 1). An experimental package containing 1 g of dry material eliminates 99–100% of leucocytes from 80 ml of fresh or preserved whole blood. Bound leucocytes are easily visible on the surface of the transparent cell wall ghosts by transmission light microscopy.

The residual white blood cell content in the filtered blood products is far below the CALL dosis and in the range of the CILL dosis. New measurements with WBC counting in a Nageotte chamber after filtration of packed red cells show that this material is capable of removing 3.49 $\log_{10}$ (residual WBC content 0.047 ± 0.06, depletion rate 99.955%).

All measured viability parameters (metabolic parameter, hemolysis, osmotic resistance, antigenicity) did not change in red blood cells after the filtration procedure of the blood components. Also their stability after subsequent storage at 4 °C was not altered. A selective linkage of certain cell types of blood to the vesicular packing material was not identifiable. At comparable experimental conditions, the material from the biomass of *Chenopodium album* L. shows a higher efficiency of leucocyte binding (Table 2) than

Table 1.

Leucocyte depletion of blood components by filtration with the vesicular packing material ($n = 12$)

	WBC		PLT	
	res. cont. (10^9/l)	depl. rate (%)	res. cont. (10^9/l)	depl. rate (%)
Fresh blood	0.035±0.02	99.1±0.8	21.4±10.4	89.5±4.2
CPD-blood				
1–2 d	0.016±0.02	99.5±0.5	68.1±12.7	61.1±15.0
7–8 d	0.004±0.01	99.9±0.2	40.0±2.6	72.5±1.5
SAGM-RCC				
7–9 d	0.012±0.02	99.7±0.6	9.0±5.9	68.9±20.8

Table 2.

Blood cell adsorption capacity of different leucocyte depletion filter material on the basis of an equal dry weight (60 mg); percentage of recovery (RBC) and depletion rate (WBC, PLT), ($n = 5$)

Material	RBC	WBC	PLT
Pectin/cellulose (Permselect)	99.8±4.4	71.4±5.5	51.7±10.0
Cellulose acetate (Erypur)	79.8±7.0	33.3±12.0	36.4±8.6
Polyester (Sepacell)	87.4±6.2	25.9±6.4	42.7±13.1
Polyester (Pall)	95.5±0.56	23.66±2.49	69.5±5.4
Cellulose (Immugard)	90.0±5.6	14.5±8.7	23.8±10.0

fibres on a cotton, cellulose, cellulose acetate or polyester basis used in commercially available leucocyte depletion filters. In preliminary experiments, we combined the two properties of the *Chenopodium* plant vesicular material [6], leucocyte depletion and the ion exchange capacity, in order to improve red blood cell preservation by a selective increase of intracellular pH: CPD-SAGM-resuspended red cell were filtered through a *Chenopodium album* L. column which was saturated with Meryman's new developed chloride free preservation solution ARC8 [7]. Figure 1 shows that the intracellular pH increases after the filtration procedure and that by this combination storage of erythrocytes in ARC8 for more than 5 weeks at 4 °C with an increased or normal content of 2,3-diphosphoglycerate can be achieved.

Selective separation from low-molecular compounds

In contrast to the *Chenopodium* material *Wolffia* plant cell material shows a smaller affinity to leucocytes. But, this material consisting of microcapsules with a thin ultrafilter membrane, enables a new form of chromatography based on diffusion and membrane separation: vesicle chromatography. With exclusion chromatography based on a process of membrane separation of hollow carriers, a stationary liquid phase in small membrane-enclosed spaces is exchanged by the principle of dialysis against an exterior mobile liquid phase. The membrane of the vesicular hollow bodies, being as thin as 1 mm, exhibits minimum diffusion resistance to the distribution of permeable substances, which enables use for separating the very large granular material, without any adverse impact upon separation quality.

The chromatography of fresh blood shows that erythrocytes, leucocytes, and platelets could be eluted without any mechanical obstruction or delay due to absorption to a volume which was equivalent to the volume of exclusion (the peak being about 30% relative to packing volume). Their behaviour was similar to that of plasma proteins and other substances above 35 kD in molar mass. Permeable low-molecular blood components,

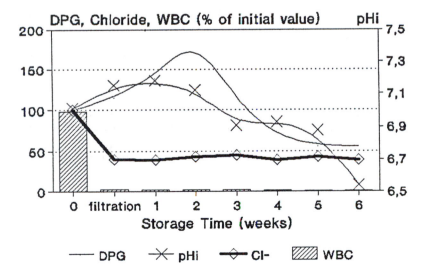

Figure 1. Red blood cell storage in ARC8 after filtration with plant packing material ($n = 3$).

such as urea, glucose and creatinine, as well as slowly dialysable substances of medium molecular weight, including myoglobin and vitamin B12, proved to be completely separable, within something between 25 and 30 min, from cells and high-molecular plasma proteins [2]. More than 90% of red blood cells, about 85% of leucocytes and 80% of platelets were recorded from the excluded fraction.

This principle can be used for the removal of cryoprotectants from cryopreserved erythrocytes or platelets [5]. In the chromatographic approach of glycerol or dimethylsulfoxide removal from erythrocytes resp. platelets after thawing the cells being eluted together with highmolecular plasma proteins. The cryoprotectants appear in the cell-free fraction and thus are separated from blood cells, without any additional steps, within 30 min from thawing of the deep-frozen samples.

CONCLUSION

With this new biotechnologically produced vesicular material an effective leucoreduction of blood components is possible. Especially, the incorporation of this material in an in-line filter — in combination with new preservation solution concepts — may be of particular interest in transfusion medicine.

There are further potential applications of these plant cell wall ghosts in other fields of medicine: (i) selective separation, extraction, purification of high molecular plasma components following the principle of exclusion dialysis in the form of group separation, using material with an increased threshold of exclusion; (ii) virus depletion of blood components by means of cascade filtration; and (iii) specific removal of toxic or pathogenic substances as well as slowly dialysable proteins from blood or liquids of biological origin.

REFERENCES

1. R. Ehwald, G. Fuhr, M. Olbrich, H. Göring, R. Knösche and R. Kleine. Chromatography based on membrane separation with vesicular packing material. *Chromatographia*, **28**, 561–564 (1989).
2. L. Mavrina, R. Ehwald, G. Matthes and G. Stamminger. Hämapherese mit Hilfe eines vesikulären pflanzlichen Trennmaterials. *Folia Haematol.*, **117**, 435–441 (1990).
3. L. Mavrina, G. Matthes and R. Ehwald. Filter zur selektiven Leukozyteneliminierung. *Patent DE 40 19*, **114** A1 (1990).
4. L. Mavrina, G. Matthes and R. Ehwald. Permeselect — ein neues Material für die Leukozyteneliminination. *Infusionstherapie*, in press.
5. L. Mavrina, S. König, A. Klein, H. Woehlecke, E. Richter, G. Matthes and R. Ehwald. Auschlußchromatographie zur Trennung kryoprotektiver Substanzen von gefrierkonservierten Blutzellen. *Folia Haematol.*, **117**, 251–258 (1990).
6. G. Matthes, L. Mavrina, E. Richter and U. Tofoté. Long-term maintained 2,3-diphosphoglycerate level in red blood cells filtered with vesicular carrier and stored in ARC8 at 4 °C. *Infusionstherapie* (in preparation).
7. H. T. Meryman, M. Hornblower and T. Keegan. Refrigerated stirage of washed cells. *Vox Sang*, **60**, 88-98 (1991).

Therapeutic Plasmapheresis (XII), pp. 923-925
T. Agishi *et al.* (Eds)
© VSP 1993

An Improved Method for Harvesting Young Red Cells

G. CHENG, X. CAO, Z. PAN, H. XU, D. XI, Y. ZHU and X. DENG

Suzhou Red Cross Blood Center, Suzhou 215006, China

Key words: erythrocyte; young; old; quality index.

INTRODUCTION

It was demonstrated that the density of young red cells is lower than that of old red cells, and the young red cells could be separated from old ones by centrifugation. Several methods using a cell separator have been used to prepare young red cell products [1, 2]. However, these methods had a higher cost. In this study, we have designed a special long bag for harvesting young red cells by centrifugation and obtained good quality young red cell products.

MATERIALS AND METHODS

Preparation of young red cells
Fresh blood was obtained from healthy donors. Whole blood (400 ml) in ACD-B was first spun at 2500 g (Beckman J 6-M) for 10 min, and 200 ml of supernatant plasma was then diverted into a sterile bag. Normal saline (approximately 50 ml) was added to the red cell concentrates and agitated for 3 min. The mixture was transferred into a special long bag and spun at 3400 g for 30 min. After centrifugation, the top 45% and the bottom 55% of red cells were divided into two populations with two forceps. The top 45% was then transferred into a sterile bag as the young red cell unit. The bottom 55% of red cells was considered to be old red cells.

EXAMINATION OF THE QUALITY OF RED CELL FRACTIONS

Reticulocyte count (Ret), mean cell volume (MCV), mean corpuscular hemoglobin concentration (MCHC), glutamic oxalacetic transaminase (GOT) and scanning electron microscopy (SEM) were selected for evaluating the quality of unseparated red cells, young red cell products and old red cells. The numbers of reticulocytes were determined by counting 2000 red cells stained with new methylene blue. MCV and MCHC were calculated after the hematocrit and the amounts of hemoglobin were measured, and the numbers of red cells were counted. The activity of GOT was assayed as previously described.

SEM was performed as follows. The red cells were fixed in glutaraldehyde and refixed in osmium tetroxide. The fixed cells were attached to glass coverslips with poly-L-lysine and then dehydrated in a graded series of alcohols. The coverslips were sputter-coated with 10 nm of gold–palladium and examined in a scanning electron microscope (Hitachi 750 type, Japan) by counting 300 red cells. Red cells were divided into two kinds according to their morphology. The biconcave erythrocytes were regarded as normal red cells and echinocytes, sphero-echinocytes were considered to be abnormal red cells.

RESULTS

The numbers of reticulocytes among unseparated red cells, young red cell products and old red cells were 0.73 ± 0.33, 2.1 ± 0.8 and $0.18 \pm 0.13\%$, respectively. It is obvious that the numbers of reticulocytes in young red cell products are much higher than those in unseparated red cells or old red cells.

MCHC of young red cell products was the lowest, but MCV is the highest among the three fractions of red cells, contrary to old red cells. These results indicate that the average volume of young red cells is bigger than that of old ones.

The activity of GOT in young red cell products is significantly higher than in unseparated red cells or old red cells. All of the results mentioned above are summarized in Table 1.

Table 1.

Fraction	Ret (%) ($n = 10$)	MCV (fl) ($n = 5$)	MCHC (%) ($n = 10$)	GOT (gHb) ($n = 10$)
Unseparated RBCs	0.73 ± 0.33	92.3 ± 2.02	29.5 ± 1.58	29.3 ± 10.10
Young RBCs	2.1 ± 0.80	101.2 ± 5.07	28.4 ± 1.4	39.5 ± 15.88
P	< 0.01	< 0.01	< 0.01	< 0.01
Old RBCs	0.18 ± 0.13	86.2 ± 2.77	31.0 ± 1.81	24.7 ± 9.33

SEM showed that the biconcave erythrocytes and the abnormal red cells in young red cell products were 80.4 and 19.6%, respectively, and that the biconcave erythrocytes in unsperated red cells and in old red cells were 72.2 and 62.8%; the anbormal red cells in the two fractions were 27.8 and 37.2%. It is apparent that the quality of young red cell products is superior to that of unseparated red cells.

In addition, we examined the numbers of while cells in four batches of young red cell products and observed that the average number of white cells in young red cell products was 1.73×10^9.

DISCUSSION

In view of the fact that the volume of red cells gradually becomes smaller and the density of red cells becomes higher during red blood cell aging, and that young red cells with lower density were separated from old ones by centrifugation, we designed a special long bag to separate young red cells. Our data showed that the packed red cell layer can be increased in the long bag and young red cells can be easily separated and harvested. After centrifugation, the packed red cell layer near the middle of the long bag was divided into two populations with two forceps. Thus, this improved technique can effectively prevent the confusion between young and old red cell populations, and can be easily controlled during the collection of hemoglobin content.

It has been reported that there are some differences in the cell volume, density and activity of enzymes between young and old red cells [3–5]. We selected five indexes to evaluate the quality of red cells before or after separation. Our results indicated that the quality of young red cell products was better than that of unseparated or old red cells.

CONCLUSIONS

In this study, we demonstrated that good quality young red cells can be easily separated in a special long bag by centrifugation. This improved method is of lower cost and greater convenience as compared with those methods using cell separators, and is suitable for patients receiving chronic blood transfusion therapy.

REFERENCES

1. R. E. Marcus *et al.* Young red cell preparation — a comparison of available methods. *Acta Haemat.*, **73**, 22–25 (1985).
2. A. W. Bracey *et al. Ex vivo* selective isolation of young red cells using the IBM–2991 cell washer. *Blood*, **61**, 1068–1071 (1983).
3. M. Magnani *et al.* Membrane-bound immunoglobulins increase during red blood cell aging. *Acta Haemat.*, **79**, 127–132 (1988).
4. J. Freedman. Membrane-bound immunoglobulins and complement components on young and old red cells. *Transfusion*, **24**, 477–481 (1984).
5. T. L. Simon, P. Sohmer and E. J. Nelson. Extended survival of neocytes produced by a new system. *Transfusion*, **29**, 221–225 (1989).

Therapeutic Plasmapheresis (XII), pp. 927-930
T. Agishi *et al.* (Eds)
© VSP 1993

Comparison of Leukocyte Depletion from Apheresis and Random Platelet Concentrates

M. K. ELIAS, J. W. SMIT,[1] M. R. HALIE,[1]
P. C. DAS and C. Th. SMIT SIBINGA

Red Cross Blood Bank Groningen-Drenthe and [1]Department of Haematology, University Hospital, Groningen, The Netherlands

Key words: leukocyte removal filter; leukocyte depletion; leukocyte immunogenic threshold; prevention of HLA alloimmunization.

INTRODUCTION

There is increasing evidence that reduction of the number of residual leukocytes in platelet concentrates (PCs) below 10 million per transfusion delays or prevents the incidence of HLA alloimmunization [1–3]. The introduction of the fourth generation leukocyte adherence filters made the preparation of leukocyte-free PCs within reach. This study was conducted to determine the performance of the two currently marketed forms of this filter: PL-100 and PL-50.

MATERIALS AND METHODS

Filtration
The Pall PL-100 filter (Pall Corp., Glen Cove, NY) was primed by inversion and squeezing the drip chamber till it was filled to about 25% of its volume, and returning it to the upright position. The PL-50 is self-priming. The flow was adjusted by gradually releasing the set clamp.

PL-100 filter. Thirteen pools of six PC units (PRP method) and 13 apheresis (Haemonetics V-50) units were filtered at gravity flow rates. Another 13 pools and 13 apheresis units were filtered at a rate of 10 ml/min or less. Pools were filtered on the day following preparation or the next day. Additionally, eight pools of 5 day old PCs were also filtered at 10 ml/min flow rate.

PL-50 filter. Thirteen pools and 13 apheresis units were filtered at the recommended flow rate of 25 ml/min.

Fraction analysis
Platelet bags were constructed in a special set-up such as to result in a mother container for the pool, connected via the filter to Y-junction tubings ending with 10 daughter containers. Pools of 10 PC units ($n = 8$) were filtered through the PL-100, at a rate of 10 ml/min. Fractions of 50 ml were separately collected and analyzed for platelet recovery and leukocyte removal.

Leukocyte counting
Pre- and post-filtration leukocyte counts were counted manually by the Bürker and Fuch's Rosenthal counting methods, as well as by the flow cytometer (FACStar, Becton–Dickinson Immunocytometry systems, Mountain View, CA), with propidium iodide labeling according to the method of Bodensteiner [4].

In vitro platelet parameters
Possible platelet activation, injury or endotoxin release by the filter, was assessed by β-thromboglobulin (βTG) release, lactic dehydrogenase leakage and endotoxin chromogenic substrate test, respectively. Platelet function and morphology before and after filtration were determined by the aggregation response to dual agonists (10 μM ADP and 2 μM epinephrine), the recovery from hypotonic shock and the morphology score.

RESULTS

Unless otherwise mentioned, all leukocyte values in the tables are those obtained by Bürker counting.

Table 1 shows the Pall filter efficiency at the rapid gravity rate versus the slow flow rate. At all flow rates, leukocyte removal and platelet recovery were greater for SDPC than for MDPC. Leucocyte depletion was lowest by filtration at gravity flow rate: the number of residual leukocytes exceeded 10 million in 3/12 SDPC (25%) and in 7/12 MDPC (58%). By reducing the filtration rate of PL-100 to 10 ml/min, leukocytes were detected in only 2/13 units of SDPC (one million in both) and in 6/13 MDPC (46%), three of which (23%) exceeded 10 million. Fifty percent of the 5 day old MDPC contained more than this threshold with only 80% platelet recovery.

The leukocyte removal percentage was greatest by PL-50 filtration at 25 ml/min flow rate: 99.997% in SDPC (only one unit contained 0.25 million leukocytes) and 99.965% in MDPC (only one unit contained 2.2 million leukocytes). Platelet recovery of SDPC was not different from PL-100, but that of MDPC improved significantly with this small filter. The only inconvenience observed with pooled PCs was the occasional clogging of the filter, necessitating stripping of the effluent line. This, however, had no apparent leukocyte fragmentation effect since this would have been depicted by the flow cytometer.

In all eight fraction analysis studies (82 measurements), the flow cytometric results correlated with those of the haemocytometer ($P < 0.001$). No leukocytes were detected by the haemocytometer in at least the first three filtered fractions; whereas the flow cytometer could identify as low as 0.1 cell/μl.

Table 2 shows the means of residual leukocytes, leukocyte removal and platelet recovery percentages per fraction. The first two fractions had the lowest platelet recovery.

Table 1.

Filtration efficiency at different flow rates

Residual leukocytes $\times 10^6$		Leukocyte removal (%)	Platelet recovery (%)
PL-100 gravity flow			
S	3.9	99.47	88.9
P	31	97.39	87.5
PL-100 at 10 ml/min			
S	0.154	99.95	96.0
P	6.13	99.0	84.3
P (5 day old)	21.9	96.03	79.2
PL-50 at 25 ml/min			
S	0.019	99.997	95.2
P	0.160	99.965	92.8

S, single donor PC; P, pools of six donor PCs. Each figure represents the mean of 3 observations.

Table 2.

Fraction analysis: Pall-100 filtration at 10 ml/min

Fraction[a]	Residual leukocytes $\times 10^6$	Leukocyte removal (%)	Platelet recovery (%)
1	0	100	70.3
2	0	100	87.3
3	0	100	93.8
4	0.8	99.93	94
5	2.2	99.75	95.5
6	5.1	99.54	95.9
7	8.6	99.24	97
8	14.2	98.67	95.1
9	15.6	98.31	97.3
10	26.7	97.57	93.5

[a] 50 ml fractions of pools of 10 PC units. Means of eight experiments.

This initial platelet loss is probably due to adhesion of platelets to the yet unoccupied filter sites.

The filtration-induced changes in *in vitro* platelet functions, morphology and pH were minimal. Activation or damage by filtration — as evidenced by the increase in βTG % release or LDH % leakage — were negligible ($P < 0.1$). All pre- and post-filtration samples were negative for endotoxin.

DISCUSSION

The PL-100 filter was shown to reduce effectively the number of residual leukocytes to far below the critical immunogenic threshold of 10 million in all SDPC units and in 77% of MDPC pools. Filtration of only five PC units would achieve this depletion level in all MDPC pools. This approach, however, is logistically not attractive. Depletion of small numbers of PC units would be at the expense of the platelet yield, since it appeared that the first two units have the lowest platelet recovery.

The PL-50 filter showed excellent results for both single and multiple donor PCs. Leukocytes were absent in more than 92% of units in both types of concentrates. The maximal leukocyte number detected after PL-50 filtration was 0.2 million in single donor platelets and 2.2 million in the pool. Moreover, PL-50 is much more efficient than PL-100 with regard to the incidence of total depletion (% of units with no detectable leukocytes).

The outcome of filtration following 5 day storage was less favourable than filtration of 1 or 2 day old PCs. Platelet activation, reaching its maximum by the end of the storage period, leads to microaggregate formation. These are retained by the filter and presumably occupy sites which otherwise would be occupied by leukocytes. This is reflected on both leukocyte removal and post-filtration platelet recovery. Moreover, membrane fragments were probably not retained by the filter as depicted by the flow cytometric distribution pattern. Whether these are platelet microparticles or leukocyte fragments remains to be investigated. It is reported [5], however, that the new generation leukocyte removal filters remove the membrane fragments as well.

No acids or endotoxins were released by the filter. Filtration does not add to platelet activation. Platelet integrity, function and morphology are well preserved in both single and multiple PCs.

Single donor platelets are better depleted and recovered after filtration than pooled multiple donor platelets. Filtration of platelets soon after preparation is preferred to filtration after storage.

REFERENCES

1. M. Fisher, J. R. Chapman, A. Tring and P. J. Morris. Alloimmunization to HLA antigens following transfusion with leucocyte-poor and purified platelet suspension. *Vox Sang*, **49**, 331–335 (1985).

2. I. Sniecinski, M. R. O'Donell, B. Nowicki and L. R. Hill. Prevention of refractoriness and HLA-alloimmunization using filtered blood products. *Blood*, **71**, 1402–1407 (1988).

3. G. Andreu, J. Dewailly, C. Leberre *et al.* Prevention of HLA alloimmunization with leucocyte-poor packed red cells and platelet concentrates obtained by filtration. *Blood*, **72**, 964–967 (1988).

4. D. C. Bodensteiner. A flow cytometric technique to accurately measure post-filtration white blood cell counts. *Transfusion*, **29**, 651–653 (1989).

5. B. D. Rawal, R. E. Davis, M. P. Bush and G. N. Vyas. Dual reduction in the immunogenic and infectious complications of transfusion by filtration/removal of leukocytes from donor blood soon after collection. *Trans. Med. Rev.*, **4**,(Suppl. 1), 36–41 (1990).

Therapeutic Plasmapheresis (XII), pp. 931-935
T. Agishi *et al.* (Eds)
© VSP 1993

Donor Plasmapheresis: A View from Scotland

J. CASH

Scotland is a small country within the United Kingdom. It has a population of only 5 million and well over 95% of our health care programmes are provided, free of charge to the population, by the Government. The national health care programme in Scotland includes a national blood transfusion service (SNBTS) which is centrally co-ordinated and managed, which relies exclusively on voluntary unpaid donors and in the late 1970s was directed to develop a programme of self-sufficiency in blood and blood products. The opportunity to achieve self-sufficiency has been much enhanced by the blood transfusion service having its own plasma fractionation centre. Thus a single organization has managerial control over both plasma acquisition and its fractionation, the former represented by five regional centres and the latter by the protein fractionation centre. Control is manifest in the context of the acquisition of market intelligence and using this in planning, the selection of appropriate options for plasma procurement, fractionation and the associated research in both these areas. In all these matters we have sought to make freely available to patients in Scotland blood and blood products of high quality and in a quantity which matches legitimate clinical demand. In most of these endeavours major contributors to programme developments are the prescribing physicians.

The primary task of blood transfusion services worldwide has traditionally been one directed towards the acquisition and issue of cellular blood components — notably, of course, red cell concentrates. In order to fulfill this task, which is of benefit to many thousands of patients, we have often asked the question: 'What is the number of blood donations that are required to meet all such cellular needs at all times?' Such a question has often been asked before and there has been a general agreement that in those countries able to make modern medicine available to all their peoples then the number of blood donations needing to be available each year is approximately $50\,000/10^6$ population. In Scotland we collect approximately $55\,000$ whole blood donations/10^6 population/year. We ought to note that should we wish, it would be possible to increase this figure substantially. In passing we should also note that in Scotland we use optimal additive solutions — a practice which enhances the quality of red cell concentrates but also enables us to acquire a maximum of approximately 300 ml of plasma from each whole blood donation processed.

These basic background facts are central to any analysis of the Scottish approach to donor plasmapheresis and will be reviewed again in that analysis. However, before this is done we need next to examine the product demands in Scotland and how they match the plasma input and associated fractionation yields.

The demand for plasma products is summarized in Table 1 and we find is best ultimately expressed as an issue of finished plasma products per 10^6 total population in the year ending March 31, 1991.

Table 1.
Plasma fractions issued in Scotland

Product	Issued per 10^6 total population in Scotland
Factor VIII (m.i.u)	1.8
Factor IX (m.i.u)	0.5
Albumin (kg $\times 10^3$)	206
IMIgG (kg $\times 10^3$)	1.0
IVIgG (kg $\times 10^3$)	8.9
Anti-Rh(D) (m.i.u)	1.5
Anti-tetanus (m.i.u)	0.25
Anti-HBV (m.i.u)	0.15
Anti-zoster (g)	5.0
Anti-rubella (i.u)	100 000
Anti-rabies (i.u)	10 000
Anti-measles (i.u)	6000
Anti-CMV (g)	600

You will have gathered that in common with so many other countries at the present time the product which is quantitatively dominating our plasma acquisition programme is factor VIII. As we then begin to consider the matching of our plasma procurement programme with product demand we must consider two critical yield questions: (i) what is our fractionation yield for factor VIII? and (ii) what is our *recovered* plasma yield?

The answer to the first question is currently a little difficult because we are engaged in the commissioning of a new manufacturing process designed to produce a high purity factor VIII concentrate. Nonetheless we can be reasonably confident that the current yield of 170 iu/kg plasma fractionated will steadily improve — but for the purposes of this talk I suggest we base our calculations on a fractionation yield of 170 iu/kg.

The answer to the second question is more readily available. We process a very high proportion of our whole blood donations; such that the average fresh plasma yield per total donation collected in 290 ml. 3500 kg is made available for direct clinical use as FFP and the rest (81 000 kg) is sent for fractionation.

A simple calculation reveals that at the present time the factor VIII concentrate made available from the recovered plasma source in Scotland is 1.8 m.i.u./10^6 total population/year. At the present time this *totally* covers the clinical demand. Anticipated increases in demand — which we believe will take place over the next 5 years — will largely be met by improvements in fractionation yields.

The total plasma procurement over the last 5 years for self-sufficiency in Scotland is summarised in Table 2. In 1991 less than 10% of this programme derived from donor plasmapheresis.

Table 2.

Total plasma procurement for
fraction in Scotland (1991)

Total plasma	= 81 300 kg
Recovered	= 90%
Source	= 10%

There will be some in the audience who will be wondering why I have come all the way from Scotland to emphasize that donor plasmapheresis plays no part in the plasma procurement programme of the SNBTS. In fact, donor plasmapheresis plays an important part in our programme but that part is small and is currently almost exclusively directed towards the procurement of hyperimmune plasma from a small number of donors. This hyperimmune plasma is fractionated to specific immunoglobulin preparation and the programme is quantitatively summarized in Table 3.

Table 3.

Specificity and quantities of hyperimmune plasma collected
in Scotland in 1991 (all by machine plasmapheresis)

Plasma specificity	Amount (kg) collected /10^6 population/year
Anti-Rh(D)	85.0
Anti-tetanus	120.0
Anti-HBV	48.0
Anti-zoster	44.0
Anti-rabies	30.0
Anti-CMV	116.0
Anti-E. coli	80.0
Total (kg)	523.0

All the donors providing this hyperimmune plasma are subject to machine plasmapheresis. The machines currently used are Haemonetics and Baxter (Haemosciences).

The operation of donor plasmapheresis in the UK is undertaken exclusively by the blood transfusion services and follows guidelines produced by the UK BTS. Specifically there is a limit of plasma obtained per annum (15 l).

It can be seen from the data presented that donor plasmapheresis is a relatively small and specialized contributor to the plasma procurement programme in Scotland. This has arisen because *in our community* the bulk of plasma needed can be acquired from existing whole blood donations that are currently the foundation of a cellular blood programme. Moreover, in our operational environment plasmapheresis has always been a significantly more expensive option than recovered plasma and that cost increment must be justified for it is a burden on all in our community. It is possible, of course, that source plasma may be competitively priced in a programme in which the primary cost centre is directed towards single donor (apheresis) platelet concentrates and the plasma is regarded as a by-product. However, this operational approach has not yet made an effective quantitative impact on our plasma procurement programmes primarily because the opportunity for justifying the use of single donor platelets is currently relatively infrequent.

The question arises then: Do we see any change in this position, specifically an increasing reliance on the use of donor plasmapheresis — source plasma?

I think we would have to respond that change in the foreseeable future is unlikely. While it is possible that new technical innovations may further reduce the unit cost of plasma acquired by the plasmapheresis option, we doubt whether this will be sufficient to significantly compete with the cost of recovered plasma. Of no less significance are the improving plasma fractionation yields which may give rise to a period of *reduced* plasma demand in many countries. Finally, whilst we take the view that the controversy over the *long-term* hazards of donor plasmapheresis — at least in terms of protein deficiency — is over and that there is no harm possible to donors if restricted to less than 15 l of plasma per annum, there remains in our minds concern that whilst donor plasmapheresis is clearly a procedure with very low morbidity and mortality, nonetheless this low level is likely to be higher than whole blood donation in appropriately matched donors. We have therefore instinctively tended to reserve plasmapheresis as an option in situations were recovered plasma procurement cannot provide an acceptable option — the procurement of hyperimmune plasma. We get the distinct impression that whilst the total plasma procurement in Europe is increasing substantially, the proportion from plasmapheresis is falling. Indeed we believe several countries in Europe are cutting back substantially on their donor plasmapheresis programmes.

But can we envisage an operational shift in the *more distant future* in which source plasma (donor plasmapheresis) becomes more attractive to those whose plasma products are derived from voluntary unpaid donors? The answer must be a tentative and qualified 'Yes' and the occasion would be if the use of a recombinant haemoglobin solution or an artificial equivalent became routine clinical practice. In this scenario the main operational pressure on the whole blood programme would be substantially reduced and the nature of blood/plasma collection programmes would have to be reviewed.

Finally, we must recognize that if there was an increase in demand for existing plasma products which outstripped the recovered plasma option, then donor plasmapheresis for routine plasma supply might be necessary. I have already indicated that this does not appear to be happening with factor VIII concentrates and any emerging pressure in this direction may well be limited by the increasing availability of recombinant factor VIII. On the other hand, if the demand for normal IVIG continues to show the dramatic increases seen in the last 5 years, this product could surplant factor VIII as the product dominating plasma procurement.

In conclusion, in those parts of the world with blood donation collection rates around 50 000 donations/10^6 population/year there seems little opportunity at the present time for major expansion in donor plasmapheresis. There is some evidence that outside the commercial plasma procurement industry donor plasmapheresis may be in decline.

The opportunities for the future remain unclear and seem likely to be heavily dependent on the intrusion of biotechnology on the practice of blood transfusion.

Therapeutic Plasmapheresis (XII), pp. 937-940
T. Agishi *et al.* (Eds)
© VSP 1993

Highly Sensitive Methods to Detect Residual Leukocytes in Leukocyte-depleted Blood Products

T. A. TAKAHASHI, M. HOSODA, Y. MOGI, H. ABE and S. SEKIGUCHI

Hokkaido Red Cross Blood Center, Sapporo, Japan

Key words: leukocyte poor blood products; platelet apheresis; leukocyte removal filter; flow cytometry; cytospin; polymerase chain reaction.

INTRODUCTION

The recent improvement of leukocyte removal filters has made it difficult to count the few remaining leukocytes in platelet concentrates using automated electronic cell counters or visual counts in hemocytometers. Also, new apheresis system, such as the COBE Spectra, produce apheresis platelets with extremely low contamination of leukocytes. The need for reliable techniques for the determination of small amounts of leukocytes in filtered blood components are increasing for the quality control of leukocyte-poor components and for the evaluation of new filters. Here we describe three methods (flow cytometry, cytospin, polymerase chain reaction) which we have developed to measure small numbers of leukocytes remaining in the apheresis platelet concentrates prepared by the COBE Spectra and the new model Fenwal CS-3000, and in both filtered platelet concentrate (PC) and red cell concentrate (RCC), including those filtered by the 6 log leukocyte removal filters.

MATERIALS AND METHODS

Flow cytometry
We used the Ortho Cytoron (Ortho Diagnostics Co. Ltd, Tokyo, Japan) flow cytometer, as this instrument incorporates a sample delivery system which delivers a defined volume of sample to the flow cell. One part of pre- and post-filtered PC and RCC were added to 7.5 parts of propidium iodide (PI) solution containing 5 mg of PI (Sigma, St Louis, MO, USA), 100 mg of RNase, 100 mg of sodium citrate and 100 μl of Triton X-100 in 100 ml of phosphate buffered saline. Stained leukocytes were measured at a flow rate of 1 μl/s for 1 min. The large numbers of leukocytes in the pre-filtered samples had first been measured in the hemocytometer and serially diluted with leukocyte-free PC or RCC prepared by repeated filtration [1].

Cytospin method
We have applied a cytocentrifuge method to count the residual leukocytes in leukocyte-depleted platelet concentrates (LDPC) using the Cytospin 2 (Shandon Southern Products Ltd, Runcorn, Cheshire, UK). Optimal conditions of cytocentrifugation were investigated for the centrifugation speed and period, for the volume of the sample. Figure 1 shows the procedure for the cytospin method [2].

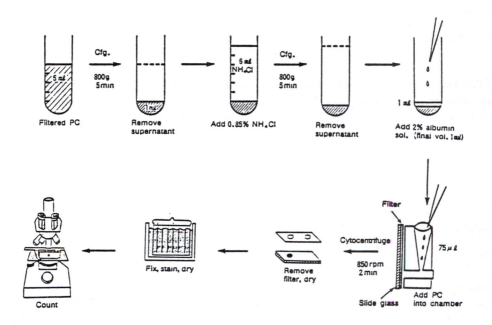

Figure 1. Procedure for the cytospin method.

Polymerase chain reaction (PCR) method

β-Globin gene was chosen as the target of the PCR because it is well characterized and considered to be a single-copy gene, and because primers could be purchased commercially. Following the extraction of DNA, the reaction was repeated 35 cycles. To detect the amplified products, a ^{32}P-labeled oligonucleotide probe was used to perform Southern blot analysis [3].

RESULTS

Flow cytometry

The number of leukocytes measured on the Ortho Cytoron as a function of cell number expected from the hemocytometer count can be expressed by the regression lines: $Y = 0.823X - 0.454$ ($r = 0.999$) for RCC and $Y = 0.801X + 0.672$ ($r = 0.999$) for PC. After correction of measurements using these regression equations, there was significant correlation between the measurement of leukocytes in PC and RCC by the Ortho Cytoron and hemocytometer in the range of 10^5–10^7 cells/ml ($r = 0.99$). When RCC and PC had been filtered with several kinds of leukocyte removal filters, the flow cytometric method could detect leukocytes to concentrations as low as 1.77×10^{-1} cells/μl. This detection sensitivity was successfully increased 10 times by concentrating samples 10 times before the analysis.

Cytospin method

Under the optimal conditions, there was a good correlation between the number of cells attached to the slide glass after cytocentrifugation (Y) and that of cells put into the sample chambers (X), expressed as the following regression line: $Y = 0.75X - 3.41$ ($r = 0.99$). When pooled PC (20 unit pool, 1 day old) were filtered through a Pall PL100 filter, neither the automated electronic cell counter (Coulter Counter model S plus IV) nor manual counting could detect leukocytes in these LDPC, but the cytocentrifuge method could detect an average of 1×10^4 lymphocytes still contaminated in them.

PCR METHOD

The PCR method could successfully detect 2.4 cells in one ml (Fig. 2). This sensitivity is 10–100-fold superior to that of the flow cytometric method. Furthermore, to avoid the use of radioisotopic materials, we developed a double PCR method, which shows similar sensitivity to that of radioisotopic PCR.

DISCUSSION AND CONCLUSION

Though various techniques have been developed quite intensively in the last few years, each method has both advantages and disadvantages. The flow cytometric method using the Ortho Cytoron flow cytometer has the advantages of easy operation, speed and high sensitivity. The cytospin method would be helpful when the flow cytometer is not available and has the advantages of defining the population of leukocytes in the filtrated blood products. The PCR method may be a promising method to detect extremely low numbers of contaminating leukocytes, and can cope with the new filters which will be developed soon to remove more leukocytes to prevent viral infection, such as HIV and HTLV-I. Figure 3 summarizes the detection sensitivity of each counting method and the number of residual leukocytes contaminated in the leukocyte-depleted blood products prepared by various filters. The combined use of these techniques should be helpful for the evaluation of new filters and for the quality control of leukocyte-poor blood components.

Mononuclear cells purified from peripheral blood using Ficoll

2.4×10^n cells / ml

n= 3 2 1 0 -1 NC NC

Position of primers on β-globin gene

	Exon1	Intron1	Exon2	

GH20   GH21

Figure 2. Sensitivity of PCR for detecting leukocytes.

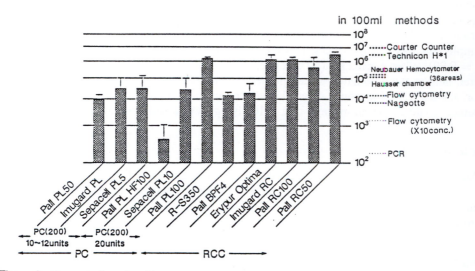

Figure 3. Concentration of residual leukocytes in 100 ml of filtered RCC or PC and the sensitivity of counting methods.

REFERENCES

1. T. A. Takahashi, M. Hosoda and S. Sekiguchi. A flow cytometric method to detect residual leukocytes in platelet and red cell concentrates. *Jpn. J. Transf. Med.*, **36**, 429–437 (1990).
2. T. A. Takahashi, M. Hosoda and S. Sekiguchi. Cytospin method for the determination of residual leukocytes in leukocyte-depleted platelet concentrates. *Jpn. J. Transf. Med.*, **35**, 497–503 (1989).
3. H. Abe, Y. Mogi, M. Hosoda *et al.* Detection of a small number of residual leukocytes in filtered blood products by polymerase chain reaction. *J. Clin. Exp. Med.*, **160**, 887–888 (1992).

23

Miscellaneous

Therapeutic Plasmapheresis (XII), pp. 943-946
T. Agishi *et al.* (Eds)
© VSP 1993

Cyclosporin-A Induced Hypertriglyceridemia: Efficacy of Plasma Exchange Cascade Filtration

L. MALFANTI, M. VALBONESI, G. LERCARI, G. FLORIO,
P. CARLIER and G. GIANNINI

Immunohematology Services, San Martino Hospital, Genova, Italy

Key words: plasmapheresis; plasma exchange; metabolic disorders; hypertriglyceridemia; cyclosporin-A; bone marrow transplantation; cascade filtration.

INTRODUCTION

Allogenic bone marrow transplantation (ABMT) is becoming a common therapy offered to different kinds of patients. Because of its complexity in terms of immunological and pharmacological management, patients with ABMT undergo a number of complications which are seldom seen in other conditions. In the last couple of years at our ABMT unit the use of steroids and cyclosporin-A (CYA) has been a very common therapeutic association. CYA was used to downregulate T_h lymphocytes along with some B cells [1, 2] by inhibiting the production of interleukin-2 and interleukin-4. Interleukin-4 and interleukin-5 appear to be responsible for the autoantibody production that in turn is responsible for the graft-versus-host-disease (GVHD). Beyond the immunological effects, which are potentiated by the contemporary administration of steroids, CYA produces several side effects, among which hypertriglyceridemia (HTG) may seldom become permanent with clinical symptoms such as retinitis, neurological compromise, and pancreatitis and disseminated intravascular coagulation. As a consequence, HTG is usually considered a benign complication that does not necessarily require discontinuation of the drug or plasmapheresis, as we described on two separate occasions [3, 4].

Since the first observation in 1988 we have been compelled to carry out four plasma exchanges and 10 cascade filtration (CF) sessions to treat seven patients with symptomatic CYA-induced HTG not responding to adjustment or discontinuation of the drug. We report here our cumulative experience.

PATIENTS AND METHODS

The study includes seven patients who underwent bone marrow transplantation because of homozygous beta-thalassemia, chronic myeloid leukemia, acute myelogenous leukemia and aplastic anemia. Their characteristics are summarized in Table 1.

After ABMT, all patients received CYA at the dose of 5 mg/kg body weight, intravenously, for GVHD prevention. CYA was given from day 1 and combined with prednisone at the dose of 1.5 mg/kg body weight when GVHD appeared. Afterwards oral CYA was maintained with a dosage depending on plasma CYA levels and kidney

Table 1.
Symptomatic patients who underwent plasmapheresis because of CYA-induced HTG after allogeneic BMT

Case no.	Diagnosis	Age/sex	Body weight (kg)	Conditioning regimen	Engraftment (day +)	GVHD (grade)
1	CML	39/M	44	TBI + CTX 200 mg/kg	+20 WBC +23 PLT	II
2	β-thalassemia	16/F	42	busulphan 14 mg CTX 200 mg/kg	+24 WBC +15 PLT	II
3	CML	35/M	57	TBI + CTX	+17 WBC +25 PLT	III
4	ANLL	42/F	51	TBI + CTX	+24 WBC +22 PLT	II
5	ANLL	34/M	62	TBI + CTX	+35 WBC +27 PLT	II
6	CML	41/F	46	TBI + CTX	+21 WBC +16 PLT	II
7	ANLL	33/F	51	TBI + CTX	+18 WBC +15 PLT	II

Engraftment for WBC > 500 granulocytes/μl and for platelets > $30 \times 10^3/\mu$l.

and liver function parameters. All patients but one developed grade II GVHD. One patient had transient grade III GVHD. When symptomatic HTG appeared, CYA was withdrawn at least 4 days before plasma exchange or cascade filtration initiation. All patients had fluctuating levels of triglycerides that only partially responded to drug adjustment or suspension prior to plasmapheresis initiation. Two patients (nos 1 and 2) were treated with continuous flow centrifugation apheresis. A Dideco S.r.l. (Mirandola, Modena, Italy) Vivacell machine was used and 3.8% albumin was employed as replacement. The mean volume of plasma exchanged at each session averaged 3.1 l. The four procedures were complicated by the fact that the buffy-coat sensor of the machines could not work properly due to the milky aspect of the plasma. As a consequence, it was necessary to proceed in the manual mode, under the visual control of the buffy-coat position. Because of these kinds of technical troubles the following 10 procedures were of the CF type and a discontinuous flow machine was preferred. A V50 cell separator was used in the semi-automated mode for plasma separation. This plasma was immediately on-line processed with an Albusave secondary filter to CF (Dideco S.r.l., Mirandola, Modena, Italy) and autologous filtered plasma was used for replacement. The sessions were carried out in the five patients we observed afterwards. At each session a mean volume of 2.68 l of plasma was collected and submitted to CF. Because of the exceedingly high levels of cholesterol and triglycerides, reverse rinsing of the secondary filter was carried out as previously described [5]. From two to five reverse rinses were necessary to maintain the filtration efficiency.

RESULTS

The biochemical results of our treatments are summarized in Table 2, along with the time of presentation of HTG. The increase in triglyceride levels was responsible for stupor or grade I–II coma in five patients and of hyperlipemic retinitis in three cases, whereas disseminated intravascular coagulation was present in a single case with pancreatitis. Two patients (nos 6 and 7) treated just because of HTG and hypercholesterolemia. In all symptomatic patients, symptoms began to subside during the first session and did not reappear afterwards despite plasma triglyceride rebound reaching levels as high as 1530 mg/ml, as we observed in patient no. 1. Two patients relapsed at 5 and 9 months intervals (patients nos 5 and 6), with triglycerides levels reaching 1630 and 1510 mg/ml, respectively. None was asymptomatic and none responded to discontinuation of the drug. A single CF session, carried out with both patients, was able to determine a rapid drop in triglycerides.

Table 2.
Effect of plasmapheresis or CF on the triglycerides and LDL cholesterol levels in patients with CYA-induced HTG

Case no.	Day of treatment after ABMT	Pre-apheresis		Post-apheresis		Type of treatment
		triglycerides (mg/dl)	LDL cholesterol (mg/dl)	triglycerides (mg/dl)	LDL cholesterol (mg/dl)	
1	+ 208	3215	414	917	217	CFC
2	+ 224	2022	347	691	185	CFC
3	+ 163	1635	442	320	178	DFC/CF
4	+ 108	1830	350	336	195	DFC/CF
5	+ 171	1970	385	470	215	DFC/CF
6	+ 205	1765	396	320	285	DFC/CF
7	+ 143	1638	515	405	266	DFC/CF

DISCUSSION

The first application of plasmapheresis for HTG is probably the one by Gerard *et al.* [6], who, in 1982, reported on the management of a patient with hyperlipemia and diabetic ketoacidosis with pulmonary odema and acute pancreatitis. As to our experience, we have successfully treated two patients with alcoholic pancreatitis and secondary hypertriglyceridemia and hyperlipemia. We have also reported two cases of therapeutic plasmapheresis in patients suffering from CYA induced HTG. After CYA therapy in ABMT a moderate elevation of triglycerides is common and does not require anything else that drug adjustment. Cases in which a symptomatic or dangerous level of triglycerides is reached are very rare and usually respond to discontinuation of the drug. When this measure is inadequate, plasmapheresis or CF may be useful to rapidly reduce the triglyceride levels and to half the progression of the symptoms or to prevent very dangerous complications such as pancreatitis or disseminated intravascular coagulation. In our cases plasmapheresis and CF were equally effective from a laboratory and clinical point of view. It is obvious, nonetheless, that apheresis treatment will remain among

therapeutic options only for a minority of cases and only until the time when a rational and adequate pharmacological therapy will be offered by an adequate pathogenic
interpretation of CYA induced hypertriglyceridemia.

REFERENCES

1. P. J. Morris. Cyclosporin-A. *Transplantation*, **32**, 349 (1981).
2. A. O. Vladutin. Effect of cyclosporin on experimental autoimmune thyroiditis in mice. *Transplantation*, **35**, 18 (1983).
3. M. Valbonesi, D. Occhini, C. Capra *et al.* Plasma exchange for the management of cyclospo-rin A-induced hypertriglyceridemia. *Intern. J. Artif. Organs*, **11**, 209 (1988).
4. M. Valbonesi, D. Occhini, R. Frisoni *et al.* Cyclosporin-induced hypertriglyceridemia with prompt response to plasma exchange therapy. *J. Clin. Apheresis*, **6**, 158 (1991).
5. M. Valbonesi, G. Lercari, G. Angelini *et al.* Cascade filtration with reverse rinse of the secondary filter. *J. Clin. Apheresis*, **3**, 240 (1987).
6. A. Gerard, F. Schooneman and J. M. Guine. Treatment by plasma exchange of a patient with hyper-lipemia and diabetic ketoacidosis with lesional pulmonary odema and acute pancreatitis. *Vox. Sang.*, **43**, 147 (1982).

Therapeutic Plasmapheresis (XII), pp. 947-948
T. Agishi *et al.* (Eds)
© VSP 1993

Ten Years of Apheresis in Canada

G. ROCK, C. HERBERT and MEMBERS OF THE CASG*

Canadian Apheresis Study Group, Ottawa, Ontario, Canada

Key words: apheresis; national registry; clinical trials.

INTRODUCTION

The Canadian Apheresis Study Group (CASG) celebrated its 10th anniversary in 1991. The CASG is a national organization representing therapeutic apheresis practice throughout Canada. Members from each of the 17 major medical centers meet annually to discuss current and proposed projects. The mandate of the CASG is to developed randomized prospective clinical trials and to provide a forum for the exchange of information concerning apheresis.

METHODS

Since 1981 the CASG has collected data on plasma exchange (PE) and cytapheresis procedures from over 30 apheresis units across the country. More than 52000 PE procedures have been carried out in this time, with approximately 6000 performed in each of the past 5 years. This levelling off in the number of procedures, and application to a more clearly defined group of patients, indicates that PE is now a basic service in most medical centers. Data on reactions to PE and on the type and amount of replacement fluid used for PE has been collected since 1985.

RESULTS

Whereas 10 years ago procedures involving hematological and neurological disorders were equivalent at 30% of the total each, the majority of procedures are now performed for neurological disorders (50%) with hematological treatments remaining at approximately 30%. The number of PEs for collagen-vascular disorders has decreased from 21% to less than 5% of the total, with no procedures now done for rheumatoid arthritis

---

*The members of the CASG are as follows: Grenfell Adams, MD, Barrett Benny, MD, Noel A. Buskard, MD, Stephen N. Caplan, MD, Robert Card, MD, William F. Clark, MD, Peter Ford, MD, John J. L. Freedman, MD, Philip Gordon, MD, John Klassen, MD, Max M. Gorelick, MD, Pierre Leblond, MD, Mariette Lepine-Martin, MD, Jack McBride, MD, Marc P. Mponté, MD, Rama C. Nair, PhD, Gail A. Rock, PhD, MD, Tsiporah Shore, MD, Kenneth H. Shumak, MD, and David M. C. Sutton, MD.

and a decline in the numbers for systemic lupus erythematosus (SLE). There has been little change in the number of PEs performed for renal disorders over the 10 year period.

The increase in the neurological category is due to a major increase in the number of procedures performed for the acute Guillain–Barré syndrome, an increase which has been consistent and has resulted in a six fold difference in the 10 year period. A doubling in the number of procedures performed for chronic inflammatory demyelinating neuropathy (CIDP) has also contributed to the increase, while myasthenia gravis totals have remained approximately the same over the 10 years. Until 1990, the fourth major contributor to the number of procedures in the neurological category was multiple sclerosis (MS). In 1985 the CASG and the Canadian Cooperative Multiple Sclerosis Study Group initiated a trial of PE in MS. These results were recently published [1] and showed no benefit to PE under the study conditions chosen. Thus, while 4 years ago 600 PE procedures were being done annually for MS, this number has been reduced to almost zero following the results of the trial.

Reactions to PE are classified as mild, moderate or severe, with a severe reaction being one in which a patient becomes clinically unstable requiring intervention by a physician and early termination of the procedure. Current data indicates that some form of reaction occurs in approximately 9% of procedures with 68% of these considered to be mild, 24% moderate and the remaining 8% severe. PE is therefore a relatively safe procedure with severe reactions occurring in seven of 1000 procedures.

In 1990, 8391 l of albumin, 3007 l of fresh frozen plasma (FFP) and 229 l of stored plasma (SP) were used for PE. The amount of SP has decreased by 50% in the last 6 years, while the amount of FFP used has increased by 15% and the albumin use has risen by only 5%.

CONCLUSIONS

A national registry permits the development of appropriate clinical trials. The CASG has coordinated or cooperated in five completed randomized clinical trials in: thrombotic thrombocytopenic purpura (TTP), rapidly progressive glomerulonephritis, multiple sclerosis, acute immune thrombocytopenic purpura and Rh disease. Currently, a Canadian cooperative multicenter study in CIDP is underway and the CASG is cooperating in an international study in SLE. A pilot study in the use of cryosupernatant as the replacement fluid in TTP is also underway. Members are kept up to date by the biannual publication of the CASG newsletter which has both national and international distribution.

The CASG has been financed by a variety of mechanisms since its initial organization. It is now largely funded by the provinces through the Canadian Blood Agency. The benefits of a national coordinating group have been apparent both in ensuring up-to-date application of new technologies and in conserving national blood resources.

REFERENCE

1. The Canadian Cooperative Multiple Sclerosis Study Group. The Canadian trial of cyclophosphamide and plasma exchange in progressive multiple sclerosis. *Lancet*, **337**, 441–446 (1991).

Therapeutic Plasmapheresis (XII), pp. 949-952
T. Agishi *et al.* (Eds)
© VSP 1993

Treatment of Systemic Amyloidosis with Dimethyl Sulfoxide and Plasma Exchange

S. YUASA, H. BANDAI, T. YURA, N. TAKAHASHI and H. MATSUO

Second Department of Internal Medicine, Kagawa Medical School, Kagawa, Japan

Key words: systemic amyloidosis; dimethyl sulfoxide; plasma exchange; prognosis.

INTRODUCTION

Systemic amyloidosis may be defined as a disease resulting from the progressive deposition of abnormal proteins in multiple organs. Although the prognosis of systemic amyloidosis depends on the type of amyloid involvement, it, in general, is characterized by a poor prognosis [1, 2]. The current treatment for amyloidosis, including alkylating agents, corticosteroids and colchicine, is not satisfactory [3, 4]. In the present study, in order to clarify the efficiency of combination treatment with dimethyl sulfoxide (DMSO) and plasma exchange, we compared the effect of combination treatment versus other conventional treatment in 12 patients with systemic amyloidosis.

PATIENTS AND METHODS

Twelve patients with systemic amyloidosis were studied (Table 1). They included three males and nine females, and their ages ranged from 24 to 92 years, with a mean of 62. Seven patients in which amyloid proteins consist of amyloid light chain, AL, included four patients with primary amyloidosis and three patients associated with multiple myeloma. The other group consisted of five patients with secondary amyloidosis due to rheumatoid arthritis and unknown disease.

Plasma exchange was usually performed once a week with a single filtration method because it has been assumed that amyloid proteins show remarkable diversity in molecular size [5]. Plasmaflo AP-05H (Asahi Medical Co., Tokyo, Japan) was used as a plasma separator and fresh frozen plasma (3.2–4.8 l each time) as replacement solution. DMSO was given percutaneously at 5–10 ml on the day before the plasma exchange therapy in patients receiving the combination treatment.

RESULTS

As shown in Table 1, anemia and nephrotic syndrome were present in 67% of 12 patients at the time of admission. Since it has been reported that anemia is not a prominent feature in the early stage of primary amyloidosis, and that the nephrotic syndrome is present in one-third of patients at the time of histologic diagnosis [6], these values

Table 1.
Summary of clinical manifestations, treatment and prognosis in 12 patients with systemic amyloidosis

| Case | Sex | Age | Amyloid protein | Anemia | NS | Organ involvement | | | | Treatment | Outcome | Duration (months) |
						heart	liver	kidney	lung			
1 CA	F	57	AA (RA)	+	+	+	−	+	+	combination	death	3
2 KO	M	59	AL (primary)	−	+	−	+	+	−	PE alone	death	4
3 SC	F	58	AL (MM)	+	−	+	−	−	−	conventional	death	7
4 CT	F	54	AL (primary)	−	+	+	+	+	−	combination	death	6
5 AN	F	71	AL (primary)	−	+	+	−	+	−	none	living	
6 KM	F	45	AA (unknown)	+	+	−	−	+	−	combination	living	
7 TM	F	92	AL (primary)	+	−	−	−	+	−	conventional	death	3
8 SF	M	82	AL (MM)	−	+	+	+	+	−	conventional	death	8
9 SU	F	66	AA (RA)	+	−	+	−	−	−	conventional	living	
10 TT	M	79	AA (RA)	+	+	+	−	+	−	combination	death	8
11 KK	F	24	AA (RA)	+	+	−	−	+	−	conventional	living	
12 YO	F	61	AL (MM)	+	−	+	+	+	−	conventional	death	6

RA, rheumatoid arthritis; MM, multiple myeloma; NS, nephrotic syndrome; PE, plasma exchange.

suggested that amyloid deposition was already extensive in our cases. Involvement of multiple organs was also present in most cases.

The combination treatment with DMSO and plasma exchange was carried out on one patient with primary amyloidosis and three patients with secondary amyloidosis (Table 1). Other conventional treatments, including alkylating agents, corticosteroids and colchicine, were performed on one patient with primary amyloidosis, three patients associated with myeloma and two patients with secondary amyloidosis. Out of four patients receiving the combination treatment, three patients died within 1 year following admission. Mortality of the patients receiving other conventional treatments was also high, and the overall mortality of 12 patients was 67%. Thus, it appeared that there were no differences in survival and progression of disease between these two groups. However, it has been found that the combination treatment delayed amyloid deposition and renal impairment in a patient with primary amyloidosis.

Case 4, a 54 year old woman, was admitted to our hospital with anorexia and weight loss. Initially, she was treated with melphalan and prednisone. However, her general condition continued to worsen despite these treatments, and a rapid deterioration of renal function was found. Therefore, she was started on a regimen of DMSO and plasma exchange, and received hemodialysis for the management of renal failure. Nausea and anorexia gradually disappeared, and renal function was stabilized after initiation of the combination treatment. However, she developed progressive cardiac failure soon after and, because of hypotension, plasma exchange was limited. Six months following admission, she died of intractable cardiac failure. A renal autopsy specimen revealed extensive amyloid deposition in glomeruli and vascular walls, but it seemed that the degree of deposition did not change when compared with a biopsy specimen.

DISCUSSION

Systemic amyloidosis is a progressive disease for which the prognosis is poor [1, 2]. Since the AL amyloid fibrils consist of the variable portions of monoclonal immunoglobulin light chains and are synthesized by plasma cells [7], attempts have been made to treat AL amyloidosis with alkylating agents and prednisone. This form of therapy has met with some degree of success, but, in general, is unsatisfactory.

Recently, DMSO has shown promise in some patients with secondary amyloidosis [8], but others found disappointing results. The use of DMSO stems from experimental observations in which it apparently could solubilize amyloid fibrils as well as prevent further deposition, thereby allowing existing deposits to be mobilized. It has been generally assumed that these proteins mobilized from the tissues are excreted in urine. However, the excretion may be insufficient in patients with impaired renal function. Therefore, in the present study, we challenged the combination treatment with DMSO and plasma exchange to achieve the effective removal of amyloid proteins.

Because amyloid deposition was already extensive at the start of therapy, significant prolongation of survival has not been documented in patients receiving the combination treatment (Table 1). However, we found that the combination treatment delayed amyloid deposition and renal impairment in a patient with primary amyloidosis. These results suggest that the combination treatment might extend the life of a patient if started at an earlier stage of the disease. Further studies with enough patients will be necessary to clarify the efficiency of this combination treatment for systemic amyloidosis.

REFERENCES

1. K. D. Brandt, E. S. Cathcart and A. S. Cohen. A clinical analysis of the course and prognosis of 42 patients with amyloidosis. *Am. J. Med.*, **44**, 955–969 (1968).

2. P. D. Gorevic and E. C. Franklin. EC, Amyloidosis. *Ann. Rev. Med.*, **32**, 261–271 (1981).

3. R. A. Kyle and P. R. Greipp. Primary systemic amyloidosis: comparison of melphalan and prednisone versus placebo. *Blood*, **52**, 818–827 (1978).

4. M. D. Benson. Treatment of AL amyloidosis with melphalan, prednisone, and colchicine. *Arth. Rheum.*, **29**, 683–687 (1986).

5. E. P. Benditt, N. Eriksen and R. H. Hanson. Amyloid protein SAA is an apoprotein of mouse plasma high density lipoprotein. *Proc. Natl. Acad. Sci. USA*, **76**, 4092–4096 (1979).

6. R. A. Kyle and E. D. Bayrd. Amyloidosis: review of 236 cases. *Medicine*, **54**, 271–299 (1975).

7. G. G. Glenner. Amyloid deposits and amyloidosis: the β-fibrillosis. *N. Engl. J. Med.*, **302**, 1283–1292 (1980).

8. M. Ravid, I. Keder and E. Sohar. Effect of single dose of dimethyl sulfoxide on renal amyloidosis. *Lancet*, **1**, 730–731 (1977).

Therapeutic Plasmapheresis (XII), pp. 953-956
T. Agishi *et al.* (Eds)
© VSP 1993

Combination Therapy of Plasma Exchange and Hemodialysis for Infants

K. TANAKA,[1] M. ITIKAWA,[1] Y. NAKAMURA,[1] K. UJIIE ,[1] M. SUENAGA,[1]
T. SHIBAMOTO,[2] T. YAMADA[3] and M. HOSHINO[3]

[1]*Hemodialysis Center, Tokyo Metropolitan Bokuto General Hospital,*
4-23-15 Koutoubashi, Sumida-Ku, Tokyo, Japan
[2]*Tokyo Medical and Dental University, Japan*
[3]*Kikukawabashi Clinic, Japan*

Key words: plasma exchange; extracorporeal circuit; infant.

INTRODUCTION

It has been reported that plasma exchange (PE) is effective for the treatment of patients
with hemolytic uremic syndrome (HUS) and Reye's syndrome (RS). When they are
complicated with renal failure, it is advisable to prescribe on-line hemodialysis (HD)
to correct electrolyte disturbances due to PE. However, combination therapy of PE and
HD (PE/HD) is often difficult to apply to small infants because of the relatively large
extracorporeal circulation volume (ECCV) to their body sizes. We attempted to reduce
the ECCV and performed PE/HD to three infants successfully.

METHODS

The patients were two cases of HUS (2 year old females) and one case of RS (3 year old
male), all complicated with acute renal failure. Each patient weighed 12, 13 and 13 kg,
respectively (Table 1). We selected Plasmacure M as a plasma separator and RA-02H as

Table 1.
Patient profiles

Case	Age (years)	Sex	Weight (kg)	Diagnosis
1	2	F	12	HUS, ARF
2	2	F	13	HUS, ARF
3	3	M	13	RS, ARF

HUS, hemolytic uremic syndrome; RS, Reye's syndrome; ARF,
acute renal failure.

Table 2.
The construction of the PE/HD circuit

	PE	HD
Membrane	Plasmacure-M	RA-02H
Surface area (m^2)	0.3	0.2
Priming volume (ml)	20	20
Tubing volume (ml)	12	10
Chamber volume (ml)	3	5

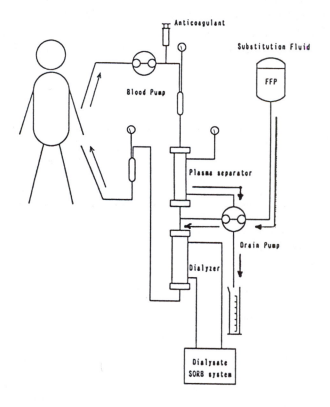

Figure 1. Flow diagram of the PE/HD circuit.

a dialyzer, the former having a surface area of 0.3 m^2 and a priming volume of 20 ml and the latter 0.2 m^2 and 20 ml. An extracorporeal PE/HD circuit was constructed by connecting them in series with narrow line tubes (inner diameter of 3 mm). The exception for that was the section in the roller pump which had a somewhat wider inner diameter of 3.3 mm. The volume of the arterial chamber was 3 ml and that of the venous chamber was larger, 5 ml, for the sake of avoiding air embolisms. The total ECCV of the circuit became about 70 ml (Table 2). Blood was drawn from and returned to the double lumen catheter indwelt in a femoral vein. The blood flow rate was between 30 and 50 ml/min, a quarter of which was set for the plasma flow rate. The dialysate was supplied from the SORB system at the rate of 200 ml/min. According to each patient's illness, 500–1000 ml of the patient plasma was exchanged for the same amount of fresh frozen plasma in each procedure (Fig. 1).

RESULTS

Two cases of HUS had experienced three and two procedures of PE/HD and were re-covered after another six and eight HD sessions, respectively. The case of RS had experienced three procedures of PE/HD and was lost after another 12 HD sessions due to intractable encephalopathy (Table 3). The blood pressure was stable during all proce-dures of PE/HD and there were no remarkable hypotension episodes leading to treatment failure (Fig. 2). As might be expected, no symptoms of electrolyte disturbances were observed. The mean reduction rate of serum urea nitrogen was 30% for one PE/HD procedure.

Table 3.
Results

Case	PE/HD	HD	Prognosis
1	3	6	recovered
2	2	8	recovered
3	3	12	died

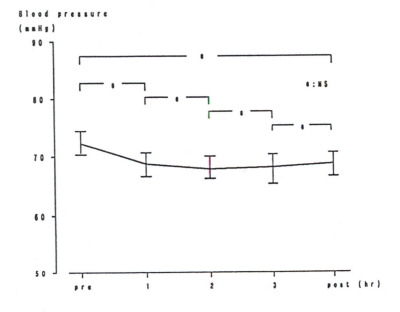

Figure 2. Mean blood pressure during PE/HD.

DISCUSSION

It has been reported that PE is effective for the treatment of patients with HUS and RS. Since renal complication is often the case, there are some risks of electrolyte disturbances, such as hypocalcemia and hypernatremia, in performing PE. So it is safe to prescribe HD simultaneously by an on-line system. However, because HUS and RS often attacks small infants, it is difficult to apply PE/HD to them without life threatening hypotension episodes due to large ECCV. In order to get rid of that dilemma, we attempted to reduce the ECCV by minimizing the extracorporeal circuit component size. If the whole blood volume was 8% of the body weight in such infants, the final ECCV amounted to only 7% of it, which was small enough to perform PE/PD successfully. Finally, we must point out some problems in relation to using that technique. First, the tube length between the catheter and a pump or a chamber was so short that some sedative procedure was needed to protect the circuit connection against actively moving patients. Secondly, because of the same reason, ordinary bed side monitoring devices could not be used. To resolve those problems, we hope to get more sophisticated devices that enable us to make more suitable circuits for small infants.

CONCLUSION

(i) We performed PE/HD on two HUS infants and one RS infant, all being complicated with acute renal failure.

(ii) We attempted to reduce the ECCV by minimizing the extracorporeal circuit component size. The final ECCV amounted to only 7% of the whole blood volume of the patients.

(iii) Two HUS patients were recovered and one RS patient was lost. The blood pressure was stable during all PE/HD procedures and there were no remarkable hypotension episodes leading to treatment failure.

Author Index